D1541285

# PHYSICIAN'S GUIDE TO TERRORIST ATTACK

# PHYSICIAN'S GUIDE TO TERRORIST ATTACK

*Edited by*

## MICHAEL J. ROY, MD, MPH, FACP

*Department of Medicine*
*Uniformed Services University of the Health Sciences*
*Bethesda, MD*

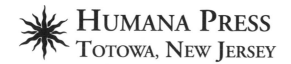
HUMANA PRESS
TOTOWA, NEW JERSEY

© 2004 Humana Press Inc.
999 Riverview Drive, Suite 208
Totowa, NJ 07512

www.humanapress.com

The content and opinions expressed in this book are the sole work of the authors and editors, who have warranted due diligence in the creation and issuance of their work. The publisher, editors, and authors are not responsible for errors or omissions or for any consequences arising from the information or opinions presented in this book and make no warranty, express or implied, with respect to its contents.

Due diligence has been taken by the publishers, editors, and authors of this book to assure the accuracy of the information published and to describe generally accepted practices. The contributors herein have carefully checked to ensure that the drug selections and dosages set forth in this text are accurate and in accord with the standards accepted at the time of publication. Notwithstanding, as new research, changes in government regulations, and knowledge from clinical experience relating to drug therapy and drug reactions constantly occurs, the reader is advised to check the product information provided by the manufacturer of each drug for any change in dosages or for additional warnings and contraindications. This is of utmost importance when the recommended drug herein is a new or infrequently used drug. It is the responsibility of the treating physician to determine dosages and treatment strategies for individual patients. Further it is the responsibility of the health care provider to ascertain the Food and Drug Administration status of each drug or device used in their clinical practice. The publisher, editors, and authors are not responsible for errors or omissions or for any consequences from the application of the information presented in this book and make no warranty, express or implied, with respect to the contents in this publication.

Cover design by Patricia F. Cleary.

Cover photo: BrandX Pictures.

For additional copies, pricing for bulk purchases, and/or information about other Humana titles, contact Humana at the above address or at any of the following numbers: Tel.: 973-256-1699; Fax: 973-256-8341, E-mail: humana@humanapr.com; or visit our Website: www.humanapress.com

This publication is printed on acid-free paper. ∞
ANSI Z39.48-1984 (American National Standards Institute) Permanence of Paper for Printed Library Materials.

Printed in the United States of America. 10 9 8 7 6 5 4 3 2 1

**Library of Congress Cataloging-in-Publication Data**

Physician's guide to terrorist attack / edited by Michael J. Roy.
       p. ; cm.
    Includes bibliographical references and index.
    ISBN 1-58829-207-X (alk. paper) -- ISBN 1-59259-663-0 (e-ISBN)
    1. Terrorism--Health aspects. 2. Disaster medicine. [DNLM: 1. Disaster Planning--organization & administration.
  2. Emergency Medical Services--organization & administration. 3. Terrorism--prevention & control. 4. Biological
  Warfare--prevention & control. 5. Chemical Warfare Agents--toxicity. 6. Decontamination--methods. 7. Nuclear
  Warfare. WX 185 P5785 2004] I. Roy, Michael J., 1962-
  RC88.9.T47P48 2004
  362.18--dc21
                                                                                                  2003008190

*This book is dedicated to the survivors of the terrorist attacks that occurred on September 11, 2001, and of the anthrax attacks that followed that fall, as well as to the families and friends who lost loved ones as a result of these horrors. Let us hope and pray that we will be able to prevent such senseless loss of life in the future.*

# PREFACE

Terrorists seek to maximize economic, political, and psychological disruption through their actions. To capture media attention for their cause, terrorists often engage in one-upmanship, acting in a more horrific and spectacular manner than has been previously seen, from the Olympic Village attack in Munich in 1972, to the airliner crashes into the World Trade Center and the Pentagon in 2001. The use of biological, chemical, or nuclear weapons has been contemplated by many terrorists, and even carried out with some success on occasion, but the medical community justifiably fears that we are likely to see more calamitous use of such agents for terrorist means in the future.

Terrorist events in the fall of 2001—the attacks upon the World Trade Center and the Pentagon on September 11, followed by dissemination of anthrax through the US mail-painfully emphasized the need for physicians to be able to diagnose and manage individuals suffering injuries as a result of exposures to biological, chemical, and nuclear, as well as explosives. *Physician's Guide to Terrorist Attack* is intended to prepare physicians and other health care workers to respond knowledgeably and confidently to a terrorist event. Whether you are a first responder working with emergency personnel amid the chaos of a disaster scene or at a hospital receiving mass casualties, a provider in the community responding to an anxious patient fearful of exposure to a biological agent, or a primary care provider or mental health specialist helping patients and their family members to cope with the psychological aftermath, this book will provide the information you need, in an easy-to-follow, clinically relevant, case-based format.

Dr. Smoak, a veteran of the US Embassy bombing in Nairobi, Kenya, reviews lessons learned from previous events with regard to the initial response. Dr. Geiling, who was chief of medical services at the Pentagon on September 11, 2001, details the impact that a terrorist event is likely to have on the medical system, providing valuable guidance on what to expect and how to prepare for a future event. Drs. Yeskey and Morse of the Centers for Disease Control and Prevention outline the approach that a community provider should take, from the initial suspicion of a terrorist event, to the involvement of public health authorities.

Dr. Murray reviews the historical use of biological, chemical, and nuclear agents, from ancient times through the present, putting into perspective recent concerns, and providing an introduction to the ensuing chapters, which provide an agent-by-agent review for the clinician. A number of the world's leading infectious diseases experts on potential biological agents focus on the key aspects of diagnosis and therapy for the 13 most feared bacteria, viruses, and toxins. A comparable field of experts then reviews the diagnostic and therapeutic approach to various chemical agents. Many of the authors have been involved in various aspects of evaluation and management of biological and chemical threats, in homeland defense efforts to combat terrorism, and in a variety of educational endeavors to help fellow clinicians prepare to diagnose and treat victims promptly should an event come to pass.

The subsequent three chapters provide critically important information as well. A chapter on blast injuries, written by leading authorities on this subject, is significant because conventional explosives are still far more likely to be used by terrorists than anything else. A chapter on nuclear and radiological weapons, written by experts at the Armed Forces Radiobiologic Research Institute, covers the gamut from a "dirty bomb" to the use of a high-powered nuclear device. Last but not least, members of the Department of Psychiatry at Uniformed Services University, internationally recognized for their disaster response experience, review the immediate and late psychological effects of terrorist events. This is particularly salient, since no matter how severe and numerous the physical casualties, it is safe to assume that they will be exceeded by those suffering from psychological traumatization.

Although it would be nice to think that physicians need not know the information that is covered here, the reality is that it is critically important for physicians to prepare themselves by acquiring the knowledge and skills necessary to cope effectively with a major terrorist event now, rather than learning through painful experience.

*Michael J. Roy, MD, MPH, FACP*

# CONTENTS

# CONTRIBUTORS

NAOMI E. ARONSON, MD, FACP • *Colonel, Medical Corps, US Army; Director, Division of Infectious Diseases, Associate Professor of Medicine, Uniformed Services University of the Health Sciences, Bethesda, MD*

STEVEN I. BASKIN, PharmD, PhD, FCP, FACC, DABT, FATS • *Division of Pharmacology, US Army Medical Research Institute of Chemical Defense, Aberdeen Proving Ground, MD*

DAVID M. BENEDEK, MD • *Major, Medical Corps, US Army; Associate Professor of Psychiatry, Uniformed Services University of the Health Sciences, Bethesda, MD*

DAVID L. BLAZES, MD, MPH • *Lieutenant Commander, Medical Corps, US Navy; Assistant Professor of Medicine, Uniformed Services University of the Health Sciences; Infectious Diseases Service, National Naval Medical Center, Bethesda, MD*

TIMOTHY H. BURGESS, MD, MPH • *Lieutenant Commander, Medical Corps, US Navy; Naval Medical Research Center, Silver Spring, MD*

STEVEN J. DURNING, MD, FACP • *Major, Medical Corps, US Air Force; Director, Clinical Concepts Course, Assistant Professor of Medicine, Uniformed Services University of the Health Sciences, Bethesda, MD*

JAMES A. GEILING, MD, FACP, FCCP • *Colonel, Medical Corps, US Army (Retired); Department of Medicine, VA Medical Center, White River Junction, VT; Assistant Professor of Medicine, Dartmouth Medical School, Hanover, NH*

THOMAS W. GEISBERT, PhD • *US Army Medical Research Institute of Infectious Diseases, Fort Detrick, MD*

DAVID L. HOOVER, MD • *Colonel, Medical Corps, US Army; Department of Bacterial Diseases, Walter Reed Army Institute of Research, Silver Spring; Professor of Medicine, Uniformed Services University of the Health Sciences, Bethesda, MD*

DUANE R. HOSPENTHAL, MD, PhD, FACP • *Lieutenant Colonel, Medical Corps, US Army; Chief, Infectious Disease Service, Brooke Army Medical Center, San Antonio, TX*

PETER B. JAHRLING, PhD • *US Army Medical Research Institute of Infectious Diseases, Fort Detrick, MD*

NIRANJAN KANESA-THASAN, MD, MTMH • *Lieutenant Colonel, Medical Corps, US Army; Medical Division, US Army Medical Research Institute of Infectious Diseases, Fort Detrick, MD*

JONATHAN S. KURCHE, BS • *Research Fellow, Division of Pharmacology, Oak Ridge Institute for Science and Education (ORISE); US Army Medical Research Institute of Chemical Defense, Aberdeen Proving Ground, MD*

TIMOTHY J. LACY, MD • *Lieutenant Colonel, Medical Corps, US Air Force; Assistant Professor of Psychiatry and Family Medicine, Uniformed Services University of the Health Sciences; Program Director, National Capital Consortium Combined Residency in Psychiatry and Family Practice, Uniformed Services University of the Health Sciences, Bethesda, MD*

JAMES V. LAWLER, MD • *Lieutenant Commander, Medical Corps, US Navy; Infectious Diseases Service, National Naval Medical Center, Bethesda, MD*

EDWARD LUCCI, MD, FACP • *Lieutenant Colonel, Medical Corps, US Army; Chief, Emergency Medicine Service, Walter Reed Army Medical Center, Washington, DC*

BEVERLY I. MALINER, DO, MPH, FABFP • *Colonel, Medical Corps, US Army; Division of Chemical Casualty Care, United States Army Medical Research Institute of Chemical Defense, Aberdeen Proving Ground, Aberdeen, MD*

AILEEN M. MARTY, MD, FACP • *Commander, Medical Corps, US Navy; Associate Professor of Medicine, Uniformed Services University of the Health Sciences, Bethesda, MD*

R. SCOTT MILLER, MD • *Chief, Department of Immunology, US Army Medical Component of the Armed Forces Research Institute of the Medical Sciences, Bangkok, Thailand*

STEPHEN A. MORSE, MSPH, PhD • *Deputy Director, Bioterrorism Preparedness and Response Program, National Center for Infectious Diseases, Centers for Disease Control and Prevention, Atlanta, GA*

CLINTON K. MURRAY, MD • *Major, Medical Corps, US Army; Infectious Diseases Service, Brooke Army Medical Center, San Antonio, TX*

LEWIS S. NELSON, MD, FACEP, FACMT • *Director, Medical Toxicology Fellowship, New York City Poison Control Center; Department of Emergency Medicine, New York University School of Medicine, New York, NY*

JONATHAN NEWMARK, MD, FAAN • *Colonel, Medical Corps, US Army; Consultant to the Army Surgeon General for Chemical Casualty Care; Division of Chemical Casualty Care, US Army Medical Research Institute of Chemical Defense, Aberdeen Proving Ground, MD*

CHRISTIAN F. OCKENHOUSE, MD, PhD • *Colonel, Medical Corps, US Army; Walter Reed Army Institute of Research, Silver Spring, MD*

RAFAEL E. PADILLA, MD • *Clinical Instructor, Brown University School of Medicine, Providence, RI*

MICHAEL J. ROY, MD, MPH, FACP • *Lieutenant Colonel, Medical Corps, US Army; Director, Division of Military Internal Medicine, Associate Professor of Medicine, Uniformed Services University of the Health Sciences, Bethesda, MD*

THOMAS M. SEED, PhD • *Radiation Casualty Management Team, Radiation Medicine Department, Armed Forces Radiobiology Research Institute, Bethesda, MD*

VIJAY K. SINGH, PhD • *Radiation Casualty Management Team, Radiation Medicine Department, Armed Forces Radiobiology Research Institute, Bethesda, MD*

PHILIP A. SMITH, PhD • *Commander, Medical Service Corps, US Navy; Division of Occupational and Environmental Health, Assistant Professor of Preventive Medicine and Biometrics, Uniformed Services University of the Health Sciences, Bethesda, MD*

BONNIE L. SMOAK, MD, PhD, MPH • *Colonel, Medical Corps, US Army; Director, Division of Tropical Public Health, Associate Professor of Preventive Medicine and Biometrics, Uniformed Services University, Bethesda, MD*

RICHARD J. THOMAS, MD, MPH • *Captain, Medical Corps, US Navy; Assistant Professor of Preventive Medicine and Biometrics, Uniformed Services University of the Health Sciences; Director, Occupational and Environmental Residency Program, National Capital Consortium, Uniformed Services University of the Health Sciences, Bethesda, MD*

JENNIFER C. THOMPSON, MD, MPH, FACP • *Major, Medical Corps, US Army; Infectious Diseases Service, William Beaumont Army Medical Center, El Paso, TX*

BARRY A. WAYNE, EMT-T, MD, FAAEM, FACFE • *Assistant Professor of Military and Emergency Medicine, Uniformed Services University of the Health Sciences, Bethesda, MD*

SAGE W. WIENER, MD • *Fellow, Medical Toxicology, New York City Poison Control Center; Department of Emergency Medicine, New York University School of Medicine, New York, NY*

JOHN M. WIGHTMAN, EMT-T/P, MD, MA, FACEP, FACFE • *Associate Professor of Emergency Medicine, Wright State University School of Medicine, Dayton, OH*

GLENN WORTMANN, MD, FACP • *Lieutenant Colonel, Medical Corps, US Army; Infectious Diseases Service, Walter Reed Army Medical Center, Washington, DC*

KEVIN YESKEY, MD • *Captain, US Public Health Service; Adjunct Associate Professor, Department of Military and Emergency Medicine, Uniformed Services University of the Health Sciences, Bethesda, MD*

# VALUE-ADDED
# EBOOK/PDA ON CD-ROM

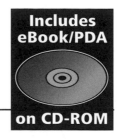

This book is accompanied by a value-added CD-ROM that contains an Adobe eBook version of the volume you have just purchased. This eBook can be viewed on your computer, and you can synchronize it to your PDA for viewing on your handheld device. The eBook enables you to view this volume on only one computer and PDA. Once the eBook is installed on your computer, you cannot download, install, or e-mail it to another computer; it resides solely with the computer to which it is installed. The license provided is for only one computer. The eBook can only be read using Adobe Reader 6.0, which is available free from Adobe Systems Incorporated at www.Adobe.com. You may also view the eBook on your PDA using the Adobe PDA Reader that is also available free from Adobe.com.

**You must follow a simple procedure when you install the eBook/PDA that will require you to connect to the Humana Press website in order to receive your license. Please read and follow the instructions below:**

1. Download and install Adobe Reader 6.0
   You can obtain a free copy of Adobe Reader 6.0 at www.adobe.com
   *Note: If you already have Adobe Reader 6.0, you do not need to reinstall it.
2. Launch Adobe Reader 6.0
3. Install eBook
   Insert your eBook CD into your CD-ROM drive
   **PC**
   Click on the "Start" button, then click on "Run"
   At the prompt, type "d:\ebookinstall.pdf" and click "OK"
   *Note: If your CD-ROM drive letter is something other than d: change the above command accordingly.*
   **MAC**
   Double click on the "eBook CD" that you will see mounted on your desktop.
   Double click "ebookinstall.pdf"
4. Adobe Reader 6.0 will open and you will receive the message
   "This document is protected by Adobe DRM"
   Click "OK"
   *Note: If you have not already activated Adobe Reader 6.0, you will be prompted to do so. Simply follow the directions to activate Adobe Reader 6.0 and continue installation.*
   Your web browser will open and you will be taken to the Humana Press eBook registration page.
   Follow the instructions on that page to complete installation.

If you require assistance during the installation, or you would like more information regarding your eBook and PDA installation, please refer to the eBookManual.pdf located on your cd. If you need further assistance, contact Humana Press eBook Support by e-mail at ebooksupport@humanapr.com.

# I

# RESPONDING TO AN INCIDENT

# 1

# Mass Casualty Events

*Lessons Learned*

## *Bonnie L. Smoak, MD, PhD, MPH, and James A. Geiling, MD, FACP, FCCP*

### CONTENTS

## 1. INTRODUCTION

Each week news headlines from around the world announce another disaster. Scores of people are killed or injured in occurrences ranging from floods or earthquakes to man-made catastrophes, such as train derailments or airplane crashes. Some of these tragedies can be characterized as mass casualty incidents, and the number of injured and killed exceeds the capacity of existing medical resources. Today, we are being called on to address new mass casualty threats posed by terrorists using conventional weapons, such as bombs, and unconventional weapons, such as "dirty bombs," small nuclear devices, and chemical and biological agents. These "weapons of mass destruction" pose new challenges to the medical community in preparing and potentially caring for the injured. Medical providers must care for the victims of such agents while protecting themselves from these same hazards. Emergency response planning becomes even more essential to mitigate the effects of unconventional terrorist acts on the lives of all those involved.

The provision of medical services is not the only response to mass casualties in a disaster; a myriad of other components are involved, including security, transportation, supplies, logistics, finance, communication, and support services for the responders and

From: *Physician's Guide to Terrorist Attack*
Edited by: M. J. Roy © Humana Press Inc., Totowa, NJ

survivors. Mass casualty response depends on communication and interaction between government agencies at the local, state, federal, and sometimes international levels. Planning is also essential to a successful response. Coordinating and establishing responsibilities and authorities prior to incidents is critical. Lessons learned from previous events are instrumental in this process. This chapter examines recurring themes from past terrorist attacks, focusing on the initial response.

Clinical care providers play a pivotal role in the response to a mass casualty incident, regardless of the cause. Rapid response and intervention can determine who survives and the quality of their future lives. In the realm of unconventional threats, the clinician's understanding and recognition of chemical or biological agent exposure is critical to identifying an incident, as well as initiating medical intervention. It was an astute infectious disease physician with laboratory support who diagnosed and reported the initial case of inhalational anthrax in 2001, alerting a nation to become vigilant for future cases (1).

Few medical providers are trained to recognize the signs of unconventional weapon exposure and to know the appropriate treatment strategies for radiological, biological, or chemical casualties. Providers need to be familiar with such threats, as well as with conventional emergency medical response requirements. As part of the first line of local responders, they may be required to perform their duties independently for many hours after an attack until outside resources are mobilized and available for consultation or assistance. As part of a larger emergency response, it is important that physicians understand how their activities integrate into the total scene. Understanding one's role in the complex response process is as important as providing hands-on intervention.

## 2. OVERVIEW OF TERRORIST INCIDENTS

In the last 10 years, hundreds of terrorist acts occurred worldwide, and many of these resulted in mass casualties. In this chapter, we focus on just a few of those high-profile terrorist incidents to illustrate critical concepts in mass casualty planning, response, and training. To orient the reader, a short description of the terrorist events used as examples in this chapter follows.

### 2.1. New York City, New York; 1993

In 1993, the first of the World Trade Center (WTC) attacks took place. The WTC complex was located on 5 acres of land in downtown Manhattan. It was composed of two 110-story office towers (Buildings One and Two), a 22-story hotel (Building Three), and four other buildings ranging in height from 8 to 47 stories. Immediately below the complex was one of the largest shopping malls in Manhattan. It was estimated that 60,000 people worked in the complex (2).

On February 26, a truck bomb exploded in the underground parking structure of Building Three, damaging five levels. Six people were killed and 1043 people sought medical help. Over 50,000 people had to be evacuated from the complex. The acute response was completed in 12 hours, and the recovery phase lasted 22 days (2,3).

### 2.2. Matsumoto, Japan; 1994

Late in the evening of June 27, members of the Aum Shinrikyo, a religious cult, released the nerve gas sarin into a residential neighborhood from a truck using a heater and fan. Several judges who were to rule on a case involving the cult lived in the area.

Seven people died, and 58 victims were admitted to five hospitals. The gas affected approximately 600 people, including rescuers. The evacuation period took 5 hours *(4)*.

### 2.3. Oklahoma City, Oklahoma; 1995

A truck bomb composed of 4800 lbs of ammonium nitrate and fuel oil exploded in front of the Alfred P. Murrah Federal Building on the morning of April 19. The blast caused the partial collapse of the nine-story building and damaged hundreds of other buildings. A total of 168 people were killed, and over 800 people were injured *(5)*. The last live rescue occurred 13 hours after the explosion, and the search and recovery phase lasted 21 days *(6)*.

### 2.4. Tokyo, Japan; 1995

During rush hour on the morning of March 20, members of the Aum Shinrikyo cult released sarin in five different subway trains on three separate subway lines. All the trains were heading to a central area of government buildings in the heart of the city *(7)*. Eventually, 15 subway stations were affected. The attack killed 12 persons, and more than 5500 individuals sought medical attention at more than 200 hospitals and clinics within hours of the incident *(8)*.

### 2.5. United States Embassies, Nairobi, Kenya and Dar es Salaam, Tanzania; 1998

Mid-morning on August 7, near-simultaneous truck bombings occurred outside the American Embassies in the capital cities of Kenya and Tanzania. In Tanzania, 12 people were killed and 85 injured. The bombing in Nairobi caused a much greater number of casualties. The Ufundi Cooperative House, a seven-floor building adjacent to the Embassy, collapsed. Massive damage occurred within the Embassy and other buildings within a two-block radius. Over 200 people were killed, including 12 Americans and 32 Kenyan employees of the American Embassy. Over 4000 people were injured, and 524 were admitted to local hospitals *(9)*. Twenty-five injured Embassy personnel were air-evacuated to other counties for medical treatment.

### 2.6. New York City, New York; 2001

On September 11, a hijacked airplane was flown into the North Tower (Building One) of the WTC. Approximately 20 minutes later, a second hijacked aircraft struck the South Tower. A few hours into the emergency response, both towers collapsed. Other buildings in the WTC complex were seriously damaged, and a third building, Building Seven, collapsed after burning. Over 1100 people were treated at five hospitals within Manhattan during the first 48 hours *(10)*. By August 16, 2002, 2726 death certificates had been issued *(11)*.

### 2.7. Arlington, Virginia; 2001

An hour after the first plane struck the North Tower of the WTC in New York City, a third hijacked plane crashed into the west side of the Pentagon, destroying three of the five concentric building rings on that side of the structure. One hundred eighty-nine deaths occurred. Local hospitals treated 106 persons, and 49 of these patients required admission. The search and rescue/recovery phase of the response lasted 10 days *(12)*.

### 2.8. U.S. Anthrax Incidents; 2001

Anthrax disseminated through the postal system in envelopes caused 22 cases of illnesses from October 4 to November 20. Cases were diagnosed along the East Coast in seven locations—New York, New Jersey, Florida, Pennsylvania, Virginia, Connecticut, Maryland, and the District of Columbia. Eleven of the cases were inhalational anthrax, and five of these were fatal *(13)*. The public health response required to identify exposed individuals and to offer chemoprophylactic drugs to those at high risk of acquiring disease was massive. Over 10,000 persons were offered antimicrobial prophylaxis *(14)*.

### 2.9. Bali, Indonesia; 2002

On the evening of October 12, two bombs exploded in the resort town of Kuta. First, a small bomb was detonated outside of Paddy's Bar, and then a bomb-laden van carrying ammonium nitrate exploded 30 meters away at the Sari Nightclub. The thatched roof of the club ignited, causing a large fire. The capacity for an emergency response was limited, with few fire engines or ambulances available. The explosion killed 185 people, most of them foreign tourists. Three hundred sixteen people were hospitalized, and 120 of these were later evacuated from the island *(15)*.

## 3. LESSONS LEARNED

### 3.1. Incident Confirmation

At the time of the incident, most people at the scene and even the initial responders did not recognize the event as a terrorist attack. This has been true for high explosive attacks as well as chemical and biological attacks. During the 1993 WTC attack, responders initially thought a transformer had exploded *(2)*. Neither of the first-reported, large-scale chemical or biological attacks was recognized as a terrorist incident at the time they occurred. During the fall of 1984, a large community outbreak of *Salmonella typhimurium* affecting 751 persons occurred in The Dalles, Oregon. After an epidemiological investigation, public health officials concluded that the outbreak was caused by a single strain of bacteria associated with various foods at several restaurants served at varying times. However, they were unable to explain how transmission of the bacteria could have occurred. It was only later, during a criminal investigation into the activities of a religious group led by Bhagwan Shree Rajneesh, that investigators learned that some members had intentionally contaminated food at several restaurants in an attempt to influence voter turnout on an election day *(16)*.

In a similar manner, the nature of the attack and the use of a nerve gas were not considered during the terrorist attack in Matsumoto, Japan. The emergency responders thought that the first victims evacuated were ill from food poisoning, contaminated water, or natural gas. Although organophosphate poisoning was suspected on clinical grounds, none of the responders considered the toxic agent to be a nerve gas, and no decontamination procedures were performed. Sarin was identified from environmental samples 7 days after the incident *(4)*. Just 2 years later, in the 1995 Tokyo attack, the possibility of a nerve agent was again not appreciated until 3 hours into the response, when a government laboratory identified sarin as the agent. This information was disseminated slowly to hospitals, and decontamination procedures were delayed *(17)*.

Failure to consider the possibility of a terrorist attack as a cause of a biological or chemical incident probably contributed to further casualties in the above situations. Even when a terrorist attack is suspected, failure to consider terrorist tactics can result in more victims. Terrorist tactics could include the simultaneous use of two or more weapons of mass destruction. Following the 2001 attacks in New York and Washington, there was concern that a biological attack might have occurred. Syndromic surveillance systems were established in New York emergency departments. These systems classified patient medical evaluations into several clusters of clinical signs, symptoms, and diagnoses reflecting illnesses and symptoms associated with diseases caused by biological agents. An increase in the number of patients presenting with these clusters might provide an early warning that an exposure to a biological agent had occurred (18). An existing system, ESSENCE, in the Washington DC area was placed on heighten alert (19).

During their initial assessment of any mass casualty situation, emergency responders must evaluate the possibility that it could be the result of a terrorist act. The use of secondary bombs, booby traps, or combinations of a conventional explosive with hazardous material or chemical agents should be considered when a terrorist act is suspected. Initial responders must approach all mass casualty situations with caution. Responders to the disaster or casualties may even themselves be targeted. On the afternoon of October 7, 1996 in Lisburn, Northern Ireland, a car bomb exploded in the parking lot of Thiepval Barracks, the headquarters of the British Army. Twelve minutes later, as medical personnel were attending to casualties, a second car bomb exploded outside the treatment rooms, creating more casualties (20).

### 3.2. Command and Control

Confusion reigns at disaster sites until emergency responders establish command and control elements at the scene. The most important element is a location near the disaster site where individuals with the authority over resources can coordinate the response. During smaller emergency responses, this site is frequently called an incident command center (ICC), and one individual, the incident commander, is responsible for decision making. During a terrorist event, numerous agencies and organizations respond. A unified command center is created from the individuals representing agencies with different jurisdictional responsibilities and authority. Decisions are made through joint planning and information sharing. During the response to the Oklahoma bombing, an ICC was initially established, followed by the creation of a Multi-Agency Coordination Center, as the number of agencies increased (21). Similarly, the Arlington County Fire Department established an ICC at the Pentagon site, and later, a unified command team, composed of representatives from the police, fire department, Federal Bureau of Investigation (FBI), Department of Defense, and Federal Emergency Management Agency, was created (12). Responses to both the 1993 and 2001 terrorist attacks in New York City also used this model of control (3,22).

Another critical control element is the quick establishment of a secure perimeter around the incident. This is needed for accountability of rescue personnel and to direct resources better. During the Oklahoma City bombing, police were unable to secure the perimeter during the early response phase. Hundreds of individuals were at the site, and more kept coming to the 20-city-block disaster scene. Rumors of a second bomb 1 1/2 hours after the first explosion helped to clear the area of all personnel. Only then was the site secured and rescue efforts able to proceed in a safe and organized manner (21).

The ability to establish a perimeter quickly relates to the geographic location of the attack. Both the Pentagon attack in 2001 and the Murrah Building attack in 1995 occurred in urban areas and were similar in scale. However, the response at the Pentagon was facilitated by the fact that the building already had limited traffic access and was surrounded by large spaces. Establishing a perimeter there was easier than in Oklahoma City, where there were no physical landmarks to help delineate the scene *(23)*. Although a perimeter was quickly created, controlled access to the Pentagon site was difficult to establish during the early phase. The police were unable to distinguish which persons were authorized to enter the site until an identification card system was in place *(12)*. Part of planning an emergency response for high-risk targets should include identifying possible perimeters that could be easily and quickly established. Once a secure perimeter is in place, it is possible to have a full accountability of who is at the site. Identification cards should be issued to limit access to the scene to only those responders who should be there *(21)*.

Confusion over control issues has occurred not only among the multiple responding agencies, but also among units within individual agencies themselves. This was reported after the Oklahoma City bombing and the 2001 WTC and Pentagon attacks *(12,22)*. During the 2001 WTC attack, dispatched firefighting units failed to report to staging areas and instead proceeded directly to the site. As a result, the command center did not know the location of all the responding units. Furthermore, these units did not receive important safety information before arriving at the scene *(22)*.

For a safe and efficient response to occur, one agency must establish control of the incident scene quickly. In the United States, the local fire department is the responsible agency. Disaster planning, written agreements, and regular mass casualty exercises can lessen coordination problems with other responding agencies.

### *3.3. Communication*

Information in mass casualty events is critical. In order to respond to the incident effectively, responders need to know the extent of damage to buildings, the number and type of casualties, and the security and safety of the scene. This information must be gathered, verified, and disseminated throughout the response chain. For years after, action reports cite communications as one of the most problematic areas of the response *(3,12,22)*.

The enormity of the emergency responses created strains on the communication systems within single agencies. During the 1993 WTC bombing, the incident commander needed the ability to communicate with 156 firefighting units and 56 chiefs. There were insufficient communication resources to handle this task *(3)*. Communication difficulties among the 200 firefighting units and 100 ambulances also hindered the New York City Fire Department's (FDNY) response during the 2001 WTC attack *(22)*.

Communication failures among different responding agencies have happened in most past terrorist incidents. Land lines and cell phones were overloaded with calls from citizens trying to obtain information about the disaster or trying to locate their loved ones. Radio channels were oversaturated. Adding to the difficulties of establishing control at the scene, communication equipment and systems were not compatible among all the responding organizations. During both the Tokyo gas attack and the Oklahoma bombing, communication was lost between the hospitals and the ambulances at the scenes. Responders were unable to tell the hospitals the condition of transported patients, and they had no way of knowing which hospital was able to receive more patients *(21,24)*. Communications between the FDNY and New York City Police Department were limited during the acute emergency phase in 2001, hindering coordination of that response *(22)*. To compensate for the loss of electronic means of communication, runners were used to pass information during many of these disasters *(12,21,25)*.

Clearly, communications is one area that needs substantial improvement. Financing communication equipment and upgrades, along with ensuring the interoperability of systems, is paramount. Planning and adherence to agreed-on procedures will also improve communications during a response.

### 3.4. Initial Responders

Traditionally, initial responders are defined as local police, firefighters, and emergency medical technicians or paramedics. These professionals train to assist the public during catastrophic events and they do so on a daily basis. Recent terrorist attacks have usually occurred in densely populated urban areas. These acts created a scale of devastation that had not previously been seen, resulting in large numbers of casualties and the destruction of many buildings. During these incidents, other professionals were needed at the scene. Ruptured gas and water pipes, broken power lines, falling debris, and unstable structures necessitated the presence of utility workers, construction workers, and engineers to ensure that rescue and recovery efforts could proceed safely. Mental health workers were also at the response site as they mingled with other responders to help them cope with the sights, sounds, and smells of the tragedy. Local, state, and national government officials were present, along with workers from relief organizations, churches, and social support groups. All these professionals were initial responders working at the incident sites, and they were exposed to all the hazards and horrors associated with it. Care of the victims was only one piece of the entire disaster-response puzzle.

Many of these people were thrust into new roles and did not have the proper training or equipment to perform their jobs safely. Many needed respiratory protection for smoke and other hazardous substances *(12,21,23)*. Most had never been in situations in which they would have witnessed violent deaths or body parts lying among debris. They had not received training to develop coping skills, and many of their organizations did not have the psychological support structure to help them process and recover from their experiences.

Certain workers might benefit from specialized response training for terrorist events, such as those employed at major high-threat events or public sites. Ticket agents, guides, and custodial workers are just a few of the types of workers that might be the first to respond to a terrorist attack on a public building. A lack of knowledge about the potential effects of chemical and biological agents could be lethal to them. In fact, two of the fatalities during the Tokyo attack were subway workers who cleaned up the liquid spill without protective gear, not suspecting that it was a nerve agent, even though people were clearly becoming ill *(17)*.

Response plans for large terrorist attacks should recognize the need for many types of workers at a disaster site and should incorporate all potential workers into protocols, guidelines, and training scenarios. Likewise, each of the professional groups that typically do not respond to emergencies should identify, educate, and train specific individuals to work with other initial responders during a large terrorist attack.

Emergency responders, despite their training, have died or been injured while performing their jobs. During the 1993 WTC bombing, 124 emergency responders were injured *(3)*. In the Oklahoma City bombing, a nurse was killed from falling debris during the early response, and, during the 2001 WTC attacks, 450 emergency responders died when the buildings collapsed unexpectedly *(23)*.

The rate of injuries among responders is very difficult to determine because the denominator data (total duration of time at the site for all responders) must be crudely estimated. During the Oklahoma City bombing, an injury rate of 0.0015 injuries per hour was estimated for firefighters and a rate of 0.0012 for members of the Urban Search and Rescue Teams. Most of the injuries were minor, the most common being strains and sprains (21.4%), eye injuries (19.4%), and lacerations/crush/puncture wounds (18.4%) *(26)*. During the first 24 hours after the WTC attacks, 240 New York firefighters and emergency medical service personnel (FDNY rescue workers) sought medical attention. Most were for eye and/or respiratory irritation. Among these injuries, 28 FDNY rescue workers required hospitalization. Most were for fractures, and three individuals had life-threatening inhalation injuries. Approximately 1 year after the attack, 363 FDNY rescue workers remained on emergency leave or light duty assignment because of respiratory illness *(27)*.

The risk of injury to rescue workers will probably be higher in a chemical attack. During the response in Matsumoto, 34.6% (18/52) of the emergency workers experienced symptoms of nerve gas toxicity. One required hospitalization. As noted earlier, the emergency responders did not suspect a terrorist attack or the use of a nerve gas, and no personal protection measures were taken *(28)*. During the second sarin attack in Japan, 9.9% (135/1364) of the emergency medical technicians were affected by the nerve agent. Respiratory protection was not used because the nature of the attack was not appreciated until several hours into the response *(24)*.

A potential factor for the risk of acquiring injuries is nonfamiliarity with the incident site or facility. Pentagon responders unfamiliar with the building layout were unable to communicate their location when asking for assistance and were not able to evacuate the building rapidly when structural threats required quick egress *(12)*.

These reports indicate that rescuers are potentially at high risk for injuries and that some of these injuries are preventable if appropriate personal protection equipment, such as eye protection or respirators, is worn. Identifying hazards in the early phases of the response and informing all the responders is important. However, following the 2001 WTC attack, some responders complained that they had received too much or conflicting information about hazardous conditions. Hazards were identified without conveying the health risks to rescuers and without stating what protective measures were needed and available to mitigate the hazard. Responders from one organization might wear some type of respiratory protection whereas a worker next to him from another organization wore nothing. This was attributed to different groups providing different risk assessments, different recommendations for respirators by different organizations, and no one enforcing the use of safety equipment *(23)*.

Clearly the proper use and appropriate level of personal protection equipment should be a high priority for responders. Although responders may be willing to accept some risk to save a life, responders' safety and health should be a critical concern after the immediate emergency phase has passed. Management of the scene should include enforcement of organizational guidelines for personal protection equipment. The failure to provide the proper protective equipment and to follow safety guidelines will result in more injuries and possibly the death of responders.

### 3.5. *Volunteers and Donations*

Volunteers, even though well intentioned, have often created problems. Most were not familiar with the emergency command and control systems and were not trained in recognizing potentially hazardous situations. Many did not have medical training and even if they did, it was difficult for trained responders to verify their credentials. During the 2001 WTC response, officials had the burden of dedicating a considerable amount of scarce resources to verifying the credentials of volunteers *(22)*.

Establishing control at past terrorist sites was made more difficult by hundreds of well-meaning volunteers, off-duty policemen and firefighters, and family members looking for relatives who had flooded the area. Suddenly, emergency responders had to spend their time corralling and redirecting these people, instead of focusing on the rescue effort *(21,22)*. It was estimated that by mid-afternoon on the day of the attack, there were more than 3000 people (volunteers and professionals) at the Pentagon, making control of the scene very difficult *(12)*. During the 1993 WTC bombing, self-dispatched firefighters from neighboring cities responded on their own and had to be turned away by the FDNY *(3)*.

Physicians and other health care providers have appeared at an incident scene and established their own treatment and triage areas *(22)*. At the Pentagon, incident commanders were not initially aware that military medical providers had set up triage sites within the Pentagon health facility and at other sites around the building perimeter. An accurate account of the number of victims treated and their disposition was delayed *(12)*.

Disaster response plans need to account for a large number of people volunteering their help. All volunteers should report to a designated site, away from the disaster. When possible, their skills and expertise should be verified. When needed, the volunteers should be assigned to specific duties and locations by the command center, helping to ensure their safety and a coordinated response. Self-dispatching activities of professional responders greatly impede the ability of the incident commander to gain control at the scene, which endangers lives. Procedures for the recall and utilization of emergency personnel when they are not involved in the immediate response should be established.

During past terrorist events, the public also reacted to the tragic images on television with massive donations of goods and services. Unfortunately most of the donations were unsolicited and not needed. In Oklahoma City, donations added to the chaos and were a major logistical problem, requiring identification, cataloguing, distribution, and storage of the items. The donations were also a security issue when individuals left unidentified boxes at police stations and hospitals *(21)*.

One item that is frequently donated, but rarely needed, is whole blood from distant communities. Most immediate blood requirements are met through donations from the affected community. During the Nairobi bombing, over 200 units of blood were delivered by international responding agencies, although blood was never requested and local hospitals did not have the capacity to store it *(25)*.

To prevent the problems arising from donations of physical items, the public should be encouraged to donate cash to private, nonprofit relief organizations. Press releases approved by the appropriate government agencies should inform the public if specific items are needed. Donation coordinators should be designated along with a specific location and central phone number or web site.

### 3.6. Victims

At most disasters, victims left the scene and sought medical care on their own or with the help of passing good Samaritans before emergency responders arrived. At the 1993 WTC bombing, one-third of the 1043 victims sought medical care on their own. Emergency medical services at the site evaluated 632 patients; 176 of them were treated and released at the scene (2). During the Oklahoma City bombing, most people walked to the nearest hospital, overwhelming their initial response capacity (21). A similar situation occurred during the Tokyo sarin attacks. It was estimated that 35% of the more than 5000 victims walked to the closest hospitals, 25% took a taxi, and 14% were transported in private vehicles (24). At the 2001 WTC incident, victims left the scene even after triage points had been established (23).

There has never been the rapid establishment of a centralized database containing the identification of victims from all the responding medical sites during a large terrorist attack. This makes it difficult to identify, track, and report systematically the status of the injured victims. Family members were often forced to go from hospital to hospital looking for their loved ones (21). Privacy issues of the patient conflicted with the frantic attempts of their loved ones to find them. During the 2001 WTC attack, the patient-tracking system of the emergency medical services was manual and was quickly overwhelmed (22).

The Bali nightclub bombing made extensive use of the Internet to find potential victims of this tragedy. Friends and family members sent emails to a central internet site, inquiring if anyone knew where and when a particular individual was last seen. This appeared to be a very successful and efficient way to gather and disseminate information (29).

In many terrorist attacks, tracking patients with minor injuries was difficult. In Oklahoma City, it was estimated that the visits of 10–20% of patients treated and released by health care facilities were not recorded (30). Medical charting in the emergency room at St. Luke's Hospital during the Tokyo attack was also chaotic, and information from mildly affected patients was lost (31).

An extensive body of literature exists describing types of injuries seen after conventional terrorist bombings (32). The patterns of injuries and death observed in conventional attacks were generally related to the type and size of the explosive material used, building construction, surrounding structures, and whether there was associated structural collapse (33). Death rates increased dramatically whenever a building collapsed. In the Oklahoma bombing, people located in the collapsed region of the building were significantly more likely to die than in other areas affected by the explosion (30).

Most deaths in past conventional attacks occurred at the time of the explosion. Most victims who survived the initial detonation suffered physical injuries that were survivable. In Arlington County, authorities noted that the expected glut of injuries after the Pentagon attack was never realized. Despite 189 deaths, only 106 people were treated at local hospitals, with 49 requiring hospitalization. The Arlington County responders were involved in the initial evaluation of less than half of these cases (12).

### 3.7. Psychological Effects

Responders are exposed to many factors that can cause severe psychological stress—areas of mass destruction, victims with grotesque injuries, and mangled bodies are just a few. After the collapse of the towers at the WTC in 2001, eight FDNY rescue workers sought emergency medical care for acute stress reaction (27). To address immediate psychological needs during the response, mental health providers have been at the site of terrorist attacks to mingle and talk with the responders. Other stress mitigation programs included short briefings prior to shift changes about conditions at the site and critical incident stress debriefings after the response (12,22).

Psychological issues can persist long after buildings have been rebuilt and the community life has returned to normal. In past disasters, persons at risk for long-term psychological effects were identified as those sustaining physical injuries, persons with underlying psychological concerns or mental illness, and personnel exposed to the grotesque and mortally injured. All initial responders, from firefighters to utility workers, fall into this latter category (34). During the 11 months following the attacks on the 2001 WTC, 1277 stress-related illnesses were reported among New York City rescue workers, representing a 17-fold increase from the 11 months preceding the tragedy (27).

Responders may experience fewer long-term consequences from the psychological stress of a bombing than victims of the blast. After the Oklahoma City bombing, the prevalence of post-traumatic stress disorders was significantly lower among responding firefighters (13%) than among male victims of the bomb (23%) (35). Long-term counseling support services are needed for initial responders, as well as the victims and others in the community. The use of unconventional weapons during the Tokyo sarin attack and the U.S. anthrax incident created unique psychological stresses among the public. In both instances, hundreds of people sought medical care even though they had no symptoms and had not been exposed to the agents (17,36). These healthy but anxious people taxed existing medical resources at a time when others needed care. The fear generated by the use of chemical or biological agents should not be underestimated. Public education campaigns are needed to alleviate these concerns and to give the public some means of evaluating their true needs. Emergency response plans must include methods for communicating with the public and for safely triaging the anxious well in order to maintain a functional medical response.

### 3.8. Mortuary Affairs

Terrorist events with high fatality rates presented unique problems. The capacities to handle bodies and conduct death investigations were taxed. Temporary morgues were established, and additional refrigeration space and supplies, such as body bags, were required. Often, inexperienced personnel worked with remains, and even experienced personnel had problems coping.

Volunteers on mortuary support teams may require specific preventive medicine support, such as immunization against hepatitis B. Medical teams at the Pentagon disaster provided such support to several team members who arrived to work without this necessary precaution (37).

The rapid identification of victims who have died is an important issue, not only for surviving friends and relatives, but also for law, insurance, and relief agencies. Death certificates require positive identification and are needed to obtain aid for bereaved families and to avoid fraudulent claims. The identity of some will be difficult because the explosive blast may have blown off clothes and identification cards. Others have major distinguishing feature destroyed, or only body parts remain. A variety of methods have been used for positive identification. In the Oklahoma City bombing, fingerprints and/ or dental X-rays were used to identify most victims. Matching pre- and post-disaster radiological findings, such as degenerative changes in joints or healed fractures, aided in the positive identification of six victims *(38)*. DNA analysis may be the only way to provide positive identification.

In the Oklahoma City bombing, unavoidable delays in official death notifications added emotional trauma to bereaved families. Delays were partly caused by the lengthy recovery process at the scene. Furthermore, there was a legal requirement to autopsy all victims and a need to collect physical evidence from the bodies *(5)*.

The creation of family assistance centers following an event helped people who had missing relatives and friends *(21)*. These centers were places where people could wait and where information about the missing was released when it became available. Members of the clergy, mental health professionals, medical examiners, and relief organizations, such as the Red Cross, staffed the centers.

### *3.9. Duration of Event*

Local firefighters and emergency medical services are organized to respond to events lasting minutes to hours. The rescue, search, and recovery phases following terrorist attacks have lasted for weeks, and in the case of the 2001 WTC attacks, for months. The prolonged duration of the rescue and recovery phases strained the equipment, resources, and personnel of responding organizations in past terrorist attacks. Supplies were rapidly depleted. During the 2001 WTC attack, there were insufficient stocks of such items as boots, batteries, respirators, safety glasses, and gloves. Furthermore, once supplies were obtained, the enormous geographic area of the devastation made distribution difficult. The 2001 WTC site was divided into multiple regions in order to stage supplies near the workers *(23)*. At the Pentagon, the Arlington County responders did not have ready access to a cache of medical supplies large enough to respond to the incident. Supplies from ambulances were taken, leaving these units ill equipped to transport patients. Fortunately, the number of expected casualties did not materialize *(12)*.

The logistical planning of supplies is important in large disasters. Stockpiles of needed items can be prepositioned for geographic regions at high risk of attack; plans for smaller communities should include contact information of businesses and relief organizations that can rapidly provide supplies and equipment.

The prolonged period of search and recovery meant that the work time of emergency responders had to be managed carefully. This included ensuring that off-duty emergency responders did not self-dispatch themselves to the site, so that they would be able to replace others when their regular duty started. It also required that only the necessary number of emergency responders needed were dispatched, maintaining a capacity to respond to other emergencies that might occur. Finally, regular work shifts had to be instituted as soon as the acute search and rescue phase was over *(12,22)*.

### *3.10. Criminal Investigation*

One of the major differences between a natural disaster response, such as an earthquake, and a response to a terrorist act is that the latter is considered a crime scene. When an event within the United States meets the federal definition of a terrorist act, the FBI will assume jurisdiction. Emergency responders to a terrorist act must focus on saving lives and preventing further injury, as well as be concerned with preserving evidence. During the Oklahoma City bombing, the priorities were " (1) save lives, maintain safety, find bodies; (2) secure the crime scene and protect the evidence." *(21)* Medical emergency responders help protect the evidence by only touching and removing items when necessary, minimizing the number of personnel, and recognizing that articles removed from victims could be evidence. Initial responders may also help law enforcement by carefully observing the scene as they first approach the rescue and reporting their impressions at a later time. Important observations could be debris that indicates an explosion or suspicious casualties *(39)*. After the Nairobi bombing, one of the bombers was caught while seeking medical care *(25)*.

### *3.11. VIP Visits*

Once the immediate phase of the emergency response was completed, politicians, celebrities, and other public figures often visited the site and offered their thanks to the rescuers. The timing of these visits sometimes interfered with ongoing recovery efforts; however, emergency responders had little control over the occurrence of these visits *(12,23)*.

### *3.12. Media*

The media has been a mixed blessing during responses to terrorist attacks. Initially, it provided the only source of information about the incident to hospitals and responding agencies, especially when communication lines failed *(21)*. Media reports were a prime source of information for hospitals and medical staff on alert as a result of the Pentagon attacks, compensating for a lack of information from authorities at the crash site *(12)*.

However, in an effort to provide information quickly, some items were not verified and were not true, adding to the confusion of the response. After the Oklahoma bombing, the media pointed to Middle Eastern terrorist groups as being the perpetrators, although an American was ultimately convicted of the crime *(6)*. During this same incident, the media, without an official request from responding agencies, told all available doctors to report to hospitals. This was not necessary and added to the confusion at the hospitals *(21)*.

The media has served an important role in providing emergency information to the public. During the Pentagon attack, there was fear that a second plane would crash in the area and the media was instrumental in informing the public to evacuate all federal buildings. The media has also served to educate the public about potential risks. During the anthrax incidents, the public was educated about the potential illnesses associated with infection, the risk of secondary infections, and prophylaxis options.

An ongoing public information operation is necessary following terrorist attacks to prevent rumors and to provide information to the public about the incident. If needed, emergency information about personal protection, evacuation, or decontamination can be disseminated through the media using principles of risk communication. As early as possible, a site should be designated for the media where information can be passed to them. It should be close to the incident without interfering with the emergency response.

## 4. TERRORIST ATTACKS
## AGAINST UNITED STATES INTERESTS OVERSEAS

Terrorist attacks directed at U.S. government installations overseas are not a new development but are a growing concern in light of today's political environment. The recent increase in the use of large explosive devices by terrorist groups makes it imperative that all U.S. interests overseas be prepared to deal with the consequences of a possible attack. Many of the issues in dealing with a mass casualty situation in the United States are similar to those faced by U.S. responders overseas; however, there are some unique differences. This section describes some lessons learned from the Embassy bombing in Kenya *(25)* and the situations that differ from a domestic response.

One of the most crucial differences in responding to an attack overseas is that the initial responders will often not get help from U.S. resources for at least 24 hours. The success of a response to mass casualty events overseas is dependent on the host nation infrastructure and on the existing resources at the affected site. During the Nairobi bombing, the first international search and rescue team arrived 22 hours after the bombing, and the American Fairfax County Urban Search and Rescue Team arrived 41 hours after the blast *(9)*. All the injured personnel from within the Embassy had been rescued within 8 hours of the explosions, and all but three of the thousands that were injured outside the Embassy had been rescued by local responders before these teams arrived. Planning, preparation, and training in these situations become even more critical to saving lives and avoiding additional injuries

Command and control issues differ from domestic incidents. The U.S. ambassador, as the President's personal representative, has the responsibility and authority over all U.S. assets within the country. Command and control of the incident scene, however, is the responsibility of the local government, who might or might not have the resources to respond adequately. Emergency medical services are often rudimentary in developing countries. At the time of the bombing, Nairobi did not have municipal emergency medical services. Despite the best efforts of State Department personnel to establish triage points and organize an orderly transport of casualties to local hospitals after the Nairobi bombing, most casualties were taken by bystanders to the nearest medical treatment center. Accountability of Embassy personnel was lost. It would take days of repeated physical searches of medical facilities and morgues to find all the injured or dead Embassy personnel.

As in domestic terrorist acts, the FBI is the lead U.S. investigative agency, but overseas they must work in cooperation with local law authorities. All laws and regulations of the host nation must be followed. This includes regulations regarding the evacuation of patients, as well as the return of remains. The host country generally requires local death certificates before bodies can be returned to their final burial places. Unfortunately, this may take some time. Local forensic medical examiners can be few in number, and the country simply may not have the capacity to perform the required examinations and paperwork quickly on all the fatalities. At the time of the Nairobi bombing, there was only one forensic pathologist serving as medical examiner for Kenya.

As in domestic incidents, it is difficult to determine just what has happened. Overseas the attack could well be part of a political coup d'état. Communications, as in domestic attacks, are critical in determining what happened and the scope of the incident. In most developing countries, communication systems are antiquated and do not have the capacity to handle even the daily load. Emergency response planners overseas must develop alternate communication systems. During the Nairobi bombing, landlines were unusable, and the communication control system for the radio network was destroyed in the blast. Consequently, everyone had equal assess to the single radio channel that remained, and priority messages could not be broadcast.

Overseas terrorist acts expose U.S. government personnel caught in such incidents to unique psychological stresses. As the intended targets of such attacks, they are victims; however, they also must be the principal rescuers and responders. In Nairobi, Embassy personnel even performed the duties of a mortuary team, collecting, identifying, and storing their friends' bodies until they could be flown back to the United States or buried in Kenya. After the immediate response, Embassy personnel had to re-establish operations within the host nation and continue day-to-day services with a minimum of resources.

The community as well as the individual suffers psychological trauma. Domestically, a strong community response helps individuals to cope with the tragedy on a short-term as well as a long-term basis. Overseas, the immediate Embassy community response is strong, but the long-term community support rapidly disappears as individuals are reassigned to other missions or return to the United States. Within a year of the Nairobi bombing, over 80% of the U.S. personnel had left Kenya.

Planning for the evacuation of injured should be an early consideration. Even where levels of acute care are adequate, local medical services and personnel can be overtaxed quickly. Prior to the arrival of the first U.S. air evacuation plane, Embassy employees occupied 10 of the 11 intensive care beds at the Nairobi Hospital. Evacuating U.S. casualties allowed these scarce resources to be used by others.

In an overseas terrorist attack, local media relationships can be strained. In a domestic incident the responders are viewed as heroes, but overseas the U.S. responders can be seen as responsible for the devastation to the host country. After all, if U.S. personnel were not there, the bombing would not have occurred. Sometimes the terrorist incident can be used to further the political agenda of groups opposed to the United States. A daily newspaper in Nairobi portrayed the efforts to establish a secure perimeter around the Embassy as an act of aloofness, deliberately intended not to help Kenyan civilian casualties.

## 5. CONCLUSIONS

Just as there is a "fog of war," there is also a "fog of disaster" when terrorists strike, producing large areas of devastation and mass casualties. As the size of the destruction increases, the difficulties in managing the emergency response increase. Communication failures and lack of coordination among responding agencies and individuals add to the confusion. Our knowledge about managing of the consequences of terrorist attacks safely and effectively has improved in recent years because of the publication of critical analyses of past terrorist events. These articles are more than just historical recordings. They allow us to examine and validate our assumptions about disaster responses and, hopefully, help us to spend our limited disaster response budgets more wisely.

The full coordination of local, state, and national agencies will only be achieved by having large-scale disaster drills in which all aspects of the attack and response are played out. Such drills have been instrumental in coordinating the response in past terrorist incidents. Responders at the Oklahoma bombing have repeatedly emphasized how important it was to establish face-to-face contacts with the people with whom they later had to coordinate activities *(21)*. Communication difficulties, chain of command, and areas of responsibilities can all be worked on prior to an event. A successful outcome to a disaster is made more likely when there is a plan that has been repeatedly practiced and personnel who have been repeatedly trained.

As military, political, and symbolic buildings and structures have strengthened their security measures, terrorists are able to produce mass casualty situations by attacking "softer" targets. The nightclub bombing in Bali reminded us that most communities have potential targets for terrorists. Terrorist attacks will continue. Physicians, as part of a community emergency response, must train and prepare for possible biological, chemical, radioactive, and high-explosive terrorist acts. By reviewing past incidents and using their lessons, hopefully we won't repeat past mistakes.

## REFERENCES

1. Hughes JM, Gerberding JL. Anthrax bioterrorism: lessons learned and future directions. Emerg Infect Dis 2002;8:1013–1014.
2. Maniscalco PM. Medical operations at the World Trade Center bombing—March 1993. In: Christen H, Maniscalso PM, eds. The EMS Incident Management System. EMS Operations for Mass Casualty and High Impact Incidents. Prentice-Hall, Upper Saddle River, NJ, 1998, pp. 149–159.
3. The World Trade Center Bombing: Report and Analysis. United States Fire Administration. Technical Report Series. Report 076. (Accessed 10 January 2003 at http://www.usfa.fema.gov/downloads/pdf/publications/tr076.cfm)
4. Okudera H, Morita H, Iwashita T, et al. Unexpected nerve gas exposure in the city of Matsumoto: report of rescue activity in the first sarin gas terrorism. Am J Emerg Med 1997;15:527–528.
5. Responding to terrorism victims. Oklahoma City and beyond. U.S. Department of Justice, Office of Justice Programs, Office for Victims of Crime, Washington, DC, 2000. (Publication number: NCJ 183949.)
6. Buck G. Overview of terrorism. In: Buck G, ed. Preparing for Terrorism. An Emergency Services Guide. Delmar Publishers, Albany, NY, 1998, pp. 1–41.
7. Okumura T, Takasu N, Ishimatsu S, et al. Report on 640 victims of the Tokyo subway sarin attack. Ann Emerg Med 1996;8:129-35.
8. Sidell FR. Chemical agent terrorism. Ann Emerg Med 1996;28:223–224.
9. Macintyre AG, Weir S, Barbera JA. The international search and rescue response to the US Embassy bombing in Kenya: The medical team experience. Prehosp Disaster Med 1999;14:215–221.
10. Centers for Disease Control and Prevention. Rapid assessment of injuries among survivors of the terrorist attack on the World Trade Center—New York City, September 2001. MMWR 2002;51:1–5.
11. Centers for Disease Control and Prevention. Deaths in World Trade Center terrorist attacks–New York City, 2001. MMWR 2002;51(special issue):16–18.
12. After-Action Report on the Response to the September 11 Terrorist Attack on the Pentagon. Arlington County Fire Department, Arlington, VA, 2002. (Accessed 10 January 2003 at http://www.co.arlington.va.us/fire/edu/about/docs/aar.htm)
13. Jernigan DB, Raghunathan PL, Bell BP, Brechner R. Investigation of bioterrorism-related anthrax, United States, 2001: epidemiologic findings. Emerg Infect Dis 2002;8:1019–1028.
14. Shepard CW, Soriano-Gabarro M, Zell ER, et al. Antimicrobial postexposure prophylaxis for anthrax: adverse events and adherence. Emerg Infect Dis 2002;8:1124–1132.
15. Accessed on 5 February 2003 at http://www.indo.com/bali121002.
16. TörÖk TJ, Tauxe RV, Wise RP. A large community outbreak of salmonellosis caused by intentional contamination of restaurant salad bars. JAMA 1997;278:389–395.
17. Pangi R. Consequence Management in the 1995 Sarin Attacks on the Japanese Subway System. BCSIA Discussion Paper 2002-4, ESDP Discussion Paper ESDP-2002-01: John F. Kennedy School of Government, Harvard University, 2002.
18. Centers for Disease Control and Prevention. Syndromic surveillance for bioterrorism following the attacks on the World Trade Center—New York City, 2001. MMWR 2002;51(special issue):13–15.
19. Lewis MD, Pavlin JA, Mansfield JL, et al. Disease outbreak detection system using syndromic data in the greater Washington DC area. Am J Prev Med 2002;23:180–186.
20. Vassallo DJ, Taylor JC, Aldington DJ, Finnegan AP. Shattered illusions—the Thiepval Barracks bombing, 7 October 1996. J R Army Med Corps 1997;143:5–11.
21. Oklahoma City—Seven Years Later. Lessons for Other Communities. Oklahoma City National Memorial Institute for the Prevention of Terrorism, Oklahoma City, OK, 2002.

22. McKinsey Report—Increasing FDNY's Preparedness. New York Fire Department, New York, 2002. (Accessed 10 January 2003 at http://www.nyc.gov/html/fdny/html/mck_report/index.html).
23. Protecting emergency responders: lessons learned from terrorist attacks. RAND Science and Policy Institute, Santa Monica, CA, 2002.
24. Okumura T, Suzuki K, Fukuda A., et al. The Tokyo subway sarin attack: disaster management, Part 1: Community emergency response. Acad Emerg Med 1998;5:613–617.
25. Smoak BL. Personal observations during Nairobi bombing, 1998.
26. Dellinger A, Waxweiler R, Mallonee S. Injuries to rescue workers following the Oklahoma City bombing. Am J Ind Med 1997;31:727–732.
27. Centers for Disease Control and Prevention. Injuries and illnesses among New York City Fire Department rescue workers after responding to the World Trade Center attacks. MMWR 2002;51(special issue):1–5.
28. Nakajima T, Sato S, Morita H, Yanagisawa N. Sarin poisoning of a rescue team in the Matsumoto sarin incident in Japan. Occup Environ Med 1997;54:697–701.
29. Accessed 10 January 2003 at http://News.bbc.co.uk/1/hi/in_depth/asia_pacific/2002/bali.
30. Mallonee S, Shariat S, Stennies G, Waxweiler R, Hogan D, Jordan F. Physical injuries and fatalities resulting from the Oklahoma City bombing. JAMA 1996;276:382–387.
31. Okumura T, Suzuki K, Fukuda A, et al. The Tokyo subway sarin attack: disaster management, Part 2: Hospital response. Acad Emerg Med 1998;5:618–624.
32. Wightman JM, Gladish SL. Explosions and blast injuries. Ann Emerg Med 2001;37:664–678.
33. Stein M, Hirshberg A. Medical consequences of terrorism. The conventional weapon threat. Surg Clin North Am. 1999;79:1537–1552.
34. Norwood AE, Ursano RJ, Fullerton CS. Disaster psychiatry: principles and practice. Psychiatr Q 2000;71:207–226.
35. North CS, Tivis L, McMillen JC, et al. Psychiatric disorders in rescue workers after the Oklahoma City bombing. Am J Psychiatry 2002;159:857–859.
36. Mott JA, Treadwell TA, Hennessy TW, et al. Call-tracking data and the public health response to bioterrorism-related anthrax. Emerg Infect Dis 2002;8:1088–1092.
37. Geiling J. Personal observation during Pentagon response, 2001.
38. Nye PJ, Tytle TL, Jarman RN, Eaton BG. The role of radiology in the Oklahoma City bombing. Radiology 1996;200:541–543.
39. Dolan NJ, Maniscalco PM. Crime scene operations, In: Maniscalco PM, Christen HT, eds. Understanding Terrorism and Managing the Consequences. Prentice Hall, Upper Saddle River, NJ, 2002:253–266.

# 2

# Hospital Preparation and Response to an Incident

## *James A. Geiling, MD, FACP, FCCP*

The opinions and assertions contained herein are those of the author and are not to be construed as official or as necessarily reflecting the views of the Department of the Army, the Department of Defense, or the Department of Veterans Affairs.

### CONTENTS

*If supposedly civilized nations confined their warfare to attacks on the enemy's troops, the matter of defense against warfare chemicals would be a purely military problem, and therefore beyond the scope of this study. But such is far from the case. In these days of total warfare, the civilians, including women and children, are subject to attack at all times.*

—Colonel Edgar Erskine Hume, Medical Corps, US Army, 1943

## 1. INTRODUCTION AND BACKGROUND

Hospital-based physicians normally at some time their career study, prepare, and practice skills required to treat mass casualties. The focus traditionally centers on the

From: *Physician's Guide to Terrorist Attack*
Edited by: M. J. Roy © Humana Press Inc., Totowa, NJ

presentation of many patients appearing at the Emergency Department (ED) door with multitrauma as a consequence of a conventional weapon or explosion or a natural disaster. The events of September 11, 2001 (hereafter called 9/11) and the subsequent anthrax cases that year demonstrate that acts of terrorism, including those of chemical or biological agents, have come to the forefront of our daily lives. Current governmental reports predict repeated events over time. Only through intensive education and training can physicians and medical facilities adequately prepare to meet the medical challenges imposed by chemical, biological, radiological, nuclear, and explosive (CBRNE) weapons of terror, commonly knows as weapons of mass destruction (WMD). Much work lies ahead, for over 70% of hospitals may not be prepared to handle such incidents *(1)*, and only 20% have any plans for handling biological or chemical incidents *(2)*.

## 2. DISASTERS AND MASS CASUALTY INCIDENTS

Disasters occur when normal, basic services of a society become disrupted to such an extent that widespread human and environmental losses exceed the community's emergency management capacity *(3)*. Disasters normally imply involvement of a large geographic area with many casualties. However, "disasters" should be distinguished from "mass casualty incidents" (MCIs), defined as "... events resulting in a number of victims large enough to disrupt the normal course of emergency and health care services of the affected community" *(4)*. Disasters, then, typically result in MCIs but encompass a broad range of calamities to society beyond high numbers of patients or casualties.

Disasters and MCIs in the medical literature have typically been described as arising from internal (that is from within the health care facility) or external causes. Terrorism is a man-made, external disaster and serves as the focus for this study.

## 3. DISASTER RESPONSE IN THE UNITED STATES

Recent disaster response in the United States dates to the 1964 earthquake in Alaska, when needs far exceeded local capabilities. Governmental review led to development of the Disaster Relief Act in 1974 that outlined the law and procedures for state governors to request formally federal assistance. As a follow-on, the Federal Emergency Management Agency (FEMA) was created in 1979 primarily in response to the needs of the Cold War; by 1989, however, it became empowered and funded to focus its efforts on other disaster responses as well. The current basis for federal disaster response in the United States is PL 93-288 (and later amended in PL 100-707), the Robert T. Stafford Disaster Relief and Emergency Assistance Act (most commonly known as the *Stafford Act) (5)*.

Under the guidance of FEMA, the response to a federally declared disaster within the United States, known as the Federal Response Plan (FRP), is divided into 12 functional areas called Emergency Support Functions (ESFs; *see* Table 1). Hurricane Andrew in 1992 saw the first use of the FRP. In such a disaster, FEMA provides overall direction to the lead and support agencies within each ESF. However, fundamental to the federal disaster response is that the federal assets deploy to assist and coordinate with the state government, which maintains overall responsibility for any disaster within its boundaries *(5)*.

Beginning in 1980 as the Civilian-Military Contingency Hospital System (CMCHS), the national response for mass medical needs was designed to increase the number of beds available to the military health care system in times of emergency. Following a 1981 review of the federal disaster response to the eruption of Mt. St. Helens, the National

Table 1
The 12 Emergency Support Functions

| Function | Lead agency |
| --- | --- |
| 1. Transportation | Department of Transportation |
| 2. Communication | National Communication System |
| 3. Public works/engineering | Deptartment of Defense (U.S. Army Corps of Engineers) |
| 4. Fire fighting | Department of Agriculture |
| 5. Information/planning | Federal Emergency Management Agency (FEMA) |
| 6. Mass care | American Red Cross |
| 7. Rescue support | General Services Administration |
| 8. Health and medical services | Department of Health and Human Services (now Department of Homeland Security) |
| 9. Urban search and rescue | FEMA |
| 10. Hazardous material | Environmental Protection Agency |
| 11. Food | Department of Agriculture |
| 12. Energy | Department of Energy |

From ref. 5.

Disaster Medical System (NDMS), under the lead of the Office of Emergency Preparedness (OEP) in the Department of Homeland Security (DHS) (formerly in the Department Health and Human Services; DHHS), replaced and updated the CMCHS. NDMS also includes the Department of Defense (DOD), the Department of Veterans Affairs (DVA), and FEMA. OEP, in addition to providing overall direction to NDMS, also oversees the development, training, and implementation of Disaster Medical Assistance Teams (DMATs) and other specialty teams. DOD assists in transportation and medical support, DVA provides physical facilities and medical supplies at the disaster site, and FEMA aids with personnel, training, and funding *(5)*.

Under ESF 8, DHS/OEP has responsibility for:

1. Assessment of health and medical needs
2. Surveillance of health care issues
3. Acquisition and distribution of medical personnel
4. Acquisition and distribution of health and medical equipment and supplies
5. Medical evacuation
6. Inpatient care
7. Food/drug/medical-device safety
8. Worker health and safety
9. Radiological monitoring
10. Chemical or Hazmat monitoring
11. Biological monitoring
12. Mental health assessment
13. Development and dissemination of public health information
14. Vector control
15. Water and sewage management
16. Victim identification and mortuary services *(5)*.

The 61 DMATs and specialty teams that OEP supervises come from across the United States, each normally sponsored by a local civilian agency, such as a regional trauma center. Approximately 35 volunteer medical and support personnel are deployed with each team. When designated "on call" through a rotating schedule, team members must be prepared to deploy within 12–24 hours of notification, be self-sustaining for 72 hours, treat 250 patients, and remain on location for 10–14 days. In addition to providing both general surgical and medical capabilities, several specialty teams (e.g., burns, pediatrics, and so on) can also be generated and deployed. During the mission, team members become federal employees, although their task is primarily to interface with and support local medical systems (5).

## 4. DISASTER EFFECTS ON HOSPITALS

### 4.1. Historical Data

Mass casualties, particularly from sudden impact explosions or detonations, result in a predictable set of injuries and circumstances surrounding the event. Many of the lessons learned from previous disasters were discussed in Chapter 1 of this guide. Review of these historical precedents will prove to be invaluable in preparing physicians and facilities for the medical consequences of a terrorist event.

One major study from 1988 reviewed 14 reports of terrorist bombings from 1969 to 1983 (6). The review included information on 220 worldwide incidents that caused 3357 casualties. In these events, the average number of victims was 15.3 casualties/incident. Four hundred twenty-three (12.6%) persons died before receiving any medical care. However, 2934 (87%) of the victims survived the immediate event; of these, 881 (30%) were admitted. Forty (1.4%) of the immediate survivors eventually died. Of the 1339 casualties with sufficient data to review, 18.7% were deemed critical (range 7.6–34%), and 45.5% were admitted. Overtriage (defined in this paper as the "proportion of noncritically injured survivors hospitalized for immediate care") was 59% (range 8.3–80%). Conversely, there was only one single case of possible undertriage. Head injuries were the predominant cause of immediate (71%) and late (52%) deaths. Records of 812 survivors showed that the surgical procedures were categorized as soft tissue in 67%, bone in 17.5%, abdominal in 5.5%, head in 2%, and miscellaneous in 8%.

The impact of these types of terrorist bombings on hospitals has most recently been described in the Oklahoma City bombing which occurred on April 19, 1995. A detailed retrospective review of medical examiner records, hospital records, physician surveys, and building occupant and survivor surveys, as well as ambulance dispatches, media reports, and several other sources were used in one study to look at the injury and fatality patterns from the blast. The blast injured a total of 759 persons, of whom 167 died (case fatality ratio of 22%); 162 deaths occurred at the scene, three persons were dead on arrival at the emergency room, and two persons died of wounds on days 2 and 23 following admission. Of the remainder, 509 were treated as outpatients and released (67% of the injured or 86% of the immediate survivors), and 83 were hospitalized (11% of the injured or 14% of the immediate survivors). The injuries were primarily soft tissue lacerations, abrasions, contusions, and punctures (74% to the extremities, 48% to the head, 45% to the face, and 35% to the chest) and musculoskeletal injuries (the most common fracture sites were the extremities, face and neck, back, chest, and pelvis) (7).

Another study that looked at the Oklahoma City bombing evaluated the impact on the EDs in the city through a retrospective review of 388 available medical records at 13 hospitals (8). Following the explosion, the median time to arrival at the emergency department was 91 minutes, with most making it by 3 hours. Patients who eventually were admitted to the hospital took longer to get to the ED than those who were treated and released. The mode of transportation was 56% by privately owned vehicle, 33% by emergency medical services, 10% by walking or being carried, and 1% by other means.

Most (64%) of the patients who were treated in the field were admitted to the hospital: 28% to the operating room, 24% to a ward, and 9% to the intensive care unit; 3% were dead on arrival. Once a patient was seen in the ED, the contact time was approximately 1 hour. The five most common procedures conducted in the ED were wound care, tetanus immunization, intravenous line placement, pulse oximeter use, and the administration of analgesics. For patients discharged from the ED, the most common diagnoses were laceration (30%), contusion (9%), fracture (8%), strain (6%), head injury (6%), and abrasion (6%).

Most of the literature surrounding the medical effects of terrorism focuses on the more frequently used conventional weapons or explosions. The most publicized use of chemical agents for terrorism occurred in Tokyo in the middle 1990s when on two occasions the Aum Shinrikyo Japanese religious cult released sarin gas. The first release came on June 27, 1994 in the city of Matsumoto and resulted in 600 persons being exposed; 58 of them were admitted and 7 died *(9)*. The more famous and larger event took place in Tokyo on March 20, 1995, when the cult released sarin gas in the subway, resulting in the deaths of 11 commuters and medical evaluation of 5000 persons *(10)*.

### 4.2. Current Assessment of Hospital Preparedness

Although fortunately no terrorist-related MCI occurred at the 1996 Atlanta Olympic Games, "unprecedented" preparations took place to prepare the community for any medical consequences of a terrorist attack involving WMD. Most local, state, and federal (including military) assets involved in the plan focused on prehospital assessment, diagnosis, decontamination, and treatment. Examples included the establishment of a Federal Bureau of Investigation (FBI) team specializing in the rapid assessment of an incident site, the development of a multiagency Science and Technology Center to provide multidisciplined consultation, the stockpiling of antimicrobials and antidotes, enhanced surveillance, and specialized first-responder training. In addition, augmented clinical capabilities included 30 specially trained DMATs, the U.S. Marine Corps Chemical and Biological Incident Response Force (CBIRF), and the newly developed Metropolitan Medical Strike Teams (MMSTs). In addition to some stand-alone capability, these organizations could also augment or support local medical facilities, many of which developed and exercised their own medical response plans *(11)*.

Since 9/11, the entire nation and the health care infrastructure have embarked on ambitious programs designed to provide medical support to the populace in the event of significant disaster, to include a terrorist-dispersed WMD. Prior to 9/11, lack of hospital preparedness for a chemical or biological terrorist attack was somewhat understandable. In May 2001, fewer than 20% of 186 EDs from four northwestern states had plans for biological or chemical weapons events. Forty-five percent had some decontamination capability, but only 29% could provide enough atropine for 50 sarin nerve agent casualties *(12)*.

Although plans since 9/11 have moved forward with fervor, as reported in November 2001 *(1)*, hospitals continue to believe they are unprepared for such an event. Of 30 hospitals in FEMA Region III (Pennsylvania, West Virginia, Maryland, the District of Columbia, and Virginia) that responded to a survey, 73% believe they are completely incapable of handling a biological or chemical incident; only urban hospitals (26% of the total) felt somewhat prepared for these scenarios. Preparation for a nuclear weapon was identical, with the exception of a hospital in close proximity to a nuclear power plant. Only 73% of respondents were prepared for patient decontamination (one room only). WMD preparedness was incorporated into the emergency preparedness plans in 27% of the facilities. Finally, only 23% of the respondents reported that their staff had received any WMD training (all lecture-based), and only one metropolitan hospital had conducted mandatory training for its clinical personnel.

Hospital disaster preparedness typically falls under the purview of emergency medicine staff. Hospital and inpatient-based physicians such as intensivists, have only recently begun to expand their role outside the resource-rich intensive care unit into settings that may require triage. MCIs involving terrorism, or more common Hazmat incidents, will necessarily involve these physicians and may require them to play a role in the triage and prioritization of limited inpatient resources. Unfortunately, "training in disaster management, including Hazmat incidents, is not part of training guidelines for intensivists" *(13)*.

## 5. PREPARATION

### *5.1. Disaster Response Plans*

Disaster medicine has its own literature that, through an evidence-based approach, may be useful in disaster planning. The consequences of disasters, particularly those resulting from explosive devices, are often predictable, based on information such as that given in Subheading 4.1. above. However, the use of that information to prepare a medical response often becomes problematic, particularly as the response broadens and crosses departmental and agency boundaries. "Most disaster response problems are not failures of the individual. More often they are *system problems*. That is, the usual organizational systems (procedures, management structures, and designation of responsibilities) established by various organizations to cope with routine, daily emergencies are not well adapted for use in disasters" *(14)*.

Unfortunately, little has been written about such system faults. Coordination among agencies and their communication of information is usually the biggest problem facing a multiagency disaster response. For example, when a mock extortionist threat to detonate a nuclear device at the Summer Olympics in Atlanta was used in a multiagency exercise in 1994, major weaknesses were identified in the cooperation between agencies whose priorities and incentives conflicted. In this exercise, the FBI focused its efforts on identifying and capturing the terrorists, whereas the Department of Energy and DOD were most concerned with disabling the bomb *(15)*.

Sudden impact disasters, such as a terrorist bombing, can be thought of as occurring in a time sequence of five phases: (1) interdisaster; (2) predisaster or warning; (3) impact or detonation; (4) emergency response or relief; and (5) rehabilitation or reconstruction *(16)*. Development of a comprehensive response plan should take place following such a disaster, during the rehabilitation phase, or prior to the next one (the interdisaster phase). The interest in generating such a plan is "… proportional to the recency and magnitude of the last disaster" *(14)*. Notably, this is also the best time to submit plans for funding.

Unfortunately, once the reconstruction is well under way, such planning begins to wane. "People are unlikely to give priority attention to an unlikely future disaster when there are fifteen tasks to be accomplished by Friday" *(14)*. This perspective, in the current setting of limited governmental resources, often results in an apathetic response to disaster planning. Thus, to accomplish such a task, disaster preparedness proposals must be cost-effective.

Planning in detail for a disaster and all its possible outcomes is an overwhelming task that is doomed to incompletion. In contrast, disasters of moderate size have a better chance of funding, are more likely to be rehearsed, and have a higher probability of occurring. Such model disasters should include approximately 120 casualties, for disasters of this magnitude will pose most of the interorganizational dilemmas that occur in larger events. Ideally, the plan and management structure should allow for a modular expansion of response "… as the incident (and the number of resources that need to be coordinated) grows in size" *(14)*.

Hospital disaster planning often faces significant challenges because the task is complex, time-consuming, and often relegated as an "additional duty." Designated persons tasked to develop a hospital plan need experience, patience, and a detailed understanding of the organizational personalities in order to foster cooperation in developing the plan. Additionally, the planner must ensure that the anticipated workload is appropriately divided for optimal use of critical specialties *(17)*.

## 5.2. Notional Plans

Once the intent to develop a plan matures and becomes a priority for an organization, what ensures its successful application when the disaster occurs? Unfortunately, planning for a disaster response is merely an illusion unless "… it is based upon valid assumptions about human behavior, incorporates an inter-organizational perspective, is tied to resources, and is known and accepted by the participants" *(14)*. The written product, although a template for action, fails to demonstrate adequate preparation unless it is accompanied by training. Through training, the plan validates what people are "likely" to do rather than what they "should" do *(14)*.

Although disaster planning is fraught with a multitude of challenges, "… the *process* of planning is more important than the written product that results" *(14)*. The personal contacts and familiarity of individuals within the organizations participating in the disaster planning all contribute to a modicum of success. Unfortunately, with the frequent turnover of individuals within the organizations, particularly at the federal level, the mistakes of past disaster responses often recur.

The medical literature pertaining to disaster preparedness planning is primarily focused on the community level. However, principles of good preparedness planning that apply to the prehospital environment are also valid for hospital disaster plans. A common 10-point approach includes the following *(18)*:

1. View disasters as quantitatively and qualitatively different from accidents and minor emergencies.
2. Plan as a continuing process rather than focusing on an end product such as a written plan.
3. Look at a multihazard, generic plan rather than an agent-specific plan.
4. Focus on the coordination of emergent resources rather than a fixed command and control structure.

5. Look at general principles rather than specific details.
6. Assume that potential victims (and staff) will react well during a crisis.
7. Emphasize the need for intra- and interorganizational integration during the development of the plan.
8. Anticipate likely problems and possible solutions.
9. Plan according to disaster data rather than personal anecdotes or "war stories."
10. Plan according to phase (mitigation, preparedness, response, and recovery).

## 6. DISASTERS VS EMERGENCIES

Every organization plans for, and often experiences, a variety of emergencies, yet disasters usually stress normal organizational structure and procedures beyond their design capabilities. Table 2 delineates some common differences between routine emergencies and disasters.

## 7. INTERAGENCY COOPERATION

Interagency communication and coordination challenge normal emergency responses in disasters. Most agencies tend to model their organizational and emergency responses along the typical military model of command and control, that is, centralized control under a single commander and decentralized execution. However, "... realistic disaster management in a country with a decentralized government such as the United States, with its traditional preferences for local control and private enterprise, probably cannot be accomplished using a military model, rather, coordination among various independent responding organizations needs to be based on negotiation and cooperation" *(14)*.

The cooperation needed in disasters is best demonstrated in the development of predisaster planning with parties of all agencies, emergency operations centers, and the Unified Command structure of the Incident Command System or Hospital Emergency Incident Command System (HEICS). Efficient disaster response and multiagency cooperation develop by conducting joint planning and training, coordinating the division of labor and responsibilities, agreeing to common communication terminology and procedures, and fostering informal contacts. Knowledge and comfort with others in the disaster-response team promotes an opening of communication regarding glitches in terminology, equipment, and, most importantly, the desire to share critical information ("who else needs to know?"). It is these less-formal procedures that advance an effective disaster response; pre-existing personal, political, and jurisdictional disputes (more commonly known as "turf" or "sandbox" issues) impede multiagency cooperation *(14)*.

## 8. EXERCISING THE PLAN

Rehearing the disaster plan helps to identify potential areas needing improvement or revision and increases the likelihood of success in a real event. Exercises can range from simple desktop discussions to community-wide drills; the more involvement and interagency cooperation, the more meaningful the event. Unfortunately, these drills tend to infrequently, occur without full participant involvement, and fail to test the plan fully; in effect, a false sense of security develops *(17)*.

Hospitals in Israel often run vigorous rehearsals in order to improve their response efforts to frequent, recurring disasters. Between 1986 and 1994, 30 detailed chemical practice drills were conducted in 21 major hospitals. Each exercise involved the treatment

Table 2
Differences in Disasters

| Routine emergencies | Disasters |
|---|---|
| Interaction with familiar parties | Interaction with unfamiliar parties |
| Familiar tasks/procedures | Unfamiliar tasks/procedures |
| Intraorganization coordination | Intra- and interorganization coordination |
| Intact communications, roads, and so on | Disrupted communications, blocked roads, and so on |
| Intraorganizational communications | Interorganizational communications |
| Familiar terminology | Unfamiliar, organization-specific terminology |
| Local press attention | National/international media attention |
| Management adequate for resources | Resources overwhelm management capacity |

From ref. *14.*

of 100–400 simulated patients and included the use of personal protective equipment and decontamination with 25% of the patients including children and adults who required intensive care and ventilatory support. Hospital- and community-wide plans that arose from this exercise included the following principles:

1. Hospital designation: specific hospitals remote from the event should be designated to receive only chemical casualties
2. Optimal use of manpower
3. Preventing hospital contamination
4. Blocking free access to the hospital
5. Triage: using experienced emergency personnel according to chemical, age, and medical criteria
6. Extension of nurses' authority: expanding diagnosis and treatment using established treatment protocols *(19)*

## *8.1. Roles*

The urgency of disasters or MCIs coupled with medical providers' desire to serve and care for the injured potentially leads to conflicts in roles and responsibilities. Health care providers possess a unique skill set, based on their core training and subsequent experiences. These competencies affect how each responds to the stressful event played out in an MCI. In general, providers should care for the victims of a disaster in the environment in which they normally practice medicine. Although each disaster is unique, requiring innovation and adjustment, several basic rules of role assignment apply:

1. Prehospital medics, corpsmen, EMTs, and others should perform the initial assessment, triage, stabilization, and evacuation to the casualty collection and treatment point, where the first physician should intervene.
2. Only physicians, nurses, and other providers specially trained to work in the field, prehospital environment should do so.
3. Only if excess physicians or hospital-based providers exist should they move forward to the disaster scene.
4. Medics or prehospital personnel are poor replacements for nurses or hospital-based providers.
5. Physicians and nurses are better prepared than most to care for the public health needs of the affected population *(20).*

## 9. PERSONAL PROTECTIVE EQUIPMENT

No universal personal protective equipment (PPE) recommendations can be made for all potential scenarios. However, PPE recommendations can be standardized by category. Level C protection, that, is full-face mask with a powered or nonpowered canister filtration system and associated chemical barrier suit, is probably adequate for most health care workers. This especially applies to those workers remote from the scene whose only exposure will be to those agents that remain on skin and clothing of the exposed victims *(31)*. Specific biological and infectious control measures have been detailed elsewhere *(34)*.

## 10. PUBLIC RELATIONS

Problems with the media often result from failure to plan for their presence and involvement. They will be present, so failing to plan for media relations predisposes to problems that could disrupt the disaster response. Normally the media will always want the same information, i.e., casualty information, property damage, disaster response and relief activities, other characteristics of the crisis, and theories on the cause of the disaster *(14)*.

Effective media management in a disaster follows several important concepts. The first is that both the media and the public view silence, or not releasing information, with suspicion. Information must be released as soon as feasible, especially within the first 24 hours. Once the site is safe, access to it becomes a goal for the media and needs to be granted as soon as possible. Speculation and opinion by spokesmen results in mistrust by the media and their audience; questions that cannot be truthfully answered should be researched before release. Finally, after the media begin to release their story, the leadership of the response effort must monitor both the truthfulness of the story and the reaction by the audience *(21)*.

## 11. FACILITIES

The baseline hospital preparation for a terrorist event will most likely be compliance with those standards of disaster preparedness established by the Joint Commission on the Accreditation of Healthcare Organizations (JCAHO). The JCAHO disaster preparedness requirements fall mostly under the Environment of Care (EC) standards. EC 1.4 requires that plans address four major disaster phases: mitigation, preparedness, response, and recovery. It also requires plans to address evacuation of the facility while establishing alternate care sites. Finally, it mandates a plan that is integrated with other efforts in the community *(22)*.

Hospitals need to approach disaster planning on a regional level to ensure that all patients receive appropriate care within the constraints of community capabilities. Civilian hospitals should communicate with military treatment facilities (MTFs) and develop a cooperative planning relationship. In addition to added treatment capabilities, MTF staffs have often undergone extensive training in preparing for the care of victims of a WMD event and can aid in community preparation. They often also have designated teams specially prepared to handle such MCIs. Capabilities may include agent detection, decontamination, trauma management (which can be rapidly exported), evacuation, mental health support, and communications or logistical support.

Civilian hospitals may also have well-established relationships with local Veterans Health Administration (VHA) facilities. Although normally viewed as a resource accessible only to military veterans, these clinics and hospitals will most certainly be used in times of disaster. The VHA has four statutory missions that clearly transcend boundaries in time of need: provide medical care to eligible veterans, train health professionals, conduct research, and support the Departments of Defense and Health and Human Services during times of national emergency. Additionally, the VHA could assist local WMD preparedness planning by:

1. Providing WMD and disaster health professional training
2. Assessing and assisting local and regional planning efforts through the use of its VHA Area Emergency Managers
3. Planning to deliver direct health care in its fixed or mobile facilities, assisting with decontamination and patient staging, and giving other support to often fiscally strapped private hospitals
4. Assisting in the storage and distribution of national stocks of pharmaceuticals, vaccines, and so on
5. Cooperate with other local, state, and federal disease surveillance systems, which may prove useful in detecting a bioterrorism event
6. Conducting ongoing research and implementing proven treatment or preventive strategies in such disaster-related topics as post-traumatic stress disorder and environmental hazards *(23)*

Finally, hospitals can best plan and prepare for disasters by following several selected principles. The first is to develop strategies that overcome the normal resistance to preparedness. This may best be handled by planning for what is likely in the hospital's location, and then, in order to prepare for the less likely, developing procedures for planned improvisation. Second, the hospital and its Emergency Operations Center (EOC) need to ensure that the medical response facilities (or capabilities) will survive and function. Third, the hospital must participate in community-wide disaster planning and training. Communication reliability is always threatened in disasters, so communications strategies not involving the telephone must be planned and exercised. All plans should allow for modular expandability. As so often happens, the plan must consider large numbers of unsolicited volunteers and donations. Finally, especially in a WMD release, the hospital must know how to integrate into state and federal response plans *(24)*.

## 12. EDUCATION AND TRAINING

The events of 9/11 have clearly changed the focus and expanded the requirements for education on the effects of WMD. Nevertheless, to date, medical education has been unprepared for such events. In 1998, 76 emergency medicine residency program directors noted in a survey that 53% of their residencies did include formal training in bioweapons, but most of that was in lecture format. More (84%) included training in Hazmat or chemical agent release, but, again, most of that education took place in lecture format. Rarely did their training for these events include practical or "field" exercises, and only half the respondents knew about personal protective equipment in the ED *(25)*.

Formalizing medical training for WMD events, for all levels of providers, will greatly prepare health care workers and facilities to respond to such events. Prior to the 9/11 tragedies, a task force of health care professionals looked at this need and reported their recommendations for such training. These awareness and performance objectives provide a framework on which facilities and educational organizations can base their education and training program *(26)*. Awareness objectives of the educational program included:

1. Terrorism
2. Event types
3. Index of suspicion and event recognition
4. Response systems and communications
5. Key elements of a WMD response
6. Personal protection and safety.

These awareness objectives were then matched to performance objectives, tailored to the way the learners will use the information in their roles. Recommended performance objectives included:

1. Event recognition
2. Unified incident command/management structure
3. Response support
4. Safety and protection
5. Decontamination
6. Isolation and containment
7. Evidence preservation
8. Psychological effects
9. Communication and agency interaction
10. Triage
11. Treatment
12. Transportation
13. Recovery operations
14. Fatality management.

## 13. RESPONSE

### *13.1. Assessment*

Explosive or conventional weapons, and most chemical weapons, will result in the immediate influx of victims and (especially with chemical weapons) even greater numbers of "worried' well." Interaction with law enforcement agencies as well as first responders will give hospital personnel good information regarding the event and potential agent. Release of a bioweapon, on the other hand, will probably result in a latency period of hours to days, whereupon patients will begin to appear at EDs as well as clinics and offices. Initial identification will require a process known as *syndromic surveillance* until laboratory confirmation. For example, the Department of Health in Maryland asks that physicians maintain a high level of suspicion for:

1. Gastroenteritis of any apparent infectious etiology
2. Pneumonia with the sudden death of a previously healthy adult
3. Widened mediastinum in a febrile patient without another explanation
4. Rash of synchronous vesicular/pustular lesions
5. Acute neurological illness with fever
6. Advancing cranial nerve impairment with progressive generalized weakness *(27)*.

## 13.2. Command And Control Issues

All phases of a disaster require direction and oversight. Once a disaster has occurred, hospitals and other health care facilities must establish an EOC. The function, leadership, access, communications procedures, and so on must be clearly identified. The size, location, interaction with reporting staff, and ongoing patient receiving and treatment activities must be coordinated in order to support, not interfere with or complicate, the response effort. A typical composition includes the hospital director, chief of staff, senior nursing supervisor, and representative staff from such organizations as public affairs, engineering, public safety, and secretarial staff (as found in HEICS). In addition to coordinating internal facility operations, the EOC must oversee and direct communications with outside agencies and authorities. Finally, the EOC must be in a secure location and prepared with emergency supplies for continuous operations. In a WMD release, this will require special attention to weather conditions, decontamination operations, and building security *(28)*.

## 13.3. Security

Hospital security becomes pivotal in maintaining clinical operations in the event of a WMD release. The initial wave of victims or "worried well" that appear at a facility may unknowingly bypass precautionary measures for contaminated casualties until the nature of the event has been clarified. Thereafter, more incoming patients, worried family members, hospital staff on recall, and volunteers will challenge any imposed security measures. In addition, normal police or other security support may be occupied at the scene or elsewhere in the community.

## 13.4. Intelligence

Prior warning of an event will clearly aid facility and provider response. Although limited by the available intelligence capabilities of law enforcement and other government agencies, sharing of information with medical authorities may not occur, even if valuable information is known. Prior integration of medical planners into local, state, and federal emergency planning and operations organizations builds the necessary trust and familiarity that becomes crucial to effective medical response in time of need. Medical providers and organizations must become familiar with these agencies' operations and must fully understand the sensitive nature of the intelligence information in order to maintain and further encourage incorporation of medical planning into an overall community response to a WMD event.

## 13.5. Detection

Detection will probably rely on agencies and organizations outside the medical treatment facility itself. The Centers for Disease Control and Prevention (CDC) plan to integrate the surveillance for illness and injury as a consequence of the release of a chemical or biological weapon into other U.S. disease surveillance systems. This will result in a partnering of the CDC with state and local health agencies as well as hospital clinics and EDs, poison control centers, and other health care facilities. In addition, the CDC, the Association of Public Health Laboratories, and their partners will create a multilevel Laboratory Response Network (LRN) for bioterrorism to analyze biological agents; it will also partner with other federal agencies such as the U.S. Environmental Protection Agency to diagnose chemical agent exposure *(29,30)*.

Unless it is specifically trained and maintained, a hospital-directed detector will probably slow treatment and decontamination procedures. Most treatment will be ongoing while confirmatory tests continue, thus making this equipment best suited to nonhospital agencies *(31)*.

### *13.6. Decontamination*

Ideally, health care facilities should have decontamination capability in preparation not only for a biological or chemical terrorist event, but also the more common Hazmat events. Outdoor shower-like capability best suits most scenarios, obviating the need for ventilation and permitting the influx of large numbers of patients. With additional provisions for inclement weather, maintaining patient privacy, and securing patients' personal effects, these facilities can permit most patients to conduct self-decontamination with a series of showers and soapy water. This setup frees medical personnel to care for injured patients or those incapable of self-decontamination. Plain soap and water rather than 0.5% hypochlorite is the best material for most scenarios. Simply having the patients disrobe may remove 75–90% of any residual agent. Finally, most facilities and government agencies do not require wastewater containment, although water utilities should be notified *(31)*.

### *13.7. Triage*

MCIs caused by a conventional weapon will result in large numbers of wounded patients suddenly appearing at the ED. Experienced surgeons or other physicians who regularly treat trauma victims should meet the ambulances (or other vehicles, realizing that most victims will arrive by their own means) and immediately triage patients. Stein and Hirshberg *(32)* recommend simple division into urgent and nonurgent categories, with additional providers beginning advanced trauma life support for urgent patients. They advocate dividing surgical care into two phases: (1) the initial phase, when casualties arrive, chaos is maximal, and the exact numbers of casualties remain unknown; and (2) the definitive phase. Notably, they recommend that all patients be thoroughly evaluated for the often missed phonal (tympanic membrane) and ocular trauma.

Depending on the nature of the event and surgical demands placed on the receiving hospital, redistribution of patients to other facilities may be considered. This transfer may be to a facility of higher capability or to one with lesser means that can aid in more time-consuming processes such as wound debridement or orthopedic fixation. Blast injuries will also require matching patients in need of ventilatory support with institutions capable of supporting mechanical ventilation and intensive care support *(32)*.

Early in a bioweapon release, triage categories my differ significantly from those of a conventional weapon. One proposed mechanism expands on the triage categories found in conventional epidemics. The SEIR categories include:

1. *S*usceptible individuals (including those with incomplete or unsuccessful vaccination)
2. *E*xposed individuals (those who are infected, incubating, and noncontagious)
3. *I*nfectious individuals (those who are symptomatic and contagious)
4. *R*emoved individuals (those who are no longer sources of infection, i.e., they survive or die from the illness, and their remains are not contagious)

5. Vaccinated successfully (those with confirmed "take" or who have completed a course for immunity" *(27)*.

Most disasters, and especially those involving WMD, can be expected to result in fatalities. In addition to the difficult challenge of declaring patients as "expectant" during multiple stages of triage, handling of the remains must be considered and planned. Remains held at on-scene locations and those in hospital morgues may require special handling and close coordination with law enforcement agencies, for these events will probably be considered as crimes. In addition, normal sensitivities to family members searching for their loved ones, infection control issues, hazardous or contaminated remains, and media inquiries will also require detailed planning *(17)*.

### 13.8. Infection Control

Until the nature of the event has been defined, a WMD release, particularly a bioterrorism event, may involve infectious patients. Such an event will require external triage to assist in mitigating the effects on hospital personnel and previously admitted patients, as well as isolation of victims themselves *(22)*. Planning for the infection control of such an event will also be required by JCAHO. For example, the hospital's infection control plan must incorporate or separately identify the infection prevention and control measures that will be implemented in an MCI *(33)*. The Association for Professionals in Infection Control and Epidemiology (APIC), in concert with the CDC Hospital Infections Program Bioterrorism Working Group, has developed detailed infection-control plans, templates, and health care facility checklists *(34,35)*.

### 13.9. Logistic Support

MCIs involving a WMD release will exponentially increase the logistic support necessary to support the medical effort. Planning processes, communications equipment, decontamination equipment and supplies, antibiotics, antidotes, and many other consumables will place significant burdens on individual facilities and communities. Cooperation will be required with a rapid influx of resources from state and federal sources. Such efforts require pre-event planning, coordination, and exercise. The American Hospital Association estimates that an urban hospital called on to treat 1000 biological or chemical casualties will require $3 million in additional funds and supplies during the first 48 hours; a rural hospital responding similarly to 200 patients may still require $1.5 million *(22)*.

### 13.10. Personnel Issues

Supporting the response effort will require close attention to many personnel issues. These will include attention to the mental and physical health of the workers, attending to the needs of their families, and providing them with the necessary food, clothing or supplies, rest, and respite from the operations. Medical workers will probably continue sustained operations well after the acute event, and hence planning and implementing this "marathon" response becomes critical to maintaining the health of the community.

### 13.11. Handling Evidence

WMD events will probably involve a criminal act and hence will attract a multitude of agencies for the investigations. At times, the roles, responsibilities, and agendas may conflict and appear to impede the medical response effort. However, looking at the event from a community response, all agencies must cooperate for the greater good, health, and survival of the community. Medical authorities must plan, understand, rehearse, and implement their actions in concert with law enforcement agencies in order to assist in this process.

## 13.12. Aftermath

### 13.12.1. RECOVERY

Once an event transpires, recovery operations will begin shortly. Foremost will be the need to resume a sense of normalcy for patients and staff. Depending on the scenario, potentially contaminated areas will need to be reinspected to ensure that the areas are safe to reoccupy. The author's personal experience with the Pentagon disaster on 9/11 revealed a host of other environmental or recovery issues that will inevitably require attention:

1. Air quality
2. Worker's current health as a baseline for future workers' compensation inquiries
3. Personal stress issues for the staff
4. Disseminating information using basic principles of risk communication.

### 13.12.2. MENTAL HEALTH SUPPORT

As discussed in Subheading 4.1., in their detailed review of disasters in the surgical literature, Frykberg and Tepas (6) focused primarily on the injury patterns sustained in 220 bombings from 1969 to 1983. However, they noted in their "Lessons Learned" that these events also revealed a great need for mental health support following the disaster. WMD events will only add to that need. Details of this support are given in Chapter 26 and elsewhere in this book. Nevertheless, hospitals and local health care facilities need to be aware of their role in such support, both for acute needs and to prevent long-term sequelae. The actions and resources needed must be planned, rehearsed, and then implemented, with particular attention to the rescuers and health care workers, in addition to victims of the attack (36).

## 13.13. Community Quarantine

Should a large-scale bioweapon release of an infectious agent occur, large-scale community quarantine may become necessary. Local hospitals, clinics, and individual health care providers will certainly play a role in this event. Fortunately, recent history has not required such action; no large-scale quarantine has occurred in the United States in over 80 years. However, failure to execute—or even rehearse—the procedures for a quarantine has put our processes in jeopardy. A recent national exercise, TOPOFF 2000, revealed the many political, ethical, and administrative challenges that face implementation. It is essential to plan for the possibility of a quarantine that will involve action on the part of local health care facilities in concert with local, state, and federal public health agencies (37).

## 14. SUMMARY

Future terrorist events will most commonly take place in the community at locations or events that will maximize the effect of the terrorist's action on the public. Although health care facilities and their employees may be the primary target, they will continue to support the victims in the role they ordinarily play. Health care workers and their institutions have historically provided the life saving and support needed for victims of all disasters, sometimes jeopardizing their own personal safety and well-being. Such support will require additional education, planning, training, and capability expansion, but it can be achieved. This *Physician's Guide to Terrorist Attack* aids in this process.

## ACKNOWLEDGMENTS

The author would like to thank LTC Michael Roy, Director, Division of Military Internal Medicine and Associate Professor of Medicine, Uniformed Services University and the U.S. Army Soldier and Biological Chemical Command, (SBCCOM), Aberdeen Proving Ground, for their support and assistance in this endeavor.

## REFERENCES

1. Treat KN, et al. Hospital preparedness for weapons of mass destruction incidents: an initial assessment. Ann Emerg Med 2001;38:562–565.
2. Wetter DC, Daniell WE, Treser CD. Hospital preparedness for victims of chemical or biological terrorism. Am J Public Health 2001;19:710–716.
3. SAEM Disaster Medicine White Paper Subcommittee. Disaster medicine: current assessment and blueprint for the future. Acad Emerg Med 1995;2:1068–1076.
4. Briggs S, Leong M. Classic concepts in disaster medical response in humanitarian crises. In: Leaning J, Briggs S, Chen L, eds. Humanitarian Crises, the Medical and Public Health Response. Harvard University Press, Cambridge, MA, 1999, pp. 69–79.
5. Roth PB, Gaffney JK. The federal response plan and disaster medical assistance teams in domestic disasters. Emerg Med Clin North Am 1996;14:371–382.
6. Frykberg ER, Tepas JJ. Terrorist bombings; lessons learned from Belfast to Beirut. Ann Surg 1988;208:569-576.
7. Mallonee S, et al. Physical injuries and fatalities resulting from the Oklahoma City bombing. JAMA 1996;276:382–386.
8. Hogan DE, et al. Emergency department impact of the Oklahoma City terrorist bombing. Ann Emerg Med 1999;34:160–167.
9. Okudera H, et al. Unexpected nerve gas exposure in the city of Matsumoto: report of rescue activity in the first sarin gas terrorism. Am J Emerg Med 1997;15:527–528.
10. Okamura T, et al. Report on 640 victims of the Tokyo subway sarin attack. Ann Emerg Med 1996; 28:129–135.
11. Sharp T, et al. Medical preparedness for a terrorist incident involving chemical and biological agents during the 1996 Atlanta Olympic Games. Ann Emerg Med 1998;32:214–223.
12. Wetter DC, Daniell WE, Treser CD. Hospital preparedness for victims of chemical or biological terrorism. Am J Public Health 2001;91:710–716.
13. Kvetan, V. Critical care medicine, terrorism, and disasters: are we ready? Crit Care Med 1999;27: 873–874.
14. Auf der Heide E. Disaster Response: Principles of Preparation and Coordination. CV Mosby, St. Louis, 1989.
15. Stern J. The Ultimate Terrorist. Harvard University Press, Cambridge, MA, 1999.
16. Noji EK. The nature of disaster: general characteristics and public health effects. In: Noji EK, ed. The Public Health Consequences of Disasters. Oxford University Press, New York, 1997, pp. 3–20.
17. Waeckerle JF. Disaster planning and response. N Engl J Med 1991;324:815–821.
18. Quarantelli EL. Ten criteria for evaluating the management of community disasters. Disasters 1997;21:39–56.
19. Tur-Kaspa I, et. al. Preparing for toxicological mass casualty events. Crit Care Med 1999;27:1004–1008.
20. Bissel RA, Becker BM, Burkle FM. Health care personnel in disaster response, reversible roles or territorial imperatives? Emerg Med Clin North Am 1996;14:267–288.
21. Church RE. Effective media relations. In Noji EK, ed. The Public Health Consequences of Disasters. Oxford University Press, New York, 1997, pp. 122–132.

22. Schultz CH, Mothershead JL, Field M. Bioterrorism preparedness: I: The emergency department and hospital. Emerg Med Clin North Am 2002;20:437–455.
23. Kizer KW, Cushing TS, Nishimi RY. The Department of Veterans Affairs' role in federal emergency management. Ann Emerg Med 2000;36:255–261.
24. Auf der Heide E. Disaster planning. Part II, Disaster problems, issues, and challenges identified in the research literature. Emerg Med Clin North Am 1996;14:453–480.
25. Pesik N, Keim M, Sampson TR. Do US emergency medicine residency programs provide adequate training for bioterrorism? Ann Emerg Med 1999;34:173–176.
26. Waeckerle JF, et al. Executive summary: developing objectives, content, and competencies for the training of emergency medical technicians, emergency physicians, and emergency nurses to care for casualties resulting from nuclear, biological, or chemical incidents. Ann Emerg Med 2001;37:587–601.
27. Burkle FM. Mass casualty management of a large-scale bioterrorist event: and epidemiological approach that shapes triage decisions. Emerg Med Clin North Am 2002;20:409–436.
28. Lewis CP, Aghababian RV. Disaster planning part I, overview of hospital and emergency department planning for internal and external disasters. Emerg Med Clin North Am 1996;14:439–452.
29. CDC Strategic Planning Workgroup. Biological and chemical terrorism: strategic plan for preparedness and response. Recommendations of the CDC Strategic Planning Workgroup. MMWR 2000;49(RR-4).
30. Pavlin JA, et al. Diagnostic analyses of biological agent-caused syndromes: laboratory and technical assistance. Emerg Med Clin North Am 2002;20:331–350.
31. Macintyre AG, et al. Weapons of mass destruction events with contaminated casualties. Effective planning for healthcare facilities. JAMA 2000;283:242–249.
32. Stein M, Hirshmerg A. Medical consequences of terrorism; the conventional weapon threat. Surg Clin North Am 1999;79:1537–1552.
33. English J. Utilization of JCAHO standard for disaster management. Presented at Chest 2002, Annual Symposium of the American College of Chest Physicians, San Diego, CA, November, 2002.
34. Association for Professionals in Infection Control and Epidemiology Bioterrorism Task Force and CDC Hospital Infections Program Bioterrorism Working Group, 13 April, 1999. Bioterrorism readiness plan: a template for healthcare facilities. Accessed at www.apic.org/bioterror, 8 November, 2002.
35. Association for Professionals in Infection Control and Epidemiology and The Center for the Study of Bioterrorism and Emerging Infections (CSB&EI), Saint Louis University School of Public Health, 1 October 2001. Mass casualty disaster plan checklist: a template for healthcare facilities. Accessed at www.apic.org/bioterror, 8 November, 2002.
36. Benedek DM, Holloway HC, Becker SM. Emergency mental health management in bioterrorism events assistance. Emerg Med Clin North Am 2002;20:393–407.
37. Barbera J, et al. Large-scale quarantine following biological terrorism in the United States; scientific examination, logistic and legal limits, and possible consequences. JAMA 2001;286:2711–2717.

# 3

# Physician Recognition
# of Bioterrorism-Related Diseases

*Kevin Yeskey, MD,*
*and Stephen A. Morse, MSPH, PhD*

## CONENTS

## 1. INTRODUCTION

In October 2001, the United States experienced an unprecedented bioterrorist attack associated with the intentional release of *Bacillus anthracis* through mailed letters and packages *(1)*. Five deaths and 17 other cases of anthrax were confirmed. Clinicians and clinical laboratories had a primary role in the response to this attack. One of the most important lessons has been the recognition that the capacity to respond effectively depends largely on the local efforts, particularly among clinicians, hospitals, and the public health departments. The Centers for Disease Control and Prevention (CDC) is working to strengthen the local response by helping to ensure that all frontline clinicians have a baseline set of information to recognize and treat bioterrorism-related diseases and to exclude these diseases as part of the differential diagnosis. Furthermore, it is important that physicians recognize their role as first responders in a covert bioterrorism attack.

From the public health perspective, bioterrorism can be defined as the deliberate release of pathogens and their toxins into a population for the purpose of causing illness or death. Bioterrorism events can be characterized by two types of scenarios: overt (announced) and covert (unannounced). Because of their terrorism training, traditional "first responders" (e.g., firefighters or law enforcement) are the most likely to respond to an announced release of a biological agent or, more likely, to a hoax. In the context of the recent anthrax attack, an example of an overt attack would be the letter received and opened in a Senator's office in the Hart Senate Office Building. The envelope contained

From: *Physician's Guide to Terrorist Attack*
Edited by: M. J. Roy  © Humana Press Inc., Totowa, NJ

a letter stating that it contained anthrax spores and that the opener was going to die. First responders were called, the presence of spores of *Bacillus anthracis* was confirmed, and exposed individuals were placed on antimicrobial prophylaxis. To date, no one in the Hart Senate Office Building has developed anthrax.

We currently lack the ability to conduct real-time environmental monitoring for a covert release of a biological agent in all our cities. A covert release would probably go unnoticed, with those exposed leaving the area long before the act of terrorism became evident. Because of the incubation period, the first signs that a biological agent has been released may not become apparent until days or weeks later, when individuals become ill and seek medical care. Thus, the "first responders" to a covert bioterrorism event will probably be the astute clinician or laboratory or public health worker who recognizes the index case or identifies the responsible agent *(2)*.

Biological agents may enter the body via several routes *(3)*: (1) the inhalational route (entering the lungs as an aerosol); (2) the oral route (ingested in food or water); (3) the percutaneous route (injected through the skin); and (4) the dermal route (absorbed through the skin or mucous membranes). The inhalational or aerosol route is considered to be the most important by the military when planning defenses against biological warfare *(4)*; however, all these routes could be used to introduce biological agents into civilian populations. From the medical perspective, it is important to remember that symptoms will often vary depending on the route of infection. Moreover, many agents can cause similar initial symptoms when delivered by the same route. For example, patients with inhalational anthrax, pneumonic plague, and pneumonic tularemia will initially present with nonspecific clinical symptoms such as high fever, chills, headache, and malaise *(5–7)*, which could be difficult to diagnose and recognize as a biological attack. Diseases caused by most of the agents (Table 1) considered likely candidates for use by a bioterrorist are rare, uncommonly seen in a routine medical practice, and would be considered reportable through the public health system. Practicing physicians should be familiar with the syndromes that can result from infection with the agents of public health concern (Table 2). With a covert biological attack, the most likely first indicator of an event would be an increased number of patients presenting with clinical features caused by the disease agent. However, with few exceptions, an epidemiological investigation would be needed to differentiate a naturally occurring outbreak from a bioterrorism event.

## 2. EPIDEMIOLOGICAL INDICATORS OF A COVERT BIOLOGICAL EVENT

Routine medical surveillance may reveal unusual patterns of disease presentation that would indicate a potential bioterrorism event. Some of these diseases may first appear in non-human animal populations, providing evidence of a terrorist's use of a biological agent. In some cases it may be extremely difficult to determine whether a disease is naturally occurring or introduced intentionally to cause disease. Medical surveillance is essential in the early detection of a covert release. What are the features that may indicate a covert intentional release of a biological agent? Lists of occurrences have been developed that would raise suspicion of an intentional release *(9)*. In the case of smallpox, the mere presence of a single case would indicate that terrorism was responsible. The last human cases of smallpox were in Birmingham, England in 1978 *(10)*, and the only publicly acknowledged stores of smallpox virus are in World Health Organization (WHO) reference laboratories in the United States and Russia *(11)*.

## Table 1
## The Critical Biological Agents[a]

| Category | Description | Agents (Reference) |
|---|---|---|
| **Category A** | High-priority agents are those that:<br><br>1. Can be easily disseminated or transmitted from person to person;<br>2. Cause high mortality, with potential for major public health impact; and<br>3. Might cause public panic and social disruption; and<br><br>4. Require special action for public health preparedness. | Category A agents include:<br><br>*Bacillus anthracis* (anthrax) (7)<br>*Yersinia pestis* (plague) (5)<br>*Francisella tularensis* (tularemia) (6)<br>*Clostridium botulinum* neurotoxins (botulism) (15)<br>Variola major (smallpox) (11,14)<br>Filoviruses: Ebola, Marburg (Ebola/Marburg hemorrhagic fever) (16)<br>Arenaviruses: Lassa, Junin (Lassa fever, Argentine hemorrhagic fever) (16) |
| **Category B** | The second highest priority agents include agents that:<br><br>1. Are moderately easy to disseminate;<br>2. Cause moderate morbidity and low mortality; and<br>3. Require specific enhancements of the CDC's diagnostic capacity and disease surveillance. | Category B agents include but are not limited to:<br><br>*Coxiella burnetti* (Q-fever)<br>*Brucella* spp. (brucellosis)<br>*Burkholderia mallei* (glanders)<br>Alphaviruses: VEE, EEE, WEE (Venezuelan, Eastern, and Western encephalomyelitis)<br>Ricin toxin from *Ricinus communis* (castor beans)<br>Epsilon toxin from *Clostridium perfringens*<br>Staphylococcal enterotoxin B |
| A subset of Category B agents includes: | Pathogens that are spread by food or water. | These pathogens include but are not limited to:<br>*Salmonella* spp.<br>*Shigella dysenteriae*<br>*Escherichia coli* "0157:H7"<br>*Vibrio cholerae*<br>*Cryptosporidium parvum* |
| **Category C** | Emerging pathogens that could be engineered for mass dissemination in the future because of:<br><br>1. Availability;<br>2. Ease of production and dissemination; and<br>3. Potential for high morbidity and mortality and major public health impact. | Category C agents include but are not limited to:<br>Nipah viru<br><br>Hantaviruses<br>Tickborne hemorrhagic fever viruses<br>Tickborne encephalitis viruses<br>Yellow fever virus<br>Multidrug-resistant *Mycobacterium tuberculosis* |

[a]Modified from ref. 8.

Table 2
Syndromes Potentially Resulting from Bioterrorism

| Syndrome | Agents |
| --- | --- |
| Encephalitis | Eastern equine encephalomyelitis virus |
| | Venezuelan equine encephalomyelitis virus |
| | Western equine encephalomyelitis virus |
| Hemorrhagic mediastinitis | *Bacillus anthracis* |
| Pneumonia with abnormal | *Yersinia pestis* |
|   liver function tests | *Francisella tularensis* |
| | *Coxiella burnetii* |
| | *Burkholderia mallei* |
| | *Burkholderia pseudomallei* |
| Papulopustular rash | Variola major virus |
| Hemorrhagic fever | Ebola virus |
| | Marburg virus |
| | Junin virus |
| | Lassa |
| Descending paralysis | *Clostridium botulinum* neurotoxins |
| Nausea, vomiting and/or | *Salmonella* spp. |
|   diarrhea[a] | *Shigella dysenteriae* |
| | *Escherichia coli* 0157:H7 |
| | Staphylococcal enterotoxin B |

[a]Nausea and vomiting can also occur as part of the early-phase symptoms of inhalational anthrax or the prodrome of smallpox.

Individually, the clues listed below would not directly confirm a terrorist event. They must be evaluated within the context of a full epidemiological investigation. In many cases, other possible causes must be considered, such as travel to an endemic area or re-emergence of an uncommon infectious disease. An astute clinician or an effective surveillance system will detect the presence of a disease, but the skilled epidemiologist will determine the potential source of the outbreak.

## 2.1. Unusual Illness in a Population

The appearance of a rare or extremely uncommon disease appearing in the population would raise suspicion of a covert release, particularly if those with the disease do not have a history of travel to an endemic area or recent exposure to others who have traveled to areas where the disease may be endemic. An example of this was the outbreak of West Nile fever in New York in 1999 *(12)*. This disease had never been seen before in the United States, and although the outbreak was not the result of bioterrorism, its emergence has caused concern.

## 2.2. Number of Patients

Epidemics are unusually large numbers of patients with a specific disease. Presentation of a large number of patients seeking health care for the same disease is not, in itself, enough to warrant investigations as a covert bioterrorism event. There are many naturally occurring epidemics each year; however, this may be the first indication of a release, and, in an epidemic situation, one should look for other indicators. The possibility of an intentional release should be considered in the context of a common source of exposure when there are large numbers of patients with the same disease. Large numbers of people seeking treatment at the same time is suggestive of a common source of exposure to a disease with a fixed incubation period. This would be uncommon in a naturally occurring event. An endemic disease (e.g., plague) that suddenly becomes epidemic suggests either a change in the agent (i.e., genetic modification/mutation), a change in the population's exposure pattern, or exposure of a naive subpopulation.

### 2.3. Unusual Presentations

Only rarely do medical conditions defy explanation, and almost always, a cause of death can be determined. Unexplained syndromes could be caused by a very rare disease that goes unrecognized, a disease agent that has been genetically engineered, or a combination of different illnesses not commonly seen together. Rare or unusual diseases in the United States could indicate intentional introduction by a terrorist or, more likely, unintentional introduction through foreign travel or contact with an animal reservoir.

An unusual geographic distribution or seasonal occurrence of cases can represent an important clue. For example, plague is endemic in the Western United States. A case of plague in the Eastern United States would suggest either the intentional introduction of the agent or a history of travel to an endemic area. An unusual seasonable distribution of cases could suggest an intentional introduction (e.g., influenza during the summer months) outside the normal period of communicability or a new strain of the infectious agent.

Laboratory methods have been used to generate a "genetic fingerprint" that can be used to identify specific strains by comparisons with other strains of the same agent; similar methods have been used to detect genetic manipulation of the agent. Unusual strains or genetic manipulation could indicate that the agent was intentionally released.

Many agents can be transmitted to humans by one or more routes of infection (e.g., droplet, water, food). Moreover, infectious agents usually have a typical presentation, which is related to the route of transmission. An atypical route of transmission or atypical presentation of a disease is highly suggestive of an intentional exposure. For example, cutaneous anthrax is endemic in many parts of the world and is the most common form of human anthrax. The pulmonary form of anthrax (inhalational anthrax) is rare, and its presentation in the United States would be highly suspicious of an intentional release *(1)*.

### 2.4. Unusual Response to Treatment

Antibiotic resistance or an increase in virulence may occur as the result of spontaneous mutations or through the natural acquisition of genetic material. However, they can also occur as a result of intentional genetic manipulation. Unexpected resistance to frontline antibiotics, more severe illness, or higher mortality rates should raise suspicion.

## 3. RECOMMENDATIONS FOR PHYSICIANS

In the wake of the terrorist attacks of September 11, 2001, the Johns Hopkins Center for Civilian Biodefense Strategies identified a number of key actions that physicians could take in preparation for a response to bioterrorist attacks *(13)*:

- Develop an increased awareness of the ongoing threat of bioterrorism.
- Develop a working knowledge of the CDC Category A agents (Table 1).

Table 3
Selected Bioterrorism-Related Websites

- Bioterrorism Watch in Harrison's online textbook:
  www.harrisononline.cm/amed_news/news_article/281.html. Chapters from the book,
  specific links to the *New England Journal of Medicine* and extensive links to other
  primary sources and major websites.
- CDC's bioterrorism website:
  www.bt.cdc.gov. Includes extensive links, patient information sheets, downloadable
  presentations, and indexed press releases/advisories There is a separate site
  (www.cdc.gov/mmwr/indexbt.html) listing MMWR reports on bioterrorism agents.
- *Medical Aspects of Chemical and Biological Warfare. Textbook of Military Medicine.*
  Office of the Surgeon General, Washington, DC 1997 (Zajtchuk R, Bellamy RF, eds.):
  www.nbc-med.org/SiteContent/HomePage/WhatsNew/MedAspects/contents.html.
  Detailed chapters on biological and chemical weapons. Chapters on specific agents
  complement those in other major infectious diseases texts.
- Johns Hopkins Center for Civilian Biodefense Studies website:
  www.hopkins-biodefense.org. Policy, congressional testimonies, debates, excercises, and
  medical information.
- American Society for Microbiology website:
  www.asmusa.org. Public policy and links to other sites. Emphasis is on microbiological
  aspects.
- Infectious Diseases Society of America bioterrorism website:
  www/idsociety.org/BT/ToC.htm. Resources for the practicing physician. Images, diagnosis
  and management, postexposure prophylaxis and treatment, epidemiology, public health
  and laboratory issues, pathology.
- World Health Organization:
  www.who.int/emc/deliberate_epi.html. This website contains information for the general
  public; online publications include the 2nd edition of *Health Aspects of Biological and
  Chemical Weapons.*
- Center for the Study of Bioterrorism and Emerging Infections, St. Louis University
  School of Public Health:
  www.bioterrorism.slu.edu. Provides links to primary sources as well as downloadable
  presentations.
- Center for Disaster Preparedness, University of Alabama at Birmingham:
  www.bioterrorism.uabedu/. Differential diagnosis of bioterrorist agents. Bioterrorism
  continuing education module.
- Department of Epidemiology, UCLA School of Public Health:
  www.ph.ucla.edu/epi/bioter/bioterrorism.html. Links to county, state, national, and
  international sites on public health preparedness and response to bioterrorism. Course
  offerings on bioterrorism.

- Become familiar with relevant lines of communication, as well as important and emergency phone numbers [e.g., hospital epidemiologist, state epidemiologist, local health
  department (may be city or county), and the CDC emergency number (770-488-7100)].
- Maintain a high index of suspicion for unusual disease presentations, health care
  utilization patterns, and clusters of disease in clinics and offices. Immediately notify the
  appropriate authorities if you suspect an unusual event or need medical guidance.

- Refer questions to your local or state health departments, or to the CDC public inquiry phone number (404-639-3534 or 800-311-3435) regarding infectious diseases and bioterrorism preparedness response efforts.
- Have referral numbers for mental health and support services.
- Be prepared to handle requests for antibiotic prescriptions in the event of a bioterrorist attack. The CDC maintains a National Pharmaceutical Stockpile containing large quantities of antibiotics and other medical supplies that will be distributed in the event of an epidemic brought on by an act of bioterrorism. State health departments are developing local distribution strategies.

## 4. RESOURCES

Physicians should be familiar with important websites that provide current information. Some of them are listed in Table 3. The bioterrorism website of the Infectious Diseases Society of America (IDSA) is particularly relevant to practicing physicians. It has information on the clinical presentations and syndromic differential diagnoses of Category A agents, treatment recommendations, contact information, and additional resources.

## 5. SUMMARY

The alertness, open-mindedness, and sound clinical judgment of physicians and other health care professionals will be crucial in a successful public health response to future acts of bioterrorism.

## REFERENCES

1. Jernigan JA, Stephens DS, Ashford DA, et al. Bioterrorism-related inhalational anthrax: the first 10 cases reported in the United States. Emerg Infect Dis 2001;7:933–944.
2. Centers for Disease Control and Prevention. Notice to readers: ongoing investigation of anthrax— Florida, October 2001. MMWR 2001;50:877.
3. Mims C, Playfair J, Roitt I, et al. Medical Microbiology, 2nd ed. Mosby, London, 1998.
4. Eitzen EM. Use of biological weapons. In: Sidell FR, Takafuji ET, Franz DR, eds. Textbook of Military Medicine: Medical Aspects of Chemical and Biological Warfare. Borden Institute, Washington, DC, 1997, pp. 437–450.
5. Inglesby TV, Dennis DT, Henderson DA, et al. Plague as a biological weapon. Medical and public health management. JAMA 2000;283:2281–2290.
6. Dennis DT, Inglesby TV, Henderson DA, et al. Tularemia as a biological weapon. Medical and public health management. JAMA 2001;285:2763–2773.
7. Inglesby TV, O'Toole T, Henderson DA, et al. Anthrax as a biological weapon, 2002. Updated recommendations for management. JAMA 2002;287:2236–2252.
8. Khan AS, Morse S, Lillibridge S. Public-health preparedness for biological terrorism in the USA. Lancet 2000;356:1179–1182.
9. Noah D, Sobel A, Ostroff S, Kildew J. Biological warfare training: infectious disease outbreak differentiation criteria. Mil Med 1998;163:198–201.
10. Shooter RA. Report of the investigation into the cause of the 1978 Birmingham smallpox occurrence. London: Her Majesty's Stationery Office, 1980.
11. Breman JG, Henderson DA. Diagnosis and management of smallpox. N Engl J Med 2002;346: 1300–1308.
12. Centers for Disease Control and Prevention. Outbreak of West Nile-like viral encephalitis—New York, 1999. MMWR 1999;48:845–849.
13. Johns Hopkins Center for Civilian Biodefense Strategies: http://www.hopkins-biodefense.org/ interim.htm.

14. Henderson DA, Inglesby TV, Bartlett JG, et al. Smallpox as a biological weapon. Medical and public health management. J.A.M.A. 1999;281:2127–2137.
15. Arnon SS, Schechter R, Inglesby TV, et al. Botulinum toxin as a biological weapon. Medical and public health management. JAMA 2001;285:1059–1070.
16. Borio L, Inglesby TV, Peters CJ, et al. Hemorrhagic fever viruses as biological weapons. Medical and public health management. JAMA 2002;287:2391–2405.

# 4

# Introduction to Biological, Chemical, Nuclear, and Radiological Weapons

## With a Review of Their Historical Use

## Clinton K. Murray, MD

The opinions and assertions contained herein are those of the author and are not to be construed as official or as representing the position of the Department of the Army or the Department of Defense.

## CONTENTS

INTRODUCTION
BIOLOGICAL WARFARE
CHEMICAL WEAPONS
NUCLEAR AND RADIOLOGICAL WEAPONS
SUMMARY
REFERENCES

## 1. INTRODUCTION

History will record 2001 as a watershed year for the role of organized medicine in the national response to terrorism. Significant terrorist events on U.S. soil, highlighted by the use of explosive weapons and biological agents, has heightened concern for future widespread use of chemical, biological, radiological, nuclear, and explosive materials. The total number of international terrorist attacks in 2001 declined to 346, down from 426 in 2000. However, these attacks were more deadly. There were 3547 deaths and 1080 injuries in 2001, compared with 409 deaths and 796 injuries in 2000 *(1)*.

Although no one definition completely describes terrorism, the U.S. Government generally defines terrorism as premeditated, politically motivated violence perpetrated against noncombatant targets by subnational groups or clandestine agents, usually intended to influence an audience. The *Code of Federal Regulations* defines terrorism as "… the unlawful use of force and violence against persons or property to intimidate or coerce a government, the civilian population or any segment thereof, in furtherance of political or social objectives" (28 C.F.R. Section 0.85). The Federal Bureau of Investigation (FBI) further delineates terrorism into either international or domestic categories

From: *Physician's Guide to Terrorist Attack*
Edited by: M. J. Roy © Humana Press Inc., Totowa, NJ

*(2)*. Domestic terrorism involves groups or individuals who operate entirely within the United States or its territories without foreign guidance. Traditionally, terrorist counter-measures have focused on the most active domestic terrorist groups such as the Animal Liberation Front (ALF) and the Earth Liberation Front (ELF). However, the role of international terrorists and the scope of their reach were accentuated on September 11, 2001. International terrorism is defined as a violent act, whether aimed at U.S. citizens or not, intended to influence or intimidate governments by perpetrators who normally operate or seek asylum outside the United States. Currently, 33 international terrorist groups are recognized by the Secretary of State as Foreign Terrorist Organizations *(1)*. The countries most frequently shielding and/or supporting terrorists are Iran, Iraq, North Korea, Libya, Syria, Sudan, India, Pakistan, and Egypt. These countries have been described by the Central Intelligence Agency as attempting to acquire technology relat-ing to weapons of mass destruction and advanced conventional munitions. The key suppliers include Russia, North Korea, China, and miscellaneous western countries *(3)*.

Chemical, biological, radiological, nuclear, and explosive materials are attractive weapons for potential terrorists *(1–4)*. Such arsenals can induce significant fear not only in actual use but also in threatened use. Based on the material used and the means of dissemination, these weapons can be inexpensive, difficult to detect, and have a delayed onset of action. Their disadvantages are accidents during deployment, lack of control during dissemination, and the persistence of some agents. In addition, as shown with the unity and the aggressive retaliation of the American people after the terrorist events of September 11, use of these agents engenders a strong desire for severe retribution against the terrorists and cements public patriotism, boosting government power.

Our current focus on terrorism and weapons of mass destruction has been dictated by such events as the bombing of the Murrah Federal Building, the discovery of the advanced biological weapons programs in Iraq and the former Soviet Union, the nerve gas attack in the Tokyo subway, the attacks with large "explosive weapons" against the World Trade Center and Pentagon, and the anthrax contamination of letters. These events increase the likelihood that weapons of mass destruction will be used in the future. Clinicians must be aware of potential agents and how to respond to them. Health care professionals are obliged to maintain a heightened sense of awareness of these agents in order to detect events early, providing an opportunity to prevent further attacks and to minimize further dissemination of the agents. The distribution of anthrax-laden letters revealed the impor-tance of prompt responses and rapid, adequate communication among physicians, health departments, the media, and other experts integral to an effective response. This chapter introduces weapons of mass destruction (chemical, biological, radiological, and nuclear) that are of concern to practicing physicians, with an emphasis on historical use.

## 2. BIOLOGICAL WARFARE

The threat of biological weapons has been a real concern recently, as there has been an escalation of anthrax hoaxes over the last decade. However, the threat of biological attack came to fruition in 2001. Anthrax-contaminated letters released in the United States led to 5 deaths and 11 confirmed inhalation cases *(5)*. At least 10,000 individuals were advised to undergo prophylaxis for possible anthrax exposure after the release of these letters *(6)*. Anthrax fears were heightened when we learned of the perpetrator's ability to manipulate anthrax spores to a small enough diameter to allow them to pass through unopened envelopes. In addition, our own postal system's letter sorting process aerosolized the spores contained in the letters, exposing postal workers and cross-contaminating the mail. National attention focused on medication stockpiles and vaccine availability, as both were in short supply or unavailable to the public. The threat of anthrax attack persists, as there is continued concern that terrorists may have the capability to employ this agent, and the perpetrator of the initial letters has not been apprehended.

Historical use of biological weapons in one form or another dates back centuries; however, substantiating their use is problematic. Limitations include confirming allegations of biological attacks, the lack of reliable microbiological and epidemiological data regarding alleged or attempted attacks, the use of allegation of biological attack for propaganda, and, finally, the secrecy surrounding biological weapons programs. Despite these obstacles, it is still informative to evaluate the past uses of biological armaments to determine possible future deployment methods, likely agents, and medical measurements needed to combat their use including prevention and management. The following historical overview is a compilation of reports from numerous sources *(7–13)*.

Filth, cadavers, and animal carcasses are the classic means of biological warfare. The earliest reports date back to the 6th century BC when Assyrians poisoned enemy wells with rye ergot. Subsequently, Scythian archers attempted to increase the lethality of their arrows by placing blood and manure or decomposing flesh on them in 400 BC. In a unique approach to biological warfare, Hannibal hurled venomous snakes onto the enemy ships of Pergamon at the battle of Eurymedon in 190 BC, purportedly resulting in victory for Hannibal.

A more remarkable endeavor in biological warfare occurred in 1346 when plague broke out in the Tartar army during its siege of Kaffa. The Mongol attackers hurled the corpses of their own troops who died from plague over the city walls. The plague epidemic that followed in the fortified city forced the defenders to surrender. Some escaped the city by sea, an escape that some historians consider to have begun the Black Death pandemic that spread through Europe. This tactic of spreading disease to enemy armies has been repeated frequently throughout history, but always with questionable benefit.

In 1495, the Spanish spiked the enemy's wine with the blood of leprosy patients while combating the French near Naples. In 1650, a rabid dog's saliva was placed into hollow spheres that were fired against the enemy. Smallpox has been used on several occasions. Pizarro is reported to have presented South American natives with variola-contaminated clothing in the 15th century. During the French and Indian War, the English, led by Sir Jeffery Amherst, gave smallpox-laden blankets Indians loyal to the French. Subsequently, Native American Indians defending Fort Carillon suffered epidemic casualties from smallpox, resulting in the loss of the fort to the English.

During the Civil War, retreating Confederates in Mississippi poisoned wells and ponds with dead animals to deny water sources to the Union troops. Other agents possibly employed in the Civil War included yellow fever- and smallpox-laden clothes.

Compared with chemical agents, biological agents were rarely employed during World War I. Most of the reports entail German use of glanders in the United States and attempts at releasing plague in St. Petersburg, Russia in 1915.

A new era of biological warfare was fostered with the advance of biochemistry and microbiology in the 1930s and 1940s. The Japanese set out on an ambitious biological warfare program in 1930s with production complexes such as Unit 731, located 40 miles south of Harbin, Manchuria, which continued to operate until it was burned in 1945. A post-World War II investigation revealed the extent of activities undertaken by the Japanese. Their research included such agents as cholera, anthrax, shigella, and typhoid, frequently in human studies utilizing prisoners of war. Reportedly, approximately 1000 autopsies were performed at Unit 731, predominantly victims exposed to aerosolized anthrax. Some estimate there were as many as 3000 human deaths, mostly prisoners and Chinese nationals. Intelligence also describes a plague epidemic in China and Manchuria after overflights by Japanese planes suspected of dropping plague-infected fleas. By 1945, the Japanese program had stockpiled 400 kg of anthrax to be used in a specially designed fragmentation bomb.

A more inspiring event occurred during World War II when research into vaccine and serological testing was used as biological defense instead of biological warfare. Traditionally, the German army avoided deporting populations with epidemic typhus by screening the populations with the Weil-Felix reaction for evidence of disease. Parts of occupied Poland used this information to inoculate local residents with a formalin-killed *Proteus* OX-19. This vaccine induced a biological false-positive test for typhus, averting deportation of Polish residents to concentration camps.

Offensive biological warfare research in the United States was initiated in 1941 in response to a perceived German biological warfare program threat, in ignorance of the extent of Japanese activity. This research was conducted at Camp Detrick, Maryland. Research incorporated numerous agents and focused on the feasibility of dissemination. Numerous volunteers known as white coats, predominantly Seventh Day Adventists, were exposed to these agents to learn about pathogenesis, disease, treatment, and prevention. The vulnerability of the U.S. population was illustrated by the release of the benign agents *Serratia marcescens* off the coast of San Francisco in the 1950s and *Bacillus globii* in a New York subway in 1966. Although significant strides were made in the offensive biological warfare arena, President Nixon stopped all offensive biological and toxin weapons research and production by executive order in 1969. Between May 1971 and May 1972, all stockpiles of biological agents and munitions were destroyed in the presence of monitors. Agents destroyed included *Bacillus anthracis*, botulinum toxin, *Francisella tularensis*, *Coxiella burnetti*, Venezuelan equine encephalitis virus, *Brucella suis*, and staphylococcal enterotoxin B. The United States Army Medical Research Institute of Infectious Diseases (USAMRIID) was begun in 1953 as a medical defensive program. USAMRIID continues today at modern-day Fort Detrick, Maryland.

In 1972, the United States, the United Kingdom, and the USSR signed the Biological Weapons Convention, formally known as the Convention on the Prohibition of the Development, Production and Stockpiling of Bacteriological (Biological) and Toxin Weapons and on Their Destruction. Over 140 countries have since added their ratification. This treaty prohibits the research and stockpiling of biological agents. However, there have been several cases of suspected or actual use and/or research into offensive biological weapons by signers of the convention.

Among the most notorious of these infractions were the yellow rain incidents in Southeast Asia, the use of ricin as an assassination weapon in London in 1978, and the accidental release of anthrax spores at Sverdlovsk in 1979. In the late 1970s, reports describe an aerosol release over inhabitants of Laos and Cambodia by planes and helicopters. People and animals exposed to the aerosols became disoriented and ill, and a small percentage died. The working explanation was that trichothecene toxins (in particular, T-2 mycotoxin) were the cause of the yellow rain. Fascinatingly, an alternative theory proposes that the effect was owing to feces produced by swarms of bees. In 1978, a Bulgarian exile named Georgi Markov was killed in London by a tiny pellet filled with ricin toxin, introduced into the subcutaneous tissue of his leg with a device disguised in an umbrella. The Bulgarian secret service obtained the technology to achieve this act from the former Soviet Union.

The extent of the former Soviet Union's active biological warfare research came to light in April 1979, when an anthrax outbreak in a Russian city surfaced. Residents living in a narrow zone extending 4 km downwind of a Soviet military microbiology facility in Sverdlovsk developed high fevers and difficulty breathing, resulting in approximately 66 fatalities *(13)*. The Soviet Ministry of Health initially blamed the deaths on the consumption of meat contaminated with anthrax, although this was highly improbable based on the scientific data available. In 1992, Russian President Boris Yeltsin acknowledged that the Sverdlovsk incident was in fact related to military developments at the microbiology facility. Further evidence of the former Soviet Union's activities was revealed when a senior biological warfare program manager defected from Russian in 1992 and outlined a remarkably robust biological warfare program. This program included research into genetic engineering, binary biologicals, and chimeras, as well as the industrial capacity to produce such agents. The instability of the Russian government and the availability of large financial resources to terrorist groups make it possible that these agents and/or the scientific experts could be acquired by foreign countries.

Further examples of the use of biological agents include the contamination of Tylenol packages with cyanide, which ushered in the era of tamper-proof packaging. In 1984, the Rajneesh cult in Oregon tried to influence an election by contaminating local salad bars with *Salmonella* to prevent voters from reaching the polls. This incident resulted in 751 cases of enteritis and 45 hospitalizations. Although the Aum Shinrikyo cult is known for the sarin attack of the Tokyo subway, they allegedly also conducted research with *Bacillus anthracis*, *Clostridium botulinum*, and *C. burnetti*. They purportedly launched eight unsuccessful biological attacks in Japan using *Bacillus anthracis* and botulinum toxin. They went so far as to send cult members deploying to the former Zaire in 1992 to obtain Ebola virus for weapons development.

The United Nations inspections of Iraq's biological warfare capabilities exposed the extent of research undertaken by that country *(14,15)*. Representatives of Iraq have announced active research into the offensive biological warfare agents *Bacillus anthracis*, botulinum toxins, and *Clostridium perfringens* (one of the toxins). In 1995, United Nations inspectors uncovered active research on anthrax, botulinum toxins, *Clostridium perfringens*, aflatoxins, wheat cover smut, and ricin. The Iraqi government also field-tested *Bacillus subtilis* (a simulator for anthrax), botulinum toxin, and aflatoxin. The research included testing various delivery systems such as rockets, aerial bombs, and spray tanks. Overall, Iraq produced 19,000 L of concentrated botulinum toxin (nearly 10,000 L put into munitions), 8500 L of concentrated anthrax (6500 L put into munitions) and 2200 L of aflatoxin (1580 L put into munitions) prior to or during the time of the Persian Gulf War. In December 1990, the Iraqis had filled 100 R400 bombs with botulinum toxin, 50 with anthrax, and 16 with aflatoxin. In addition, 13 SCUD warheads were filled with botulinum toxin, 10 with anthrax, and 2 with aflatoxin. These weapons were deployed in January 1991 to four locations, although they were never used during the war. An alarming report in January 1998 revealed that Iraq had sent approximately a dozen biological warfare researchers to Libya. The reported goal was to assist Libya with the development of a biological warfare complex disguised as a medical facility in the Tripoli area.

Biological agents include living organisms or the materials derived from those organisms that cause disease in or harm to humans, animals, or plants, or cause deterioration of material. They can be in numerous forms including liquid, droplets, aerosols, or dry powders *(16)*. The characteristics of biological agents vary based on the properties and means of release. These characteristics include the potential for massive number of casualties, ability to produce lengthy illnesses requiring prolonged and extensive care, ability to spread via contagion, paucity of adequate detection systems, presence of an incubation period that enables victims to disperse widely, and ability to complicate diagnosis by producing nonspecific symptoms or mimicking endemic infectious disease. The impact of biological weapons has been assessed by the World Health Organization using hypothetical attacks of 50 kg of differing agents by aircraft along a 2-km line upwind of a population center of 500,000 *(16)*. Anthrax had the greatest impact, with 95,000 dead and 125,000 incapacitated. Tularemia resulted in 30,000 dead and 125,000 incapacitated. The other agents described included Q fever, resulting in 150 dead and 125,000 incapacitated, brucellosis, resulting in 500 dead and 125,000 incapacitated, typhus, resulting in 19,000 dead and 85,000 incapacitated, tickborne encephalitis, resulting in 9500 dead and 35,000 incapacitated, and Rift Valley fever, resulting in 400 dead and 35,000 incapacitated.

The threat of biological agents is not limited to humans. The natural foot and mouth disease outbreak in the United Kingdom resulted in the slaughter of 3.1 million animals and drastically impacted on the economy. A terrorist could perpetrate a similar incident with catastrophic results.

After the release of anthrax in the United States, significant efforts were made to control the future use of biological agents. The Centers for Disease Control and Prevention has described categories for biological threat agents (Table 1) and agents within those categories (Table 2) (www.cdc.bt.gov). This system is based on numerous factors such as morbidity and mortality, ease of production, ease of dissemination, ability to diagnosis, and ability to induce fear and panic in a population. Although these are the likely agents, a group or individual with resources and expertise might use other agents not on this list. Recent debate has centered on the release of the genetic genomes of potential biological agents *(17)*. In addition, other agents could be designed to decimate only animal or plant populations.

Management of biological agents is dependent on many factors including means of dissemination, host immunity, and agents used. Each agent must be diagnosed quickly and then specific procedures followed based on the agent used in the attack. Significant discussion has been undertaken to approach mass immunizations, large-scale quarantine, and models for preparing for such events *(18)*.

## 3. CHEMICAL WEAPONS

The information highway has provided the necessary components to support chemical terrorism through instant access to critical information, precursor chemicals, and delivery systems. Chemical warfare includes incendiaries, poison gases, and other chemical substances. The utility of chemical terrorism has been demonstrated by the Japanese cult Aum Shinrikyo, which released Sarin on the Tokyo subway system in 1995, resulting in

Table 1

Centers for Disease Control and Prevention's Biological Disease/Agent Categories[a]

Category A diseases/agents. The US public health system and primary health care providers must be prepared to address various biological agents, including pathogens that are rarely seen in the United States. High-priority agents include organisms that pose a risk to national security because they

1. Can be easily disseminated or transmitted from person to person
2. Result in high mortality rates and have the potential for major public health impact
3. Might cause public panic and social disruption
4. Require special action for public health preparedness

Category B diseases/agents. The second highest priority agents include those that

1. Are moderately easy to disseminate
2. Result in moderate morbidity rates and low mortality rates
3. Require specific enhancements of the CDC's diagnostic capacity and enhanced disease surveillance

Category C diseases/agents. The third highest priority agents include emerging pathogens that could be engineered for mass dissemination in the future because of

1. Availability
2. Ease of production and dissemination
3. Potential for high morbidity and mortality rates and major health impact

[a]See www.cdc.bt.gov.

12 deaths and injuries more than 5500 people. Investigations revealed a stockpile of enough chemicals to kill 4.2 million people. The advantage of chemical weapons over other weapons of mass destruction was accented when investigations demonstrated that significant financial resources (approximately $30 million annually) were used to develop and subsequently release biological weapons such as anthrax and botulinum toxin but without successful results.

History is a tool to evaluate past mistakes and allow us to anticipate the type and mode of chemical attack in the future. Although incomplete, this review highlights some chemical agents that have been employed. The data presented here were mostly collected from the references given in refs. 20 and 21. Chemical warfare dates back to ancient times. The earliest acts involved throwing burning oil and fireballs by both defenders and attackers of fortified cities. The most primitive form of a flamethrower was used as early as the 5th century BC. The Chinese designed stink bombs of poisonous smoke and shrapnel. In approximately 423 BC, allies of Sparta and the Spartan army in the Peloponnesian War took an enemy fort by directing smoke from lighted coals, sulfur, and pitch through a hollowed-out beam into the fort.

Early use of chemical warfare also included naval operations. Around the 7th century AD, Greek fire, floating rosin, sulfur, pitch, naphtha, lime, and saltpeter were used against enemy ships. In the 15th and 16th centuries, Venice employed unspecified poisons in hollow explosive mortar shells or sent chests of poison to its enemy.

The development of modern inorganic chemistry in the late 18th and early 19th centuries and organic chemistry during the following century fostered increased interest in chemical warfare. During this time significant debate surfaced as to the morality of

Table 2
Centers for Disease Control and Prevention's List of Biological Diseases/Agents by Category[a]

Category A
    Anthrax (*Bacillus anthracis*)
    Botulism (*Clostridium botulinum* toxin)
    Plague (*Yersinia pestis*)
    Smallpox (variola major)
    Tularemia (*Francisella tularensis*)
    Viral hemorrhagic fevers: filoviruses (e.g., Ebola, Marburg) and arenaviruses (e.g., Lassa, Machupo)

Category B
    Brucellosis (*Brucella* species)
    Epsilon toxin of *Clostridium perfringens*
    Food safety threats (e.g., *Salmonella* species, *Escherichia coli* O157:H7, *Shigella*)
    Glanders (*Burkholderia mallei*)
    Melioidosis (*Burkholderia pseudomallei*)
    Psittacosis (*Chlamydia psittaci*)
    Q fever (*Coxiella burnetii*)
    Ricin toxin from *Ricinus communis* (castor beans)
    Staphylococcal enterotoxin B
    Typhus fever (*Rickettsia prowazekii*)
    Viral encephalitis: alphaviiruses (e.g., Venezuelan equine encephalitis, eastern equine encephalitis, western equine encephalitis)
    Water safety threats (e.g., *Vibrio cholerae*, *Cryptosporidium parvum*)

Category C
    Emerging infectious disease threats such as Nipah virus, hantavirus
    Tickborne hemorrhagic fever viruses
    Tickborne encephalitis viruses
    Yellow fever
    Multidrug-resistant tuberculosis

[a]*See* www.cdc.bt.gov.

chemical warfare. Early stances among British admiralty rejected the use of burning, sulfur-laden ships as a prelude to marine landings in France in 1812 as "against the rules of warfare." In 1854 the British War office condemned Sir Lyon Playfair's proposal to use cyanide-filled shells to break the siege of Sebastopol during the Crimean War as being inhumane and as bad as poisoning the enemy's water supply. Governments also began to convene meetings to control the use of these agents during military campaigns. Early examples include The Brussels Convention of 1874 and the Delegates to the Hague Conventions in 1899 and 1907. These attempts either to eliminate poisons in combat or to control their use resulted in little more than feeble and loosely worded resolutions.

The First World War demonstrated the lethality of chemical warfare. Chlorine and mustard gas produced 1 million casualties and 90,000 fatalities. During World War I, Germany used portable flamethrowers and, along with the French, riot control agents. These riot control agents were the first to be used on the modern battlefield, but they were largely ineffective. Germany with its heavily developed industries, was the first large-scale user of chemical agents during the war. Germany released approximately 150 tons of chlorine gas near Ypres, Belgium in 1915. Although the gas caused 800 deaths, the more devastating effect was psychological, resulting in the retreat of 15,000 Allied troops. This overwhelming effectiveness caught the Germans unprepared to take advantage of the victory. The British began to respond in kind with chlorine after the initial attack, and both sides later added phosgene and chloropicrin to their arsenals. To provide protection against these agents, which primarily afflict the pulmonary system, masks were developed. Additional agents were subsequently developed, including diphosgene by the Germans and hydrogen cyanide by the French. The face of chemical warfare again changed near Ypres, Belgium in 1917. German artillery shells delivered sulfur mustard, resulting in 20,000 casualties. This persistent agent caused more widespread damage to organ systems such as the lungs, eyes, and skin. In addition, a latent period of up to several hours meant that immediate clues to exposure, were seen with the previous agents, were lacking. Protective equipment now had to protect not only the airway but also the skin and eyes. Management of mustard injuries also overwhelmed the medical system. Although fewer than 5% of the casualties who reached medical treatment stations died, the injuries were slow to heal and requireded convalescent periods averaging more than 6 weeks.

Further attempts to control chemical warfare were sought in the 1925 Geneva Protocol, which was ratified by all the major powers except the United States and Japan. Although it implied the prohibition of the first use of chemical and biological weapons, it did not prevent development, possession, or retaliatory use. Some countries such as Russia and Germany expanded offensive and defensive chemical agent programs from the late 1920s through the mid-1930s. Outrage against chemical warfare prevented these activities in other countries, such as the United States. Between the Great Wars, numerous other agents were developed including nitrogen mustard and toxic organophosphate compounds such as tabun and sarin.

Although the threat of chemical warfare was even greater during World War II, no nation during World War II used broadly recognized chemical agents on the battlefield, with the possible exception of Japan during attacks on China. Nazi Germany weaponized thousands of tons of nerve agents. These agents were not used during the war in combat; however, their horrific use was employed in the Holocaust. It has been proposed that Adolph Hitler was a casualty of mustard attacks during World War I, which moved him not to use the agent during World War II. Other factors that may have prevented their use include the lack of German air superiority and concern that the Allies had their own nerve agent program for retaliation, an inaccurate assumption. The most notable chemical event during World War II was not the offensive use of chemical agents. In 1943, Germany bombed Bari Habor, Italy where the *John Harvey*, an American ship loaded with 2000 100-pound mustard bombs, was anchored. Over 600 military casualties and an unknown number of civilian casualties resulted. Casualties included inhalation of mustard-laden smoke and widespread systemic poisoning following ingestion of—and skin exposure to—mustard-contaminated water by sailors attempting to keep afloat in the harbor.

More recent examples include the Yemen War of 1963–1967, when Egypt probably employed mustard bombs in support of South Yemen against royalist troops in North Yemen. The United States used defoliants and riot control agents in Vietnam and Laos. The United States Government believes the Geneva Protocol in 1975 did not apply to defoliants or riot control agents; therefore, their official position is that they did not use chemical warfare. Further reports include the release of chemical weapon against Cambodian refugees and the Hmong tribesmen of central Laos; however, these reports were never confirmed. The Soviet Union was also accused of using chemical agents in Afghanistan. Iraq used chemical agents against Iran during the 1980s; as a consequence, approximately 100 Iranian soldiers underwent treatment in European hospitals. A United Nations investigation confirmed the use of the vesicant mustard and the nerve agent GA. Further reports of nerve agent use and retaliation by Iran against Iraq have been described. In 1988, Iraqi airplanes released nerve agents, cyanide, and mustard against the village of Halabja to control the Kurdish citizens within Iraqis own borders. During the Gulf War, stockpiles of nerve agents and mustard gas were found at Al Muthanna, 80 km northwest of Baghdad.

Chemical stockpiles exist throughout the world in countries such as the former Soviet Union, Libya, and France, and two dozen other nations may have the capability to manufacture offensive chemical weapons. Currently the United States stockpile includes nerve agents (GB and VX) and vesicants (primarily mustard H and HD). Many of the agents are obsolete and are currently being destroyed. Approximately 60% of the stockpiles are in bulk storage containers and 40% are stored in munitions.

Chemical weapons are designed to injure, kill, or incapacitate personnel and may be used to deny access or use of an area, facility, or material. Agents can be harassing, incapacitating, or lethal and come in solid, liquid, or gas form (21,22). Lethal agents include choking agents, blood agents, vesicant agents, and nerve agents. Agents can be persistent, such as vesicant mustard and VX nerve agents, which evaporate slowly and stay on terrain, material, and equipment for prolonged periods. Nonpersistent agents, such as phosgene, cyanide, and the G series nerve agents, evaporate quickly. There are seven major categories—blister/vesicants, blood, choking/blood/pulmonary, incapacitating, nerve, riot control/tear, and vomiting (Table 3) (www.cdc.bt.gov).

Clinical manifestations are based on the chemical agent dispersed and the form of dispersal—solids, liquids, gases, aerosols, or vapors. A local effect may be produced on the eyes and skin (and by inhalation), but absorption has subsequent systemic effects. Liquid agents may persist on materials and continue to be a hazard until decontamination occurs. Penetration of fragments or clothing contaminated with liquid chemical agents of any type may lead to intramuscular exposure and subsequent systemic effects. The effect of chemical weapons occurs within minutes to hours rather than days, as is typically the case with biological weapons.

Management generally involves decontamination with fresh air, copious water irrigation, hypochlorite, and/or removal of affected material (21,22). Specific antidotes for certain agents are available, including intravenous sodium nitrate and sodium thiosulfate for cyanide poisoning, atropine, pralidoxime chloride, and diazepam for nerve agents and physostigmine for incapacitating agents (21,22).

## 4. NUCLEAR AND RADIOLOGICAL WEAPONS

The nuclear age was ushered in by the discovery of nuclear fission in late 1938 and the 1941 theory proposing the development of an atomic bomb. The ultimate power of nuclear weapons was revealed with the 1945 bombing of Hiroshima and Nagasaki, Japan, with a fission (plutonium) bomb resulting in approximately 200,000 deaths. After World Word II, the cold war propelled the nuclear arsenals of the United States and the Soviet Union. The destructive capacity of these weapons progressed to the development of the fusion (hydrogen) bombs, about 25 times the power of the plutonium bomb dropped on

Table 3
Categories of Chemical Agents[a]

Blister/vesicants

Distilled mustard (HD)
Lewisite (L)
Mustard gas (H)
Nitrogen mustard (HN-2)
Phosgene oxime (CX)
Ethyldichloroarsine (ED)
Lewisite 1 (L-1)
Lewisite 1 (L-2)
Lewisite 1 (L-3)
Methyldichloroarsime (MD)
Mustard/Lewisite (HL)
Mustard/T
Nitrogen mustard (HN-1)
Nitrogen mustard (HN-3)
Phenodichloroarsine (PD)
Sesqui mustard

Blood

Arsine (SA)
Cyanogen chloride (CK)
Hydrogen chloride
Hydrogen cyanide (AC)

Choking/lung/pulmonary damaging

Chlorine (CL)
Diphosgene (DP)
Cyanide
Nitrogen oxide (NO)
Perflurorisobutylene (PIIIB)
Phosgene (CG)
Red phosphorous (RP)
Sulfur trioxide-chlorosulfonic acid (FS)
Teflon and perflurorisobutylene (PHIB)
Titanium tetrachloride (FM)
Zinc oxide (HC)

Incapacitating

Agent 15
BZ
Canniboids
Fentanyls
LSD
Phenothiazines

Nerve

Cyclohexyl sarin (GF)
GE
Sarin (GB)

Table 3 (*Continued*)
Categories of Chemical Agents[a]

Nerve (*continued*)
   Soman (GD)
   Tabun (GA)
   VE
   VG
   V-gas
   VM
   VX

Riot control/tear
   Bromobenzylcyanide (CA)
   Chloroacetophenone (CN)
   Chloropicrin (PS)
   CNB (CN in benzene and carbon tetrachloride)
   CNC (CN in chloroform)
   CNS (CN and chloropicrin in chloroform)
   CR
   CS

Vomiting
   Adamsite (DM)
   Diphenylchloroarsine (DA)
   Diphenylcyanoarsine (DC)

[a]*See* www.cdc.bt.gov.

Nagasaki. Although no military use of nuclear weapons has occurred since 1945, the world teetered on the brink of nuclear war during the Berlin crisis in 1961 and the Cuban missile crisis of 1962.

As the arms race increased the lethality and number of nuclear weapons, the worldwide use of nuclear energy also expanded. More than 425 nuclear power reactors were operating in over 30 countries by the mid-1990s. In addition to commercial nuclear power plants, there are many nuclear engineering departments in universities with small experimental reactors in densely populated urban areas. These nuclear power reactors are possible sites of terrorist attacks. Although the accident at the Chernobyl nuclear power plant was not the result of a terrorist attack, significant lessons can be learned from it.

Radiological weapons, also known as "dirty bombs" or radioactive dispersal devices, combine conventional high explosives and radioactive materials (e.g., spent fuel rods from a nuclear reactor) to contaminate an area with radioisotopes *(23)*. This may not result in the short-term lethality of a traditional nuclear fusion or fission bomb, but it may lead to long-term contamination and public panic. The combination of an explosive device with radioactive material allows for greater dispersal of radioactive material. It also contaminates conventional wounds with radioactive material.

Certain low-level radioactive devices such as smoke detectors, isotopes used in research, and nuclear medicine radiopharmaceutical agents could induce significant "radiation" fear without the use of explosives or complications of radiation exposure. However, other more highly radioactive sources could be dispersed with or without conventional explosives to cause complications of radiation exposure. These agents include radiotherapy machines that use cobalt-60 and cesium-137 or industrial radiographic devices that use cesium-137 and iridium-192. These sources are usually metallic, but a few devices contain powder in a capsule that could be effortlessly dispersed, resulting in a radioactively contaminated area.

The most destructive forces of traditional thermonuclear weapons are the winds and pressure, the thermal pulse, and secondary fires. Resulting injuries include blast injury (blast wave overpressure forces and indirect blast wind drag forces), wounds with poor healing owing to radiation contamination, thermal injuries, and burn injuries transformed into more severe burns secondary to radiation and eye injuries. The effects of fallout and radiation are usually limited to significant long-term effects, but minimal short-term effects. Other medical complications include acute and chronic stress disorders.

Radiation exposure can result in localized or whole-body exposure and in internal or external contamination *(23,24)*. Table 4 describes the different radioactive materials *(24)*. The clinical manifestations depend on the extent of penetration and the absorbed dose in various tissues. Ionizing particles include alpha particles that are relatively large and are halted by the dead layers of the skin or a uniform. They only cause damage if an individual is contaminated internally. Beta particles can penetrate to the basal stratum of the skin and cause a "thermal burn" in large doses. Radiation from a nuclear detonation or fallout includes gamma particles that are like X-rays. Their high penetrability can result in whole-body exposure. Neutrons are released during a nuclear detonation but not fallout. Like gamma particles, they can result in whole-body exposure; however, neutrons can cause 20 times the damage of gamma particles. If exposure to significant doses of radiation occurs, an acute radiation syndrome develops, with three corresponding phases of illness. The two most radiosensitive systems of the body are the hematopoietic and the gastrointestinal. Manifestations depend on individual radiation sensitivity, type of radiation, and radiation dose absorbed *(24)*. Symptoms will be more profound, and the phases more brief, with increasing doses of radiation. Nausea, vomiting, and malaise mark the prodromal phase of radiation sickness. The latent period is a relatively unremarkable period. The length of the latent phase lasts from a few hours in central nervous system disease to many weeks in hematopoietic system disease, depending on the dose of radiation. The final phase is the manifest phase, which correlates with dose of radiation and organ system involvement (central nervous, gastrointestinal, or hematopoietic). The important aspects of minimizing the effects of radiation are time, distance, and shielding *(23,24)*.

Management consists of treatment of symptoms, supportive care, including aggressive prevention of infections, treatment of conventional injuries associated with trauma, and psychological support *(23,24)*. Internal contamination with plutonium or americium may respond to chelating agents. Other experimental agents are being evaluated to counteract the effect of radiation.

## 5. SUMMARY

The increasing lethality of terrorists' activities, and their use of biological and explosive weapons, have heightened our awareness of possible future biological, chemical, nuclear, radiological, and explosive weapons. History is replete with the use of weapons of mass destruction. Analysis of these events enhances our analysis of future deployment, likely agents, and medical management. It is through seeking knowledge of these agents

Table 4
Radioactive Materials of Terrorist Importance

| Radioactive material | Characteristics |
| --- | --- |
| Americium | $^{241}$Am is a decay daughter of plutonium and an alpha emmiter. It is used in smoke detectors and other instruments. It is found in fallout from a nuclear weapon. Large quantities can cause whole-body irradiation. |
| Cesium | $^{137}$Ce is found in medical radiotherapy devices. It emits both gamma rays and beta radiation. It can cause whole-body irradiation. |
| Cobalt | $^{60}$Co is used in medical radiotherapy devices and commercial food irradiators. It generates gamma rays and beta rays. It can cause primary whole-body irradiation and acute radiation syndrome. |
| Depleted uranium | DU emits limited alpha, beta, and some gamma radiation. DU does not cause a radiation threat. Inhaled uranium compounds and DU fragments in wounds can result in whole-body distribution, particularly to bone and kidney. |
| Iodine | $^{131, 132, 134, 135}$I is found after reactor accidents and following the destruction of a nuclear reactors. Radioactive iodine is a normal fission product found in reactor fuel rods. Most of the radiation is beta rays with some gamma. Primary toxicity is the thyroid gland. |
| Phosphorus | $^{32}$P is found in research laboratories and in medical facilities. It has strong beta rays. |
| Plutonium | $^{239, 238}$Pu is produced from uranium in reactors. It is the primary fissionable material in nuclear weapons and is the predominant radioactive contaminant in nuclear weapons accidents. Primary radiation is from alpha particles. Toxicity is primarily from inhalation. |
| Radium | $^{226}$Ra is used in the former Soviet Union as instrument illumination, in industry and in older medical equipment. Primary radiation is alpha particles but daughter products emit beta and gamma rays. |
| Strontium | $^{90}$Sr is the direct fission product (daughter) of uranium. It and its daughters emit beta and gamma rays. |
| Tritium | $^{3}$H is used in nuclear weapons, luminescent gun sights, and muzzle-velocity detectors. It is a beta emitter. |
| Uranium | $^{238, 235, 239}$U is found (in order of increasing radioactivity) in DU, natural uranium, fuel rods, and weapons-grade material. Uranium and its daughters emit alpha, beta, and gamma radiation. DU and natural uranium are not serious irradiation threats. Used fuel rods and weapons-grade uranium emit significant levels of gamma radiation. |

Data from ref. *21*.

and responding appropriately with comprehensive communication that the impact of future use can be minimized.

## REFERENCES

1. Patterns of global terrorism 2001. United States Department of State, May 2002. Accessed at: www.state.gov/s/ct/rls/pgtrpt/2001/.
2. Terrorism in the United States 1999. Counterterrorism threat assessment and warning unit counter-terrorism division. Federal Bureau of Investigation. Accessed at: www.fbi.gov/publications/terror/terror99.pdf.
3. Unclassified report to Congress on the acquisition of technology relating to weapons of mass destruction and advanced conventional munitions, 1 January through 30 June 2001. Accessed at: www.odci.gov/cia/publications/bian/bian_jan_2002.htm.

4. Henderson DA. The looming threat of bioterrorism. Science 1999;283:1279–1282.
5. Inglesby TV, O'Toole T, Henderson DA, et al. Anthrax as a biological weapon, 2002, updated recommendations for management. JAMA 2002;287:2236–2251.
6. Brookmeyer R, Blades N. Prevention of inhalational anthrax in the U. S. outbreak. Science 2002;295:1861.
7. Robertson AG, Roberston LJ. From asps to allegations: biological warfare in history. Mil Med 1995;160:369–373.
8. Christopher GW, Cieslak TJ, Pavlin JA, Eitzen EM. Biological warfare: a historical perspective. JAMA 1997;278:412–417.
9. Sidell FFR, Franz DR. Overview: defense against the effects of chemical and biological warfare agents. In: Sidell FR, Takafuji ET, Franz DR, eds. Textbook of Military Medicine: Medical Aspects of Chemical and Biological Warfare. Borden Institute, Washington, DC, 1997, pp. 1–8.
10. Smart JR. History of chemical and biological warfare: an American perspective. In: Sidell FR, Takafuji ET, Franz DR, eds. Textbook of Military Medicine: Medical Aspects of Chemical and Biological Warfare. Borden Institute, Washington, DC, 1997, pp. 9–87.
11. Eitzen M, Takajufi ET. Overview of biological warfare. In: Sidell FR, Takafuji ET, Franz DR, eds. Textbook of Military Medicine: Medical Aspects of Chemical and Biological Warfare. Borden Institute, Washington, DC, 1997, pp. 415–424.
12. Franz DR, Parrot CD, Takafuji ET. The U. S. biological warfare and biological defense programs. In: Sidell FR, Takafuji ET, Franz DR, eds. Textbook of Military Medicine: Medical Aspects of Chemical and Biological Warfare. Borden Institute, Washington, DC, 1997, pp. 425–436.
13. Meselson M, Guillemin J, Hugh-Jones M, et al. The Sverdlovsk anthrax outbreak of 1979. Science 1994;266:1202–1207.
14. Kortepeter M, Christopher G, Cieslak T, et al., eds. USAMRIID's Medical Management of Biological Casualties Handbook. USAMRIID, Fort Detrick, MD, 2001.
15. Zilinskas RA. Iraq's biological weapons: the past as future. JAMA 1997;278:418–424.
16. WHO Group of Consultants. Health Aspects of Chemical and Biological Weapons. World Health Organization, Geneva, 1970.
17. Read TD, Parkhill J. Restricting genome data won't stop bioterrorism. Nature 2002;417:379.
18. Barbera J, Macintyre A, Gostin L, et al. Large-scale quarantine following biological terrorism in the United States scientific examination, logistic and legal limits, and possible consequences. JAMA 2001;286:2711–2717.
19. O'Toole T, Mair M, Inglesby TV. Shining light on dark winter. Clin Infect Dis 2002;34:972–983.
20. Joy RTJ. Historical aspects of medical defense against chemical warfare. In: Sidell FR, Takafuji ET, Franz DR, eds. Textbook of Military Medicine: Medical Aspects of Chemical and Biological Warfare. Borden Institute, Washington, DC, 1997, pp. 87–110.
21. Chemical Casualty Care Division, eds. Medical Management of Chemical Casualties Handbook, 3rd ed. U.S. Army Medical Research Institute of Chemical Defense, Aberdeen Proving Ground, MD, 2000. Available on-line at ccc.apgea.mil/products/handbooks/mmccthirdeditionjul2000.pdf.
22. Evison D, Hinsley D, Rice P. Chemical weapons. BMJ 2002;324:332–335.
23. Mettler FA, Voelz GL. Major radiation exposure—what to expect and how to respond. N Engl J Med 2002;346:1554–1561.
24. Jarrett DG. Medical Management of Radiological Casualties Handbook. Armed Forces Radiobiology Research Institute, Bethesda, MD, 1999.

# II    BIOLOGICAL AGENTS

# 5

# Anthrax

*Steven J. Durning,* MD, FACP
*and Michael J. Roy,* MD, MPH, FACP

The opinions or assertions contained herein are the private views of the authors and are not to be construed as official or as representing the opinion of the Department of the Army, the Department of the Air Force, or the Department of Defense.

## Contents

## 1. INTRODUCTION

The September 11, 2001 terrorist attacks, followed shortly thereafter by the dissemination of anthrax through the U.S. mail, has drawn considerable attention in both the medical and lay communities to the risks of bioterrorism. The word *anthrax* has caused hysteria in the minds of many Americans in recent months, as evidenced by the many hoaxes and false alarms dealt with by fire departments and other authorities. Anthrax remains a leading bioterrorism threat to military troops engaged in combat, as well as to civilian populations targeted by terrorists.

Although anthrax probably achieved greater international attention in 2001 than ever before, this was not by any means the first time that anthrax has been implicated as a biological weapon. The Soviets officially denied having a biological warfare program, but this was belied by the 1979 accidental release of anthrax in the city of Sverdlovsk that resulted in at least 77 cases (66 deaths) of inhalational anthrax (*1*). The Japanese sect Aum Shinrikyo unsuccessfully attempted to spread anthrax and botulism before fatally releasing the nerve agent sarin in Matsumoto and in the Tokyo subway system (*2*). Among many other threats and hoaxes, a package sent to the international headquarters of B'nai

From: *Physician's Guide to Terrorist Attack*
Edited by: M. J. Roy © Humana Press Inc., Totowa, NJ

B'rith, in Washington, DC, in April 1997, is notable *(3)*. In this case, a package claimed to have anthrax but in fact had a related but far less pathogenic species, *Bacillus cereus*. What was remarkable about this case was that this credible hoax led to the cordoning off of two blocks in the center of downtown Washington for 9 hours while authorities were trying to determine the contents of the package, resulting in major traffic disruptions throughout the city.

## 2. BACKGROUND

*Bacillus anthracis* is a spore-forming, Gram-positive bacteria found in soil throughout the world. Anthracis is derived from the Greek *anthrakis*, or coal, as cutaneous disease leads to a characteristic black or "coal-like" lesion. This bacteria infects both wild and domesticated animals, as well as humans. Anthrax spores demonstrate remarkable resistance to environmental conditions such as heat and light. Anthrax spores can last for decades in the soil; spores released during explosives testing on Gruinard Island during World War II remained viable for over 30 years following the conclusion of testing *(4)*.

Anthrax has considerable historical significance. It is suspected to represent the cause of the Fifth and Sixth Plagues of Egypt described in Exodus, the first disease for which Koch established a microbial origin in 1876, and for which Pasteur developed an effective live vaccine for in 1881 *(1)*. Although cutaneous anthrax has been described for centuries, the first cases of inhalational anthrax were not identified until the late 1800s, in association with sorting wool from infected animals, perhaps representing the first instance of occupational respiratory infectious disease *(1)*.

Inhalational anthrax represents a leading bioterrorism threat because of ready access (high prevalence in soil throughout the world), high infectivity (i.e., transmitted by opening mail), ability to form an odorless and invisible aerosol, and high lethality. The Biologic Weapons Convention, signed by many nations in the 1970s *(5)*, prohibited bioterrorism weapons research or production. Despite this treaty, several nations are believed to have biological weapons, and some have subsequently acknowledged having anthrax programs, including Iraq and the Soviet Union. Indeed, the largest epidemic of inhaled anthrax in this century occurred after spores were accidentally released from a military research facility in Sverdlovsk, Russia in 1979, resulting in 66 reported deaths *(6)*. Fortunately, many experts agree that manufacturing what the media touts as "weapons grade" anthrax such as that used in the 2001 United States Postal Service incident, may be beyond the capacity of many terrorist groups, who lack access to advanced biotechnology equipment or funding to support such activities *(7)*. ("Weapons grade" anthrax is a controversial term implying that the powder of *B. anthracis* has been milled to minimize electrostatic charges, providing uniform particle size and reduced clumping and ensuring high spore concentration.) For example, Aum Shinrikyo attempted to use anthrax on several occasions, fortunately largely without success *(2)*. Al Quaeda has also attempted to acquire biological weapons, but as of this writing there is no evidence that they have been successful.

Anthrax is the first disease to be deliberately disseminated through the U.S. mail. There were 11 confirmed cases of inhalational anthrax, 7 confirmed cases of cutaneous anthrax, and 4 additional suspected cases of cutaneous anthrax resulting from this incident in the fall of 2001 *(8)*. At least 20 of the 22 cases were linked to five letters contaminated with a single strain of anthrax that were mailed from Trenton, New Jersey *(9)*. Five of 11 cases of inhalational anthrax resulted in death, and thousands of people received prophylactic antibiotics after possible exposure to anthrax spores.

We have made significant strides in our understanding of inhalational anthrax from both the U.S. Postal Service incident and the Sverdlovsk outbreak, as only 18 other cases of inhalational anthrax, all owing to occupational exposure, have occurred in the United States during the 20th century. Despite this understanding, however, we must rely primarily on conjecture in considering the potential impact of a large-scale inhalational anthrax bioterrorism attack, and the efficacy of proposed post-attack measures remains largely unknown. The handful of cases that resulted from the U.S. mail incident pale in comparison with estimates of the potential effect of the intentional dissemination of anthrax from an airplane over an urban area. Indeed, a 1993 report by the U.S. Congressional Office of Technology Assessment estimated that up to 3 million deaths would follow the aerosolized release of 100 kg of weapons grade anthrax spores over the Washington, DC area, a lethality on the order of a hydrogen bomb *(10)*.

This chapter reviews the pathogenesis, clinical manifestations, and key considerations in the diagnosis and treatment of anthrax infection in humans. Particular attention is paid to the diagnosis and therapy of inhalational anthrax, the form of anthrax infection that carries the highest lethality and the greatest bioterrorism threat. This discussion includes clinical clues to assist the heath care provider with differentiating inhalational anthrax from influenza, influenza-like illness, and community acquired pneumonia and addresses treatment issues such as postexposure prophylaxis and the anthrax vaccine.

## 3. PATHOGENESIS

A brief review of the pathogenesis of *B. anthracis* can greatly facilitate understanding of this organism's clinical manifestations as well as the options for diagnostic testing and therapy.

*B. anthracis* has three known virulence factors: an antiphagocytic capsule and two protein toxins. The antiphagocytic capsule is composed of poly-D glutamic acid *(1)*. The capsule provides resistance to phagocytosis and may also contribute to the resistance of anthrax to lysis by serum cationic proteins *(11)*. Anthrax strains that lack this capsule have been shown to be avirulent *(1)*. Indeed, the sterile filtrate-based anthrax vaccine employed by the U.S. military and the live attenuated vaccine that has been developed and administered in the former Soviet Union both use strains of anthrax that lack this capsule *(12)*.

The two protein exotoxins are commonly known as edema factor and lethal factor. The names were derived after they were shown to lead to edema and death, respectively, when injected into experimental animals. Each toxin requires the presence of another protein, called protective antigen, for virulence. Protective antigen binds to the host cell's surface, allowing the action of these two exotoxins. This antigen is the target of our current vaccine *(13)*.

After spores are introduced into the host, they are ingested at the exposed site by macrophages, probably leading to destruction of some spores. Surviving spores then germinate into vegetative forms, which produce virulence factors. Spores germinate in an environment that is conducive to replication, where there is an abundance of amino acids, nucleosides, and glucose, such as is found in the bloodstream and lymph nodes; spore formation, on the other hand, is promoted by exposure to air or environments unsuitable for replication *(14)*. The trigger(s) responsible for the transformation of spores to the vegetative state are not fully understood *(15)*. Once transformation to the vegetative state occurs, clinical manifestations rapidly follow.

Protective antigen binds to a receptor on the surface of host cells and is subsequently cleaved by a protease on the cell surface. This cleavage of protective antigen creates a binding site to which the lethal factor or the edema factor can bind with high affinity *(11)*. This complex subsequently undergoes endocytosis by the host cell, allowing the toxins to express activity. Edema toxin impairs leukocyte function and affects water homeostasis, causing edema *(7)*. Lethal toxin causes release of tumor necrosis factor-$\alpha$ (TNF-$\alpha$) and interleukin-1$\beta$, factors that are believed to cause sudden death in anthrax infection *(16)*. These toxins lead to the distinctive clinical findings with anthrax: edema, hemorrhage, tissue necrosis, and a relative lack of leukocytes *(1)*.

For example, in inhalational anthrax, spores enter the tracheobroncheal tree and are ingested by alveolar macrophages, probably leading to destruction of a portion of the spores. Remaining viable spores are next transported to regional tracheobronchial lymph nodes, germinating within these macrophages to vegetative forms that produce virulence factors. Exotoxin production at this site leads to the hallmark of inhalational anthrax: massive edema, hemorrhage, and necrotizing lymphadenitis and mediastinitis, producing the characteristic widened mediastinum on chest X-ray as seen in the clinical vignette. Importantly, the timing of germination of spores to the vegetative (toxin-producing) state can vary widely after exposure, leading to the need for prolonged antibiotic therapy to ensure killing of all vegetative forms, which, unlike spores, are antibiotic-sensitive. Indeed, viable spores have been demonstrated from lymph nodes of an experimental monkey 100 days after inhalational anthrax exposure and a long course of antibiotic therapy *(17)*.

### Case Vignette

Albert Brown, a 33-year-old news editor at CNN headquarters in Atlanta, reported feeling well until yesterday morning when he awoke feeling feverish, sweaty, and very tired despite having had a good night's sleep. He took some Tylenol and called in sick to work yesterday, but the fever, fatigue, and general ill feeling persisted, with some nausea and not much appetite. He felt like he had "the flu" but reported having had a flu shot this year. This morning, he developed a dry cough with some chest discomfort, difficulty breathing, and a feeling that he couldn't get enough air, prompting him to present for evaluation. His joints were not painful, but he had a diffuse throbbing headache, and his muscles felt tired and achy all over. He did not have a runny nose or a sore throat. None of his household contacts were ill.

Upon further questioning, he reported that his eyes were a little sensitive to light and his chest felt tight, with a continuous dull aching pain behind the sternum. He had had some soup and crackers for dinner last night and a little cereal and orange juice in the morning. This seemed to make his nausea a little worse, and he had some abdominal discomfort within an hour or so of eating but had not vomited. His temperature last night was 102.4°F and was 101.3°F this morning before leaving home. He had some chills and despite several blankets felt that he could not get warm at these times.

Mr. Brown lives in a single-family home with his wife, who is a law professor at Emory University, and his 6-year-old son. Mr. Brown traveled to Europe on business about a month ago, and he and his wife vacationed in the Bahamas for a week about 2 months ago. He was not ill on either trip but did have a cold about a week after returning from the Bahamas. He has never had a pneumonia vaccination.

Mr. Brown drinks 1–2 beers or glasses of wine several times a week, does not smoke, and denies the use of any recreational drugs. He takes no prescription medications, herbals, or homeopathic preparations. He denied allergies to medications. He takes Tylenol or Motrin for occasional headaches and has had migraines in the past that responded well to sumatriptin or Fiorinal.

Mr. Brown and his wife like to eat out and enjoy ethnic restaurants (especially Mexican, Japanese, Indian, and Vietnamese). He rarely cooks at home, calling himself a master of the microwave. He reported doing a lot of work on the computer and has contact with a lot of other employees; as far as he knew none of them have been ill. He sometimes handles mail for some of the CNN news anchors.

On physical exam, Mr. Brown appeared tired and in some discomfort, with labored, somewhat rapid breathing. His temperature was 101.5°F, with a respiratory rate of 22, blood pressure of 102/60, and heart rate of 118. When asked to touch his chin to his chest, he had no restrictions in head movement but complained of the muscles in his neck and shoulders feeling achy; head and neck exam was otherwise unremarkable. Lung exam revealed a slight dullness at both bases, with crackles throughout the lower right lung field.

Cardiac exam yielded tachycardia, without murmurs, rubs, or gallops. Abdominal exam revealed normal bowel sounds, with slight diffuse tenderness. There were no rebound tenderness, distention, or masses. There were no skin lesions or rashes. Neurological exam was unremarkable.

Laboratory studies showed a white blood cell count of 12.4 [80% polymorphonuclear leukocytes (PMNs), 12% band forms], hematocrit 42%, and platelets 105,000. Chemistries were notable for sodium 132 mmol/L, potassium 5.4 mmol/L, chloride 100 mmol/L, bicarbonate 28 mmol/L, and glucose 47 mg/dL. Liver function tests showed mild elevations of aspartate aminotransferase (AST; 60 U/L) and alanine aminotransferase (ALT; 58 U/L), with a moderate depression of the serum albumin to 3.0 g/dL. Upon lumbar puncture, opening pressure was normal, there were 6 white blood cells and 211 red blood cells per high powered field (differential of 50% PMNs, 50% lymphocytes), protein was 68, and glucose was 45. The chest X-ray is displayed in Fig. 2.

What clinical findings suggest inhalational anthrax infection?
What clinical features help you differentiate this diagnosis from influenza?
How do you make this diagnosis?
What treatment(s) should be instituted and for how long?
What public health measures should be taken if this represents a case of anthrax?

## 4. CLINICAL PRESENTATION

Three clinical presentations have been described with anthrax infection in humans: cutaneous, gastrointestinal, and inhalational. Given the rarity of human anthrax infection in the United States, with the last occupational case of inhalational anthrax being reported in the 1970s *(18)*, any case of inhalational anthrax should be considered to be caused by bioterrorism until proved otherwise. Cases of cutaneous anthrax without clear occupational risk should also raise a concern for possible terrorist attack.

### *4.1. Cutaneous Anthrax*

Historically, this has been the most common form of anthrax, representing 95% of anthrax cases seen in the United States in the 20th century *(16)*. Exposed areas of skin such as the face, neck, hands, and forearms are most commonly involved, particularly at the site of prior cuts or abrasions. A case report from the U.S. Postal Service incident revealed that cutaneous anthrax can occur without antecedent cutaneous injury, as the patient had no reported evidence of prior visible cuts, abrasions, or lesions at the site where cutaneous infection developed *(19)*. The initial skin lesion is most often seen 1–6 d after exposure, with reports as late as 12 d after the accidental release of anthrax in Sverdlovsk, Russia *(6)*. Initially, a pruritic red papule or macule up to 1–2 cm in diameter is usually seen and may be mistaken for a mosquito or spider bite. However, unlike the typical presentation of insect bites, the lesion rapidly evolves and satellite lesions can also develop, so that by the next day, 1–3-mm vesicles containing clear to hemorrhagic fluid (Fig. 1A) often appear. The vesicles subsequently rupture, and the mixture of blood and necrotic skin produces the classic leathery, depressed, painless black eschar (Fig. 1B) that falls off within 1–2 wk, most often without even leaving a scar. Edema of the surrounding tissues often accompanies the eschar phase *(9)*, and, when present, is nearly pathogno-monic for cutaneous anthrax.

The clinical manifestations of cutaneous anthrax are predicted by the pathophysiology of infection. Spores come in contact with the host and then germinate into vegetative forms at the site of infection, with subsequent production of virulence factors after a variable period of time (explaining, in part, the range in latency period). Owing in part to toxin-mediated impairment of leukocyte function, the vesicles are typically filled with bacteria. As in inhalational and gastrointestinal infection, the toxins cause surrounding tissue necrosis and edema. In a minority of cases, spores migrate to lymph nodes and subsequently germinate, leading to associated necrosis and edema. Unlike the primary cutaneous site, necrosis and edema of lymph nodes are often painful and may conse-quently lead to fatal systemic infection in up to 20% unless effective treatment has been initiated; on the other hand, with antibiotics, death owing to cutaneous anthrax is rare *(20)*. Recently, bioterrorist-related cutaneous anthrax in an infant was complicated by the development of a severe microangiopathic anemia, thrombocytopenia, and coagulopathy.

The differential diagnosis of cutaneous anthrax includes brown recluse spider bite, carbuncle, cellulitis, cowpox, bullous erysipelas, cat-scratch disease, tularemia, orf (a viral disease of sheep and goats that is transmittable to humans), rat bite fever, ecthyma gangrenosum, vasculitides, and rickettsial spotted fever *(1,9)*. Key clinical clues for making this diagnosis include the lack of pain, rapid evolution, occasional massive edema, and the near pathognomonic black eschar. Recognition of cutaneous anthrax is important, not only in terms of considering possible terrorist attack if clear occupational risk factors are not present, but also as institution of appropriate antibiotic therapy dra-matically reduces the mortality of this form of *B. anthracis* infection *(19)*.

## 4.2. Gastrointestinal Anthrax

Classically, gastrointestinal anthrax has been reported after ingestion of infected meat that has not been sufficiently cooked, with the presumption that symptoms follow the deposition and germination of spores in the upper and/or lower gastrointestinal tract. Other authorities believe that gastrointestinal anthrax results from ingestion of high quantities of vegetative forms *(7)*, as bowel transit would probably not permit germina-tion of spores to the vegetative form.

Gastrointestinal anthrax can present as two distinct syndromes: oropharyngeal and abdominal. As in inhalational and cutaneous anthrax, common features of gastrointesti-nal anthrax include edema and hemorrhagic necrosis. In the abdominal form, disease

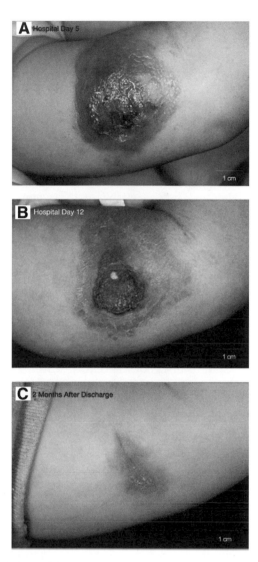

**Fig. 1.** Seven-month old infant with cutaneous anthrax. (Reprinted, with permission, from Freedman A, Afonja O, Chang WU, et al. Cutaneous anthrax associated with microangiopathic hemolytic anemia and coagulopathy in a 7-month-old infant. JAMA 2002;287:869–874. Copyright 2002, American Medical Association.)

frequently involves the terminal ileum or cecum *(21)*, and can involve the bowel wall as well as mesenteric lymph nodes. Presenting symptoms frequently include nausea, vomiting, fever, and severe abdominal pain. Not surprisingly, patients can also present with hematemesis, hematochezia, melena, and/or ascites *(1)*. Primary gastrointestinal anthrax has not been reported in the United States. However, hematogenous seeding of the gastrointestinal tract may occur with cutaneous anthrax and is especially common with inhalational anthrax. In 39 of the 42 fatal cases of inhalational anthrax in Sverdlovsk, gastrointestinal lesions were identified *(21)*. As opposed to cases resulting from ingestion, hematogenous dissemination to the gastrointestinal tract typically afflicts the submucosa but not Peyer's patches or the mesenteric lymph nodes.

Oropharyngeal disease also occurs after ingesting infected meat. Presenting features can include severe sore throat, ulcer, lymphadenitis, fever, and edema. Dysphagia and respiratory distress have also been reported with oropharyngeal disease *(1)*. Mortality rates as high as 50% have been reported with gastrointestinal anthrax *(1)*.

### *4.3. Inhalational Anthrax*

Given the high infectivity and lethality of anthrax, terrorists would probably attempt to aerosolize anthrax spores, resulting primarily in inhalational anthrax, the most fatal form. This is one of the most feared bioterrorism scenarios; even with the administration of appropriate antibiotics, many might still die, and the medical system could quickly become completely overwhelmed. Indeed, even with the recent mail-related, small-scale anthrax attack at the U.S. Capitol, available medical resources were heavily burdened.

Anthrax spores are 1–2 μm in diameter, enabling them to pass easily into the alveoli, where they are deposited, taken up by alveolar macrophages, and transported to the mediastinal and peribronchial lymph nodes *(1)*. Spores may germinate immediately, or germination may be delayed; animal studies suggest that germination can be delayed for as much as 2–3 mo *(17)*. Once germination does occur, however, the rapidly multiplying bacteria release toxins that induce a hemorrhagic mediastinitis, with marked edema and necrosis—the hallmark of inhalational anthrax infection that is often appreciated as a widened mediastinum on chest X-ray *(7)*. It is important to remember that the infection is within the lymph nodes; anthrax does not classically cause a true pneumonia, although there may be a localized region of hemorrhagic necrosis similar to the Ghon complex of tuberculosis, and some of the cases seen in the Fall of 2001 had pulmonary infiltrates on chest radiograph.

None of the 42 patients who underwent autopsy in Sverdlovsk had evidence of true pneumonia, and 11 had evidence of a focal, hemorrhagic, necrotizing lesion analogous to the Ghon complex *(21)*. Furthermore, these findings are similar to other human case series as well as animal studies of inhalational anthrax *(7,22,23)*. It remains unclear why germination in the lymph nodes is sometimes delayed for weeks to months. Indeed, at Sverdlovsk, cases of inhalational anthrax occurred up to 43 d after exposure *(6)*, and cases of fatal inhalational anthrax have reportedly occurred up to 58 d after exposure in experimental monkeys *(15)*. In the recent U.S. mail-related outbreak, the incubation period was 4–6 d for 9 of the 11 cases of inhalational anthrax with a known time of exposure *(24)*.

Inhalational anthrax is often described as having a biphasic clinical course. The initial phase features nonspecific influenza-like symptoms such as fever, chills, diaphoresis, headache, cough, nausea, vomiting, diarrhea, abdominal pain, and malaise. The presence of two symptoms, however, should raise the suspicion for anthrax: dyspnea and chest pain *(24,25)*. A chest X-ray may also show pathognomonic mediastinal widening induced by anthrax, which is not seen in upper respiratory viral infections (Fig. 2). Of the 11 cases of inhalational anthrax spread through the U.S. mail in October and November of 2001, the initial chest X-ray was interpreted as normal in only three cases, but more careful review by radiologists identified abnormalities in every case *(24,25)*. Two patients had pulmonary infiltrates without mediastinal widening, with the others having at least hilar or paratracheal fullness, but more commonly frank mediastinal widening. Furthermore, all 11 cases had pleural effusions. Hemorrhagic pleural effusions are also prominent in other series *(6)*, including Sverdlovsk.

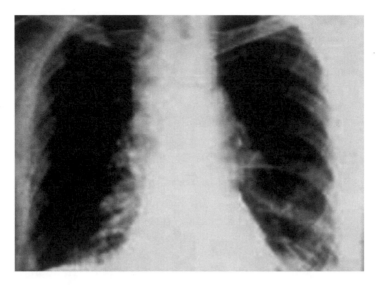

**Fig. 2.** Chest X-ray of inhalational anthrax, demonstrating marked mediastinal widening and a small parenchymal infiltrate. (Reprinted, with permission, from Friedlander AM. Anthrax. In: Zajtuch R, Bellamy RF, eds. Textbook of Military Medicine: Medical Aspects of Chemical and Biological Warfare. US Dept. of the Army, Surgeon General, and the Borden Institute, Washington, DC, 1997, pp. 467–478.)

Although it was generally not seen in the recent bioterrorism-related cases, historical reports document that some patients may paradoxically have transient improvement in their symptoms after a day or two. Regardless, a fulminant downhill course (the second phase) rapidly ensues that is consistent with septic shock, manifest by severe dyspnea, hypoxia, hypotension, and death. In Sverdlovsk, the median duration of this second phase was 1 d, and all cases resulted in death *(6)*.

The minimal effective dose of spores leading to inhalational anthrax is not presently known. Suprisingly few workers in high-risk occupations developed inhalational anthrax prior to mandatory anthrax vaccination. A study at a Pennsylvania goat hair mill demonstrated that workers were inhaling up to 510 anthrax particles per 8-h shift. Despite this concentration of spores, no cases of inhalational anthrax occurred *(12,26)*. In the past 100 yr, only 18 cases of occupationally related inhalational anthrax have been reported in the United States, with the most recent case in 1976 *(18,27)*. Thus, *every* case of inhalational anthrax should be assumed to be due to bioterrorism until proved otherwise. Poor data from monkey studies suggested that the $LD_{50}$ (lethal dose sufficient to kill 50% of individuals exposed) is somewhere between 2500 and 55,000 inhaled anthrax spores *(28)*. However, the meaning of these experimentally induced primate findings for infection in humans is not clear. The fatal inhalational anthrax cases in New York City and Connecticut in the recent U.S. Postal Service outbreak suggest that the minimal dose of spores needed to cause infection is small, and recent studies in monkeys suggest that the minimal dose may be as little as 1–3 spores *(29)*. These cases also suggest that the very young and very old may have a lower threshold for developing infection after exposure, which is presumably related to reduced immune system activity.

Meningitis complicates about half the cases of inhalational anthrax, although it also may occur with cutaneous or intestinal anthrax *(1)*. Rarely, it has been reported to occur without a clinically apparent primary focus of infection *(1)*. In the Sverdlovsk outbreak, 21 of 42 autopsies showed evidence of hemorrhagic meningitis *(21)*. Bedside findings are indistinguishable from other forms of bacterial meningitis—nuchal rigidity and other signs of meningismus, delirium, and, if untreated, obtundation that can progress to coma and is almost invariably fatal. Pathological features include widespread edema and hemorrhage into the leptomeninges *(16,21)*. Anthrax should be considered in cases of meningitis with high cerebrospinal fluid (CSF) red blood cell counts (RBCs).

## 5. DIAGNOSIS OF ANTHRAX

### *5.1. Cutaneous Anthrax*

Cutaneous anthrax should be suspected in individuals who present with painless, pruritic papules, vesicles, or ulcers—especially if accompanied by prominent edema and/ or development of a black eschar. Patients with cutaneous anthrax often have systemic symptoms including fever, malaise, and headache, which can assist in making the diagnosis. A black eschar with massive edema is virtually pathognomonic for cutaneous anthrax *(1)*. Gram stain and/or culture of the skin lesion will usually reveal the diagnosis. However, the yield of cultures from the skin lesion is dramatically decreased when antibiotics have been given for more than 24 h *(9)*. If clinical suspicion is high and the Gram stain is negative, or if the patient is taking antibiotics, punch biopsy with immunohistochemical staining and/or polymerase chain reaction (PCR) is recommended *(30)*.

### *5.2. Inhalational Anthrax*

The symptoms of the initial phase of inhalational anthrax infection are nonspecific and are easily mistaken for common viral syndromes such as influenza. Unfortunately, if treatment is not initiated during this phase, the infection will almost certainly be fatal. Therefore, it is imperative that physicians have a high index of suspicion under the appropriate circumstances, which can be broken down into suggestive clinical signs and symptoms, suggestive epidemiologic findings, and laboratory and radiographic clues.

Clinical symptoms and signs that suggest anthrax as opposed to influenza or other respiratory viruses include the presence of more concerning symptoms such as dyspnea and chest pain in patients presenting with a suspected viral respiratory illness. Dyspnea and chest pain were reported in 9/11 and 7/11 cases, respectively, of mail-related inhalational anthrax cases in 2001 *(31)*. On the other hand, dyspnea and chest pain are rare in laboratory-confirmed influenza and influenza-like illness, occurring in less than 30% of cases. Nausea or vomiting were seen in 9/11 cases of inhalational anthrax in 2001 *(31)*. These symptoms are also uncommon in influenza and influenza-like viral upper respiratory infections and can serve as important clues to the diagnosis of inhalational anthrax. Drenching sweats were also prominent in U.S. inhalational anthrax cases (7/10); this symptom is rarely seen in occupation-related inhalational anthrax cases, influenza, or influenza-like illness. Clinical symptoms and signs reported less frequently with inhalational anthrax than in laboratory-confirmed influenza or influenza-like illness included headache, myalgias, and (especially) sore throat and rhinorrhea (Table 1).

Epidemiological findings that suggest inhalational anthrax include probable exposure history to spores (i.e., mail handler), recent case(s) of confirmed inhalational and/or cutaneous anthrax, sudden appearance of multiple cases of severe flu-like illness with high mortality, unexplained respiratory failure, unexplained sepsis and/or death following acute febrile illness, and influenza-like illness in summer months *(9)*.

## Table 1

Comparison of Presenting Symptoms and Signs and Laboratory Findings in 11 Cases of Inhalational Anthrax (IA, 2001 U.S. Postal Service Outbreak) Versus Patients With Influenza-Like Illness (ILI) and Hospitalized Patients With Community-Acquired Pneumonia (CAP)[a]

| Symptom and sign | IA | ILI | p value[b] | CAP | p value[c] |
| --- | --- | --- | --- | --- | --- |
| Tachycardia | 9/11(82) | 58/422 (14) | 0.0001 | 320/649 (49) | 0.04 |
| Presence of: | | | | | |
| Nausea or vomiting | 9/11 (32) | | | 227/649 (35) | 0.002 |
| Chest pain | 7/11 (54) | | | 202/650 (31) | 0.04 |
| Lack of:[d] | | | | | |
| Sore throat | 9/11 (32) | 166/684 (24) | 0.0001 | | |
| Nasal symptoms | 8/11 (73) | 131/684 (19) | 0.0002 | | |
| Headache | 6/11 (55) | 97/684 (14) | 0.002 | | |
| Myalgias | 4/11 (36) | 60/684 (9) | 0.01 | | |
| Lab findings[e] | | | | | |
| Leukocytosis | 3/11 (27) | 47/697 (7) | 0.04 | 393/645 (61) | 0.03 |
| High AST | 8/9 (89) | 122/687 (18) | <0.0001 | 77/269 (29) | 0.0004 |
| High ALT | 8/9 (89) | 219/687 (32) | 0.0008 | 54/185 (29) | 0.0005 |
| Hyponatremia | 8/10 (30) | 63/687 (9) | <0.0001 | 222/636 (35) | 0.005 |
| High BUN | 4/8 (50) | 23/630 (4) | <0.0002 | | |
| Low platelet count | 2/9 (22) | 26/660 (4) | 0.05 | | |
| High hemoglobin | 4/11 (36) | 40/670 (6) | 0.004 | | |
| High bilirubin | 3/8 (33) | 38/682 (6) | 0.009 | | |
| Hypoalbuminemia | 6/9 (67) | 12/686 (2) | <0.0001 | | |
| Hypocalcemia | 8/8 (100) | 303/687 (44) | 0.002 | | |

[a]Data are number/total, with percentages in parentheses. Only findings with p value <0.05 are shown.

[b]IA vs ILI.

[c]IA vs CAP.

[d]Presence of abdominal pain, diarrhea, nausea or vomiting, chest pain, dyspnea, and chills not available for patients with influenza-like illness (other studies suggest that presence of chest pain and/or dyspnea can assist with discriminating IA from ILI).

[e]Creatinine, platelet count, hemoglobin, bilirubin, potassium, albumin, and calcium levels not available for patients with CAP. Modified from ref. 31.

Ideally, there would be a reliable laboratory test to confirm the diagnosis of anthrax promptly. Blood cultures for *Bacillus* are positive almost universally within 24 h in patients with inhalational anthrax as well as in cutaneous and gastrointestinal infection that has spread systemically *(7,9,32)*, and cultures should be obtained promptly before starting antibiotics. However, definitive diagnosis of *B. anthracis* requires specialized testing at reference laboratories, as standard hospital laboratories do not identify the *anthracis* species by blood culture. Definitive diagnostic options include *B. anthracis* PCR, immunohistochemistry, gamma phage lysis, and gas liquid chromatography *(9)*. In the United States, a Laboratory Response Network (LRN) has been established, and the 81 laboratories in the LRN can definitively diagnose anthrax and other bioterrorism agents *(7)*.

In the Sverdlovsk outbreak of inhalational anthrax, blood cultures were positive for *B. anthracis* in all cases in which patients did not receive antibiotics prior to presentation, as well as for patients who had received antibiotics for less than 21 h *(9,32)*. Interestingly, antibiotic administration for more than 24 h prior to obtaining cultures virtually precluded recovery of anthrax from culture samples obtained from any site *(9,32)*. A presumptive diagnosis of *B. anthracis* can be made if Gram-positive, sporulating, rods that are nonmotile, nonhemolytic, and encapsulated (the latter usually demonstrated by India ink examination) are identified *(9)*. A "curled hair" peripheral edge colony morphology can also provide assistance in making the diagnosis of anthrax as well as seeing Gram-positive rods in the buffy coat.

Other laboratory findings that can assist in making a diagnosis of inhalational anthrax include (percent of cases in U.S. Postal Service outbreak appears in parentheses): leukocytosis and/or a left shift (100%), hyponatremia (80%), hypoalbuminemia (67%), elevated transaminases (67%), and elevated hemoglobin (36%) *(24,31)*. Severe hypoglycemia, hyperkalemia, and hypocalcemia have been described in animal studies but were not observed in the U.S. Postal Service outbreak *(24,36)*. Thrombocytopenia has also been reported in animal studies and has occurred in 22% of cases in the recent U.S. outbreak.

Kuehnert et al. *(31)* recently compared the clinical features that can help differentiate inhalational anthrax from influenza-like illness and community-acquired pneumonia (Table 1). Investigators compared data from the 11 reported U.S. Postal Service inhalational anthrax cases with data from 691 patients at an ambulatory clinic who had influenza-like illness (473 had laboratory-confirmed influenza) and 650 patients who had community-acquired pneumonia. Compared with ambulatory patients who had influenza-like illness, patients with inhalational anthrax were significantly *more likely* to have tachycardia, high hematocrit, hypoalbuminemia, and hyponatremia and *less likely* to have sore throat, nasal symptoms, headache, and myalgias. Compared with patients with community-acquired pneumonia, patients with inhalational anthrax were *more likely* to have nausea or vomiting, chest pain, tachycardia, elevated transaminases, hyponatremia, and normal white blood cell counts. They also created a multivariate discrimination model using these key differentiating features *(31)*.

The following variables were used for comparing inhalational anthrax with influenza-like illness (2 points assigned to features with greatest discriminating ability) *(31)*:

> *2 points each*: tachycardia, hypoalbuminemia, lack of nasal symptoms
> *1 point each*: hyponatremia, high hematocrit, lack of headache, no myalgias

A score of 4 or more captured all 11 patients with inhalational anthrax (100% sensitivity); a score of less than 4 had a specificity of 96%. The following variables were used for discriminating inhalational anthrax from community-acquired pneumonia *(31)*:

*1 point each*: nausea or vomiting, tachycardia, elevated transaminases, hyponatremia, normal white blood cell count

A score of 2 or more had a 100% sensitivity for inhalational anthrax, and a score of less than 2 had a 48% specificity. These models may assist with differentiating inhalational anthrax from influenza-like illness and community-acquired pneumonia. However, caution should be used when these models are employed; given the small number of inhalational anthrax cases and the lack of validation of their model on a separate population, these results may not be applicable to future cases.

Serology is generally useful only for making a retrospective diagnosis. Antibody to protective antigen or the capsule is seen in over two-thirds of cases of cutaneous and orophanygeal anthrax *(1)*. Sputum Gram stains and culture are unlikely to be positive, as bronchopneumonia has not been reported following inhalational anthrax exposure *(1,9)*.

A chest radiograph should be promptly obtained when inhalational anthrax is expected. Importantly, all cases of inhalational anthrax in the recent U.S. outbreak had chest radiograph findings, including mediastinal widening in 70% and pleural effusions in 80% *(24)*. Mediastinal widening with or without pleural effusions, in a previously healthy individual with evidence of respiratory failure or sepsis, is highly suggestive of inhalational anthrax infection. Likewise, hemorrhagic necrotizing lymphadenitis and/or hemorrhagic necrotizing mediastinitis in a previously healthy adult is virtually pathognomonic of inhalational anthrax *(21)*. Chest computed tomography (CT) was obtained in 8 of 10 cases in the Postal Service outbreak and likewise showed abnormalities in 100% of cases, detecting highly characteristic hyperdense or hemorrhagic mediastinal and hilar lymph nodes, mediastinal adenopathy, and pleural effusions *(9)*.

It is essential to keep in mind that the patient is unlikely to survive unless appropriate antibiotics have already been initiated prior to the return of results, so cultures should only be used to confirm the presumptive diagnosis. More rapid diagnostic tests using enzyme-linked immunosorbent assay (ELISA) and PCR techniques can be helpful, but unfortunately are not yet widely available *(7,9)*.

In patients who have a credible exposure history to inhalational anthrax but have no symptoms, nasal swabs of each nostril should be performed. Nasal swabs that are positive for *B. anthracis* confirm exposure, not infection. Gram stain of nasal swabs in this setting is of very limited value and is not recommended for excluding the diagnosis of inhalational anthrax in symptomatic patients.

Meningitis due to anthrax can be seen with inhalational anthrax cases. Meningitis due to anthrax is not clinically distinguishable from meningitis owing to other causes. However, an important clue can be the presence of blood in the CSF; meningitis owing to anthrax is hemorrhagic in up to 50% of cases *(1,21)*. Gram-positive rods are often seen in the CSF, aiding in making this diagnosis. Indeed, a high number of RBCs and Gram-positive rods in the CSF prompted the diagnosis of the index case of anthrax in the 2001 U.S. postal service outbreak *(33)*. Meningitis owing to *B. anthracis* can be confirmed by identifying the organism in the CSF by culture.

Inhalational anthrax can be confused with viral respiratory infections, especially in the early stages, which can delay initial diagnosis. However, even without initial bedside clues, the rapidity of progression, severity of illness, unusual radiographic findings, and high likelihood of identifying bacteria in individuals who are not receiving antibiotics (by Gram stain and culture) should lead to proper identification of inhalational anthrax infection. Again, the following features appear to be particularly helpful in distinguishing inhalational anthrax from other forms of pulmonary infections:

1. *Presence* of certain symptoms and signs including chest pain, dyspnea, drenching sweats, nausea or vomiting, and tachycardia
2. *Absence* of typical clinical findings such as rhinorrhea, sore throat, headache, and myalgias
3. Link to epidemiological source (i.e., mail carrier or index case already identified)
4. Laboratory findings—positive Gram stains and/or cultures, hemorrhage (i.e., hemorrhagic pleural effusions, hemorrhagic meningitis), hyponatremia, hypoalbuminemia, elevated transaminases, high hematocrit
5. Chest radiograph and/or CT findings such as mediastinal widening and pleural effusions
6. High discrimination model score.

## 6. TREATMENT

Inhalational anthrax is unique among potential bioterrorist agents in combining the following features: effective treatment is readily available, it is imperative to initiate treatment immediately, and it is arguably the biological agent most likely to be used by terrorists. There are no clinical studies of the treatment of inhalational anthrax; in humans, treatment guidelines are largely the result of limited case series of inhalational anthrax in humans, extrapolation from animal data, in vitro studies, and expert opinion. Treatment issues include antibiotic therapy for symptomatic disease, prophylaxis (postexposure antibiotic therapy and active immunization), and public health measures such as infection control and decontamination.

The importance of notifying public health and law enforcement agents after a case of anthrax has been diagnosed cannot be overemphasized. Furthermore, the laboratory should be notified when suspected cases of anthrax are encountered to ensure that *Bacillus* species can be properly identified on culture results (many laboratories do not identify species of *Bacillus*, as it most often represents a contaminant, *B. cereus*, in nonbioterrorism cases) and so that laboratories can institute proper safety precautions in handling patient specimens.

### 6.1. Antibiotic Therapy in Patients With Symptoms

Although ciprofloxacin is widely believed to be the most efficacious antibiotic against anthrax, it achieved this status largely by chance. When the U.S. military prepared for the possibility that Iraq might use anthrax as a biological weapon in the 1990–1991 Gulf War, military planners were concerned that the Iraqis might genetically engineer anthrax strains resistant to common antibiotics such as penicillin and doxycycline—a concern that had been raised in scientific reports *(34)*. Ciprofloxacin was the new wonder drug at the time, leading to its selection as the treatment of choice in the Gulf War, since it was extremely unlikely that the Iraqis would have been able to engineer resistance against it. In fact, the anthrax utilized in the 2001 mail-disseminated cases was sensitive to multiple antibiotics, including penicillin, doxycycline, rifampin, and ciprofloxacin. However, anthrax produces an inducible β-lactamase, meaning that it may not be susceptible to β-lactamase inhibitors if a high volume of bacteria is present. Therefore, penicillin should not be used as a single agent when a high microbial load is suspected (in fact, in such an instance, monotherapy with any agent is not advisable) *(9)*. Doxycycline is considered to be as effective as ciprofloxacin against anthrax, and in particular has been shown to be effective against cutaneous disease. Additionally, doxycycline is inexpensive and has few side effects. Clindamycin is active against anthrax in vitro and has the potential advantage of stopping protein toxin synthesis, demonstrated in studies with *Streptococcus pyogenes (9)*.

It is important to remember that cephalosporins, often used for treatment of pneumonia, are not effective against anthrax, as *B. anthracis* produces a cephalasporinase. In addition, the mortality rate from inhalational anthrax is exceedingly high if therapy is delayed until pathognomonic diagnostic findings (e.g., widened mediastinum on chest radiograph) develop. Indeed, studies suggest that delaying the institution of antibiotic therapy by just a few hours can substantially reduce the chances of survival *(1,35)*. As a result, many authorities recommend treating all patients with fever or other evidence of systemic disease for anthrax in an area where anthrax cases are occurring until the disease is excluded *(7,9)*.

Patients with suspected inhalational anthrax should be admitted to a hospital and started on multiple iv antibiotics *(1,7,9)*. Currently, the CDC recommends initially using ciprofloxacin or doxycycline plus one to two other iv antibiotics (Table 2) *(36)*. Conversion to oral antibiotics is feasible upon stabilization, to complete a course totaling at least 60 d *(36,37)*. Some authorities recommend combination therapy with penicillin or chloramphenicol in cases of anthrax meningitis, because of concerns over adequate CNS penetration of ciprofloxacin and doxycycline. Additionally, some experts recommend use of clindamycin as a part of the intravenous regimen due to its ability to inhibit toxin production in static culture *(9)*. Other antibiotics that are usually effective in vitro include macrolides, aminoglycosides, and vancomycin.

Once clinically stable enough to take oral medications, a patient may be transitioned to single-regimen oral antibiotic therapy, preferably with ciprofloxacin or doxycycline. The duration of therapy remains controversial. Recent CDC recommendations regarding duration of therapy give the following three options: 60 d of antibiotics with close clinical follow-up, 100 d of antibiotics alone, or 100 d of antibiotics with vaccination against anthrax (three doses at 2-wk intervals) *(36–38)* (Table 2). These recommended durations are based largely on studies in monkeys. Five of 29 monkeys treated with antibiotics for 30 d after exposure to aerosolized anthrax relapsed after therapy was discontinued, resulting in death that was not seen when a 60-d course of antibiotics was provided *(15)*. The 100-d recommendation is based in part on the finding of the persistence of anthrax spores in the lungs of monkeys 100 d after inhalational exposure *(17)*. Interestingly, in these studies, monkeys did not develop protective antibodies and thus died on subsequent rechallenge with inhalational anthrax spores, providing some rationale for incorporating vaccination in the treatment plan. Given the long course of therapy, after the antibiotic susceptibility of the index case has been determined, the most widely available, efficacious, least costly, and least toxic oral antibiotic should be considered *(7)*.

Additional treatment issues may include fluid resuscitation, intensive monitoring, and correction of electrolyte abnormalities (more common in animal studies), and in some cases pressors and ventilator support. The CDC recommends considering corticosteroids in patients with severe mediastinal edema as well as in patients with meningitis *(36)*. Other actions that should be taken after possible exposure include immediate isolation of any potential source of anthrax spores, removal and isolation of clothing or other items

Table 2
Pharmacological Therapy for Anthrax Infection[a]

| Route | Treatment | Postexposure Prophylaxis (PEP) |
|---|---|---|
| Inhalational[b] | iv, **ciprofloxacin** 400 mg q12h[c] | **po ciprofloxacin** (500 mg bid)[d] |
| | iv, **doxycycline** 100 mg q12h[e] | **po doxycycline** (100 mg bid)[f] |
| | Additional iv medications[g] | |
| | iv penicillin | po amoxicillin (500 mg tid) |
| | iv levofloxacin | po levofloxacin |
| | iv ofloxacin | po ofloxacin |
| | iv rifampin | |
| | iv gentamicin | |
| | iv erythromycin | |
| | iv chloramphenicol | |
| | iv tetracycline | |
| | Continue therapy for 60 d[h] | Continue therapy for 60 d[h] |
| | (oral and iv therapy combined) | |
| Gastrointestinal | **Same as inhalational** | None |
| | Continue therapy for 60 d[h] | |
| | (oral and iv therapy combined) | |
| Cutaneous[i] | **po ciprofloxacin** (500 mg bid) | None |
| | **po doxycycline** (100 mg bid) | |
| | po amoxacillin (500 mg tid) | |
| | po levofloxacin | |
| | po ofloxacin | |
| | Continue therapy for 60 d[h] | |
| | (oral and iv therapy combined) | |

[a]Pregnant and lactating women and immunocompromised adults: same recommendations. The recommended drugs per CDC guidelines are in bold; oral antibiotic regimens should include one drug.

[b]Combination therapy with iv ciprofloxacin or doxycycline + one to two additonal antibiotics. Patients should be transitioned to oral antibiotics once stable (at PEP dose).

[c]10 mg/kg iv q12h in children (maximum of 400 mg per dose).

[d]15 mg/kg q12h in children (maximum of 500 mg per dose).

[e]Weight > 45 kg: 100 mg iv q12h; weight ≤ 45 kg: 2.2 mg/kg q12h (in children).

[f]Weight > 45 kg: 100 mg po bid; weight ≤ 45 kg: 2.2 mg/kg po bid.

[g]Additional iv medications should only be used in addition to bold medications.

[h]Duration of therapy should be at least 60 d with close clinical follow up. Other options approved by the CDC include: (2) 100 d of antibiotic therapy; or (3) 100 d of antibiotic therapy + vaccination (3-shot series, given at 2-wk intervals).

[i]Combination therapy with iv ciprofloxacin or doxycycline + one to two additonal antibiotics is recommended if systemic signs or symptoms are present.

Modified from ref. 36.

that might have been exposed, and hand washing followed by showering with soap and water. Importantly, there is no evidence of person-to-person transmission of anthrax.

Prior to the 2001 U.S. Postal Service anthrax outbreak, the mortality rate of inhalational anthrax was exceedingly high; 16/18 (89%) U.S. occupational cases and 68/79 (86%) Sverdlovsk cases resulted in death. In the U.S. Postal Service outbreak, 5/11 (45%) inhalational anthrax cases resulted in death (7). The etiology of the improved survival in 2001 has not been specifically confirmed; however, experts believe that several factors were probably involved. First, diagnosis was frequently prompt; all four patients exhibiting late-stage (phase 2 or fulminant) signs prior to antibiotic administration died *(24)*. In addition, improved elements of care, which may have improved outcome, include the advent of critical care units, improved ventilator support, and the use of multidrug antibiotic regimens. It is also important to mention that a recent analysis of Sverdlovsk data suggests that the number of inhalational anthrax cases and deaths was probably under-reported, with potentially as many as 250 cases and 100 deaths, respectively *(39)*. Furthermore, it appears that Sverdlovsk patients who had onset of symptoms more than 30 d after spore release had a higher survival rate *(7)*.

The treatment of cutaneous anthrax helps prevent progression to systemic disease and death. It does not, however, prevent the development and evolution of the eschar. The current recommendation for treatment of cutaneous disease with systemic involvement, extensive edema, or lesions on the head and/or neck is the same as for inhalational anthrax. For patients who do not have one or more of these findings, the recommended treatment is oral ciprofloxacin or doxycycline for at least 60 d, as cutaneous anthrax may be associated with inhalational anthrax exposure (Table 2). Only one case of cutaneous anthrax was reported in the United States in the 1990s *(40)*, leading to the need to consider possible concomitant inhalational anthrax owing to bioterrorism in patients who present with cutaneous disease. Corticosteroid therapy is recommended by some experts in patients with massive edema. Topical therapy is not helpful.

Like inhalational anthrax, gastrointestinal anthrax should be treated with large doses of two to three iv antibiotics until stabilization occurs and the transition to oral antibiotics can be accomplished. The same antibiotic agents that are recommended for inhalational anthrax should be considered in cases of gastrointestinal anthrax (Table 2) *(36)*,

### 6.2. Postexposure Prophylaxis

The rationale for postexposure prophylaxis after potential inhalational exposure is to prevent rapidly progressing inhalational anthrax. Experimental evidence suggests that treatment with antibiotics within 24 h after exposure to a lethal dose of inhalational anthrax can significantly reduce the risk of death *(1)*. Furthermore, animal studies suggest that combining antibiotics with active immunization may provide the greatest reduction in mortality *(1)*.

Determining who should receive postexposure prophylaxis therapy based on possible inhalational exposure is determined by several features, including known clinical cases, environmental conditions at the time of exposure, environmental cultures, and nasal cultures. Patients who have a credible exposure history, especially if identified as positive on nasal swabs, should receive at least 60 d of treatment, and perhaps up to 100 d, with consideration given to administration of anthrax vaccine *(41)*.

Patients with a likely exposure history but no symptoms should have nasal swabs obtained, and antibiotic prophylaxis with either ciprofloxacin 500 mg po bid or doxycycline 100 mg po bid should be strongly considered. It is reasonable to limit the prescription to 7–10 d of therapy, to allow for adequate time for testing and informing numerous patients of results. If nasal and/or environmental swab results are positive and/or the patient was in the space of a known inhalational exposure area, treatment should be continued for at least 60 d. Importantly, a negative nasal swab does not rule out anthrax exposure; further diagnostic studies and therapy should be based on all clinical information. An experimental model suggests that the yield of nasal specimens is dramatically reduced with increasing time after exposure to nasal specimen, to the point where they are almost universally negative more than 24 h after inhalational anthrax exposure *(42)*. Unfortunately, a patient from the U.S. Postal Service anthrax incident who had a negative nasal swab died from inhalational anthrax *(43)*. Indeed, the CDC recommends that the nasal swab should not be used to rule out inhalational anthrax infection.

Importantly, person-to-person transmission of inhalational anthrax has not been reported, so family members and other contacts who are concerned about secondary exposure should be educated and reassured.

### 6.3. Antibiotic Therapy for Special Groups

Ciprofloxacin and other fluoroquinolones are not generally recommended during pregnancy owing to their association with arthropathy in children. Furthermore, the teratogenic effects of ciprofloxacin in pregnancy are unknown, although animal studies have not demonstrated teratogenicity with this antibiotic. Doxycycline has been associated with hepatotoxicity in pregnant women and fetal toxic effects including retarded skeletal growth. Given the lethality of inhalational anthrax, however, at least one consensus panel of expert physicians *(7)* still recommends either ciprofloxacin or doxycycline as first-line therapy in pregnancy and in breast-feeding mothers (Table 1). If the latter is used, liver function tests should be regularly monitored.

As fluoroquinolones have occasionally been linked to the development of arthropathy in children, many experts would recommend using a penicillin derivative (e.g., amoxicillin) for children if susceptibility testing allows. The American Academy of Pediatrics discourages use of doxycycline in children under age 9 yr because the drug can result in retarded skeletal growth in infants and discolored teeth in infants and children *(44)*. Again, given the lethality of inhalational anthrax infection, several experts still recommend ciprofloxacin or doxycycline as first-line therapy *(9)*.

There have been no reports of anthrax infection in immunocompromized adults or children or in corresponding animal models; many authorities therefore recommend the same schedule of antibiotics favored for immunocompetent adults and children *(36)*.

### 6.4. Immunization

The anthrax vaccine currently used by the U.S. military contains no whole bacteria; it is an inactivated cell-free product *(45)*. It is made from a filtrate of an attenuated strain of *B. anthracis*, targets protective antigen, and is produced by the Bioport Corporation of Michigan. This vaccine has been safely and routinely administered to at-risk mill workers, veterinarians, laboratory workers, and livestock handlers for decades. The military administers the vaccine in a series of six shots over 18 mo, and hundreds of thousands of military service members have received the vaccine, although production problems interrupted initial plans to vaccinate all military service members fully. Although local reactions at the site of inoculation, such as tenderness, erythema, edema, or pruritis have occurred in up to 30% of men and 60% of women, serious side effects, such as allergic reactions requiring hospitalization, have been uncommon *(46)*. The most frequently reported systemic adverse event is headache, which occurs in 0.4% of shots. Local reactions are reported to occur in approximately 3–4% of cases *(7)*. The vaccine has been shown to be effective in monkeys exposed to inhalational anthrax. Postal workers exposed to anthrax in late 2001 were offered the vaccine, but most elected not to receive it. A live, attenuated vaccine has been used for humans in Russia.

## 6.5. Infection Control

Standard barrier isolation precautions are recommended for hospitalized patients—no patient-to-patient transmission of anthrax has ever been reported to occur. Cremation of individuals who have died of anthrax is probably the best way to prevent further transmission of the disease *(7)*. If autopsy is performed, all instruments and materials should be autoclaved or incinerated.

The greatest risk to human health occurs following initial aerosolization of anthrax spores, so-called primary aerosolization. The duration that spores remain airborne and the distance that they travel prior to falling to the ground depends largely on meteorological conditions and properties of the spores. Under optimal conditions, this period would probably last hours to a day at most *(7)*. It is impossible to state with certainty whether secondary aerosolization resulting in clinical disease occurs, as conflicting evidence on this matter exists. Prior to the U.S. postal service incident, all inhalational anthrax cases in humans, including the Sverdlovsk incident, suggested that this does not occur. However, the Environmental Protection Agency attempted to assess the risk of secondary aerosolization in the Hart Building by placing blood agar gel plates around the office and then simulating normal office activity. Ninety-four percent of these plates grew anthrax, demonstrating that "usual" activities in a highly contaminated environment could potentially lead to significant secondary aerosolization of spores and possible infection. Also, the cost of decontamination to decrease the slight risk of secondary aerosolization is not small; it is estimated that approximately 23 million dollars were spent on decontamination of the Hart Building *(47)*.

Anthrax is a rare infection in humans—the physician should assume that inhalational anthrax is due to bioterrorism until proved otherwise. Consideration of bioterrorism should also be entertained in patients presenting with cutaneous anthrax. The vignette demonstrates many features that should raise one's suspicion of anthrax: epidemiological factors (handles mail and had influenza vaccine), findings from the history (chest pain, shortness of breath, prominence of gastrointestinal symptoms, and absence of sore throat and rhinorrhea), and physical examination findings (tachycardia and dullness to percussion consistent with pleural effusion). Also, this patient's laboratory results (hyponatremia, hypoalbuminemia, elevated transaminases, hyperkalemia, hypoglycemia, and high CSF RBCs) and radiographic findings (widened mediastinum) suggest anthrax infection. Diagnosis is dependent on having a high initial index of suspicion, supported by consistent laboratory and radiological findings; it can be subsequently confirmed by nearly 100% positive blood culture results in individuals who have not received prior antibiotics. Local and state health departments, the CDC, and hospital laboratory workers should be notified immediately when one suspects a case of inhalational anthrax. Treatment of anthrax should be continued for at least 60 d using ciprofloxacin or doxycycline. Anthrax vaccination has been shown to be safe and effective, and no case of anthrax has resulted from person-to-person transmission.

## REFERENCES

1. Friedlander AM. Anthrax. In: Sidell FR, Takafuji ET, Franz DR, eds. Textbook of Military Medicine: Medical Aspects of Chemical and Biological Warfare. Borden Institute, Washington, DC, 1997, pp. 467–478.
2. WuDunn S, Miller J, Broad W. How Japan germ terror alerted the world. New York Times May 26, 1998;A1,6.

3. Carus SW. Bioterrorism and Biocrimes: The Illicit Use of Biological Agents in the 20th Century. Center for Counterproliferation Research, National Defense University, Washington, DC, 1998.

4. Manchee RJ, Stewart WD. The decontamination of Gruinard Island. Chem Br 1988;July:690–691.

5. Monterey Institute for International Studies (chemical and biological weapons resource page). Chemical and Biological Weapons. Monterey Institute for International Studies, Monterey, CA, 2001.

6. Meselson M, Guillemin J, Hugh-Jones M, et al. The Sverdlovsk anthrax outbreak of 1979. Science 1994;266:1202–1208

7. Inglesby TV, O'Toole T, Henderson DA, et al. Anthrax as a biological weapon, 2002 updated recommendations for management. JAMA 2002;288:2236–2252.

8. Centers for Disease Control and Prevention. Update: investigation of bioterrorism-related anthrax Connecticut, 2001. MMWR 2001;50:1077–1079.

9. Bartlett JG, Inglesby TV, Borio L. Management of anthrax. Clin Infect Dis 2002;35:851–859.

10. Office of Technology Assessment, US Congress. Proliferation of Weapons of Mass Destruction. US Government Printing Office, Washington, DC, 1993, pp. 53–55. Publication OTA-ISC-559.

11. Keppie J, Harris-Smith PW, Smith H. The chemical basis of the virulence of *Bacillus anthracis*, IX: Its aggressins and their mode of action. Br J Exp Pathol 1963;44:446–453.

12. Inglesby, et al. Anthrax as a biological weapon. Medical and public health management. JAMA 1999;281:1735–1745.

13. Brachman P, Friedlander A. Anthrax. In: Plotkin S, Orenstein W, eds. Vaccines, 3rd ed. WB Saunders, Philadelphia, 1999, pp. 629–637.

14. Titball RW, Turnbull PC, Hutson RA. The monitoring and detection of *Bacillus anthracis* in the environment. J Appl Bacteriol. 1991;70(suppl):9S–18S.

15. Friedlander AM, Welkos SL, Pitt MLM, et al. Postexposure prophylaxis against inhalational anthrax. J Infect Dis 1993;167:1239–1242.

16. Dixon TC, Meselson M, Guillemin J, Hanna PC. Anthrax. N Engl J Med 1999;341:815–826.

17. Henderson DW, Peacock S, Belton FC. Observations on the prophylaxis of experimental pulmonary anthrax in the monkey. J Hyg 1956;54:28–36.

18. Brachman PS. Inhalational anthrax. Ann NY Acad Sci 1980;353:83–93.

19. Freedman A, Afonja O, Chang WU, et al. Cutaneous anthrax associated with microangiopathic hemolytic anemia and coagulopathy in a 7-month-old infant. JAMA 2002;287:869–874

20. Lew D. *Bacillus anthracis* (anthrax). In: Mandell GL, Bennett JE, Dolan R, eds. Principles and Practices of Infectious Disease. Churchill Livingstone, New York, 1995, pp. 1885–1889.

21. Amramova FA, Grinberg LM, Yampolskaya O, Walker DH. Pathology of inhalational anthrax in 42 cases from the Sverdlovsk outbreak in 1979. Proc Natl Acad Sci USA 1993;90:2291–2294.

22. Ross JM. The pathogenesis of anthrax following the administration of spores by the respiratory route. J Pathol Bacteriol 1957;73:485–495.

23. Dalldorf F, Kaufmann AF, Brachman PS. Woolsorter's disease. Arch Pathol 1971;92:418–426.

24. Jernigan JA, Stephens DS, Ashford DA, et al. Bioterrorism-related inhalational anthrax: the first 10 cases reported in the United States. Emerg Infect Dis 2001;7:933–944.

25. Barakat LA, Quentzel HL, Jernigan JA, et al. Fatal inhalational anthrax in a 94-year-old Connecticut woman. JAMA 2002;287:863–868.

26. Dahlgren CM, Buchanan LM, Decker HM, et al. *Bacillus anthracis* aerosols in goat hair processing mills. Am J Hyg 1960;72:24–31.

27. Borio L, Frank D, Mani V, et al. Death due to bioterrorism-related inhalational anthrax: report of two patients. JAMA 2001;286:2554–2559.

28. Defense Intelligence Agency. Soviet Biological Warfare Threat. Publication DST-161OF-O57-86. US Department of Defense, Washington, DC, 1986.

29. Peters CJ, Hartley DM. Anthrax inhalation and lethal human infection. Lancet 2002;359:710–711.

30. Investigation of bioterrorism-related anthrax and interim guidelines for clinical evaluation of persons with possible anthrax. MMWR 2001;50:941–948.

31. Kuehnert MJ, Doyle TJ, Hill HA, et al. Clinical features that discriminate inhalational anthrax from other acute respiratory illnesses. CID 2003;36:328–336.

32. Grinberg LM, Abramova FA, Yampolskaya OV, et al. Quantitative pathology of inhalational anthrax I: Quantitative microscopic findings. Mod Pathol 2001;14:482–495.

33. Bush LM, Abrams BH, Beall A, Johnson CC. Index case of fatal inhalational anthrax due to bioterrorism in the United States. N Engl J Med 2001;345:1607–1610.

34. Stepanov AV, Marinin LI, Pomerantsev AV, Staritsin NA. Development of novel vaccines against anthrax in man. J Biotechnol 1966;44:155–160.

35. Lincoln R, Klein F, Walker J, et al. Successful treatment of monkeys for septicemic anthrax. Antimicrobial Agents and Chemotherapy, 1964. American Society for Microbiology; 1965, pp. 759–763.
36. Centers for Disease Control and Prevention. Update: investigation of bioterrorism-related anthrax and interim guidelines for exposure management and antimicrobial therapy. MMWR 2001;50:909–919.
37. Centers for Disease Control and Prevention. Update: investigation of bioterrorism-related anthrax and interim guidelines for clinical evaluation of persons with possible anthrax. MMWR 2001;50:941–948.
38. Centers for Disease Control and Prevention. Additional options for preventive treatment for exposed persons to inhalational anthrax. JAMA 2002;287:579.
39. Brookmeyer R, Blades N, Hugh-Jones M, Henderson D. The statistical analysis of truncated data: application to the Sverdlovsk anthrax outbreak. Biostatistics. 2001;2:233–247.
40. Centers for Disease Control and Prevention. Human anthrax associated with an epizootic among livestock North Dakota, 2000. MMWR 2001;50:677–680.
41. Centers for Disease Control and Prevention. Evaluation of postexposure antibiotic prophylaxis to prevent anthrax. MMWR 2002;51:59.
42. Hail AS, Rossi CA, Ludwig GW, et al. Comparison of noninvasive sampling sites for early detection of *Bacillus anthracis* spores from rhesus monkeys after aerosol challenge. Mil Med 199;164:833–837.
43. Borio L, Frank D, Mani V, et al. Death due to bioterrorism-related anthrax. JAMA 2001;286:2554–2559.
44. American Hospital Formulary Service. AHFS Drug Information. American Society of Health System Pharmacists, Bethesda, MD, 1996.
45. Office of the Surgeon General, United States Army, Falls Church, VA. www.anthrax.osd.mil.
46. Surveillance for adverse events associated with anthrax vaccination. MMWR 2000;49:341–345.
47. Hsu SS. Cost of anthrax cleanup on Hill to top $23 million, EPA says. Washington Post, March 7, 2002:A7.

---

# 6 Plague

## Jennifer C. Thompson, MD, MPH, FACP

The opinions expressed here are the private views of the author and should not be construed as official or as representing the opinion of the Department of the Army or the Department of Defense.

### CONTENTS

### Case Vignette

On July 25, a 13-year-old girl, who spent considerable time outdoors, handled and then released a wild chipmunk. On July 27, she complained of a sore throat and tenderness in her right groin, and she reportedly had a temperature of 40°C (104°F). On July 29, she saw a physician who noted an oral temperature of 38.3°C (101°F), pharyngeal erythema, tender cervical lymph nodes, and a 1 by 2-cm tender right inguinal lymph node. Laboratory tests, including complete blood count, urinalysis, and throat culture, as well as tests for mononucleosis, were done, and oral penicillin was prescribed. Three days later she was seen again, still febrile and with expanding right inguinal nodes. Her white blood count was 20,500/mm³, and a chest X-ray was normal. Because of her history of residence in a plague-enzootic area, a diagnosis of plague was considered. She was hospitalized and given parenteral streptomycin. By the following morning, she was tachypneic and producing bloody sputum. She appeared moribund. She was transferred to a large, regional medical center where,

From: *Physician's Guide to Terrorist Attack*
Edited by: M. J. Roy © Humana Press Inc., Totowa, NJ

despite intensive supportive care and therapy with intravenous chloramphenicol, she developed overwhelming sepsis and died on August 2. A chest radiograph taken before death revealed extensive pulmonary infiltrates. Antemortem aspiration of the right inguinal lymph node demonstrated Gram-negative bipolar staining bacilli on Giemsa stain. Both the aspirate and multiple cultures of blood yielded *Yersinia pestis*. In addition, fluorescent antibody stains for *Y. pestis* were positive in blood smears, culture material, and pulmonary secretions *(1)*.

## 1. INTRODUCTION

Plague, the disease caused by *Yersinia pestis*, has been responsible for millions of deaths across the world and through the ages. The name alone engenders fear and apprehension and has come to describe any disease of wide prevalence or excessive mortality *(2)*. After three devastating pandemics and numerous outbreaks dating back to antiquity, it can be argued that no other single disease has so shaped the course of global history. Although possible references to plague are evident in the bible *(3)*, the first clearly documented plague pandemic occurred in AD 541–543. This first great pandemic is reported to have killed up to one-fourth of the population of the Roman Empire *(4)*, with losses throughout North Africa, Europe, and central and southern Asia. The influence on history is obvious: after this pandemic and subsequent epidemics, the invincibility of Rome was eroded, and the Roman Empire was never re-established. The second plague pandemic occurred in 1346 and earned the familiar yet formidable epithet Black Death or Great Pestilence because of its devastating cost in terms of human life. It is estimated that up to one-third of the population of Europe may have succumbed, with a death toll that possibly exceeded 42 million *(4)*. The impact of this extensive depopulation on the religious, sociocultural, and economic milieu of 14th century Europe was far-reaching and unprecedented *(4,5)*. The pandemic finally ended in 1720 partly because of such factors as improvement in general standards of personal hygiene, as well as ecological changes that did not favor the primary flea vector or rat host *(6)*. The third plague pandemic began in the 19th century in China and, facilitated by modern transportation, spread to every inhabited continent. The death toll was in excess of 12 million in India alone, with unknown but extensive losses in other parts of the world *(6)*. Today, outbreaks of plague occur periodically in various parts of the world *(7–10)*. However, with the advent of effective antibiotic therapy as well as the development of an understanding of the epidemiology and modes of transmission of the infection, future naturally occurring pandemics are unlikely, and the total death toll in recent outbreaks has not approached historically established rates. Even so, mortality rates as high as 60% continue to be seen under certain circumstances *(11)*.

## 2. HISTORY AND POTENTIAL AS A BIOTERRORIST AGENT

The devastating morbidity and mortality associated with plague and its potential for defeating an enemy through intentional transmission have been recognized throughout history. An early example is described in an account of the 14th century conflict between the Tartars and the Genoese in the city of Caffa (now Feodosia, Ukraine). The Tartars had sustained severe losses from plague but tried to use this to their advantage by catapulting the cadavers of their dead over enemy lines. An outbreak of plague subsequently occurred among the Genoese, and the city of Caffa was surrendered shortly afterwards *(12)*. The perception of the disease and its tremendous impact are summarized in contemporary accounts of this event: "one infected man could carry the poison to others and infect people and places with the disease by look alone. No one knew, or could discover, a means of defense" *(13)*. Since the flea vector of plague abandons an infected corpse as it cools, the cadavers are unlikely in reality to have been the only source of the subsequent plague outbreak among the Genoese *(6)*.

More recently, plague was one of several diseases that were studied intensively in Unit 731, a Japanese biological warfare research facility that was in existence during World War II *(14)*. Field testing from this unit was associated with the aerial dissemination of 5 kg of plague-infected fleas among the Chinese population of a seaside resort *(15)*. Although hundreds of people died as a result of these tests and the subsequent recurring epidemics, there was dissatisfaction with the efficiency of this method of dispersal. Other efforts included dropping flasks of plague-infected fleas into wells and other water sources and also scattering fleas directly into rice and wheat fields *(15)*. Over time, methods were developed that did not require the flea vector at all, and at least one suspicious outbreak of wartime human plague occurred after the aerial dispersal of various forms of particulate matter from an aircraft over China *(6)*.

One can only speculate on the full impact today of the effective aerosolization of viable plague organisms in a bioterrorist effort. It has been predicted that most of the resulting cases would be pneumonic plague *(16,17)*, since this is the form of the disease that is the most transmissible and would be associated with the highest mortality. One report has estimated that the aerosolized release of 50 kg of *Y. pestis* over a city with a population of 5 million would result in 150,000 clinical cases and up to 36,000 deaths. In this hypothetical scenario, an additional 80,000–100,000 people would require hospitalization and/or isolation as a result of primary exposure, and secondary cases might occur in up to 10% of the remaining population *(18)*. In an exercise to assess the response to an act of bioterrorism, a fictional scenario was devised that involved the release of *Y. pestis* into the performing arts center in Denver, Colorado. The result was 3700 notional cases of pneumonic plague with 950 deaths by the fourth day of the exercise. Also of particularly grave concern were the potential problems in leadership and decision making as well as the confusion regarding distribution of resources that were highlighted by the exercise *(19)*.

## 3. ETIOLOGICAL AGENT

Alexandre Yersin and Shibasaburo Kitaso discovered *Yersinia pestis*, the etiological agent of plague, almost simultaneously during the Hong Kong plague epidemic in 1894. The organism has undergone several changes in nomenclature since its initial identification: *Bacterium pestis* until 1900, then *Bacillus pestis* until 1923, followed by *Pasturella pestis*, and finally *Yersinia pestis* in 1970 *(5)*. The genus *Yersinia* belongs to the family Enterobacteriaceae and contains two other species that are also pathogenic in humans: *Y. pseudotuberculosis* and *Y. enterocolitica*. *Y. pestis* is a pleomorphic, Gram negative, nonmotile, non-spore-forming, non-lactose-fermenting coccobacillus that exhibits bipolar, "safety pin" staining with Giemsa, Wright's or Wayson staining *(20)* (Fig. 1). The organism is an obligate parasite that grows aerobically on most culture media, including blood agar or MacConkey agar. The optimal temperature for growth is 28°C; extended incubation at 37°C tends to produce smaller, mucoid-appearing colonies *(21)*.

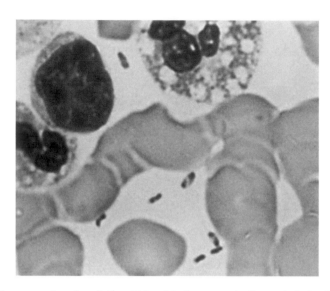

**Fig. 1.** Wright-Giemsa stain of peripheral blood in bacteremic *Y. pestis* infection demonstrating the characteristic bipolar ("safety pin") staining. (Courtesy of the Centers for Disease Control and Prevention.)

*Y. pestis* possesses several virulence factors that have been characterized genetically and implicated in its pathogenesis. Fraction 1 (F1) antigen, a component of the capsular envelope, resists phagocytosis *(5)*. The plasmid-mediated V and W antigens have been shown to play a role in intracellular survival and replication. Other virulence factors include a lipopolysaccharide endotoxin as well as coagulase enzyme *(22)*.

## 4. EPIDEMIOLOGY

Plague is a zoonosis that is usually transmitted among animals by fleabites. Natural enzootic cycles are established in multiple rodent species and occur worldwide, particularly in Asia and Africa. These cycles are associated with periods of intense infection within the rodent population, resulting in dramatic die-offs. Human populations in such areas are at high risk for infection after these die-offs because the flea vector actively searches for an alternative host after the death of the rodent. This is the basis for most of the outbreaks of sylvatic plague that occur in endemic areas. Plague outbreaks can also occur in urban settings, usually in the context of crowding, poor sanitation, and heavy infestation with peridomestic rats *(21)*.

Historically, the oriental rat flea (*Xenopsylla cheopis*) has been the vector most commonly associated with natural transmission, with domestic rats such as the black rat, *Rattus rattus*, or the brown rat, *R. norvegicus*, often serving as host reservoirs *(22)*. However, any type of flea should be considered a potential vector in plague endemic areas, and, in fact, the human flea, *Pulex irritans*, was implicated during the Black Death *(6)*. There are also a variety of host species that can either serve as reservoirs or amplify the infection. Reservoir hosts such as deer mice and ground squirrels are only partially susceptible to infection, but they are able to harbor infected fleas that can then transmit infection to more susceptible animals. Highly susceptible animals such as prairie dogs may acquire a very high bacteremic burden, which can result in amplification of infected

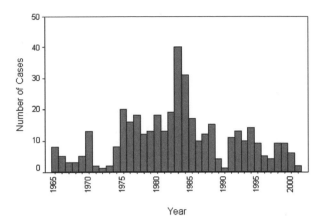

**Fig. 2.** Yearly incidence of human plague in the United States, 1965–2001. (Compiled from data courtesy of Russell Enscore and Katherine Feldman, Bacterial Zoonosis Branch, Division of Vector-Borne Infectious Diseases, Centers for Disease Control and Prevention.)

fleas. Most carnivores such as domestic dogs are resistant to infection, but they too can harbor infected fleas that can transmit the infection to other hosts. Larger animals such as camels and goats that may live in close proximity to humans may be susceptible to plague and have also been implicated in human epidemics *(23)*.

In the United States, males and females are equally affected by plague *(22)*, with most cases occurring in the endemic areas of New Mexico, Arizona, Colorado, California, and Utah during the months between April and October. Among the 401 cases reported to the Centers for Disease Control and Prevention (CDC) between 1965 and 2001, bubonic plague comprised the vast majority, and 14% of all cases were fatal (Russell Enscore, Centers for Disease Control and Prevention, personal communication). The yearly incidence of plague in the United States is illustrated in Fig. 2.

## 5. PATHOGENESIS

The cycle of infection with *Y. pestis* begins when a flea takes a blood meal from a bacteremic animal that is infected with the organism. *Y. pestis* produces a coagulase that causes blood to clot in the foregut of the flea, and the clotted blood becomes a nidus for the replication of the bacteria *(22)*. The blood clot causes obstruction of the proventriculus such that the flea is unable to swallow. When the flea attempts to take another blood meal from an uninfected host, the obstruction causes it to regurgitate a heavy burden of *Y. pestis* organisms into the skin of the host.

After inoculation, the bacteria migrate to regional lymph nodes, where they undergo phagocytosis by polymorphonuclear and mononuclear cells of the host. At this early stage, the bacteria are highly susceptible to phagocytosis because the growth conditions within the flea promote the expression of only a small amount of envelope antigen (fraction 1 or F1). However, the bacteria are able to resist intracellular killing owing to the presence of V and W antigens. The result is that the bacteria multiply aggressively intracellularly, and eventually the phagocytic cell is destroyed. Progeny cells that are formed within the mammalian host elaborate larger quantities of F1 antigen and are resistant to subsequent phagocytosis *(5)*. The lymph node becomes enlarged and increasingly inflamed, with areas of hemorrhage and necrosis. Ultimately, the release of a large burden of organisms can quickly cause bacteremia in the host. At this stage, endotoxemia results in clinical manifestations such as hypotension and end-organ dysfunction that are characteristic of Gram-negative sepsis. In terminal cases, *Y. pestis* can be isolated from almost all host tissues, and there is characteristically a particularly high bacterial burden in the bloodstream, lymph nodes, and spleen *(21)*.

## 6. CLINICAL MANIFESTATIONS OF DISEASE

There are three primary forms of the disease: bubonic, septicemic, and pneumonic. Other manifestations that have been reported, such as meningitis, usually represent complications of one of the primary forms.

### *6.1. Bubonic Plague*

Bubonic plague is the most common manifestation of infection, accounting for over 75% of naturally occurring cases *(21)*. This is the form of the disease that usually develops after a fleabite or after inoculation of infected material. Symptoms generally develop within 2–8 d of exposure. Typically the patient will develop fever, headache, and tender lymph nodes (buboes) proximal to the site of inoculation (Fig. 3). Buboes frequently occur in the inguinal or femoral area owing to the frequency of fleabites on the lower extremities. Persons who acquire plague by other mechanisms, such as handling infected cats, may be more likely to develop axillary or cervical lymphadenopathy *(24)*, and any lymph node site may be involved, depending on the site of inoculation. Mediastinal lymphadenopathy has been reported, particularly in pediatric cases *(25)*, but this finding is much more commonly associated with inhalation anthrax. There may only be severe pain and tenderness at the lymph node site before the node becomes visibly or palpably enlarged. Ultimately, buboes typically become exquisitely tender and may enlarge to up to 10 cm in diameter. There may be a single ovoid, nonfluctuant mass or a cluster of nodes and associated edema. The bubo will usually recede with administration of appropriate antibiotic therapy, and incision and drainage are generally not required. However, the development of a fluctuant mass may be a manifestation of secondary bacterial infection, and incision and drainage might be warranted under such circumstances. Although there is often associated erythema, ascending lymphangitis is unusual. The presence of a prominent lymph node is by no means pathognomonic for plague; the differential diagnosis will depend on the clinical situation and may include staphylococcal or streptococcal lymphadenitis, tularemia (*Francisella tularensis*), cat scratch disease (*Bartonella henselae*), lymphogranuloma venereum (*Chlamydia trachomatis*), or chancroid (*Haemophilus ducreyi*).

### *6.2. Septicemic Plague*

Although often considered a separate entity, septicemic plague probably represents a fulminant manifestation of bubonic disease, in which either the systemic symptoms dominate before formation of a bubo occurs, or the lymph node enlargement occurs abdominally or is intrathoracic and not readily apparent. Septicemic plague is characterized by manifestations of hypotension and multiorgan dysfunction that are indistinguishable from Gram-negative sepsis associated with other pathogens. Disseminated intravascular coagulation (DIC) is sometimes reported *(6)*, and this has been associated with dramatic and potentially devastating complications such as acral necrosis (Fig. 4).

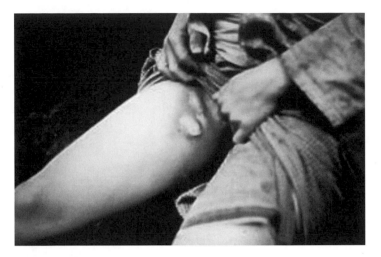

**Fig. 3.** Femoral bubo in a patient with bubonic plague. (Courtesy of the Centers for Disease Control and Prevention.)

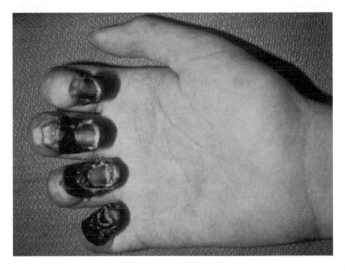

**Fig. 4.** Gangrene of the digits in a patient with septicemic plague. (Courtesy of the Centers for Disease Control and Prevention.)

Septicemic plague is typically associated with high-grade bacteremia and a greater likelihood of gastrointestinal symptoms such as abdominal pain or diarrhea (26). The mortality of septicemic plague has approached 50% in some series (5). This has been attributed to a delay in diagnosis owing to the absence of the suggestive bubo, and the fact that empiric antibiotic therapy that may be administered for sepsis typically is not effective against *Y. pestis*.

### 6.3. Pneumonic Plague

Pneumonic plague can occur via hematogenous spread during the bacteremic phases of either bubonic or septicemic plague, or, alternatively, it can be acquired as a primary infection after inhalation of the organism during contact with a patient or animal with plague pneumonia. Patients with secondary plague pneumonia typically develop respiratory symptoms such as cough, hemoptysis, or chest pain after initially presenting with signs and symptoms of bubonic or septicemic plague. In primary plague pneumonia, the illness typically begins with cough and shortness of breath within 24 h of exposure. Sputum may be blood-tinged and purulent and often reveals Gram-negative rods of *Y. pestis* on Gram stain *(27)*. There is no pathognomic or characteristic chest X-ray finding in pneumonic plague; alveolar infiltrates, consolidation, and cavitary disease have all been reported *(28,29)*.

## *6.4. Meningitis*

Plague meningitis is an uncommon manifestation of the infection that may occur in 0.2–7% of cases *(30)*. It is likely that the meninges are seeded during the bacteremic phase of the infection, but clinical meningitis often only becomes evident after several days of illness *(31)*. Patients typically have fever, headache, and signs of meningeal irritation that are indistinguishable from other forms of bacterial meningitis. The cerebrospinal fluid demonstrates a pleocytosis with Gram-negative rods evident on Gram stain. There is a slight association between the presence of axillary or cervical buboes and the development of plague meningitis, but this is not a consistent finding *(30)*. Inadequate treatment of other forms of plague may predispose to the development of meningeal disease, particularly if agents that do not penetrate the cerebrospinal fluid are used *(22)*.

## *6.5. Pharyngitis*

Plague can also present as an acute tonsillitis associated with cervical lymphadenopathy. Fever is typically present in these cases, and *Y. pestis* can usually be recovered from the pharynx, but evidence of systemic infection may be minimal. It is believed that pharyngeal plague is acquired via inhalation or ingestion of viable organisms. A syndrome of asymptomatic pharyngeal carriage of plague has also been reported *(32)*. In these instances, the organism was cultured from the pharynx of healthy individuals who had contact with a patient with clinical plague. Interestingly, these patients appeared to clear the colonization without sequelae even in the absence of antibiotic therapy.

## 7. DIAGNOSIS

Making the diagnosis of plague usually is not difficult when the patient presents with a prominent bubo. However, in the absence of the bubo, the manifestations of the infection are nonspecific and can be associated with a variety of other syndromes. Septicemic plague is often indistinguishable from other forms of Gram-negative bacteremia until a microbiological diagnosis is made. Pneumonic plague is easily confused with other fulminant forms of pneumonitis. When the differential diagnosis includes natural plague infection, it is critical to determine whether exposure to fleas, rodents, or other animals has occurred, particularly if there has been travel to enzootic areas such as the western United States. Exposure to a sick cat with plague is a clear risk factor for pneumonic disease in humans *(24)*. These epidemiological clues may raise early suspicion so that appropriate therapy can be initiated while one awaits laboratory results.

Laboratory confirmation of plague requires the isolation of the organism from blood or other body fluids or tissues. Two to four sets of blood cultures should be obtained on any patient in whom plague is suspected. Depending on the clinical findings, sputum and cerebrospinal fluid should be sent to the microbiology laboratory for analysis. Scrapings from skin lesions may also be cultured to yield the diagnosis *(5)*.

If a bubo is present, it should be aspirated. Buboes usually do not contain pus, so it is necessary to inject saline into the lymph node in order to aspirate a specimen. This can be achieved by using a 20-gage needle attached to a 10-mL syringe containing 1 mL of sterile, nonbacteriostatic saline (21,22). The sterile saline is injected into the lymph node and immediately reaspirated a few times to obtain specimens for microscopic slides and for culture. Microscopic slides should be air-dried and then stained using Gram, Giemsa, Wright, or Wayson stains. Body fluid specimens should be inoculated onto blood and MacConkey plates as well as into infusion broth. Y. pestis usually grows well on most microbiology culture media, but it may take 48 h for the typically smooth, opaque bacterial colonies with irregular edges to become evident (5). Biochemical tests can be used to identify Y. pestis, but some automated microbiological identification systems may not be programmed to identify the organism.

Serological testing can also be used to confirm the diagnosis of plague retrospectively. The test available through the CDC detects the presence of anti-F1 antibodies via a passive hemagglutination assay. The test is performed using paired serum with acute and convalescent, or convalescent and postconvalescent, specimens. A fourfold or greater increase or decrease in titer or a single titer of 1:16 or greater is presumptive evidence of plague infection (22).

There are other methods by which the diagnosis of plague can be made, but these techniques tend to be limited to research laboratories or other highly specialized facilities. F1 antigen or serum antibodies to F1 can be measured by enzyme-linked immunosorbant assay (ELISA). DNA hybridization techniques have also been used, but they are limited by extensive time requirements and low sensitivity. Polymerase chain reaction (PCR) has promise as a diagnostic technique that is both rapid and sensitive (33).

High clinical suspicion will be paramount for the diagnosis of plague during a bioterrorist incident. Victims of the attack would probably present with symptoms initially indistinguishable from other severe respiratory illnesses (17), making an early diagnosis particularly challenging. The identification of plague might be suggested by the development of rapidly progressive pneumonia associated with hemoptysis and ultimately with high mortality. Clusters of such cases should definitely raise the clinical suspicion of a bioterrorist event, and inhalation anthrax as well as pneumonic plague should be considered under those circumstances. Once a diagnosis of plague is confirmed or suspected, several features should raise the question of a possible bioterrorist attack: occurrence in a non-enzootic area and the absence of travel to enzootic areas, or the inability to identify obvious occupational risk factors. Even within an enzootic area, the occurrence of multiple human cases in the absence of an antecedent rodent die-off should also raise concern, particularly if pneumonic plague is prevalent.

Once the suspicion of plague is raised, it is critical to notify the hospital's infection control practitioner and the local health department. This will help to ensure that appropriate diagnostic testing is arranged and completed through the state reference laboratory and/or the CDC.

## 8. THERAPY

Streptomycin has traditionally been the treatment of choice for plague, since the drug has a strong historical track record. However, there are no controlled trials documenting its efficacy. The usual dose is 30 mg/kg administered im in two doses per day for 10 d, with a maximum dose of 2 g/d. Even though patients may show clinical improvement and become afebrile within 4–5 d, it is generally recommended that a full 10-d course of therapy be completed, since viable organisms may remain sequestered in buboes for several days *(21)*. Gentamicin has also been used with good results and is now considered an alternative agent, but there are few available data on the use of other aminoglycosides. Gentamicin is administered at a dose of 5 mg/kg im or iv once daily. Alternatively, a loading dose of gentamicin 2 mg/kg can be given, followed by 1.7 mg/kg im or iv three times per day *(17)*.

When neither streptomycin nor gentamicin is available, or when nephrotoxicity or ototoxicity precludes the use of an aminoglycoside, doxycycline is an appropriate alternative agent. The dose of doxycycline is 100 mg iv twice daily or 200 mg iv once daily. This drug can also be used to complete the 10-d course of therapy when there has been clinical improvement with the aminoglycoside. Ciprofloxacin 400 mg iv twice daily is also recommended as an alternative agent by some authorities *(17)*.

Chloramphenicol has also been shown to be effective in the treatment of plague. Because this drug achieves good penetration of the cerebrospinal fluid, it is strongly recommended for the treatment of plague when meningitis is suspected or confirmed. The dose of chloramphenicol is 25 mg/kg iv four times per day.

Sulfonamides have been studied as a treatment for plague; although they are effective, these drugs appear to be associated with a higher rate of complications, and currently they should be considered second-line agents in most instances *(17)*.

## 9. SPECIAL POPULATIONS

### *9.1. Pregnant and Breast-Feeding Women*

Plague is a potentially life-threatening infection in any patient, and it presents particular challenges for the patient who is pregnant. In addition to the risk of a severe, systemic illness during pregnancy, potential fetal toxicities are associated with the usual therapies for plague. Aminoglycosides such as streptomycin and gentamicin are potentially associated with fetal ototoxicity. Tetracyclines may result in enamel hypoplasia and dental discoloration in the fetus. Given the life-threatening potential of plague, the risks associated with these highly effective therapies need to be balanced against the risk of an inadequately treated infection. A few cases of plague in pregnant patients have been reported *(34–36)*. In each of these cases, the mother was treated with a standard regimen for plague and had an uneventful recovery from the illness, and the infant did not appear to sustain any sequelae either from the mother's illness or from the therapy that was administered. The current recommendation is for pregnant or breast-feeding women to receive gentamicin as the drug of first choice for plague, with doxycycline or ciprofloxacin as alternatives if gentamicin is unavailable or when oral therapy is appropriate *(17)*.

### *9.2. Children*

Historically, children have accounted for a large proportion of the cases of natural plague *(37)*, but the diagnosis in pediatric patients can be particularly challenging owing to unusual presentations of the illness. Meningitis has been more common among pediatric patients in some series *(30,31)*, and unusual manifestations such as Reye's syndrome have also been described *(38)*. Although survival of infants as young as 5 d of age has been reported *(37)*, delay in diagnosis owing to absence of a bubo in very young children can result in unfortunate outcomes *(39)*.

The current recommendation is for children to receive either streptomycin or gentamicin as first-line therapy for plague, with doxycycline, ciprofloxacin, or chloramphenicol as alternative agents *(17)*. The total duration of therapy should be at least 10 d, as for adult patients. The dose of streptomycin in children is 15 mg/kg im twice daily with a maximum daily dose of 2 g. Gentamicin is administered at 2.5 mg/kg im or iv three times daily. For children who weigh more than 45 kg, the adult dose of doxycycline may be used. For children weighing less than 45 kg, the dose is doxycycline 2.2 mg/kg iv twice daily, with a maximum daily dose of 200 mg. The dose of ciprofloxacin is 15 mg/kg iv twice daily. The dose of chloramphenicol is 25 mg/kg iv four times per day.

### 9.4. Immunocompromised Individuals

There are no data on the manifestations or outcomes of plague in immunocompromised individuals. The current recommendation is for such patients to be treated using the same guidelines that are available for immunocompetent adults and children *(17)*.

## 10. ANTIMICROBIAL RESISTANCE

Failure of therapy owing to antimicrobial resistance in *Y. pestis* has not been a problem to date, but naturally occurring strains with multidrug resistance have been isolated, and the potential for genetic manipulation of the organism for use in a bioterrorist attack is unknown. In 1997, the first clinical isolate of *Y. pestis* with high-level resistance to multiple antibiotics, including streptomycin, tetracycline, and chloramphenicol, was reported *(40)*. Of concern, antibiotic resistance was mediated via a plasmid that was transferable in vitro to other strains of *Y. pestis*. A second clinical isolate with high-level resistance to streptomycin has now been described *(41)*. The clinical implications of these developments remain unclear, but it seems evident that increased surveillance for possible treatment failures will need to be undertaken, with the goal of excluding antimicrobial resistance as a cause.

## 11. PREVENTION

### 11.1. Infection Control

Plague pneumonia may be transmitted person-to-person via respiratory droplets if an infected individual is coughing. For this reason it is recommended that droplet precautions and isolation be implemented for all patients with known or suspected plague until pneumonic infection has been ruled out, or until the patient has received at least 72 h of effective therapy and has made clinical improvement *(42)*. Droplet precautions require the use of a disposable surgical mask when approaching within 2 m of an infected patient. The need for N95 respirators and a negative pressure environment (as for pulmonary tuberculosis) has been the subject of some debate *(43)*. However, there is no evidence for the formation of droplet nuclei in pneumonic plague, and several authorities, including the CDC and the Working Group on Civilian Biodefense, have concluded that surgical masks provide adequate protection *(44)*. Eye protection in the form of goggles or face shields should also be used to reduce the risk of conjunctival innoculation, since ocular plague has been reported after exposure to pneumonic plague patients *(45)*.

Once the patient has received 72 h of effective therapy and is clinically improved, standard precautions alone may be implemented. However, droplet precautions and eye protection should be in use during aspiration of buboes or other procedures that may result in the dispersal of infected material *(42)*.

There is clear evidence that plague can be transmitted to microbiology laboratory workers via occupational exposure *(46)*. The hospital microbiology laboratory should be alerted whenever specimens from a known or suspected case of plague are being sent for identification, and biosafety level 2 conditions should be implemented. Biosafety level 3 is required if aerosol-generating procedures such as grinding, centrifugation, and so on are planned, but such procedures should be avoided if possible.

The bodies of patients who have succumbed to plague should be handled with standard precautions by trained personnel. Aerosol-generating procedures associated with autopsy should be avoided if possible *(17)*. If such procedures are unavoidable, they should be conducted in a negative-pressure environment by personnel wearing N95 respirators *(42)*.

It is not necessary to take special measures to decontaminate the environment beyond standard precautions after a case of plague. *Y. pestis* does not form spores and therefore cannot survive for extended periods outside the host *(17)*.

## 11.2. Postexposure Prophylaxis

When a case of pneumonic plague has been diagnosed, it is necessary to identify individuals who have had close contact with the patient (defined as coming within 2 m of the index case) prior to the completion of 72 h of effective therapy. This group of individuals, which may include household contacts and hospital employees, should receive postexposure antibiotic prophylaxis for 7 d. Doxycycline 100 mg orally twice per day or ciprofloxacin 500 mg orally twice per day are recommended regimens, with chloramphenicol 25 mg/kg orally four times per day as an alternative *(17)*. For children who require postexposure prophylaxis and weigh more than 45 kg, the adult dose of doxycycline may be used. For children weighing less than 45 kg, the dose is doxycycline 2.2 mg/kg orally twice daily, with a maximum daily dose of 200 mg. The dose of ciprofloxacin is 20 mg/kg orally twice daily. If chloramphenicol is to be used, the dose is 25 mg/kg orally four times per day.

Close contacts who are receiving postexposure prophylaxis should be monitored for fever, development of cough, or other signs of illness. Should such signs or symptoms develop, the patient should receive immediate medical attention with treatment for pneumonic plague on a presumptive basis until or unless this diagnosis can be definitively excluded.

## 11.3. Vaccination

There is no plague vaccine currently available. A killed, whole cell vaccine that was previously available in the United States was discontinued by its manufacturer, Greer Laboratories (Lenoir, NC), in 1999 because of financial considerations. The vaccine was recommended for use only in high-risk persons such as laboratory personnel working with viable *Y. pestis*, and field workers in endemic areas *(47)*; it was also routinely administered to military personnel. There are, however, no controlled clinical trials to evaluate the efficacy of the vaccine. Only circumstantial evidence exists, and this is derived from the experience with military personnel serving in Vietnam. From 1961 to 1971, the attack rate of plague among Vietnamese civilians was 333 cases/$10^6$ person-years of exposure. This is compared with an attack rate of 1 case/$10^6$ person-years of exposure among immunized U.S. service members. Murine typhus is spread by the same vector (*Xenopsylla cheopis*) as plague, but the incidence of this infection was comparable in the two groups, suggesting that the servicemen were protected from plague despite extensive exposure to the vector *(48)*. This indirect evidence, in conjunction with several animal studies demonstrating protection from bubonic plague, was used to justify the continued use of the vaccine.

It is unclear whether the previously available vaccine conferred adequate protection in the setting of aerosolized exposure to plague. Pneumonic plague has been reported in previously vaccinated individuals *(47)*, but there is evidence that the clinical course of the subsequent infection may have been attenuated *(49)*. The vaccine also had other limitations, including a short duration of immunity and increasing rates of local reactions with successive doses *(50,51)*.

In light of these shortcomings, strategies for a new vaccine against plague are clearly warranted. Live attenuated preparations and subunit vaccines are currently under study *(52,53)*, as are vaccines that utilize a variety of routes of administration *(54)*. The role of mucosal immunity in conferring protection against pneumonic plague is an intriguing question that is currently being explored *(52,55)*.

### *11.4. Vector and Reservoir Control*

Each case of human plague that is reported to the CDC is subject to a systematic investigation to determine the continued risk to other persons in the vicinity. The first step is often to educate the community on the use of personal protective measures and the avoidance of sick or dead animals. Serological surveys of wild and peridomestic hosts can help to characterize the nature and extent of the epizoological problem. Based on this assessment, flea-directed insecticides can be applied around homes and to pets. Measures to reduce rodent infestation should also be implemented, including reducing the amount of food and shelter that are available to rodents as well as using rodenticides where appropriate. In any effort to achieve rodent control, it is critical for the flea vector to be the first target, since a severe die-off of rodents will result in the release of potentially infected fleas that will seek alternative hosts, including humans. Measures such as using insecticides and rodenticides are more effective in the management of urban plague; sylvatic plague is often associated with a widespread and inaccessible rodent reservoir that is not amenable to intervention.

## REFERENCES

1.  Centers for Disease Control and Prevention. Plague—South Carolina. MMWR 1983;32:417–418.
2.  Stedman's Medical Dictionary, 24th ed. Williams & Wilkins, Baltimore, 1982:1092.
3.  The Holy Bible. New International Version. International Bible Society, Colorado Springs, CO, 1984, I Samuel 5:6, 9.
4.  Aker F, Cecil JC. The influence of disease upon European history. Mil Med 1983;148:441–446.
5.  Perry RD, Fetherston JD. *Yersinia pestis*-etiologic agent of plague. Clin Microbiol Rev 1997;10:35–66.
6.  McGovern TW, Friedlander AM. Plague. In: Sidell FR, Takafuji ET, Franz DR, eds. Textbook of Military Medicine: Medical Aspects of Chemical and Biological Warfare. Borden Institute, Washington DC, 1997, pp. 479–502.
7.  Centers for Disease Control and Prevention. Fatal human plague—Arizona and Colorado 1996. MMWR 1997;48:617–620.
8.  Centers for Disease Control and Prevention. Human plague—India 1994. MMWR 1994;43:689–691.
9.  Ruiz A. Plague in the Americas. Emerg Infect Dis 2001;7:539–540.
10. Boisier P, Rahalison L, Rasolomaharo M, et al. Epidemiologic features of four successive annual outbreaks of bubonic plague in Mahajanga, Madagascar. Emerg Infect Dis 2002;8:311–316.
11. Gradon JD. Plague pneumonia. Curr Infect Dis Rep 2002;4:244–248.
12. Derbes VJ. De Mussis and the great plague of 1348: a forgotten episode of bacteriological warfare. JAMA 1966;196:179–182.

13. Wheelis M. Biological warfare at the 1346 siege of Caffa. Emerg Infect Dis 2002;8:971–975.
14. Christopher GW, Cieslak TJ, Pavlin JA, et al. Biological warfare: a historical perspective. JAMA 1997;278:412–417.
15. Harris S. Japanese biological warfare research on humans: a case study of microbiology and ethics. Ann NY Acad Sci 1992;666:21–52.
16. Franz DR, Jahrling PB, Friedlander AM, et al. Clinical recognition and management of patients exposed to biological warfare agents. JAMA 1997;278:399–411.
17. Inglesby TV, Dennis DT, Henderson, DA, et al. Plague as a biological weapon: medical and public health management. JAMA 2000;283:2281–2290.
18. WHO. Health Aspects of Chemical and Biological Weapons. World Health Organization, Geneva, 1970, pp. 107–109.
19. Inglesby TV, Grossman R, O'Toole T. A plague on your city: observations from TOPOFF. Clin Infect Dis 2001;32:436–445.
20. Smego RA, Frean J, Koornhof HJ. Yersiniosis I: Microbiological and clinicoepidemiological aspects of plague and non-plague Yersinia infections. Eur J Clin Microbiol Infect Dis 1999;18:1–15.
21. Palmer D. Plague. In: Gorbach SL, Bartlett JG, Blacklow NR, eds. Infectious Diseases, 2nd ed. WB Saunders, Philadelphia, 1998, pp. 1568–1575.
22. Butler T. Yersinia species, including plague. In: Mandell GL, Bennett JE, Dolin R, eds. Mandell, Douglas and Bennett's Principles and Practice of Infectious Diseases, 5th ed. Churchill Livingstone, Philadelphia, 2000, pp. 2406–2414.
23. Christie AB, Chen TH, Elberg SS. Plague in camels and goats: their role in human epidemics. J Infect Dis 1980;141:724–726.
24. Gage KL, Dennis DT, Orloski KA, et al. Cases of cat-associated human plague in the western U.S., 1977–1998. Clin Infect Dis 2000;30:892–900.
25. Sites VR, Poland JD. Mediastinal lymphadenopathy in bubonic plague. Am J Roentgenol Radium Ther Nucl Med 1972;116:567–570.
26. Hull HF, Montes JM, Mann JM. Septicemic plague in New Mexico. J Infect Dis 1987;155:113–118.
27. Cleri DJ. Vernaleo JR, Lombardi LJ, et al. Plague pneumonia disease caused by Yersinia pestis. Semin Respir Infect 1997;12:12–23.
28. Aslofrom DJ, Mettler FA, Mann JM. Radiographic manifestations of plague in New Mexico, 1975–1980. Radiology 1981;139:561–565.
29. Florman AL, Spencer RR, Sheward S. Multiple lung cavities in a 12-year-old girl with bubonic plague, sepsis and secondary pneumonia. Am J Med 1986;80:1191–1193.
30. Becker TM, Poland JD, Quan TJ, et al. Plague meningitis—a retrospective analysis of cases reported in the United States, 1970–1979. West J Med 1987;147:554–557.
31. Martin AR, Hurtado FP, Plessala RA, et al. Plague meningitis: a report of three cases in children and a review of the problem. Pediatrics 1967;40:610–616.
32. Marshall JD, Quy DV, Gibson FL. Asymptomatic pharyngeal plague infection in Vietnam. Am J Trop Med Hyg 1967;16:175–177.
33. Engelthaler DM, Gage KL, Montenieri JA, et al. PCR detection of Yersinia pestis in fleas: comparison with mouse inoculation. J Clin Microbiol 1999;37:1980–1984.
34. Mann JM, Moskowitz R. Plague and pregnancy: a case report. JAMA 1977;237:1854–1855.
35. Wong TW. Plague in a pregnant patient. Trop Doc 1986;16:187–189.
36. Coppes JB. Bubonic plague in pregnancy. J Reprod Med 1980;25:91–95.
37. White ME, Rosenbaum RJ, Canfield TM, et al. Plague in a neonate. Am J Dis Child 1981;135:418–419.
38. Washington RL, Barkin RM, Hillman JR. Septicemic plague that mimics Reye's syndrome. Am J Dis Child 1979;133:434.
39. Leopold JC. Septicemic plague in a 14-month old child. Pediatr Infect Dis 1986;5:108–110.
40. Galimand M, Guiyoule A, Gerbaud G, et al. Multidrug resistance in Yersinia pestis mediated by a transferable plasmid. N Engl J Med 1997;337:677–680.
41. Guiyoule A, Gerbaud G, Buchrieser C, et al. Transferable plasmid-mediated resistance to streptomycin in a clinical isolate of Yersinia pestis. Emerg Infect Dis 2001;7:43–48.
42. Weber DJ, Rutalia WA. Risks and prevention of nosocomial transmission of rare zoonotic diseases. Clin Infect Dis 2001;32:446–456.
43. Levison ME. Safety precautions to limit exposure from plague-infected patients [Letter]. JAMA 2000;284:1648.

44. Inglesby TV, Henderson DA, O'Toole T, et al. Safety precautions to limit exposure from plague-infected patients [Letter]. JAMA 2000;284:1648–1649.

45. White ME, Gordon D, Polant JD, Barnes AM. Recommendations for the control of *Yersinia pestis* infections. Infect Control Hosp Epidemiol 1980;1:324–329.

46. Burmeister RW, Tigertt WD, Overholt EL. Laboratory-acquired pneumonic plague. Ann Intern Med 1962;56:789–800.

47. Centers for Disease Control and Prevention. Prevention of plague: recommendations of the Advisory Committee on Immunization Practices (ACIP). MMWR 1996CRR-14:7.

48. Cavanaugh DC, Elisburg BL, Llewellyn CH, et al. Plague immunization. V. Indirect evidence for the efficacy of the plague vaccine. J Infect Dis 1974;129(suppl):S37–S40.

49. Cohen RJ, Stockard JL. Pneumonic plague in an untreated plague-vaccinated individual. JAMA 1967;202:217–218.

50. Cieslak TJ, Christopher GW, Kortepeter MG, et al. Immunization against potential biological warfare agents. Clin Infect Dis 2000;30:843–850.

51. Reisman RE. Allergic reactions due to plague vaccine. J Allergy 1970;46:49–55.

52. Titball RW, Williamson ED. Vaccination against bubonic and pneumonic plague. Vaccine 2001;19:4175–4184.

53. Jones SM, Day F, Stagg AJ, et al. Protection conferred by a fully recombinant sub-unit vaccine against *Yersinia pestis* in male and female mice of four inbred strains. Vaccine 2001;19:358–366.

54. Eyles JE, Spiers ID, Williamson ED, et al. Analysis of local and systemic immunologic responses after intra-tracheal, intra-nasal and intra-muscular administration of microsphere co-encapsulated *Yersinia pestis* sub-unit vaccines. Vaccine 1998;16:2000–2009.

55. Baca-Estrada ME, Foldvari M, Snider M, et al. Intranasal immunization with liposome-formulated *Yersinia pestis* vaccine enhances mucosal immune responses. Vaccine 2000;18:2203–2211.

# Tularemia

*Christian F. Ockenhouse* MD, PhD

The opinions and assertions contained herein are those of the author and are not to be construed as official or as representing the position of the Department of the Army or the Department of Defense.

## CONTENTS

## 1. INTRODUCTION

A biological warfare pathogen intended to inflict massive panic, incapacitation, and ultimately death would have many of the properties characteristic of *Francisella tularensis*, the causative agent of tularemia. The intended release of as few as 10 organisms in an aerosolized and genetically engineered version of this lethal bacteria would cause a bewildering clinical syndrome indistinguishable from any one of a host of common bacterial and viral illnesses encountered by millions of Americans each year. Nonspecific symptoms such as fever and chills, headache, malaise, cough, and pneumonia resulting from infection with the pathogen coupled with difficulty in the rapid identification of the organism in blood and sputum would substantially delay diagnosis, resulting in both an increase in the numbers of patients and an increase in the severity of the illness. Furthermore, the ability of the organism not only to survive in an open hostile environment but also to re-emerge to terrorize and infect unsuspected persons months after an initial attack through aerosolization of dormant organisms from its grass and soil habitat, the ability of household pets to serve as unsuspecting reservoirs for infection, and the transmission of the pathogen through common pests such as mosquitoes and ticks would elicit fear and dread despite public health containment of a primary biological attack. The virulence of the bacterium, its transmissibility, and its capacity to induce significant morbidity make *F. tularensis* a potential biological warfare agent. In this review I sum-

From: *Physician's Guide to Terrorist Attack*
Edited by: M. J. Roy © Humana Press Inc., Totowa, NJ

marize the epidemiology, pertinent clinical findings, diagnosis, treatment, and postexposure prophylaxis associated with tularemia.

## 2. EPIDEMIOLOGY

Tularemia (rabbit fever, deer-fly fever, Ohara disease) is a zoonotic bacterial disease caused by the bacteria *Francisella tularensis*. *F. tularensis* is a small, Gram-negative, oxidase-negative, aerobic, nonmotile coccobacillus. There are two distinct subspecies, *F. tularensis*, biovar *tularensis* (type A), and *F. tularensis*, biovar *palaearctica* (type B). Type A strains, which are more virulent, are limited to North America, particularly Arkansas, Oklahoma, South Dakota, and Missouri *(1)*. Type B strains are found in the Northern Hemisphere, including North America, Europe, Russia, China, and Japan. Type B organisms produce infections that are often milder and indolent. *F. tularensis* has not been found in Africa or South America.

Approximately 200 cases of tularemia are reported in the United States per year. In the summer of 2000, an outbreak of tularemia in 15 patients occurred on Martha's Vineyard, Massachusetts; 11 of them had the pneumonic form of the disease *(2)*. That same year, a similar outbreak of tularemia occurred in 270 persons in Sweden *(3)*. After extensive epidemiological investigations of both outbreaks, the risk factors associated with disease were found to be multifactorial, including the use of a lawn mower or brush cutter [odds ratio (OR) of 9.2], mosquito bites (OR 8.8), owning a cat (OR 2.5), and farm work (OR 3.2) *(2,3)*. These risk factors have long been associated with the mechanisms known to influence acquisition of the disease. In addition, transmission of tularemia can occur by direct inoculation of contaminated animal tissue or after ingestion of contaminated meat or water, and by bites from ticks, deer flies, and mosquitoes.

An important aspect in attaining a weapons-grade pathogen for aerosolization is the infective dose required to cause disease. With *F. tularensis*, as few as 10 organisms are sufficient to initiate a virulent and potentially lethal infection *(4)*. *Francisella* can survive for extended periods in water, mud, and animal carcasses. Reservoirs for the organism in nature include many species of wild animals and birds including rabbits, muskrats, squirrels, skunks, coyotes, beavers, water rats, and domesticated cats *(5)*. Direct and indirect transmission to humans typically occurs through the bite of infected animals such as domesticated cats *(6)* or the handling of blood and/or tissue while skinning and dressing rabbits and other infected animals *(7,8)*. Tularemia can be acquired through the consumption or handling of insufficently cooked meat contaminated with the organism, drinking contaminated water, and contact with contaminated animal skins. *F. tularensis* is resistant to freezing, with rabbit meat remaining infectious after more than 3 years of freezing. Inhalation of bacteria from the dust of contaminated soil and occupational exposure from farming and landscaping have been reported and are responsible for large epidemic outbreaks *(2,9)*. In addition to infection via the respiratory route, other mucous membranes (ocular, oropharyngeal) are a potential point of entry of the organism. It is important to remember that there is no person to person transmission of this disease.

Vectors that can transmit the disease to humans include mosquitoes, deer flies (*Chrysops discalis*), and ticks (*Dermacentor andersoni, Dermacentor variabilis, Amblyoma americanum*), which are infected throughout their lifetime and can transovarially pass the organisms to their progeny. The highest incidence of tularemia occurs in the summer months when tickborne and mosquito transmission occurs. A second peak in the winter occurs, presumably from hunting wild animals such as rabbits. Transmission of the organism is not stable and can vary from year to year.

Another important mode of transmission is to clinical and research laboratory personnel who unsuspectingly may become infected with this highly infectious organism during the routine culture of clinical isolates. The danger to such personnel from aerosolized organisms without biological safety cabinets is high, as recent case reports suggest *(10)*. The confirmation of the organism and antimicrobial sensitivity testing should be referred to appropriate state public health laboratories with biosafety level 3 (BSL-3) containment facilties.

## 3. DIAGNOSIS

The criteria for the diagnosis of any infectious disease is accuracy, speed, reproducibility, and safety. Unfortunately, the current methods for the diagnosis of infections caused by *F. tularensis* are unsatisfactory. The diagnosis of tularemia by serology, both serum agglutination and enzyme-linked immunosorbent assay (ELISA), remains the method of choice *(11)*. Serum agglutination titers documenting a fourfold increase in titer between acute and convalescent sera or an absolute titer of 1:160 or higher help aid in the diagnosis of exposure to *F. tularensis* (although crossreactions with *Brucella*, *Proteus*, and heterophile antibodies are known to occur). Antibodies to the organism typically appear after the second week of infection, and it is not unusual to have negative serological agglutination tests despite acute infection *(12)*. Therefore, a presumptive diagnosis based on clinical presentation and epidemiological exposure mandate aggressive treatment in the absence of definitive diagnosis. The organism may be identified directly by fluorescent antibody assays (FA test) on specimens obtained from an ulcer exudate or lymph node aspirate. If a biopsy of a suspected lesion from a patient infected with tularemia is performed, the patient may benefit from a course of antibiotics for a potential bacteremia, which may occur as a result of the biopsy procedure.

In some rare cases, *F. tularensis* can be directly cultured from aspirates of ulcers or pleural fluid, or from blood *(13)*. However, culture of the organism should only be attempted in a BSL-3 laboratory, since laboratory personnel are at high risk for infection from this highly infectious bacteria. Special media containing cysteine or cystine for growth are required to isolate the organisms. Modified Mueller-Hinton broth, chocolate blood agar, and modified charcoal yeast extract agar have been used to isolate the bacteria *(11)*. The bacteria grow as smooth, blue-gray colonies, and identification as *Francisella* can be made by slide agglutination using commercially available antisera. Polymerase chain reaction (PCR), to identify *Francisella* rapidly and accurately from clinical specimens, has been developed but is currently a research tool not generally available in the clinical microbiology laboratory *(14,15)*.

## 4. CLINICAL PRESENTATION

The route of inoculation of the bacteria often predicts the clinical presentation of the disease, and the severity of illness depends on the virulence of the organism (type A or type B strains) *(16,17)*. Since the clinical presentation of this disease can be confused with other infectious etiologies such as plague, staphylococcal and streptococcal infections, cat-scratch fever, and sporotrichosis, accurate clinical description, rapid diagnosis, and expeditious institution of therapy are required. There are six clinical forms of tularemia: pulmonary, glandular, ulceroglandular, oculoglandular, oropharyngeal, and typhoidal.

From a biowarfare perspective, the most important clinical manifestation of intentionally released tularemia is the appearance of pneumonia. Organisms are introduced directly into the respiratory tract by the inhalation of bacteria. This is the primary route for the delivery of a weaponized form of the pathogen. However, endemic epidemics of pneumonic tularemia have provided important clues as to how the pathogen initiates infection, the natural history of the disease, the symptomatology, and the response to therapy. Pulmonary symptoms are characterized by a nonproductive cough, pleuritic chest pain, dyspnea on exertion, malaise, fever, and myalgias. Radiographic findings may be normal or may show pulmonary infiltrates that mimic other fungal and bacterial pneumonias, tuberculosis, or malignancy *(18)*. Hilar adenopathy can be seen in in 36% of cases *(9)*. Pleural effusions complicating tularemic pneumonia are rare, although pleural-based granulomatous inflammation secondary to *F. tularensis* infection has been reported and can be confused with the more common *Mycobacterium tuberculosis* infection *(17)*. The mortality rate from untreated tularemic pneumonia is high *(18)*.

The most common form of infection is classified as ulceroglandular or glandular tularemia. A localized, nonhealing, punched-out, circular ulcer with raised borders forms at the site of inoculation in small breaks in the skin, leading to lymphadenopathy and lymphadenitis in 90% of the cases. In many cases an ulcer or erythematous papule may not be clinically evident, and the only manifestation of infection is a relatively nonspecific regional lymphadenitis and systemic illness. The incubation period for the disease is approximately 3 d (range 2–10 d). Fever is the primary sign of infection, and flu-like symptoms appear prior to or concurrent with swelling and pain in regional lymph nodes. Duration of fever may be up to 3 wk in approximately 20% of cases treated with appropriate antibiotics.

The other major classification of tularemia is a systemic illness called *typhoidal tularemia*. Typhoidal tularemia is the most frequently fatal form of the disease and results from rapid dissemination of the organisms into multiple organs by hematogenous spread. This form of the disease may occur in patients with underlying illness, poor nutritional state, alcohol abuse, and chronic renal failure. Splenomegaly may be observed in 15–20% of the patients, whereas hepatomegaly is less common.

Other less common forms of tularemia include oropharyngeal tularemia resulting from the ingestion of infectious organisms, which may induce a pharyngitis, diarrhea, abdominal pain, and emesis. Oculoglandular tularemia is extremely rare and is acquired by the direct inoculation of bacteria into the conjunctival sac. Dermatological manifestations of the disease may include erythema nodosum and erythema multiforme *(16)*.

Rarely, *Francisella* can cause meningitis with cerebrospinal fluid findings of an elevated protein and a predominance of mononuclear cells *(19)*. A precise history of rabbit and cat exposure should be elicited and therapy immediately initiated, if other more common causes of meningitis are excluded.

## 5. TREATMENT

Factors to be considered in the treatment of tularemia include the natural resistance of *F. tularensis* to all penicillins and other β-lactams, the intracellular environment of the organism, the tendency to cause suppurative adenitis, and the need for both parenteral antibiotics in severe infection and oral antibiotics for localized ulceroglandular disease. When choosing an antibiotic regimen, one needs to consider whether the infection has been diagnosed with certainty, as opposed to suspecting the diagnosis based solely on the history or clinical examination. Since treatment with antibiotics that may not have adequate cellular penetration would fail to eliminate the bacteria, clinical relapse may occur. Therefore, treatment should be directed toward the elimination of both extracellular and intracellular forms of the bacteria. Factors affecting clinical relapse include underlying immunosuppression, insufficient duration of therapy, and the use of bacteriostatic versus bacteriocidal antibiotics *(18)*. An additional consideration may be the deliberate engineering of antibiotic resistance cassettes.

Treatment guidelines for tularemia that is intentionally released have recently been published *(20)*. The traditional antibiotic of choice in the treatment of tularemia is streptomycin (1 g im twice daily for 10–14 d) *(21,22)*. However, because streptomycin is not a registered antibiotic in many countries, alternative antibiotics with comparable efficacy to streptomycin, but with less potential for the adverse side effects of ototoxicity and nephrotoxicity, have been sought. Gentamicin, another bacteriocidal aminoglycoside, is an adequate alternative to streptomycin and has been successfully used to treat the disease in both the adult *(23)* and pediatric populations *(24)*, albeit with a greater relapse rate (6%) *(25)*. Caution should be exercised when using gentamicin alone because of its variability in cell penetration, higher frequency of relapses, and need to maintain high blood levels of the antibiotic. Treatment with gentamicin (5 mg/kg/d im or iv) to maintain blood levels at approximately 5 µg/mL should continue for 10–14 d. Tetracycline is efficacious, but, again, higher relapse rates occur, which may be a function of its bacteriostatic versus bacteriocidal activity. Doxycycline at 100 mg iv or po twice daily is recommended as an alternative choice of antibiotic. Quinolones, such as ciprofloxacin (400 mg iv twice daily or 500–750 mg twice daily orally for 10–30 d), have been shown to be particularly efficacious, with resolution of fever within 2 d of beginning therapy and fewer documented relapses *(25,26)*. Because of its excellent bacteriocidal activity, stability in an acidic environment, and levels of antibiotic achieved in soft tissues, ciprofloxacin is an excellent alternative in culture-proven *Francisella* infections and may become the antibiotic of choice for suspected but not proven infection. In pregnant women infected with tularemia, gentamicin, doxycycline, and ciprofloxacin have been recommended as the antibiotics of choice by the Working Group on Civilian Biodefense *(20)*.

In vitro antimicrobial susceptibility testing does not correlate with clinical response and should not be used to direct the choice of antibiotics. Cephalosporins, such as cefotaxime, ceftazidime, and ceftriaxone have in vitro activity against *Francisella* *(27)* but little to no in vivo efficacy *(28)*. For cases of suspected meningitis owing to *F. tularensis*, chloramphenicol should be added to streptomycin *(29)*. A single case report showed that imipenem (500 mg iv every 8 h for 14 d) could achieve clinical cure with no relapse *(30)*. The best indicator of response to therapy is the resolution of fever, which usually falls within 3 d of instituting therapy *(24)*.

## 6. POSTEXPOSURE PROPHYLAXIS

The Working Group on Civilian Biodefense has recommended a treatment for patients with tularemia in a mass casualty setting with specific postexposure prophylaxis for a total duration of 14 d *(20)*. The U.S. Food and Drug Administration has not approved

Table 1
Recommendations for Tularemia Treatment

| Antibiotic | Adults | Pregnant women | Children[a] |
|---|---|---|---|
| Doxycycline | 100 mg po twice daily | 100 mg po twice daily | 2.2 mg/kg po twice daily |
| Ciprofloxacin | 500 mg po twice daily | 500 mg po twice daily | 15 mg/kg po twice daily |

[a]In children > 45 kg, use doxycycline 100 mg po twice daily; ciprofloxacin should not exceed 1 g per day.

gentamicin and ciprofloxacin for this use; however, in the absence of controlled human and animal studies suitable for regulatory approval, these recommendations are the current best choice in case of intentional biological release of *Francisella* (Table 1).

In certain situations (such as possible exposure to laboratory personnel), exposed persons can be placed on a fever watch and treated if symptoms develop *(20)*. There is no licensed vaccine against tularemia. However, a live attenuated vaccine for laboratory personnel exposed to *F. tularensis* has been shown to be safe and partially efficacious, although it is important to note that in volunteer studies, not all volunteers given the live attenuated vaccine were protected against inhalational challenge with virulent organisms *(31,32)*. This vaccine is held as an Investigational New Drug by the U.S. Army Medical Research Institute of Infectious Diseases (USAMRIID), Fort Detrick, Frederick, MD.

The are several protective measures one can use to minimize contact with and infection by *F. tularensis* from naturally acquired sources. These include the need to avoid potentially contaminated drinking water and to refrain from bathing and swimming in untreated water. Wild rabbit and rodent meat must be carefully handled and thoroughly cooked; protective clothing in conjunction with insect repellents will help protect against transmission of the organism by mosquitoes, ticks, and flies. For laboratory workers who may come in contact with the bacteria, the importance of the use of gloves and masks is obvious. Although quarantine is not indicated, universal secretion precautions should be taken for infected open lesions.

Finally, two useful reviews on clinical recognition and management of patients exposed to biowarfare pathogens, including tularemia, are included in the references and should occupy a prominent place in the physician's library *(20,33)*.

## REFERENCES

1. Centers for Disease Control and Prevention. Cases of selected notifiable diseases. United States, weeks ending December 11, 1993, and December 5, 1992. MMWR 1993;42:955–958.
2. Feldman KA, Enscore RE, Lathrop SL, et al. An outbreak of primary pneumonic tularemia on Martha's Vineyard. N Engl J Med 2001;1601–1606.
3. Eliasson H, Lindback J, Nuorti JP, Arneborn M, Giesecke J, Tegnell A. The 2000 tularemia outbreak: a case-control study of risk factors in disease-endemic and emergent areas, Sweden. Emerg Infect Dis 2002;8:1–8.
4. Scriker R, Eigelsbach HT, Mitten JQ, Hall WC. Pathogenesis of tularemia in monkeys aerogenically exposed to *Francisella tularensis* 425. Infect Immun 1972;5:734–744.
5. Sanford JP. Tularemia. JAMA 1983;250:3225–3226.
6. Capellan J, Fong IW. Tularemia from a cat bite: case report and review of feline-associated tularemia. Clin Infect Dis 1993;16:472–475.
7. Francis E. Tularemia. JAMA 1925;84:1243–1250.
8. Boyce JM. Recent trends in the epidemiology of tularemia in the United States. J Infect Dis 1975;131:197–199.

9. Syrjala H, Kujala P, Myllyla V, Salminen A. Airborne transmission of tularemia in farmers. Scand J Infect Dis 1985;17:371–375.

10. Shapiro DS, Schwartz DR. Exposure of laboratory workers to *Francisella tularensis* despite a bioterrorism procedure. J Clin Microbiol 2002;40:2278–2281.

11. Stewart SJ. Francisella. In: Murray PR, Baron EJ, Pfaller MA, Tenover FC, Yolken RH, eds. Manual of Clinical Microbiology. ASM Press, Washington, DC, 1995, pp. 545–548.

12. Stralin K, Eliasson H, Back E. An outbreak of primary pneumonic tularemia. N Engl J Med 2002;346:1027–1029.

13. Provenza JM, Klotz SA, Penn RL. Isolation of *Francisella tularensis* from blood. J Clin Microbiol 1986;24:453–455.

14. Fulop M, Leslie D, Titball R. A rapid, highly sensitive method for the detection of *Francisella tularensis* in clinical samples using the polymerase chain reaction. Am J Trop Med Hyg 1996;54:364–366.

15. Sjostedt A, Eriksson U, Berglund L, Tarnvik A. Detecton of *Francisella tularensis* in ulcers of patients with tularemia by PCR. J Clin Microbiol 1997;35:1045–1048.

16. Evans ME, Gregory DW, Schaffner W, McGee ZA. Tularemia: a 30-year experience with 88 cases. Medicine 1985;64:251–269.

17. Schmid GP, Catino D, Suffin SC, Martone WJ, Kaufmann AF. Granulomatous pleuritis caused by *Francisella tularensis*: possible confusion with tuberculous pleuritis. Am Rev Respir Dis 1983; 128:314–316.

18. Gill V, Cunha BA. Tularemia pneumonia. Semin Respir Infect 1997;12:61–67.

19. Lovell VM, Cho CT, Lindsey NJ, Nelson PL. *Francisella tularensis* meningitis: a rare clinical entity. J Infect Dis 1986;154:916–918.

20. Dennis DT, Inglesby TV, Henderson DA, et al. Tularemia as a biological weapon. JAMA 2001; 285:2763–2773.

21. Enderlin G, Morales L, Jacobs RF, Cross JT. Streptomycin and alternative agents for the treatment of tularemia: review of the literature. Clin Infect Dis 1994;19:42–47.

22. Penn RL. *Francisella tularensis* (tularemia). In: Mandell GL, Bennett JE, Dolin R, eds. Principles and Practice of Infectious Diseases. Churchill Livingstone, New York, 1995, pp. 2060–2068.

23. Mason WL, Eigelsbach HT, Little SF, Bates JH. Treatment of tularemia, including pulmonary tularemia, with gentamicin. Am Rev Respir Dis 1980;121:39–45.

24. Cross JT, Schutze GE, Jacobs RF. Treatment of tularemia with gentamicin in pediatric patients. Pediatr Infect Dis J 1995;14:151–152.

25. Risi GF, Pombo DJ. Relapse of tularemia after aminoglycoside therapy: case report and discussion of therapeutic options. Clin Infect Dis 1995;20:174–175.

26. Syrjala H, Schildt R, Raisainen S. In vitro susceptibility of *Francisella tularensis* to fluoroquinolones and treatment of tularemia with norfloxacin and ciprofloxacin. Eur J Clin Microbiol Infect Dis 1991;10:68–70.

27. Baker CN, Hollis DG, Thornsberry C. Antimicrobial susceptibility testing of *Francisella tularensis* with a modified Mueller-Hinton broth. J Clin Microbiol 1985;22:212–215.

28. Cross JT, Jacobs RF. Tularemia: treatment failures with outpatient use of ceftriaxone. Clin Infect Dis 1993;17:976–980.

29. Hill B, Sandstrom G, Schroder S, Franzen C, Tarnvik A. A case of tularemia meningitis in Sweden. Scand J Infect Dis 1990;22:95–99.

30. Lee HC, Horowitz E, Linder W. Treatment of tularemia with imipenem/cilastin sodium. South Med J 1991;84:1277–1278.

31. Burke DS. Immunization against tularemia: analysis of the effectiveness of live *Francisella tularensis* vaccine in prevention of laboratory-acquired tularemia. J Infect Dis 1977;135:55–60.

32. Saslow S, Eigelsbach HT, Prior JA, Wilson HE, Carhart S. Tularemia vaccine study, II. Respiratory challenge. Arch Intern Med 1961;107:134–146.

33. Franz DR, Jahrling PB, Friedlander AM, et al. Clinical recognition and management of patients exposed to biological warfare agents. JAMA 1997;278:399–411.

# 8  Brucellosis

## David L. Hoover, MD

The opinions and assertions contained herein are those of the author and are not to be construed as official or as representing the position of the Department of the Army or the Department of Defense.

### CONTENTS

## 1. INTRODUCTION

Human brucellosis is a systemic, febrile illness with highly varied onset, course, and complications. It is caused by a nonencapsulated, non-spore-forming, small, Gram-negative, aerobic coccobacillus that is usually acquired by contact with infected food animals or unpasteurized dairy products. Of the six recognized species, four (*Brucella melitensis, B. suis, B. abortus,* and *B. canis*) are the classical causes of human disease (Table 1). Another, recently recognized species (proposed name *B. maris*) isolated from a marine mammal has also infected a human *(1)*. In animals, *Brucella* usually causes abortion or epididymitis and infertility. Although many mammals may be infected, most human cases derive from infections in cattle, goats, sheep, and pigs. The generally causative preferred hosts of each *Brucella* species are shown in Table 1, which ranks the agents in descending order of pathogenicity for humans.

The manifestations of infection by *Brucella* can be reasonably anticipated by considering its pathogenesis. A number of bacterial features permit its stealthy attack and survival in its hosts. As a facultative intracellular parasite of macrophages and placental trophoblastic cells, *Brucella* is protected from potential antimicrobial effects of antibody, complement, and therapeutic antimicrobial agents once it is ingested by its target cells.

From: *Physician's Guide to Terrorist Attack*
Edited by: M. J. Roy © Humana Press Inc., Totowa, NJ

Table 1
Typical Animal Hosts and Virulence of Brucella for Humans

| Brucella species | Usual host | Virulence for humans |
|---|---|---|
| B. melitensis | Sheep, goats | High |
| B. suis | Swine | High |
| B. abortus | Cattle, bison | Intermediate |
| B. canis | Dogs | Intermediate |
| B. maris[a] | Marine mammals | Intermediate |
| B. ovis | Sheep | None |
| B. neotomae | Rodents | None |

[a]Proposed name (62).

**Case Vignette**

A 55-year-old man presented with a 7-day history of fever to 103°F, chills, sweats, and diffuse arthralgias and a 4-day history of right lower back pain. He also noticed loss of appetite, inability to focus on his duties as a government administrator, and general weakness and malaise. He denied foreign travel, exposure to animals, or ingestion of unpasteurized dairy products or rare meat. He had attended a local conference with other high-level officials 2 weeks before his symptoms began and had discovered that half of the attendees had also become ill with flu-like symptoms. Physical examination was remarkable only for a temperature of 101°F pulse of 100/min, a few 0.5–1-cm cervical lymphy nodes, and tenderness to palpation over the right sacroiliac joint and right lower lumbar region. Complete blood cell count and urinalysis were normal. X-rays of the lumbar spine and pelvis were unrevealing. A bone scan showed increased uptake in the region of the right sacroiliac joint. Urine culture was negative after 24 hours. Blood cultures drawn at the time of presentation became positive 4 days later for a small, Gram-negative coccobacillus. Bucella serology (tube agglutination test) was positive at a titer of 1:640.

The outer membrane of the most virulent strains contains long-chain O-polysaccharides. These "smooth" strains, so called because of their appearance on agar culture, frustrate natural host defenses by inhibiting complement deposition to low levels, so the organism is phagocytosed but not killed (2). In addition, the low levels of complement deposited on the bacterial surface may not trigger a significant alarm response by macrophages. The outer membrane endotoxic component of *Brucella*, lipid A, may also contribute to the stealthy attack. *Brucella* endotoxin's potency is 1/10,000th that of *E. coli* for pyrogenicity and is 1/400th as potent for induction of tumor necrosis factor-$\alpha$ (TNF-$\alpha$) production by macrophages (3). In addition, a 25-kDa *Brucella* outer membrane protein appears to suppress endotoxin-induced TNF production (4). This reduced induction and active inhibition of TNF production may prevent the host from mounting a rapid and vigorous immune response. Finally, *Brucella* grows slowly (doubling time about 2 h, compared with 15 min for *E. coli*), so disease onset and elimination of bacteria by antimicrobial agents are not as rapid as one sees with typical Gram-negative infections.

*Brucella* enters the host through contact with mucous membranes (digestive tract, conjunctiva, respiratory tract) or skin. It is phagocytosed by macrophages at the site of entry and localizes to the regional draining lymph nodes. After a period of replication, it disseminates through the blood, possibly inside mononuclear phagocytes, throughout the mononuclear phagocyte system, including liver, spleen, bone marrow, and lymph nodes *(5)*. Fever first occurs during this period of bacteremia. In addition, persistent foci of infection may develop where blood flow is high and target host cells are present (especially synovium, epididymis, placenta, and mammary glands), resulting in localized disease or bacterial persistence and shedding. Since macrophages are ubiquitous, almost any organ can be infected, and disease can manifest if bacteria are not adequately controlled at the disseminated site. Development of an effective interferon-γ-mediated cellular immune response, which may take weeks, eventually contains the infection in most cases, even without antibiotics. Relapses can occur, however, if the bacterium can temporarily evade or inhibit the host response. The immune components required for recovery from brucellosis are not completely understood. Although interferon-γ is a *sine qua non (6,7)*, the mechanism of its action is unknown. Similarly, the role of antibodies in recovery from disease is unknown, although they clearly have some effect in preventing *de novo* infection *(8)*.

## 2. POTENTIAL USE AS A BIOTERROR OR BIOWARFARE AGENT

*Brucella* has been considered as an agent for biological warfare since the 1940s. Although it was developed as a weapon by both the former Soviet Union and the United States, it was never used. United States stocks of biological weapons, including *Brucella*, were destroyed by 1969, when the offensive biological warfare program ended. Several characteristics of the organism, however, suggest that it may still be a threat for use as an incapacitating agent. It is highly resistant to drying, easily survives aerosolization in water, and is highly infectious by multiple routes *(9)*.

Two studies have provided estimates of the consequences of an attack with *Brucella* on urban centers. Kaufmann et al. *(10)* estimated 413 deaths, 82,500 casualties, and a cost of $478 million per 100,000 persons exposed, assuming a median infective dose $(ID_{50})$ of $10^3$ colony-forming units (CFU) and that the organisms used were sensitive to antibiotics. The World Health Organization (WHO) *(11)*, using an $ID_{50}$ estimate of $10^4$ CFU, predicted that an attack on a city of 1 million in a developed country would result in 200 deaths and 50,000 ill patients. These scenarios may be optimistic. The WHO prediction of number of cases may be too low, since the $ID_{50}$ is probably lower than they assumed. The $ID_{50}$ for guinea pigs after aerosol exposure is approximately 36 CFU *(9)* and that for non-human primates is about $1.3 \times 10^3$ CFU *(12)*. A recent outbreak at a vaccine manufacturing laboratory also suggests that a high attack rate is likely following aerosol exposure *(13)*. In addition, although nearly all naturally occurring strains of *Brucella* are sensitive to commonly used antibiotics, it is not difficult to produce strains resistant to multiple antibiotics. For example, a vaccine strain resistant to tetracycline, doxycycline, rifampin, streptomycin, and ampicillin was developed in the former Soviet Union *(14)*. The cost of a bioterror attack with a drug-resistant organism would be substantially above that estimated by Kauffmann et al. *(10)*. In addition, morbidity and mortality would be increased if adequate supplies of alternate drugs and delivery systems were not readily available.

## 3. EPIDEMIOLOGY OF NATURALLY OCCURRING DISEASE

An effective animal brucellosis control program, consisting of vaccination, serological testing, and slaughter of infected herds has reduced the incidence of brucellosis in the United States to less than 150 cases per year since 1984. Highly endemic areas of the world include the Mediterranean area, Middle East, Mexico, portions of South America, Eastern Europe, and Asia. In the Middle East and Mediterranean areas, annual incidence may reach 78/100,000 population (15).

In most large case series, brucellosis is acquired by direct exposure to livestock or ingestion of unpasteurized dairy products. Animal workers (including veterinarians) who contact infected animals at parturition are particularly at risk, since the concentration of *Brucella* organisms in the placenta can reach $10^{10}$ CFU/g. Direct contact of infected animal tissues with abraded or punctured skin, splashing onto conjunctiva, or aerosolization may lead to infection. In a study of slaughterhouse workers, direct inoculation onto the skin or conjunctiva was thought to be more important than inhalation as a means of acquiring infection (17).

Ingestion of unpasteurized dairy products is responsible for most nonoccupational cases of brucellosis. Indeed, in the United States, imported foods have accounted for most recent cases (18). Soft cheeses, particularly those prepared from goat milk, are prime culprits.

The bacterium's great ability to infect by aerosol frequently leads to infections of laboratory workers; indeed, *Brucella* is the most commonly reported cause of laboratory infections. In many series of laboratory infections, no specific breach of technique or obvious accident is identified (19,20). In situations in which accidents or incorrect techniques have been documented [for example, centrifuge tube breakage (21) or handling the organism outside a biosafety cabinet (22)], numerous individuals in or near the laboratory have become infected. In a manufacturing incident, an attack rate of 17.1% occurred at a facility that produced a goat vaccine, *B. melitensis* strain Rev1, for 1 week (13). Workers whose windows opened above the exhaust of the plant had an attack rate of 39.5%. *Brucella* organisms were isolated from the air inside the facility during a subsequent production cycle. The high attack rates in these natural exposures underscore the potential risk of numerous casualties if the organism were used as a bioweapon.

## 4. CLINICAL PRESENTATION

As might be expected from the host-bacterial interactions described above, brucellosis can take many forms. Table 2 shows typical frequencies of general symptoms and signs derived from large series of cases from Spain, Peru, Kuwait, Israel, Saudi Arabia, and the United States (23–27). *B. melitensis* causes most human disease and typically causes more severe illness than the other agents. Disease onset may be sudden or gradual, with fever, chills, sweats, easy fatigability, anorexia, weight loss, myalgia, and arthralgias, but few localizing signs. Patients may also present with focal symptoms and signs of inflammation in joints, spine, or testis and epididymis (Table 3). Rarely, central nervous system disease or endocarditis may occur. Focal disease is typically, but not always, accompanied by signs of systemic illness. Other patients may gradually become ill, with lassitude, anorexia, and sweats, but little or no fever. As a result of the predilection of *Brucella* to reside in the mononuclear phagocyte system, splenic or hepatic enlargement and lymphadenopathy are found in a sizable minority of patients (Table 3).

Table 2
General Signs and Symptoms of Brucellosis

| Symptom or sign | Frequency (%) |
| --- | --- |
| Fever | 94–100 |
| Malaise | 82–95 |
| Chills | 39–95 |
| Sweating | 39–93 |
| Headache | 29–77 |
| Myalgia | 39–68 |
| Back pain | 15–73 |
| Arthralgia | 17–77 |
| Anorexia | 25–52 |
| Weight loss | 13–50 |

Data from refs. *23–27.*

Table 3
Focal Disease in Brucellosis

| System | Abnormality | Frequency (%) |
| --- | --- | --- |
| Musculoskeletal | Any | 5 37 |
| | Spondylitis | 2–13 |
| | Sacroiliitis | 7–19 |
| Mononuclear phagocyte | Hepatomegaly | 37–66 |
| | Splenomegaly | 10–60 |
| | Lymphadenopathy | 9–20 |
| | Liver enzymes | 37–49 |
| Cardiac | Endocarditis | 1–2 |
| Nervous | Meningitis | 0–1 |
| Genitourinary | Epididymoorchitis | 2–10 |

Data from refs. *23–27.*

Bone and joint infections are the most common localized manifestations of brucellosis *(26–28)*. Arthritis, often multiarticular, occurs in approximately 30% of patients. The sacroiliac joints and the spine are the most often involved, but infection of hips, knees, or almost any other joint may also occur. Physical signs are nonspecific, with swelling, tenderness, and occasional erythema. Bone scans are useful to identify sacroiliitis, especially with unilateral disease. Most often, although synovial fluid is exudative, with a predominance of mononuclear cells, *Brucella* arthritis is nondestructive. Brucellar spondylitis, which shares many similarities with tuberculous disease, is more common in patients over 50 years of age. In contrast to *Mycobacterium tuberculosis*, *Brucella* usually attacks the lumbar rather than the thoracic spine, although any level may be involved. Back pain and tenderness are frequent presenting symptoms. In early stages, plain X-rays may show anterior osteophytes, focal bone destruction, and sclerosis at the superior end plate of the vertebral body. Later, softening of the end plates and spread of infection to the next superior vertebra may cause destruction of the disk or herniation of the disk into the vertebral bodies, with eventual loss of disk space and ankylosis of adjacent vertebrae *(29)*. Computed tomography and magnetic resonance imaging (MRI) show these phenomena in more detail. Spinal cord or nerve root compression and paravertebral abscess may complicate brucellar spondylitis and are best imaged with MRI.

Males may develop epididymo-orchitis, which presents with local pain and swelling, usually unilateral. The frequency of this finding varies widely, from 6 to 28% of males in different series of patients. Ultrasonography may show hypoechoic epididymis, hydrocele, and scrotal skin thickening *(30)*. In nonpregnant women, genital tract disease is distinctly uncommon.

Central nervous system brucellosis occurs in about 1% of cases *(27)*. Subacute or chronic meningitis or meningoencephalitis is the most common manifestation. Other neurological syndromes include mono- or polyradiculitis, meningovascular disease leading to stroke or intracranial hemorrhage, myelitis, and demyelinating disease *(31–33)*. Cerebrospinal fluid has elevated protein, normal or low glucose, and a lymphocytic pleocytosis. Psychiatric abnormalities, ranging from depression, insomnia, and inability to concentrate to confusion and psychosis may occur in brucellosis. The importance of these symptoms has been emphasized by some observers *(25,34)*, but others find psychiatric abnormalities to be uncommon or unrelated to brucellosis *(24,29)*.

Endocarditis, which occurs in approximately 1% of cases of brucellosis, is the primary cause of death *(35)*. Infection occurs on the aortic valve in about 80% of patients with endocarditis. Two-thirds of cases have underlying valvular heart disease, especially prosthetic valves *(36)*. Death is usually caused by congestive heart failure.

Although *Brucella* is an important cause of abortion and fetal infection in livestock, its role in human pregnancy has been a matter of some debate. A recent study indicated that abortion occurs commonly in women with active brucellosis in the first trimester and that antimicrobial treatment greatly reduces the risk of abortion *(37)*. Seropositive women in a highly endemic area of Saudi Arabia and women with active brucellosis are more likely to abort than seronegative women *(38)*. In another study, 41% of pregnant women with brucellosis aborted, and *Brucella* organisms were recovered from abortion tissues *(29)*. These studies indicate that maternal brucellosis may cause more human abortion than is commonly recognized.

Mild thrombocytopenia is common in brucellosis, but thrombocytopenic purpura is not. This complication may, however, cause severe morbidity and mortality owing to intracranial hemorrhage *(39)*.

A number of skin manifestations, including erythematous maculopapular rash and erythema nodosum, have been described in 4–6% of cases *(27,40)*. Biopsy shows nonspecific chronic inflammation or granulomas; culture of the lesions may be positive *(40)*.

## 5. DIAGNOSIS

In naturally acquired disease, a thorough travel, occupational, and dietary history should reveal risk factors for brucellosis and lead to appropriate diagnostic tests. In the event of an undetected biological attack, an outbreak of a sustained, febrile illness with accompanying arthritis should prompt consideration of the disease.

Routine laboratory studies are not very helpful. There may be slight leukocytosis or leukopenia with a relative lymphocytosis. The erythrocyte sedimentation rate is elevated in about half of patients.

The most certain diagnosis of brucellosis is made by culture of the organism from blood or other tissue. *Brucella* bacteremia in the absence of positive serological tests has been described *(41)*. Although culture in the traditional biphasic Castenada medium may require 6 weeks for cultures to turn positive, culture in enriched medium and detection by automated systems (e.g., BACTEC 9240) may lead to detection of positive results in less than a week *(20)*. In the absence of sensitive detection systems, however, blind subculture of liquid media at 3 and 6 weeks should be performed. The frequency of bacterial isolation, however, is variable, with reports ranging from 6 to 90%. A prospective study found positive blood cultures in only 70% of patients ultimately diagnosed with brucellosis; culture of bone marrow increased this to 92% *(42)*. Positive blood cultures are more common with acute disease and may be adversely affected by prior administration of antibiotics. In addition to blood or bone marrow, culture of other clinically evident sites of infection, such as cerebrospinal fluid, joint fluid, or pus, may also yield positive results. Clinical microbiology technicians should be warned if brucellosis is suspected, since cultures of the organism should be done in a biosafety cabinet to prevent infection of laboratory personnel.

Because of the low sensitivity of culture, the diagnosis of brucellosis has usually been made by serological testing. The standard tube agglutination test (STA) determines the dilution of serum required to agglutinate a reference strain of *Brucella*. This agglutinating property is owing to antibody (mostly IgM) directed against the bacterium's outer membrane lipopolysaccharide. Treatment of serum with 2-mercaptoethanol before performance of the test eliminates the contribution of IgM and results in detection primarily of IgG. IgM agglutinins are the first to rise with infection and may persist even long after successful therapy. IgG agglutinins are more commonly found when disease is active and predict relapse of infection *(41)*. Although the STA is the most commonly agreed-on standard for diagnosis, it has drawbacks. The lower limit of normal is variable. Although 1:80 is a commonly used cutoff, either lower or higher values may be appropriate, depending on the population and the laboratory. Previous infection with *Vibrio cholera*, *E. coli* 0:157, *Francisella tularensis*, or *Yersinia enterocolitica* O:9, whose lipopolysaccharides crossreact with *Brucella*, may lead to false-positive results. In addition, performance of the STA is laborious and not easily standardized. Other tests include complement fixation, enzyme-linked immunosorbent assays (ELISAs), and competitive ELISAs *(43)* that detect antibody to lipopolysaccharide or to cytoplasmic antigens. As more experience is acquired with these tests, they may replace the STA, but control of antigens and antibodies and more extensive testing will be required. Reliance on serological tests, especially if the titer is low and the exposure history is uncertain, may make a firm diagnosis difficult.

## 6. TREATMENT

The cornerstone of treatment for brucellosis is use of an appropriate combination of antibiotics for a sufficient period. Use of a single antibiotic rather than combinations frequently leads to treatment failure. Failure can occur either because patients fail to respond initially or relapse after an apparently successful course of treatment. Patients with complicated, focal infections (e.g, abscesses, spondylitis, or endocarditis) may have a poor initial response *(27)* but are not more prone to relapse than patients with uncomplicated disease. Independent predictors of relapse include positive initial blood culture, onset of disease less than 10 d before diagnosis, fever of 38.3°C or higher, thrombocytopenia, less effective antibiotic therapy, and male sex *(44,45)*.

A number of antimicrobial treatment approaches have been tried in brucellosis. There has been most experience with tetracyclines (now mostly doxycycline) and streptomycin. For adults, a highly effective therapeutic regimen (2% initial treatment failure, 5% relapse) consists of doxycycline 100 mg po bid for 45 d plus streptomycin 1 g im qd for the first 14 d *(46)*. Gentamicin 5 mg/kg/d and netilmicin 6 mg/kg/d for the first 7 d have both been successfully substituted for streptomycin *(47,48)*, although experience with the newer drugs is limited. The streptomycin-doxycycline regimen is superior to treatment with oral rifampin 900 mg/d and doxycyline 100 mg bid for 45 d *(46)*, which leads to 8% treatment failure and 16% relapse. It is likely that the reduced efficacy of the doxycycline-rifampin combination is related to reduced blood levels of doxycycline owing to induction of hepatic microsomal enzymes by rifampin *(49)*. Despite its reduced efficacy, the oral regimen has the advantage of ease of administration and may be useful in uncomplicated cases. For focal infections, however, an aminoglycoside-doxycycline regimen should be used.

For uncomplicated infections in children under 8 yr of age, tetracyclines, including doxycycline, should be avoided to prevent tooth staining. Successful treatment regimens in children include trimethoprim/sulfamethoxazole plus rifampin for 6 wk *(50)*. Gentamicin may also be added for the first 5 d *(51)*. For serious or life-threatening infections, as described below, use of doxycycline should be considered, even in this age group *(29)*.

In pregnancy, rifampin, 900 mg/d po *(52)* or a combination of rifampin and trimethoprim/sulfamethoxazole *(29)* for 8–12 wk has been recommended.

Some manifestations of brucellosis require more aggressive therapy, including use of three drugs, prolonged treatment, and/or adjunctive surgery. Duration and choice of antibiotics must be tailored to patient response, since there are no controlled studies for guidance. Endocarditis should be treated with three drugs (streptomycin, doxycycline, and rifampin) for 4 wk and then doxycycline plus rifampin for an additional 8–12 wk *(29)*. Most authorities recommend early valve replacement, although some patients with endocarditis have been successfully treated without surgery *(53)*. Neurobrucellosis, especially meningoencephalitis, may also require longer therapy, using recovery of cerebrospinal fluid parameters to normal as a guideline for stopping drug treatment. Spondylitis may also require prolonged therapy but rarely requires surgery, except for neurological complications *(54)*.

In vitro sensitivities are of questionable value in determining a drug treatment regimen. Notably, ceftriaxone, a third-generation cephalosporin, is not effective, even though organisms appear susceptible in vitro *(55)*. Similarly, use of fluoroquinolones alone, which are active in vitro against *Brucella*, results in unacceptably high relapse rates *(56)*. Combination therapy with ciprofloxacin or ofloxacin plus rifampin has been used successfully, but data are limited *(57,58)*.

## 7. PREVENTION

Naturally acquired human disease is best prevented by an effective animal brucellosis control program. No satisfactory human vaccines are available. Dairy products should be pasteurized and meat well cooked before eating. Person-to-person transmission may occur sexually *(59)*, via the placenta to the fetus, by bone marrow transplantation *(60)*, and possibly by breast-feeding *(61)*. Breast feeding should be avoided by mothers with active disease, but other transmission can be prevented by early diagnosis and treatment of index cases. Routine bloodborne pathogen precautions are sufficient for infection control of hospitalized patients. Culture plates or tubes containing or suspected to contain *Brucella* organisms should only be opened in biosafety cabinets designed to protect the operator from aerosols. Research with live *Brucella* organisms should be done in biosafety level 3 conditions.

# REFERENCES

1. Brew SD, Perrett LL, Stack JA, MacMillan AP, Staunton NJ. Human exposure to *Brucella* recovered from a sea mammal [Letter]. Vet Rec 1999;144:483.
2. Fernandez-Prada CM, Nikolich M, Vemulapalli R, et al. Deletion of wboA enhances activation of the lectin pathway of complement in Brucella abortus and Brucella melitensis. Infect Immun 2001;69: 4407–4416.
3. Goldstein J, Hoffman T, Frasch C, et al. Lipopolysaccharide (LPS) from *Brucella abortus* is less toxic than that from *Escherichia coli*, suggesting the possible use of *B. abortus* or LPS from *B. abortus* as a carrier in vaccines. Infect Immun 1992;60:1385–1389.
4. Jubier-Maurin V, Boigegrain RA, Cloeckaert A, et al. Major outer membrane protein Omp25 of *Brucella suis* is involved in inhibition of tumor necrosis factor alpha production during infection of human macrophages. Infect Immun 2001;69:4823–4830.
5. Enright FM. The pathogenesis and pathobiology of *Brucella* infection in domestic animals. In: Nielsen K, Duncan JR, eds. Animal Brucellosis. CRC Press, Boca Raton, FL, 1990, pp. 301–320.
6. Murphy EA, Sathiyaseelan J, Parent MA, Zou B, Baldwin CL. Interferon-gamma is crucial for surviving a *Brucella abortus* infection in both resistant C57BL/6 and susceptible BALB/c mice. Immunology 2001;103:511–518.
7. Zhan Y, Cheers C. Endogenous gamma interferon mediates resistance to *Brucella abortus* infection. Infect Immun 1993;61:4899–4901.
8. Montaraz JA, Winter AJ, Hunter DM, Sowa BA, Wu AM, Adams LG. Protection against *Brucella abortus* in mice with O-polysaccharide-specific monoclonal antibodies. Infect Immun 1986;51:961–963.
9. Elberg SS, Henderson DW. Respiratory pathogenicity of *Brucella*. J Infect Dis 1948;82:302–306.
10. Kaufmann AF, Meltzer MI, Schmid GP. The economic impact of a bioterrorist attack: are prevention and postattack intervention programs justifiable? Emerg Infect Dis 1997;3:83-94.
11. World Health Organization. Health Aspects of Chemical and Biological Weapons. WHO, Geneva, 1970.
12. Elberg SS, Henderson DW, Herzberg M, Peacock S. Immunization against *Brucella* infection. IV. Response of monkeys to injection of a streptomycin-dependent strain of *Brucella melitensis*. J Bacteriol 1955;69:643–648.
13. Olle-Goig JE, Canela-Soler J. An outbreak of *Brucella melitensis* infection by airborne transmission among laboratory workers. Am J Public Health 1987;77:335–338.
14. Gorelov VN, Gubina EA, Grekova NA, Skavronskaia AG. [The possibility of creating a vaccinal strain of *Brucella abortus* 19-BA with multiple antibiotic resistance]. Zh Mikrobiol Epidemiol Immunobiol 1991;9:2–4.
15. World Health Organization. Brucellosis. Fact Sheet N173. WHO, Geneva, 1997.
16. Anderson TD, Cheville NF, Meador VP. Pathogenesis of placentitis in the goat inoculated with *Brucella abortus*. II. Ultrastructural studies. Vet Pathol 1986;23: 227–239.
17. Buchanan TM, Hendricks SL, Patton CM, Feldman RA. Brucellosis in the United States, 1960–1972; an abattoir-associated disease. Part III. Epidemiology and evidence for acquired immunity. Medicine (Baltimore) 1974;53:427–439.
18. Chomel BB, DeBess EE, Mangiamele DM, et al. Changing trends in the epidemiology of human brucellosis in California from 1973 to 1992: a shift toward foodborne transmission. J Infect Dis 1994;170:1216–1223.
19. Memish ZA, Mah MW. Brucellosis in laboratory workers at a Saudi Arabian hospital. Am J Infect Control 2001;29:48–52.
20. Yagupsky P, Peled N, Riesenberg K, Banai M. Exposure of hospital personnel to *Brucella melitensis* and occurrence of laboratory-acquired disease in an endemic area. Scand J Infect Dis 2000;32:31–35.

21. Fiori PL, Mastrandrea S, Rappelli P, Cappuccinelli P. *Brucella abortus* infection acquired in microbiology laboratories. J Clin Microbiol 2000;38:2005–2006.

22. Staszkiewicz J, Lewis CM, Colville J, Zervos M, Band J. Outbreak of *Brucella melitensis* among microbiology laboratory workers in a community hospital. J Clin Microbiol 1991;29:287–290.

23. Yinnon AM, Morali GA, Goren A, et al. Effect of age and duration of disease on the clinical manifestations of brucellosis. A study of 73 consecutive patients in Israel. Isr J Med Sci 1993;29:11–16.

24. Mousa AR, Elhag KM, Khogali M, Marafie AA. The nature of human brucellosis in Kuwait: study of 379 cases. Rev Infect Dis 1988;10:211–217.

25. Malik GM. A clinical study of brucellosis in adults in the Asir region of southern Saudi Arabia. Am J Trop Med Hyg 1997;56:375–377.

26. Gotuzzo E, Alarcon GS, Bocanegra TS, et al. Articular involvement in human brucellosis: a retrospective analysis of 304 cases. Semin Arthritis Rheum 1982;12:245–255.

27. Colmenero JD, Reguera JM, Martos F, et al. Complications associated with *Brucella melitensis* infection: a study of 530 cases. Medicine 1996;75:195–211.

28. Mousa AR, Muhtaseb SA, Almudallal DS, Khodeir SM, Marafie AA. Osteoarticular complications of brucellosis: a study of 169 cases. Rev Infect Dis 1987;9:531–543.

29. Madkour MM. Madkour's Brucellosis, Springer-Verlag, Berlin, 2001.

30. Navarro-Martinez A, Solera J, Corredoira J, et al. Epididymoorchitis due to *Brucella mellitensis*: a retrospective study of 59 patients. Clin Infect Dis 2001;33:2017–2022.

31. Al-Eissa YA. Clinical and therapeutic features of childhood neurobrucellosis. Scand J Infect Dis 1995;27:339–343.

32. Al Deeb SM, Yaqub BA, Sharif HS, Phadke JG. Neurobrucellosis: clinical characteristics, diagnosis, and outcome. Neurology 1989;39:498–501.

33. McLean DR, Russell N, Khan MY. Neurobrucellosis: clinical and therapeutic features. Clin Infect Dis 1992;15:582–590.

34. Spink WW. Clinical aspects of human brucellosis. In: Larson CH, Soule MH, eds. Brucellosis. Waverly Press, Baltimore, MD, 1950, pp. 1–8.

35. Peery TM, Belter LF. Brucellosis and heart disease. II. Fatal brucellosis. Am J Pathol 1960;36:673–697.

36. Jacobs F, Abramowicz D, Vereerstraeten P, Le CJ, Zech F, Thys JP. *Brucella* endocarditis: the role of combined medical and surgical treatment. Rev Infect Dis 1990;12:740–744.

37. Khan MY, Mah MW, Memish ZA. Brucellosis in pregnant women. Clin Infect Dis 2001;32:1172–1177.

38. Sharif A, Reyes Z, Thomassen P. Screening for brucellosis in pregnant women. J Trop Med Hyg 1990;93:42–43.

39. Young EJ, Tarry A, Genta RM, Ayden N, Gotuzzo E. Thrombocytopenic purpura associated with brucellosis: report of 2 cases and literature review. Clin Infect Dis 2000;31:904–909.

40. Ariza J, Servitje O, Pallares R, et al. Characteristic cutaneous lesions in patients with brucellosis. Arch Dermatol 1989;125:380–383.

41. Baldi PC, Miguel SE, Fossati CA, Wallach JC. Serological follow-up of human brucellosis by measuring IgG antibodies to lipopolysaccharide and cytoplasmic proteins of *Brucella* species. Clin Infect Dis 1996;22:446–455.

42. Gotuzzo E, Carrillo C, Guerra J, Llosa L. An evaluation of diagnostic methods for brucellosis—the value of bone marrow culture. J Infect Dis 1986;153:122–125.

43. Lucero NE, Foglia L, Ayala SM, Gall D, Nielsen K. Competitive enzyme immunoassay for diagnosis of human brucellosis. J Clin Microbiol 1999;37:3245–3248.

44. Ariza J, Corredoira J, Pallares R, et al. Characteristics of and risk factors for relapse of brucellosis in humans. Clin Infect Dis 1995;20:1241–1249.

45. Solera J, Martinez AE, Espinosa A, Castillejos ML, Geijo P, Rodriguez, ZM. Multivariate model for predicting relapse in human brucellosis. J Infect 1998;36: 85–92.

46. Solera J, Rodriguez ZM, Geijo P, et al. Doxycycline-rifampin versus doxycycline-streptomycin in treatment of human brucellosis due to *Brucella melitensis*. The GECMEI Group. Grupo de Estudio de Castilla-la Mancha de Enfermedades Infecciosas. Antimicrob Agents Chemother 1995;39:2061–2067.

47. Solera J, Espinosa A, Martinez AE, et al. Treatment of human brucellosis with doxycycline and gentamicin. Antimicrob Agents Chemother 1997;41:80–84.

48. Solera J, Espinosa A, Geijo P, et al. Treatment of human brucellosis with netilmicin and doxycycline. Clin Infect Dis 1996;22:441–445.

49. Colmenero JD, Fernandez GL, Agundez JA, Sedeno J, Benitez J, Valverde E. Possible implications of doxycycline-rifampin interaction for treatment of brucellosis. Antimicrob Agents Chemother 1994;38:2798–2802.

50. Khuri-Bulos NA, Daoud AH, Azab SM. Treatment of childhood brucellosis: results of a prospective trial on 113 children. Pediatr Infect Dis J 1993;12:377–381.
51. Lubani MM, Dudin KI, Sharda DC, et al. A multicenter therapeutic study of 1100 children with brucellosis. Pediatr Infect Dis J 1989;8:75–78.
52. Joint FAO/WHO Expert Committee on Brucellosis. WHO Tech Rep Ser 1986;740:1–132.
53. Cohen N, Golik A, Alon I, et al. Conservative treatment for *Brucella* endocarditis. Clin Cardiol 1997;20:291–294.
54. Solera J, Lozano E, Martinez-Alfaro E, Espinosa A, Castillejos ML, Abad L. Brucellar spondylitis: review of 35 cases and literature survey. Clin Infect Dis 1999;29:1440–1449.
55. Lang R, Dagan R, Potasman I, Einhorn M, Raz R. Failure of ceftriaxone in the treatment of acute brucellosis. Clin Infect Dis 1992;14:506–509.
56. Lang R, Rubinstein E. Quinolones for the treatment of brucellosis. J Antimicrob Chemother 1992;29:357–360.
57. Agalar C, Usubutun S, Turkyilmaz R. Ciprofloxacin and rifampicin versus doxycycline and rifampicin in the treatment of brucellosis. Eur J Clin Microbiol Infect Dis 1999;18:535–538.
58. Akova M, Uzun O, Akalin HE, Hayran M, Unal S, Gur D. Quinolones in treatment of human brucellosis: comparative trial of ofloxacin-rifampin versus doxycycline-rifampin. Antimicrob Agents Chemother 1993;37:1831–1834.
59. Ruben B, Band JD, Wong P, Colville J. Person-to-person transmission of *Brucella melitensis* [see comments]. Lancet 1991;337:14–15.
60. Ertem M, Kurekci AE, Aysev D, Unal E, Ikinciogullari A. Brucellosis transmitted by bone marrow transplantation. Bone Marrow Transplant 2000;26:225–226.
61. Palanduz A, Palanduz S, Guler K, Guler N. Brucellosis in a mother and her young infant: probable transmission by breast milk. Int J Infect Dis 2000;4:55–56.
62. Jahans KL, Foster G, Broughton ES. The characterisation of *Brucella* strains isolated from marine mammals. Vet Microbiol 1997;57:373–382.

# 9

# Q Fever

## R. Scott Miller, MD

The opinions or assertions contained herein are the private views of the authors and are not to be construed as official or as representing the opinion of the Department of the Army, the Department of the Air Force, or the Department of Defense.

## 1. INTRODUCTION

Q fever, short for *Query fever*, is a zoonotic disease caused by infection with *Coxiella burnetii*, an obligate intracellular Gram-negative bacterium of low virulence but remarkable infectivity and persistence. Distributed globally, inhalation of as little as a single rickettsia-like organism may initiate infection. In addition, a spore-like form of the organism is extremely resistant to heat, desiccation, and many standard antiseptic compounds, thus allowing *C. burnetii* to persist in the environment for weeks to months. Thus, animals or humans are usually infected indirectly from inhalation of spores in a contaminated environment, such as after parturition of an infected animal. In contrast to its marked infectivity, acute infection may be asymptomatic or relatively benign, causing a transient, incapacitating febrile illness but rare fatalities. Therefore, it is considered a low-to-moderate risk agent for bioterrorist attack.

From: *Physician's Guide to Terrorist Attack*
Edited by: M. J. Roy © Humana Press Inc., Totowa, NJ

**Case Vignette**

A 32-year-old man presented to an emergency room with gradual onset of fever, chills, headache, malaise, and a cough of 5 days' duration in May. Lung exam was normal, and no focus for the fever was identified. He was diagnosed with influenza and treated with supportive therapy with acetaminophen. The symptoms continued with progression of cough, prompting him to return for re-evaluation. Chest X-ray revealed rounded opacities in both lungs. Complete blood count revealed a normal white count with a platelet count of 155,000 platelets/mL. Liver transaminases were mildly elevated. He was diagnosed with atypical pneumonia and given a course of azithromycin. His illness resolved over 7 days. The specific etiology of his infection was never determined.

Had a travel history been obtained, it would have shown that this individual had returned 2 weeks earlier from a holiday in western Australia, where he had rented a camper van and explored the farming regions. A highlight of his trip was a stay at a sheep farm where he and his family had seen several newborn lambs and shearing of the rams. His wife had experienced no clinical illness.

*C. burnetii* remains a biological warfare threat because of its ready transmissibility and its availability from environmental sources. It had been estimated that 50 kg of dried, powdered *C. burnetii* disseminated by airplane upwind of a population center of 500,000 people would produce casualties at rates similar to those of anthrax or tularemia, although with markedly less mortality *(1)*. The United States and the Soviet Union, in fact, developed Q fever as a biological warfare agent. In the 1950s, the United States performed small-scale open-air aerosol challenges with Q fever in human volunteers (Project CD-22) at Dugway Proving Ground, Utah *(2)*. All biological warfare munitions were publicly destroyed by executive order of President Richard M. Nixon between May 1971 and May 1972 *(3)*. Unlike many other agents, Q fever has not been acknowledged in a biological warfare or bioterrorist attack to date.

## 2. HISTORICAL BACKGROUND

A zoonosis also known under the eponyms of abattoir fever or Balkan grippe, query fever (Q fever) was first described among meat workers in Queensland, Australia by Edward Derrick *(4)*. He investigated an outbreak of febrile disease among abattoir workers in Brisbane in 1935 and carefully described the syndrome, although he was unable to isolate an etiological agent. He suspected a viral etiology but sent some liver emulsion from inoculated guinea pigs to Macfarlane Burnet in Melbourne. Burnet and colleagues reproduced the disease in animals and subsequently demonstrated Gram-negative rods within intracellular vacuoles of macrophages, suggestive of a rickettsial infection *(5)*.

About the same time, Gordon Davis was collecting ticks in Montana for his study of the ecology of Rocky Mountain spotted fever (RMSF). When inoculated with ticks collected from Nine Mile, Montana, some guinea pigs showed an illness atypical of the febrile orchitis of RMSF. Davis' colleague, Herald Cox, subsequently characterized this new organism as a rickettsia and was able to successfully pass it in embryonated hen eggs *(6)*.

**Proteobacteria**                                                                    **groups**

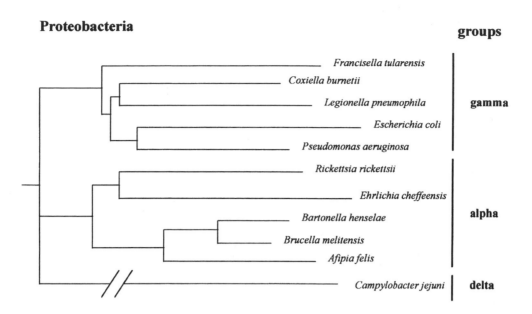

**Fig. 1.** Phylogenetic tree showing relationships of *C. burnetii* to other species of bacteria by analysis of 16S rRNA gene sequences (Reprinted with permission of Maurin M, Raoult D. Q fever. Clin Microbiol Rev 1999;12:521.)

Interestingly, these two independent efforts were connected after the laboratory-acquired infection of the director of the National Institutes of Health, Rolla Dyer, with the Nine Mile agent. Using inoculations of his own convalescent sera, he subsequently showed passive immune protection of guinea pigs to subsequent challenge with the Q fever agent *(7)*. This suggested that the Q fever agent and the Nine Mile agent were one and the same. *Coxiella burnetii*, the causative agent of Q fever, was ultimately named for the contributions of both Cox and Burnet. The most common mode of transmission, inhalational exposure to infected parturient animal tissues/secretions, was not recognized until a decade later.

## 3. THE ETIOLOGICAL AGENT

*Coxiella burnetii* is a small, obligate intracellular Gram-negative bacterium (0.2–0.4 × 0.4–1.0 μm). Despite its original classification among the Rickettsiaceae, analysis of sequences from the 16S rRNA gene has reclassified the bacterium among the γ subdivision of the Proteobacteria, not the α-1 subdivision with the *Rickettsia* genus (Fig. 1) *(8)*. *C. burnetii* is the sole member of the genus, and its closest relatives are the facultative intracellular bacteria of the genera *Legionella* and *Francisella*.

Even though *C. burnetii* is the sole member of the genus *Coxiella*, only a modest degree of heterogeneity in the *C. burnetii* genome has been described. Heinzen et al. *(9)*, using *Not*I and *Sfi*I endonucleases and pulsed-field gel electrophoresis (PFGE), identified four distinct genomic groups among strains from the United States. Over 20 different genotypes have now been described using the *Not*I endonuclease digestion and restriction length polymorphism analysis or PFGE on a geographically diverse array of isolates

*(10,11).* The actual genome varies from 1.5 to 2.4 Mb, and current evidence suggests a single linear chromosome *(12).*

Four distinct plasmid types have also been described, and the function of these 36–42-kb circular plasmids remains unknown. Many but not all *C. burnetii* isolates contain one or more of these plasmids. In some isolates without plasmids in genomic group V, DNA fragments homologous to the QpRS plasmid have been identified within the genomic DNA *(13).* Although attempts to link the heterogeneity of the genome and plasmids to human and animal pathogenicity have been described *(14,15),* these have not held up in recent larger series of *C. burnetii* strains and may reflect more a geographical clustering rather than clustering by disease manifestations *(8).*

Another unique characteristic of this bacterium is the phase variation of its antigenic lipopolysaccharide (LPS) when maintained in the laboratory *(16,17).* A major virulence determinant, the *C. burnetii* LPS contains a poorly endotoxic lipid A moiety of unique fatty acid composition. Wild-type, highly virulent *C. burnetii* displays a smooth LPS containing unique sugars in a structure that prevents antibodies access to surface proteins. Bacteria containing this LPS are designated phase I organisms, and these are resistant to complement.

After serial passages in cell cultures or embryonated cell cultures, *C. burnetii* lose much of their virulence and display a rough LPS, designated as phase II LPS. This phase results from a deletional mutation leading to a truncated LPS lacking the extended carbohydrate moiety *(17).* Thus some protein determinants are exposed to antibodies and complement. Compared with phase I organisms, this antigenic variant proves to be a weak immunogen *(18).* This antigenic variation is useful, however, in serological testing for determination between acute and chronic Q fever.

Unlike the closely related Legionellaceae, which are able to survive and multiply intracellularly or extracellularly, *Coxiella* is an obligate intracellular bacterium infecting phagocytic cells of the monocyte-macrophage lineage. In fact, *Coxiella* is unique among intracellular bacteria in that it resides and multiplies in the harsh acidic environment of the phagosome's parasitophorus vacuole, characterized as a secondary lysosome *(19).* The bacteria are internalized into an alveolar macrophage or other phagocyte by parasite-directed endocytosis. Next the *Coxiella*-containing phagosome matures into a lysosome, which contains acid phosphatase and cathepsin D and acidifies to a pH of 4.7–5.2. The organism has a unique metabolic requirement for this moderately acidic environment and replicates within this vacuole at a relatively slow rate, doubling every 8–20 h. Minimal cytopathic effects have been noted in infected cells despite prolonged infection, perhaps because of the slow replication time, which is similar to that of eukaryotic cells *(8).*

Another unique feature of *Coxiella* is the complex developmental cycle leading to spore-like small cell variants (SCVs) with a remarkable resistance to physical and chemical disruption *(20).* Viable organisms have been recovered in the laboratory after exposure to intense heat (63°C for 30 min), high salinity (10% salt solution for 180 d), physical stress (sonication for 30 min in distilled water), dessication, high and low pH, and even 0.5% formalin for 24 h *(19).* It is these persistent spore-like particles or SCVs, capable of wind dispersion and survival for weeks in nature, that make *C. burnetii* a putative biological warfare candidate.

Although the developmental cycle has not been fully elucidated, the biphasic nature of *Coxiella* development within the parasitophorous vacuole was first noted by McCaul and Williams in 1981 *(20)*. Transmission electron microscopy studies have identified electron-dense polar bodies 0.2–0.5 μm in size (the SCVs), in addition to larger, more metabolically active cells [large cell variants (LCVs)], which appear to be ultrastructurally similar to Gram-negative bacteria. Both cell forms divide by binary fission and are infectious, ultimately yielding a mixture of cell types in the new host cells *(19)*. LCVs and SCVs can be separated and purified using cesium chloride centrifugation, yielding a 95% homogenous population *(21)*.

## 3. EPIDEMIOLOGY

Q fever is a zoonosis with worldwide distribution. The range of potential reservoirs is vast, including many wild and domestic mammals, some birds, ticks, and amoebae *(8,22)*. Animals are often chronically infected, usually without clinical disease, but these animals may shed bacteria in feces, urine, and milk. Clinical infection is most often noted in pregnant females, in which massive infection of the placenta and amniotic fluid with *C. burnetii* may lead to abortion or low fetal birth weight. During birthing, over $10^9$ bacteria/g of placental tissue can be released into the environment. These organisms may persist in the local environment and be dispersed by wind, producing new infections for weeks to months afterwards.

Infection of livestock is primarily via inhalation, although chronic shedding of bacteria in the milk of infected cattle may lead to persistence of infection in a dairy herd. Huebner and Bell *(23)* showed that importation of uninfected cows into an endemic region of California resulted in 40% infection of the herd, as noted by seroconversion. Epidemiological data suggests that infected dairy cattle and goats tend to maintain a chronic infection with shedding of bacteria in milk, whereas sheep tend to clear infection initially (posing little risk to the flock after a few months) only to relapse during the immunosuppresion of pregnancy *(24)*. Household pets, such as dogs and cats, may become infected by tick bites, consumption of placentas of infected animals, or inhalation, and may thus become a domestic reservoir for human infection *(25)*.

The primary reservoir for natural human infection is livestock (sheep, goats, and cattle), particularly parturient females. Peak transmission seasons in Europe and Australia correlate with "lambing" season. Cases are usually reported sporadically, and outbreaks of Q fever are infrequently reported *(25–28)*. However, subclinical infection and the nonspecific clinical manifestations lead to under-reporting. Therefore, the disease may be endemic in areas where cases are rarely or never reported.

Q fever is an occupational hazard. Humans who work in animal husbandry (farmers, abattoir workers, and veterinarians), especially those who assist during calving or lambing, are at particular risk for infection. However, a definite risk also exists for persons who live in close proximity to, or who pass through, an area where animal birthing is occurring, even if this has occurred months previously. In a serosurvey among blood donors in France, Tissot-Dupont et al. *(29)* did not find a sex predilection for *C. burnetii* infection; however, clinical cases in hospitalized patients showed increased incidence and severity of infection among men. Other data support the notion that severity of infection may be related to inoculum size. A threefold increased seroprevalance risk of Q fever among HIV-infected individuals, mostly male drug users, suggests an enhanced susceptibility or enhanced exposure risk among this population *(30)*. HIV infection appears not to confer an increased risk of severe disease or chronic infection *(28)*.

## 4. ROUTE OF TRANSMISSION

The large majority of human transmission is via aerosol inhalation, as would also be expected with a biological warfare dispersion. The organisms are extremely infectious by this route; a single organism is capable of inducing infection and disease *(31)*. The SCVs of *C. burnetii* are taken into pulmonary alveolar macrophages and reactivate within the acidic phagolysosomes. These environmentally stable "spore-like" stages may also be carried in wind-blown dust from contaminated farms or may be aerosolized later off fomites such as contaminated clothing. Hence, many cases have no clear identifiable risk factor. Inhalation of aerosols is responsible for most laboratory-acquired cases as well.

Other routes of transmission may account for rare cases of human infection. Ingestion of high doses of infectious organisms in raw milk (cattle or goat) causes occasional infection, and may result in initial entry into the Kupffer cells of the liver, leading to granulomatous hepatitis *(27)*. Consumption of infected raw poultry eggs, common in salmonellosis, is a theoretical risk for infection. A tick bite is a rare cause of transmission *(8)*. Over 40 species of ticks are known to be naturally infected with *C. burnetii*, which multiples in the gut of the tick and is passed in large numbers in stool onto the skin during feeding *(22)*. Rare case reports of human-to-human transmission include blood transfusion or sharing of intravenous needles, sexual transmission, intradermal inoculation, congenital infections by transplacental transmission, or inhalation during autopsy or handling infected placental material *(8,32,33)*.

## 5. PATHOGENESIS

As mentioned previously, human infection is usually the result of inhalation of infected aerosols. *C. burnetii* are phagocytized by host macrophages, particularly pulmonary alveolar macrophages, and bacterial growth is triggered in the acidic environment of the phagolysozome *(19)*. Initially there is no impact on the infected cell, but eventually the lysozome becomes swollen with reproducing bacteria, rupturing the cell, and the process is repeated. Normally, there is little host response at the initial portal of entry.

As the organisms replicate within phagocytic cells, they are disseminated in circulating infected monocytes and macrophages, or possibly free in the plasma. Regardless of the mode of transmission, infection typically results in a transient bacteremia late in the incubation period and seeding of multiple organs in the body *(8)*. Typically, the incubation period lasts for 1–4 wk (average of 20 d), depending on the inoculum dose of *C. burnetii (31)*. The dose of the inoculum may also determine in part the severity of clinical symptoms.

The initial immune response is that of a polyclonal production of antibody, although the disease is eventually controlled by the cellular immune response. The humoral immune response does not control the organism's replication, and passive antibody transfer in animals did not improve splenic clearance *(34)*. However, opsonizing antibody does contribute to antibody-dependent cellular cytotoxicity later in the course of the infection *(35)*. Specific cytotoxic T-cell responses with activation of natural killer cells and activated macrophages eventually control infection, often with granuloma formation noted histopathologically. The specific cellular immune response probably does not result in organism clearance from the host in most cases, as relapse of infection is well documented from animal models of immunosuppression and a variety of human acquired immunosuppressed states including pregnancy, lymphomas and cancer, and HIV *(30,36,37)*.

Furthermore, an estimated 1% of persons, particularly those with pre-existing cardiac valvular disease or (rarely) immunosuppression at time of infection, may develop a chronic infection that can be fatal *(38)*. The host immune response in chronic infection shows a down-regulation of macrophage responsiveness to lymphokines *(39)* and reduced lymphocyte proliferation to Q fever-specific antigens *(40)*. As the organism cannot replicate extracellularly, endocarditis develops from infection of monocytes adherent to damaged endothelial tissues of the cardiac valve *(39,41)*.

## 6. CLINICAL MANIFESTATIONS

### *6.1. Acute Q Fever*

Acute infection results in an asymptomatic illness in approximately 60% of persons, as it does in nearly all animal hosts. After a 10–30 d incubation period, the remaining 40% will experience a febrile illness, and 5% of these (2% overall) may require hospitalization *(8)*. Fatal acute infections are rare. As clinical illness of Q fever is like the proverbial 'the tip of the iceberg', the need to investigate a clinical case with atypical epidemiological exposure cannot be overemphasized.

The clinical manifestations of acute infection are summarized in Table 1 and are quite diverse, thus requiring a high suspicion for diagnosis. The most common clinical syndrome is that of nonspecific, self-limited febrile illness with prominent headache. The onset of Q fever is typically abrupt, with high fever, fatigue, chills and rigors, and headache. The fever is typically sustained throughout the day, lasting for 7–14 d before resolution. Untreated, the fever may last for up to 8 wk and may be biphasic in 25% of cases. Q fever should thus be considered in the differential diagnosis of prolonged fever of unknown origin *(42)*. Older subjects tend to have a more prolonged febrile course. Headaches are typically severe, bifrontal or retro-orbital in location, and can be associated with meningismus in 5–7% of cases, warranting a lumbar puncture to exclude bacterial meningitis. Neurological symptoms include encephalopathy, hallucinations or other psychiatric symptoms, and less commonly focal neurological syndromes such as meningoencephalitis, meningitis, or myelitis *(43,44)*. Myalgias, more so than arthalgias, anorexia, and weight loss are other common generalized symptoms. A nonspecific rash, described as transient pink macular eruptions to red papules is described in 5–20% of cases *(8)*

Atypical pneumonia is another common clinical syndrome. Cough is a frequent sign, often occurring later in clinical illness, and chest pain has been reported in 10–50% of cases in various series *(8)*. Examination of the lungs is often unrevealing, with rales most frequently reported. Radiographic abnormalities vary among studies but occur in slightly over half of individuals *(43,45)*. Presentations include unilateral lobar or multilobar infiltrates, rounded opacities, increased reticular markings, and hilar adenopathy. Pleural effusion is rare.

A febrile hepatitis syndrome is also a common clinical presentation and was more common than pneumonia in a large series in France *(29)*. This is usually manifested only as elevated liver associated enzymes on biochemical testing, with typical elevations of alanine transferase (ALT), aspartate aminotransferase (AST), and alkaline phosphate to

Table 1
Signs and Symptoms of Acute Q Fever

| Clinical signs and symptoms | % of cases |
|---|---|
| Fever | 88–100 |
| Malaise or fatigue | 97–100[a] |
| Chills | 68–88 |
| Headache | 68–98 |
| Sweats or diaphoresis | 31–98 |
| Myalgias | 47–69 |
| Chest pain | 40–50 |
| Weight loss (≤ 7 kg from baseline) | 50–80 |
| Anorexia | 35–45 |
| Nausea | 22–49 |
| Diarrhea | 5–22 |
| Cough | 24–90 |
| Neurological signs | 10–35 |
| Skin rash | 5–21 |
| Myocarditis | 0.5–1 |
| Pericarditis | 1 |
| Meningoencephalitis | 1 |
| Death | 1–2 |

[a]Some report as low as 50% with malaise.
Data summarized from Maurin and Raoult (8) and Byrne (35).

two to three times normal (46). Clinical hepatitis symptoms and signs include abdominal pain, nausea and vomiting, diarrhea, and hepatomegaly. Elevated bilirubin levels occur in 10–15% of cases, but jaundice is rare. Liver biopsy typically reveals granulomatous hepatitis with characteristic doughnut granuloma (Fig. 2), and circulating autoantibodies are not infrequent (47). Massive liver necrosis and death are very rare (42).

Less common clinical manifestations include myocarditis, pericarditis, Guillain-Barré syndrome, reactive polyarthropathy, and hemolytic anemia, among others (8,48). Subacute myocarditis is probably underestimated and is detectable by abnormalities on the electrocardiogram, typically T-wave changes. Deaths in acute Q fever occur in less than 1% of clinical cases, having been associated with respiratory failure, liver failure, myocarditis/congestive heart failure, and encephalitis.

Acute Q fever in pregnancy can result in premature birth or spontaneous abortion owing to a placental infection or vasculitis, and contact with infected animals, including pet cats or dogs, should be avoided. C. burnetii can also cause direct fetal injury and has been demonstrated in fetal tissues (48). In fact, only 5 of 23 acute Q fever infections in pregnant women resulted in an uncomplicated pregnancy and delivery of a healthy, term child. The only reported case of nosocomial inhalational infection of Q fever occurred to an obstetrician who performed a dilation and curettage after spontaneous abortion secondary to Coxiella placentitis (32). C. burnetii should be added to the list of agents associated with intrauterine infection and adverse fetal outcomes, collectively grouped under the term TORCH [Toxoplasma, other (Listeria, syphilis, HIV, parvovirus B19, hepatitis B), rubella, cytomegalovirus, and herpes].

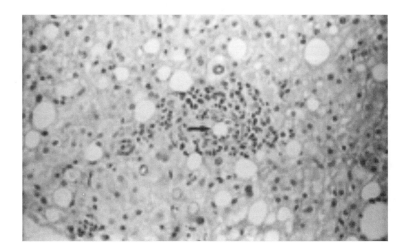

**Fig. 2.** Doughnut granuloma (arrow) in a liver section from a patient with acute Q fever hepatitis. (Reprinted with permission of Maurin M, Raoult D. Q fever. Clin Microbiol Rev 1999;12:529.)

Pregnancy is also a risk for chronic Q fever infection. The immunosuppression of late pregnancy may result in inability to clear an acute infection or a relapse of previous *Coxiella* infection, the latter of which has also been associated with fetal infection *(48)*.

### 6.2. Chronic Q Fever

Chronic Q fever usually manifests as infective endocarditis, which accounts for two-thirds of chronic *Coxiella* infection. Q fever endocarditis almost exclusively occurs in persons with underlying valvular heart disease, and *Coxiella* is the etiology of up to 5% of cases of endocarditis in highly endemic areas *(49)*. Underlying immunosuppression also appears to be a risk factor *(30)*. Endocarditis is the leading cause of mortality from *Coxiella* infection, with a 37% mortality rate in a recent compilation *(8)*. Delay in diagnosis is associated with increasing likelihood of adverse outcome. Table 2 outlines other manifestations of chronic infection including other vascular infections, osteomyelitis and osteoarthritis, and chronic hepatitis and fever without an identifiable source *(50)*.

Q fever endocarditis usually presents with fever and symptoms of heart failure secondary to valvular dysfunction. Maurin and Raoult *(8)* reported fever in 68% of cases, although fever is often less severe, even intermittent, compared with acute Q fever cases. Other common systemic symptoms include malaise, chills, headache, weakness, myalgias, and weight loss. Congestive heart failure is reported in 67% of cases with symptoms of dyspnea, acute pulmonary edema, or angina manifest. Hepatomegaly and splenomegaly (55%), clubbing of digits (37%), arterial embolic phenomena (21%), and a purpuric rash of immune complex vasculitis (19%) are not uncommon. At the time of diagnosis, common laboratory findings include an elevated erythrocyte sedimentation rate (88%), increased gammaglobulins (94%), anemia (55%), and thrombocytopenia (56%). Elevated liver-associated enzymes and microscopic hematuria are common, and antibodies associated with autoimmunity (rheumatoid factors, cryoglobulins, anti-smooth muscle antibodies, antimitochondrial antibodies, circulating anticoagulant antibodies) may be seen *(47)*.

Table 2
Prevalence of Various Manifestations of Chronic Q Fever (*n* = 313 Cases)

| Clinical signs and symptoms with endocarditis (n = 194) | % of cases |
|---|---|
| Fever | 81% |
| Hepatomegaly or splenomegaly | 42 |
| Arterial embolic phenomena | 16 |
| Thrombocytopenia | 35 |
| Elevated liver transaminases | 17 |
| Clinical manifestations | |
| Endocarditis | |
|     Pre-existing valve disease 89% | 73 |
|     Aortic 46% | |
|     Mitral 36% | |
|     Both aortic and mitral 7% | |
| Other vascular infection | 8 |
| Q fever in pregnancy | 6 |
| Osteoarthritis | 2 |
| Chronic pericarditis | 1 |
| Pseudotumors of lung or spleen | <1 |
| No foci identified | 2 |

Data summarized from Raoult et al. *(94)*.

As the bacteria will not grow on routine extracellular culture media, valvular infection with *C. burnetii* is a cause of culture-negative endocarditis and must be considered in this differential diagnosis. Furthermore, cardiac vegetations are small and are seen by transthoracic echocardiography in only 12% *(8)*. Unsurprisingly, transesophageal echocardiography will improve detection of vegetations. The diagnosis of chronic Q fever is typically confirmed by serological testing (IFA) with phase I antibody titers positive (≥ 1:800) and in higher titers than phase II antibody. Fournier et al. *(49)* have proposed a modification of Duke's criteria for the diagnosis of endocarditis to include Q fever serology as a major criterion.

Post Q-fever chronic fatigue syndrome is an often misunderstood complication of acute Q fever *(51)*. Symptoms include prolonged fatigue, myalgias/arthralgias, sweating, blurred vision, and occasionally breathlessness. Persistence of Q fever organisms after acute infection leads to obvious confusion. Furthermore, the possibility of relapse, particularly during pregnancy or acquired immunosuppression, requires vigilance to rule out Q fever endocarditis or other manifestations of chronic disease. Unlike chronic Q fever disease, the post Q-fever chronic fatigue syndrome results in a serological pattern of phase I antibodies falling to undetectable or low level titers in symptomatic persons.

## 7. DIAGNOSIS

Due to its highly infectious nature, the culture and handling of infectious material of *C. burnetii* requires experienced staff working in a biosafety level 3 laboratory. In fact, Q fever is the second most common laboratory-acquired infection *(52)*. Although *C. burnetii* has been successfully cultured in guinea pigs, mice, and embryonated hen eggs, these techniques have been largely replaced by shell-vial culture *(53)*. Human embryonic lung fibroblasts (HEL cells) are routinely used, although other human tissues may be adapted to cell monolayers in shell vials. These are inoculated with 1 mL of clinical specimen and centrifuged for 1 h at 700$g$ at 20°C to promote attachment and penetration of the bacterium into cells. Inoculated shell vials are incubated at 37°C in 5% $CO_2$ for 5–7 d. Organisms can be observed with Giemsa or Gimenez stain or direct immunofluorescence assay with polyclonal or monoclonal anti-*C. burnetii* antibodies *(54)*. Blood cultures should be obtained before initiation of antibiotics, as they will be rapidly rendered negative after drug administration *(55)*.

DNA amplification methods, such as polymerase chain reaction (PCR), and molecular detection techniques promise improved sensitivity compared with culture. These methods can be used on fresh clinical samples and shell vial cultures, as well as frozen or paraffin-embedded tissues *(56)*. PCR is the preferred method for retrospective analysis of frozen samples (best stored at –70 to –80°C). Gene targets typically amplified include sequences of the 16S or 23S rRNA gene or the repetitive element of the heat shock protein gene *htp*AB *(53,56)*. False-positive PCR results on blood samples using the *htp*AB target for amplification have been reported, and positive PCR results without other evidence of Q fever infection should be interpreted with caution *(8)*. Rapid detection systems for environmental or clinical samples using multiplex PCR technology are in development *(57)*.

A third method of direct detection of the bacteria is immunodetection in pathological specimens. The granulomatous lesions seen in the lung, liver, or bone marrow are non-specific, as are vegetations of infected heart valves. Tissue specimens, either fresh or formalin-fixed, paraffin-embedded, can be tested with immunoperoxidase staining *(41)* or monoclonal antibodies *(53)*. This technique is particularly useful for diagnosis of culture-negative endocarditis *(41)*

As direct detection techniques are employed in only a few reference laboratories, serology remains the standard method for diagnosis of *Coxiella* infection and Q fever disease. In acute Q fever, antibodies to phase II antigens predominate, and IgM antibodies are the first to appear. Unfortunately, as with many other pathogens, a detectable antibody response is not noted until 7 d to 3 wk after the onset of disease, depending on the method used. Therefore, paired acute and convalescent sera at least 2 wk apart are preferred, with a fourfold rise in titer diagnostic of an acute infection. A negative titer 45 d after illness can safely exclude Q fever as the diagnosis of acute fever *(8)*. For chronic disease, antibodies to phase I and phase II antibodies are detected, but high-titer phase I antibodies are unique to this type of infection.

The many serological methods used for antibody detection have been summarized by Fournier et al. *(53)*: complement fixation (CF), microagglutination, radioimmunoassay (RIA), indirect immunofluorescence antibody tests (IFA), Western immunoblotting, enzyme-linked immunosorbent assay (ELISA), and dot immunoblotting. Phase I and II antigens of *C. burnetii* Nine Mile strain are generally used as antigens. At present, three methods are commercially available: IFA, ELISA, and CF.

IFA remains the reference technique *(53)*. It is the simplest technique, and it has been modified to use less antigen *(58)*, but it requires experienced technicians for interpretation. This test allows determination of both phase I and phase II antibodies in the IgM, IgG, and IgA fractions. Seroconversions usually occur between d 7 and 15, and sensitivities against a reference panel by wk 3 were 91%, compared with 94% for ELISA and 78% for CF *(59)*. Rheumatoid factors can cause false positives, which can be removed with an absorbant *(53)*. Single test cutoffs for positive confirmation include titers of 1:200 or higher anti-phase II IgG or 1:50 or higher anti-phase II IgM *(58)*. For chronic Q fever infections, titers of 1:800 or higher and higher than 1:1600 anti-phase I IgG antibody have positive predictive values of 98% and 100%, respectively.

The ELISA method is very sensitive and the easiest to interpret once methods are established, making it preferred for seroepidemiological screening *(59)*. A combination IgM/IgG ELISA was recently validated for acute Q fever infection using cutoff values of 1:1024 or more for anti-phase II IgG and 1:512 or more for anti-phase II IgM *(60)*. A commercial IgM ELISA (PanBio, Brisbane, Australia) showed similar sensitivity, although occasional (12%) false positives were noted compared with IFA against a reference panel *(61)*. This can be improved with measurement of anti-phase II IgA *(62)* or a confirmation with another assay.

## 8. TREATMENT

The acidic intracellular environment in which *Coxiella* resides presents a challenge for antibiotic therapy *(63)*. As *Coxiella* cannot be grown in extracellular media, standard in vitro drug sensitivity testing cannot be performed. Embryonated egg inoculation models, animal models, and cell culture models have been tested *(64)*, and the shell vial method using infected HEL cells given a 6-d antibiotic treatment has been adopted for testing newer antibiotics *(54,64)*. A panel of 12 isolates was uniformly susceptible to trimethoprim-sulfamethoxazole (2 μg/mL), rifampin (4 μg/mL), and the tetracyclines (tetracycline, minocycline, and doxycycline at 4 μg/mL). Chloramphenicol and ceftriaxone (the only β-lactam with any activity) were bacteriostatic against most isolates. Quinolones were effective to various degrees, with sparfloxacin, levofloxacin, and moxifloxacin being the most active *(64,65)*. Erythromycin had modest activity, and azithromycin and clarithromycin are more active *(66)*.

Given the difficulties with determination of in vitro sensitivities, acquired antibiotic resistance has not been thoroughly investigated. Natural variation, especially among chronic isolates, has been noted for erythromycin, doxycycline, rifampin, and ciprofloxacin *(67)*. Moreover, doxycycline resistance has been selected for in vitro *(68)*. Mechanisms of resistance remain poorly defined, although quinolone resistance owing to mutations in gyrase A enzyme have been reported *(8)*.

Interestingly, isolates from chronically infected cell cultures (>400 d), which may more closely approximate endocarditis lesions, display more resistance to antibiotics than those infected for less than 30 d *(67)*. In fact, the lack of bactericidal activity has been noted for doxycycline, rifampin, and pefloxacin in a variety of chronic infection models *(64)*. Synergy was noted, however, with a combination of doxycycline and chloroquine, the latter increasing the pH within the phagolysosome and thus restoring bactericidal activity of the tetracycline *(63)*.

Clinically, drug trials in acute Q fever disease are hampered by the delay in diagnosis and the fact that most cases are self-limited, with resolution after a couple weeks. Powell et al. *(69)* performed a randomized placebo-controlled trial of tetracycline 500 mg po four times a day for Q fever pneumonia. If antibiotics were started with 72 h of the onset of illness, a 50% reduction in fever duration was noted. Spelman *(70)* showed the equivalence of doxycycline 100 mg twice a day compared with the same tetracycline regimen in a nonrandomized trial. Doxycycline for 14 d has become the drug of choice for its pharmacological and gastric tolerance benefits, which improve patient compliance. Shorter regimens (5–7 d) have been advocated with few supporting data.

For those unable to tolerate doxycycline or for whom it is contraindicated (pregnant women and children younger than 8 yr old), the options are less clear *(64)*. Bertrand et al. *(71)* reported successful treatment with the fluoroquinolones ofloxacin (200 mg tid) and pefloxacin (400 mg bid), for 14–21 d. As fluoroquinolones penetrate the cerebrospinal fluid, these agents should be considered in the therapy of the rare cases of Q fever meningoencephalitis *(72)*. Newer fluoroquinolone agents have not been thoroughly tested, and these are also contraindicated in pregnancy and children. Erythromycin has been effective but unreliable, and studies on clarithromycin and azithromycin are lacking. Trimethoprim-sulfamethoxazole may be an alternate, but the only available data are anecdotal and show mixed benefit.

Anecdotal reports support the addition of corticosteroids to antibiotics in Q fever hepatitis if fever persists 3 d after doxycycline is instituted *(8)*. Typical cases are elderly patients with high sedimentation rates (<100 mm/h) and autoantibodies. A prednisone burst of 40 mg daily leads to rapid defervescence, and steroids may be tapered over 1 wk.

Treatment of chronic Q fever, especially endocarditis, has been problematic owing to the lack of bactericidal agents. Single-drug therapy (doxycyclines, fluoroquinolones, rifampin, or trimethoprim-sulfamethoxazole) usually results in clinical relapse once antibiotics are withdrawn, despite an early good response. Death rates are 50–60% in these drug monotherapy trials *(64)*. Hence, combinations of antimicrobials have become standard treatment. Levy et al. *(73)* found that a combination of doxycycline-fluoroquinolone (either pefloxacin or ofloxacin) markedly improved survival compared with doxycycline alone in Q fever endocarditis. However, 50% relapse was still noted upon antibiotic withdrawal, and a minimum of 3 yr of therapy with this regimen was recommended *(64)*. A subsequent nonrandomized trial compared doxycycline-ofloxacin with doxycycline-hydroxychloro-quine in 35 patients *(74)*. Although death rates were similar (5%), clinical improvement was more prompt with a doxycycline (100 mg po bid) and hydroxychloroquine (200 mg po tid) combination, and relapse after drug withdrawal was reduced from 64% to 14%. An 18-mo initial duration of treatment with doxycycline-hydroxychloroquine is now recommended.

Therapy of Q fever endocarditis must be individualized, and consultation with an expert is recommended. Monthly clinical monitoring with complete blood count, liver-associated enzyme, and creatinine determinations and Q fever serology is recommended. Serial echocardiography should also be performed. Hydroxychloroquine levels should be monitored to be kept stable at 0.8–1.2 mg/L, and regular ophthalmologic exam to monitor for retinopathy is necessary. After treatment cessation, monitoring monthly for 6 mo, then every 2 mo for 2 yr, and yearly thereafter is recommended *(8)*. For complications of valvular dysfunction or in case of relapse, surgical replacement of an infected valve may be necessary for ultimate cure.

## 9. Q FEVER PREVENTION AND PROPHYLAXIS

Postexposure drug prophylaxis, administered to high-risk individuals after likely exposure, has given mixed results. Tigrett and Benenson *(31)* studied postexposure prophylaxis in a human challenge model with oxytetracycline 20 mg administered over 5–6 d. Prompt therapy (within 24 h) simply delayed onset of disease, presumably because of the varying incubation times of inhaled spore-like forms. Only treatment near the end of the incubation period proved to abort infection. Specific recommendations for prophylaxis of mass exposure are lacking, although some authors recommend doxycycline

100 mg po bid for 5 d starting 8–12 d after exposure *(75)*. In the author's opinion, given the self-limited nature of most cases, the risk-to-benefit ratio may favor close monitoring of potential low-risk exposures and prompt treatment for febrile illness rather than postexposure prophylaxis for all but high-risk exposures and high-risk persons (pregnancy, immunosuppression, and valvulopathies). Careful clinical screening for valvular heart disease is warranted, as the risk of endocarditis in this population following acute Q fever is greater than a third (relative risk >400 than that without valvulopathy) *(76)*. Furthermore, for those with pre-existing valvular lesions, this retrospective review advocated treatment of acute *Coxiella* infection with the combination of doxycycline and hydroxychloroquine for 12 mo as secondary prophylaxis for prevention of endocarditis, rather than doxycycline alone.

Passive immunoprophylaxis for exposed persons has not been studied recently. Protection with anti-phase I *C. burnetii* antibody was observed in mice undergoing infectious challenge *(34)*. The benefit was only seen for those animals given immunoglobulin before or at the time of challenge, not afterwards, as might be expected for an intracellular pathogen. No further testing has been performed.

Vaccination is an alternative preventive option for high-risk personnel. As *C. burnetii* is an intracellular pathogen, correlates of vaccine protection are less well established than other organisms. Evaluation consists of both antibody levels and cell-mediated immune responses, usually lymphoproliferative responses *(77)*. Most notably, skin testing after vaccination has been found to be highly predictive of protection *(78)*.

Since Q fever causes abortion and infertility in economically important domestic ungulates, initial efforts were geared toward animal vaccines. Initially, formalin-inactivated whole cell *C. burnetii* vaccines (WCVs) were tested; phase I organisms with the complete LPS were found to be more protective than phase II preparations *(79)*. In guinea pig challenge with heterologous strains, Ormsbee et al. *(79)* also demonstrated cross-protection with this preparation. More recently, chloroform-methanol extraction (CMR) vaccines have been developed and have been better tolerated in animals *(80,81)*.

In seronegative animals, vaccination has shown reduction in abortion and chronic infertility *(80,82)*. However, in previously infected animals, vaccination did not eradicate *C. burnetii* or affect persistent shedding, and it may have contributed to increased shedding in infected goat milk, leading to a human outbreak *(27,83)*. Therefore, the vaccine is considered safe and effective only in uninfected animals and is not widely used at present.

Vaccine development for humans has followed a parallel course to that of animals, with efforts focused on formalin-inactivated, purified phase I *C. burnetii* cells purified to remove some LPS residues, which are responsible for the reactogenicity *(82)*. Efforts to date have utilized a single strain of Q fever, and cross-protection against geographically diverse isolates remains to be established. A second-generation inactivated WCV, Q-Vax (Commonwealth Serum Laboratories, Melbourne, Australia), prepared from the Henzerling strain and extracted in NaCl, was licensed in 1989 and is now in use in Australia *(84)*. Efficacy has been demonstrated among abattoir workers and at-risk laboratory personnel *(84,85)*. Among 924 nonimmune abattoir workers, seroconversion was detected in two-thirds of cases, and, notably, no Q fever case was seen during 18 mo follow-up. In comparison, clinical cases of Q fever were seen in 34 of 1349 controls (2.5% case attack rate). Marmion et al. *(86)*, in a follow-up study, found 100% protection among those with sufficient time for immunity to develop after vaccination, and protection for at least 5 yr. Cell-mediated immunity as judged by lymphoproliferative assays, was also maintained for at least 5 yr. Gilroy et al. *(87)* reported no protective effect from postexposure vaccination in a small study of an abattoir outbreak in New South Wales.

Although highly immunogenic, this vaccine also demonstrates marked reactogenicity. Among nonimmunes, erythema or tenderness was commonly noted at the vaccine site. Systemic symptoms (headache, chills, or flu-like symptoms) occurred in 10–18% of subjects. Among previously exposed, local (induration, sterile abscesses, and granulomas) and systemic symptoms may be more pronounced *(82)*. Persons with a history of Q fever infection, positive serology, or a prior immunization should not be vaccinated. Intradermal skin testing with 20 ng of diluted WCV vaccine is recommended to detect sensitivity owing to prior infection. A positive test is defined as induration of more than 5 mm diameter on d 7.

A similar inactivated phase I WCV, purified by NaCl, ethanol/freon extraction, and a Brushite column, was developed at USAMRIID (Fort Detrick, MD). Production was scaled up in 1970, and the vaccine has been available for use in the United States under Investigational New Drug (IND) status since that time. Over 1000 persons have received this vaccine after prescreening for prior exposure by skin test (W.R. Byrne, personal communication). The dose is 0.5 mL administered subcutaneously. Currently, this vaccine is available as an IND product for high-risk personnel by contacting the Centers for Disease Control and Prevention (1-770-488-7100) or Commanding Officer, USAMRIID, Fort Detrick, MD.

A third-generation subfraction vaccine, developed by purification of the phase I *C. burnetii* cells using four cycles of chloroform-methanol extraction, reduced side effects while maintaining efficacy in animals *(88)*. This chloroform-methanol residue vaccine, involving four extractions of the Henzerling strain of *C. burnetii*, proved safe and effective when tested in guinea pigs with subsequent homologous aerosol challenge *(81)*. Phase I human clinical trials (0.5 mL sc) were disappointing. Reactogenicity was still marked *(89)*, and further development is ongoing at USAMRIID.

A similar vaccine, involving trichloroacetic acid extraction, was developed and tested in Czechoslovakia using the Nine Mile strain *(90)*. Local minor reactions were noted in 39% of volunteers, particularly among those with previous natural infection. This vaccine resulted in seroconversions of 55% and 74% after one and two doses, respectively, but long-term follow-up for protective efficacy was not performed. Further developmental testing has not been performed.

## 10. SUMMARY: Q FEVER AS A BIOTERRORISM AGENT

The spore-like stages of *Coxiella burnetii* make preparation, storage, and dispersal of this agent for biowarfare or bioterrorism feasible. In fact, this organism was part of the offensive biological weapons arsenal of the United States prior to the decision to destroy biological weapons munitions and stockpiles by President Richard M. Nixon in 1969. *C. burnetii* is considered an incapacitating agent, as mortality is rare from acute infection; thus it is of lower risk as an agent of bioterrorism *(91,92)*. For the same reasons, it is also an unlikely terrorist agent targeted against economically important livestock industries.

In case of intentional dispersion of infective *C. burnetii*, the route of infection would be inhalational. Thus, exposed persons would present similarly to natural infection, perhaps with shorter incubation times and a more severe illness for a substantial exposure. A cluster of undifferentiated febrile illnesses or atypical pneumonia would be the probable clinical presentation. As diagnosis by serology is delayed, public health authorities should be promptly notified of a suspicious outbreak so that samples can be collected and assayed at a reference laboratory. As clinical cases may be the 'tip of the iceberg, the extent of exposure in the population can later be assessed by seroconversion *(26)*.

Q fever infection represents low-risk infection control concern, and standard precautions for suspected exposures are generally adequate. Isolation is not required, as secondary cases are unlikely, but transmission from contaminated fomites, such as clothes, is possible. Suspected cases should be instructed to remove all clothing (preferably at a decontamination site) and store it in a plastic bag, and then shower immediately with soap and water. Suspected contaminated articles can be disinfected with 0.5% hypochlorite (1 part bleach to 9 parts water), 5% peroxide, or a 1:100 solution of Lysol *(91,93)*. Droplet precautions to health care workers involved in obstetrical procedures of infected persons or suspected postmortem cases warrant re-emphasis.

Postexposure vaccination does not appear to be effective, and postexposure chemoprophylaxis given shortly after exposure may only delay clinical presentation of illness. Given the self-limited nature of most cases, the risk/benefit ratio may favor close monitoring of low-risk exposures and prompt treatment for febrile illness rather than postexposure prophylaxis with doxycycline. Probable exposure of immunocompromised individuals and high-risk exposures warrants consideration of doxycycline postexposure prophylaxis and consultation with a public health specialist. Infection of persons with a known valvulopathy may warrant a longer regimen of doxycycline and hydroxychloroquine to prevent Q fever endocarditis *(76)*. Vaccination of high-risk individuals, such as emergency response personnel, may be warranted with the current IND product. Further guidelines are under development by the Centers for Disease Control and Prevention.

## REFERENCES

1. Report of WHO Consultants. Health Aspects of Chemical and Biological Weapons. World Health Organization, Geneva, 1970.
2. Smart JK. History of chemical and biological warfare: an American perspective. In: Sidell FR, Takafuji ET, Franz DR, eds. Textbook of Military Medicine: Medical Aspects of Chemical and Biological Warfare. Borden Institute, Washington, DC, 1997, pp. 9–86.
3. Department of the Army. U.S. Army Activity in the U.S. Biological Warfare Programs. Vol. II. Publication DTIC B19342TL. Headquarters, Department of the Army, Washington DC, 1977, Appendix 4.
4. Derrick EH. "Q" fever, new fever entity: clinical features, diagnosis and laboratory investigation. Med J Aust 1937;2:281–299.
5. Burnet FM, Freeman M. Experimental studies on the virus of Q fever. Med J Aust 1937;2:299–302.
6. Cox HR, Bell EJ. The cultivation of *Rickettsia diaporica* in tissue culture and in the tissues of developing chick embryos. Public Health Rep 1939;54:2171–2175.
7. Dyer RE. A filter-passing infectious agent isolated from ticks: IV. Human infection. Public Health Rep 1938;53:2277–2283.
8. Maurin M, Raoult D. Q fever. Clin Microbiol Rev 1999;12:518–553.
9. Heinzen RA, Stiegler GL, Whiting LL, Schmitt SA, Mallavia LP, Frazier ME. Use of pulsed field gel electrophoresis to differentiate *Coxiella burnetii* strains. Ann NY Acad Sci 1990;590:504–513.
10. Thiele D, Willems H, Kopf G, Krauss H. Polymorphism in DNA restriction patterns of *Coxiella burnetii* isolates investigated by pulsed field gel electrophoresis and image analysis. Eur J Epidemiol 1993;9:419–425.
11. Jager C, Willems H, Theile D, et al. Molecular characterization of *Coxiella burnetii* isolates. Epidemiol Infect 1998;120:157–164.

12. Willems H, Jager C, Balger G. Physical and genetic map of the obligate intracellular bacterium *Coxiella burnetii*. J Bacteriol 1998;180:3816–3822.
13. Savinelli EA, Mallavia LP. Comparison of *Coxiella burnetii* plasmids to homologous chromosomal sequences present in a plasmid-less endocarditis-causing isolate. Ann NY Acad Sci 1990;590:523–533.
14. Samuel JE, Frazier ME, Mallavia LP. Correlation of plasmid type and disease caused by *Coxiella burnetii*. Infect Immun 1985;49:775–779.
15. Valkova D, Kazar J. A new plasmid (QpDV) common to *Coxiella burnetii* isolates associated with acute and chronic Q fever. FEMS Microbiol Lett 1995;125:275–280.
16. Hackstadt K. Antigenic variation in phase I lipopolysaccharide of *Coxiella burnetii* isolates. Infect Immun 1986;52:337–340.
17. Toman R, Skultety L. Structural study on a lipopolysaccharide from *Coxiella burnetii* strain Nine Mile in avirulent phase II. Carbohydr Res 1996;283:175–185.
18. Amano KI, Williams JC. Chemical and immunological characterization of lipopolysaccharides of phase I and phase II *Coxiella burnetii*. J Bacteriol 1984;160:994–1002.
19. Heinzen RA, Hackstadt T, Samuel JE. Developmental biology of *Coxiella burnetii*. Trends Microbiol 1999;7:149–154.
20. McCaul TF, Williams JC. Developmental cycle of *Coxiella burnetii*: structure and morphogenesis of vegetative and sporogenic differentiations. J Bacteriol 1981;147:1063–1076.
21. Wiebe ME, Burton PR, Shankel DM. Isolation and characterization of two cell types of *Coxiella burnetii* phase I. J Bacteriol 1972;110:368–377.
22. Babudieri B. Q fever: a zoonosis. Adv Vet Sci 1959;5:81–182.
23. Huebner RJ, Bell JA. Q fever studies in southern California: summary of current results and a discussion of possible control measures. JAMA 1951;145:301–305.
24. Lang GH. Coxiellosis (Q fever) in animals. In: Marrie TJ, ed. Q Fever, vol I. The Disease. CRC Press, Boca Raton, FL, 1990.
25. Langley JM, Marrie TJ, Covert A, Waag DM, Williams JC. Poker players' pneumonia: an urban outbreak of Q fever following exposure to a parturient cat. N Engl J Med 1988;319:354 356.
26. Dupuis G, Petite J, Vouilloz M. An important outbreak of human Q fever in a Swiss alpine valley. Int J Epidemiol 1987;16:282–287.
27. Fishbein DB, Raoult D. A cluster of *Coxiella burnetii* infections associated with exposure to vaccinated goats and their unpasteurized dairy products. Am J Trop Med Hyg 1992;47:35–40.
28. Boschini A, Di Perri G, Legnani D. Consecutive epidemics of Q fever in a residential facility for drug abusers: impact on persons with human immunodeficiency virus infection. Clin Infect Dis 1999;28:866–872.
29. Tissot-Dupont H, Raoult D, Brouqui P, et al. Epidemiologic features and clinical presentation of acute Q fever in hospitalized patients—323 French cases. Am J Med 1992; 93:427–434.
30. Raoult D, Levy PY, Tissot-Dupont H, et al. Q fever and HIV infection. AIDS 1993;7:81–86.
31. Tigrett WD, Benenson AS. Studies on Q fever in man. Trans Assoc Am Physicians 1956;69:98–104.
32. Raoult D, Stein A. Q fever during pregnancy—a risk for women, fetuses and obstetricians. N Engl J Med 1994;330:371.
33. Milazzo A, Hall R, Storm PA, et al. Sexually transmitted Q fever. Clin Infect Dis 2001;33:399–402.
34. Humphres RC, Hinrichs DJ. Role of antibody in *Coxiella burnetii* infection. Infect Immun 1981;31:641–645.
35. Byrne, WR. Q fever. In: Sidell FR, Takafuji ET, Franz DR, eds. Medical Aspects of Chemical and Biological Warfare. Office of the Surgeon General, U.S. Army, Washington DC, 1997, pp. 523–537.
36. Syrucek L, Sobeslovsky O, Gutvirth I. Isolation of *Coxiella burnetii* from human placentas. J Hyg Epidemiol Microbiol Immunol 1958;2:29–35.
37. Raoult D, Brouqui P, Marchon B, Gastaut JA. Acute and chronic Q fever in patients with cancer. Clin Infect Dis 1992;14:127–130.
38. Raoult D, Raza A, Marrie TJ. Q fever endocarditis and other forms of chronic Q fever. In: Marrie TJ, ed. Q Fever, vol I. The Disease. CRC Press, Boca Raton, FL, 1990, pp. 179–199.
39. Mege JL, Maurin M, Capo C, Raoult D. *Coxiella burnetii*: the query fever bacterium. A model of immune subversion by a strictly intracellular organism. FEMS Microbiol Rev 1997;19:209–217.
40. Koster FT, Williams JC, Goodwin JS. Cellular immunity in Q fever: specific lymphocyte unresponsiveness in Q fever endocarditis. J Infect Dis 1985;152:1283–1289.
41. Brouqui P, Dumler JS, Raoult D. Immunohistologic demonstration of *Coxiella burnetii* in the valves of patients with Q fever endocarditis. Am J Med 1994;97:451–458.
42. Derrick EH. The course of infection with *Coxiella burnetii*. Med J Aust 1973;1:1051–1057.

43. Smith DL, Ayres JG, Blair I, et al. A large Q fever outbreak in the West Midlands: clinical aspects. Respir Med 1993;87:509–517.
44. Bernit E, Pouget J, Janbon F, et al. Neurological involvement in acute Q fever: a report of 29 cases and review of the literature. Arch Intern Med 2002;162:693–700.
45. Marrie TJ. *Coxiella burnetii* (Q fever) pneumonia. Clin Infect Dis 1995;26(suppl 3):S253–S264.
46. Marrie TJ. Liver involvement in acute Q fever. Chest 1988;94:896–898.
47. Levy P, Raoult D, Razongles JJ. Q fever and autoimmunity. Eur J Epidemiol 1989;5:447–453.
48. Stein A, Raoult D. Q fever during pregnancy: a public health problem in southern France. Clin Infect Dis 1998;27:592–596.
49. Fournier PE, Casalta JP, Habib G, Messana T, Raoult D. Modification of the diagnostic criteria proposed by the Duke endocarditis service to permit improved diagnosis of Q fever endocarditis. Am J Med 1996;100:629–633.
50. Brouqui P, Tissot-Dupont H, Drancourt M, et al. Epidemiologic and clinical features of chronic Q fever: 92 cases from France (1982–1990). Arch Intern Med 1993;153:642–648.
51. Ayres JG, Flint N, Smith EG, et al. Post-infection fatigue syndrome following Q fever. Q J Med 1998;91:105–123.
52. U.S. Department of Health and Human Services. Biosafety in Microbiological and Biomedical Laboratories, 4th ed. U.S. Government Printing Office, Washington, DC, 1999, pp. 148–149.
53. Fournier PE, Marrie TJ, Raoult D. Diagnosis of Q fever. J Clin Microbiol 1998;36: 1823–1834.
54. Raoult D, Torres H, Drancourt M. Shell-vial assay: evaluation of a new technique for determining antibiotic susceptibility, tested in 13 isolates of *Coxiella burnetii*. Antimicrob Agents Chemother 1991;35:2070–2077.
55. Musso D, Raoult D. *Coxiella burnetii* blood cultures from acute and chronic Q fever patients. J Clin Microbiol 1995;33:3129–3132.
56. Stein A, Raoult D. Detection of *Coxiella burnetii* by DNA amplification using the polymerase chain reaction. J Clin Microbiol 1992;30:2462–2466.
57. McDonald R, Cao T, Borschel R. Multiplexing for the detection of multiple biowarfare agents shows promise in the field. Mil Med 2001;166:237–239.
58. Tissot-Dupont H, Thirion X, Raoult D. Q fever serology: cutoff determination for microimmunofluorescence. Clin Diagn Lab Immunol 1994;1:189–196.
59. Peter O, Dupuis G, Peacock MG, Burgdorfer W. Comparison of enzyme-linked immunosorbent assay and complement fixation and indirect fluorescent-antibody tests for detection of *Coxiella burnetii* antibody. J Clin Microbiol 1987;25:1063–1067.
60. Waag D, Chulay J, Marrie TJ, England M, Williams JC. Validation of an enzyme immunoassay for serodiagnosis of acute Q fever. Eur J Clin Microbiol Infect Dis 1995;14:421–427.
61. Field PR, Mitchell JL, Santiago A, et al. Comparison of a commercial enzyme-linked immunosorbent assay with immunofluorescence and complement fixation tests for detection of *Coxiella burnetii* (Q fever) immunoglobulin M. J Clin Microbiol 2000;38: 1645–1647.
62. Devine P, Doyle C, Lambkin G. Combined determination of *Coxiella burnetii*-specific immunoglobulin M (IgM) and IgA improves specificity in the diagnosis of acute Q fever. Clin Diagn Lab Immunol 1997;4:384–386.
63. Maurin M, Benoliel AM, Bongrand P, Raoult D. Phagolysosomal alkanization and the bactericidal effects of antibiotics: the *Coxiella burnetii* paradigm. J Infect Dis 1992;166:1097–1102.
64. Raoult D. Treatment of Q fever. Antimicrob Agents Chemother 1993;37:1733–1736.
65. Rolain JM, Maurin M, Raoult D. Bacteriostatic and bactericidal activities of moxifloxacin against *Coxiella burnetii*. Antimicrob Agents Chemother 2001;45:301–302.
66. Gikas A, Kofteridis DP, Manios A, et al. Newer macrolides as empiric treatment for acute Q fever infections. Antimicrob Agents Chemother 2001;45:3644–3646.
67. Yeaman MR, Baca OG. Unexpected antibiotic susceptibility of a chronic isolate of *Coxiella burnetii*. Ann NY Acad Sci 1990;590:297–305.
68. Brezina R, Schramek S, Kazar J. Selection of chlortetracycline-resistant strain of *Coxiella burnetii*. Acta Virol 1975;19:496.
69. Powell OW, Kennedy KP, McIver M, Silverstone H. Tetracycline in the treatment of Q fever. Aust Ann Med 1962;11:184–188.
70. Spelman DW. Q fever: a study of 111 consecutive cases. Med J Aust 1982;1:547–553.
71. Bertrand A, Janbon F, Jonquet O, Reynes J. Infections par les rickettsiales et fluoroquinolones. Pathol Biol (Paris) 1988;36:493–495.
72. Raoult D, Marrie TJ. Q fever. Clin Infect Dis 1995;20:489–496.

73. Levy PY, Drancourt M, Etienne J, et al. Comparison of different antibiotic regimens for therapy of 32 cases of Q fever endocarditis. Antimicrob Agents Chemother 1991;35:533–537.

74. Raoult D, Houpikian P, Tissot-Dupont H, Riss JM, Arditi-Djiane J, Brouqui P. Treatment of Q fever endocarditis: comparison of 2 regimens containing doxycycline and ofloxacin or hydroxychloroquine. Arch Intern Med 1999;159:167–173.

75. Weber DJ, Rutala WA. Risks and prevention of nosocomial transmission of rare zoonotic diseases. Clin Infect Dis 2001;32:446–456.

76. Fenollar F, Fournier PE, Carrieri MP, et al. Risk factors and prevention of Q fever endocarditis. Clin Infect Dis 2001;33:312–316.

77. Izzo A, Marmion BP, Worswick DA. Markers of cell-mediated immunity after vaccination with an inactivated, whole-cell Q fever vaccine. J Infect Dis 1988;157:781–789.

78. Luoto L, Bell FJ, Casey M, Lackman DB. Q fever vaccination of human volunteers. 1. Serologic and skin test response following subcutaneous injection. Am J Hyg 1963;78:1–15.

79. Ormsbee RA, Bell EJ, Lackman DB, Tallent G. The influence of phase on the protective potency of Q fever vaccine. J Immunol 1964;92:404–412.

80. Williams JC, Peacock MG, Waag DM, et al. Vaccines against coxiellosis and Q fever. Development of a chloroform-methanol residue subunit of phase I *Coxiella burnetii* for the immunization of animals. Ann NY Acad Sci 1992;653:88–111.

81. Waag DM, England MJ, Pitt NLM. Comparative efficacy of a *Coxiella burnetii* chloroform methanol residue (CMR) vaccine and a licensed cellular vaccine (Q-Vax) in rodents challenged by aerosol. Vaccine 1994;15:1779–1783.

82. Ormsbee RA, Marmion BP. Prevention of *Coxiella burnetii* infection: vaccines and guidelines for those at risk. In: Marrie TJ, ed. Q Fever, vol I. The Disease. CRC Press, Boca Raton, FL, 1990, pp. 225–248.

83. Schmeer N, Muller P, Langel J, Krauss H, Frost JW, Wieda J. Q fever vaccines for animals. Zentralbl Bakteriol Microbiol Hyg 1987;267:79–88.

84. Ackland JA, Worswick DA, Marmion BP. Vaccine prophylaxis of Q fever: a follow-up study of the efficacy of Q-Vax (CSL) 1985–1990. Med J Aust 1994;160: 704–708.

85. Marmion BP, Ormsbee RA, Kyrkou M, et al. Vaccine prophylaxis of abattoir-associated Q fever. Lancet 1984;ii:1411–1414.

86. Marmion BP, Ormsbee RA, Kyrkou M, et al. Vaccine prophylaxis of abattoir-associated Q fever: eight years' experience in Australian abattoirs. Epidemiol Infect 1990;104:275–287.

87. Gilroy N, Formica N, Beers M, et al. Abattoir-associated Q fever: a Q fever outbreak during a Q fever vaccination program. Aust NZ J Public Health 2001;25:362–367.

88. Williams JC, Damrow TA, Waag DM, Amano KI. Characterization of a phase I *Coxiella burnetii* chloroform-methanol residue vaccine that induces active immunity against Q fever in C57BL/10ScN mice. Infect Immun 1986;51:851–858.

89. Frics LF, Waag DM, Williams JC. Safety and immunogenicity in human volunteers of a chloroform-methanol residue vaccine for Q fever. Infect Immun 1993;61:1251–1258.

90. Kazar J, Brezina R, Palanova A, Turda B, Schramek S. Immunogenicity and reactogenicity of a Q fever chemovaccine in persons professionally exposed to Q fever in Czechoslovakia. Bull WHO 1982;60:389–394.

91. Kortepeter M, ed. USAMRIID's Medical Management of Biological Casualties Handbook, 4th ed. U.S. Army Research Institute of Infectious Diseases, Fort Detrick, MD, 2001.

92. Rotz LD, Khan AS, Lillibridge SR, et al. Public health assessment of potential biologic terrorism agents. Emerg Infect Dis 2002;8:225–230.

93. Scott GH, Williams JC. Susceptibility of *Coxiella burnetii* to chemical disinfectants. Ann NY Acad Sci 1990;590:291–296.

94. Raoult D, Tissot-Dupont H, Foucault C, et al. Q fever 1985–1998. Clinical and epidemiologic features of 1,383 infections. Medicine (Baltimore) 2000;79:109-123.

95. Marrie TJ, ed. Q Fever, vol I. The Disease. CRC Press, Boca Raton, FL, 1990.

# 10 Melioidosis and Glanders

## Aileen M. Marty, MD, FACP

The opinions or assertions contained herein are the private views of the author and are not to be construed as official or as reflecting the view of the Department of the Navy or the Department of Defense.

### CONTENTS

INTRODUCTION
MELIOIDOSIS
GLANDERS
REFERENCES

## 1. INTRODUCTION

Melioidosis and glanders are diseases caused by members of the genus *Burkholderia*. These Gram-negative bacterial pathogens can produce a wide spectrum of disease in humans and other animals. *Burkholderia* are proteobacteria of the Betaproteobacteria group. Although *Burkholderia mallei*, *B. pseudomallei*, *B. cepacia*, and *B. gladioli* can all cause human disease, this chapter focuses on *B. mallei* (Löffler and Schütz, 1882; Zopf, 1885) Yabuuchi et al., 1993, the cause of glanders, and *B. pseudomallei* (Whitmore, 1913) Yabuucchi et al., 1993 *(1)*, the cause of melioidosis, because state-sponsored programs have studied, and at times used, these bacteria as agents of germ warfare.

*Burkholderia pseudomallei* and *B. mallei* cause similar illnesses and are closely related based on DNA-DNA homology, base sequence of the 16S rRNA, phenotypic character istics, and (to a lesser degree) antigen expression *(2)*. Some researchers argue that *B. pseudomallei* and *B. mallei* are pathovars of one single species *(3)*. (Pathovars are strains differentiated at the infrasubspecific level from other strains of the same subspecies.) In any case, the clinical and pathological changes caused by these agents are nearly identical, and, untreated, the acute pneumonia produced by inhalation of either organism is nearly always fatal. The *Burkholderia* are classified as biosafety level 2–3 in the United States and many European nations. Diagnosis of melioidosis or glanders in a patient in North America in the absence of travel to an endemic area, animal attack, occupational exposure, or an epidemic of clear etiology is presumptive evidence of a biological warfare attack requiring involvement of the Centers for Disease Control and Prevention (CDC) and Federal Bureau of Investigation (FBI). *Burkholderia mallei* has long been classified as a category B agent by the CDC, and, more recently *B. pseudomallei* has also

From: *Physician's Guide to Terrorist Attack*
Edited by: M. J. Roy © Humana Press Inc., Totowa, NJ

been included in this category *(4)*; use of this or another biological agent by a terrorist is coded as U01.6 (covers all biological agents used by terrorists) by the World Health Organization *(5)*.

## 2. MELIOIDOSIS

### 2.1. Definition

Melioidosis is an emerging infection caused by the bacterium *B. pseudomallei*. It has an extremely varied spectrum of clinical presentation, dependent on host-pathogen interaction. This ranges from asymptomatic seroconversion to rapidly fatal, overwhelming sepsis. Between the two extremes the infection can produce a chronic or relapsing disease or may remain dormant and essentially asymptomatic; then, after impairment of immune defenses, it can reactivate decades later and produce an acute, lethal sepsis. It is an important public health problem in endemic areas and a worthy model of bacterial pathogenesis.

Current data reveal that *B. pseudomallei* is a widely distributed environmental saprophyte and thus not a zoonosis with a reservoir in rodents, as originally described *(6)*. It is primarily endemic in soil, mud, and water of tropical and subtropical areas, affecting humans and a range of animals. Among livestock animals, goats and sheep are particularly susceptible. Pigs generally manifest asymptomatic abscesses. Other susceptible species include camels, horses, deer, alpaca, and laboratory animals. Dogs, cats, and cattle can get melioidosis, but in general they are fairly resistant to disease in the absence of an underlying immunosuppressive condition. *Burkholderia pseudomallei* can cause illness in seals and dolphins *(7)*. Cases have also been described in native Australian mammals, reptiles, and birds including wallabies, tree kangaroo, koala, crocodile, galah (rose headed cockatoo), red collared lorikeet, and a sulfur crested cockatoo *(8)*.

### 2.2. Synonyms

Whitmore disease is a synonym. Until recently, Burkholderiaceae were classified as members of the RNA group II pseudomonads organisms. Older names for *B. pseudomallei* include *Pseudomonas pseudomallei*.

### 2.3. History

The British pathologist, Captain Alfred Whitmore and his colleague C.S. Krishnaswami provided the first account of this disease among debilitated morphine addicts in Rangoon, Burma (now Myanmar) *(9)*. Whitmore went on to describe the infection in 38 patients in Rangoon *(10)*. In his honor, the disease is sometimes called Whitmore disease. The resemblance of this infection to glanders prompted doctors managing patients in Malaysia to term the infection *melioidosis*, which means "a similarity to distemper of asses" *(11)*. Although there were subsequent sporadic reports of infection *(12)*, the importance of melioidosis was largely unrecognized until the mid-20th century when reports of disease began in Thailand *(13)* and soon thereafter with the death of U.S. soldiers from melioidosis pneumonitis during the Vietnam War *(14)*.

### 2.4. Epidemiology and Transmission

Melioidosis is endemic in Southeast Asia and Northern Australia (north of 20°S and as far south as Brisbane). In Thailand, approximately 2000–5000 patients (3.6–5.5 cases per 100,000) present with melioidosis per year *(15,16)*.

The true global distribution is uncertain because neither the disease nor the organism is well known to clinicians or microbiologists, a problem compounded by absent or inadequate diagnostic laboratories in most tropical areas, inadequate serological methods, inadequate surveillance systems, and insufficient research. Although uncommonly diagnosed, sporadic outbreaks have been documented in India (Maharashtra, Kerala, Orissa, Tripura, Tamil Nadu, West Bengal, Assam, and possibly Pune), China (especially in Hainan, Guangxi, and Guangdong, Hong Kong, and Taiwan) *(17)*, Southeast Asia (Singapore, Vietnam, Malaysia, and Myanmar) *(18)*, Saudi Arabia, Africa (Egypt), and the Americas (Mexico, Panama, Ecuador, Aruba, Haiti, Brazil, Peru, Guyana, Martinique, Guadeloupe, and the U.S. states of Hawaii and Georgia as well as the territory of Puerto Rico) *(19)*. In Singapore, between 1989 and 1996 there were a total of 372 cases of melioidosis, with 147 deaths, giving a mean annual incidence rate of 1.7 per 100,000 and a case-fatality rate of 39.5% *(20)*. There are reports of melioidosis imported to the UK in infected human and non-human primates from Indonesia, the Philippines *(21)*, and Bangladesh *(22)*, implicating these countries as endemic for *B. pseudomallei.*

*Burkholderia* typically multiply in the rhizosphere (the region of soil modified as a result of the uptake and deposition of substances by growing plant roots). *Burkholderia pseudomallei* is present in contaminated soil and water, especially in stagnant waters of endemic areas. The organism is abundant in soil samples of flooded rice paddies. It is particularly common in padi fields of northeast Thailand where 80% of children have antibodies by the time they are 4 yr old. Playing barefoot in wet grass is a potential source of infection. The organism is present in sea sludge and on children's playgrounds. The interaction between *B. pseudomallei* and plants such as commonly consumed vegetables is unclear.

In Australian studies, 85% of cases develop during the rainy season; in all endemic sites the organism grows in abundance during the rainy season but it is still detectable during dry seasons from deep, moist soil samples. Recently cleared land can contain great quantities. Under optimal temperature (37–42°C), optimal pH (6.8), and optimal water content (>40%) *B. pseudomallei* survives for up to 726 d, but if temperatures drop below 21°C, *B. pseudomallei* only survives for about 18 d, though these factors vary with different strains of the organism *(23)*. Interpretation of these studies has been complicated by the recent recognition of avirulent, antigenically crossreacting environmental organisms for which the name *B. thailandensis* has been proposed *(24)*.

Infected animals excrete *B. pseudomallei* in sputum, pus, urine, and feces, so that transport of infected animals to suitable new environments can lead to the temporary or permanent establishment of new endemic foci. This was the source of the French outbreak of the mid-1970s known as the "affaire du Jardin des Plantes" *(25)*.

Inhalation and contamination of damaged (abraded, burnt, or wounded/punctured) skin or mucous membranes are the two key modes of transmission *(26,27)*. Military personnel have developed the disease in association with inhalation of dust stirred up by helicopters. Patients who acquire melioidosis by inhalation are likely to present with a primary pneumonia. Laboratory animals can acquire infection by the respiratory route. There are reports of infection via aspiration of contaminated water during near-drowning episodes *(28)*, iatrogenic inoculation *(29)*, and laboratory accidents *(30)*.

Person-to-person transmission is uncommon *(31)*. In one report a sister with diabetes became infected while serving as the caretaker for her brother, who had chronic melioidosis. Two cases of sexual transmission have been reported. Transmission in both cases was preceded by a clinical history of chronic prostatitis in the source patient. Animal-to-human transmission is rare, and there is no known animal reservoir *(32)*.

Epidemiological studies in Australia indicate that disease developed in patients ranging in age from 16 mo to 91 yr (mean of 47 yr and median of 49 yr), with children under 15 yr of age representing less than 4% of cases. Males outnumbered females by 3:1.

Factors predisposing to melioidosis include diabetes mellitus, alcoholism, chronic lung disease, chronic renal disease, and pregnancy. More recently cystic fibrosis has been proved to increase the risk of melioidosis, as it does for infection with *B. cepacia*. Malnutrition, trauma, HIV infection, cancer, and steroid and other immunosuppressive therapy, are most likely also risk factors. Lowered immunity also increases the risk for the fatal sepsis from melioidosis. The drink kava *(33)*, prepared from the powder of the root plant *Piper methysticum* and introduced to Aboriginal communities by missionaries as an alternative to alcohol, may also increase the risk for melioidosis.

There were 343 reports of melioidosis during the Vietnam War, with 36 deaths *(34)*. Additionally, serological surveys revealed mild or unapparent infection in many others, as 1–2% of healthy, nonwounded Army troops returning to the United States had positive serological results, indicating that as many as 225,000 military personnel may have had subclinical infection with *B. pseudomallei*. These individuals are at risk for recrudescence of disease, usually as cavitary pneumonia, and less often with symptoms of an acute pneumonia or septicemia, many years after primary infection.

## *2.5. Role in Biological Warfare and Terrorism*

State sponsors have studied *B. pseudomallei* and consider it a viable agent for weaponization because of its high mortality despite treatment and the lack of a vaccine. The United States studied *B. pseudomallei* as a potential biowarfare agent but never weaponized it. There is also evidence that the former Soviet Union experimented with *B. pseudomallei* as a biowarfare agent. A terrorist would most likely deliver *B. pseudomallei* as an aerosol. The chlorine tolerance of *B. pseudomallei* (and that of *B. mallei*) remains unknown; thus contamination of water with *Burkholderia* cannot be dismissed *(35)*.

## *2.6. Microbiological Characteristics*

*Burkholderia pseudomallei* are small (1–3 μm long × 0.5–1 μm wide), Gram-negative, motile, facultative intracellular, aerobic tiny rods that sometimes grow in filamentous chains. There are two serological types of *B. pseudomallei*, based on the presence of a thermostable antigen. Serotype 1 possesses the antigen and is predominantly present in Asia, whereas serotype 2 lacks the antigen and predominates in Australia and Africa *(36)*. Monoclonal antibodies can distinguish a related organism present in the soil of Southeast Asia, *B. thailandensis*, which is very similar phenotypically and serologically to *B. pseudomallei*; it differs significantly genetically, has the ability to assimilate arabinose, and is almost completely avirulent *(37)*, although at least one report indicates that it too can cause human disease, particularly in immunocompromised hosts *(38)*.

*Burkholderia pseudomallei* produces a thermolabile bactericidal substance that inhibits the growth of other bacteria such as *Bacillus anthracis*, *Brucella melitensis*, *Yersinia pestis*, *Escherichia coli*, and *Staphylococcus aureus* in the surrounding environmental area *(39)*.

Both *B. pseudomallei* and *B. mallei* have a polysaccharide biopolymer capsule that adversely affects phagocytosis. In addition, these bacteria produce harmful toxins such as pyocyanin (interferes with terminal electron transfer system), lecithinase, collagenase, lipase, and hemolysin.

## 2.7. Clinicopathologic Findings

The latency period of *B. pseudomallei* infection ranges from 2 d to 26 yr *(40,41)*. For inhalational exposure, the usual period of incubation is 10–14 d, but it may range from 2 d to many years. Melioidosis is a great mimicker, but most commonly it involves the lungs, where the bacterium can cause an abscess. Case reports disproportionately describe systemic infections, probably because blood isolates more frequently are properly identified than are isolates from other sites.

Illness ranges from an acute or localized infection, acute pulmonary infection, acute bloodstream infection, or chronic suppurative infection, to chronic granulomatous infection. Apparently asymptomatic infections are also possible. Severe urticaria develops in some patients. Even at an acute stage, this disease has a wide range of symptoms—from fever to chest pains to nausea—that can dupe doctors into the wrong diagnosis. For victims of this disease, the consequences of delayed or missed diagnosis can be fatal.

### 2.7.1. Acute, Localized Infection

This results from inoculation through a break in the skin. These patients generally manifest a localized nodule and may have fever with general muscle aches. In addition to the nodule, there is typically a secondary lymphangitis and regional lymphadenitis. Cutaneous lesions may progress to a form that resembles ecthyma gangrenosum. Some individuals may progress rapidly to septicemia.

### 2.7.2. Pulmonary Infection

The clinical picture ranges from mild bronchitis to severe necrotizing pneumonia. Typically inhalational melioidosis is an acute pyogenic process that can resemble plague. Patients have high fever (generally over 39°C), cough, chest pain, dyspnea, and cyanosis. Most have rigors, sweats, headache, widespread muscle soreness, cervical adenopathy, hepatomegaly, and splenomegaly. Chest pain is common, but a nonproductive or productive cough with normal sputum is characteristic of this form of melioidosis. Some may have blood-tinged sputum. Patients have signs and symptoms of consolidation, ordinarily in an upper lobe. Microscopic examination of the lungs reveals an acute hemorrhagic pneumonia (Fig. 1). Acute pulmonary infection can progress to acute septicemic disease, typically coupled with development of a generalized papular to pustular eruption

The typical patient with subacute or chronic pulmonary melioidosis presents with myalgias, anorexia, and weight loss. Chest X-rays disclose upper lobe infiltrates and/or cavitation that suggest the granulomatous disease visible on gross examination of the lungs (Fig. 2) *(42)*. Patients often progress to early cavitation that can mimic the pulmonary appearance of tuberculosis. The peripheral blood may have a normal or elevated leukocyte count.

### 2.7.3. Acute Bloodstream Infection

Patients with underlying illness such as HIV infection, renal failure, cystic fibrosis, and diabetes are at increased risk for septicemia, which usually progresses to septic shock. Deep inoculation of the bacterium through accidental trauma or deliberate injection increases the risk for systemic disease. Symptoms vary depending on the site of original infection but generally include respiratory distress, severe headache, fever, diarrhea, muscle tenderness, disorientation, and development of a papular to pustular eruption throughout the body.

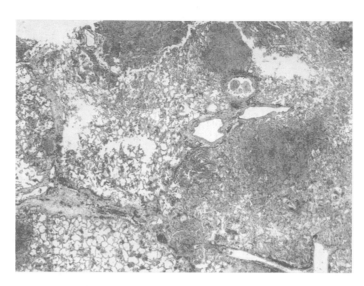

**Fig. 1.** Acute hemorrhagic pneumonia caused by *Burkholderia mallei*.

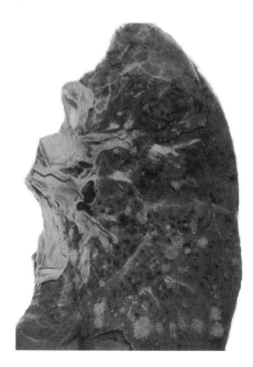

**Fig. 2.** Lung is sliced to reveal multiple granulomas causd by chronic *Burkholderia mallei*. Note most of the nodules are in the lower lobe.

### 2.7.4. CHRONIC SUPPURATIVE INFECTION

Chronic melioidosis is an infection that involves many organ systems including joints, viscera, lymph nodes (Fig. 3), skin, brain, liver, lung, bones, and spleen. Chronic melioidosis may cause osteomyelitis. It can spread from the skin through the blood to affect the heart, brain, liver, kidneys, joints, and eyes. Patients can have associated headaches, fever, chills, cough, chest pain, and/or loss of appetite.

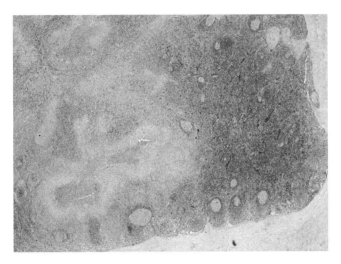

**Fig. 3.** Lymph node with suppurative granulomas caused by *Burkholderia mallei*.

### 2.7.5. NEUROLOGICAL INFECTION

Neurological melioidosis is reported most often in humans and animals in Australia; in fact, the first human diagnosed in Australia from 1950 had evidence of central nervous system involvement *(43)*. Patients with neurological melioidosis present with fever, headache, and a normal or "almost normal' initial state of consciousness. Additional symptoms may include neck stiffness, bulbar palsy, nerve VII palsy, nerve VI palsy, cerebellar signs, initial unilateral limb weakness, and (less often) initial flaccid paraparesis. Some patients require prolonged ventilation. In addition, some patients have severe peripheral motor weakness and the presence of mononuclear inflammatory cells. There seems to be a predilection for brainstem, cerebellum, and spinal cord damage. The cerebrospinal fluid shows a predominant mononuclear pleocytosis. Microabscesses form in the brain. Neurological damage may be toxin-mediated demyelination, or neurological changes could result from direct invasion *(44)*.

### 2.7.6. OTHER SITES

The melioidosis literature abounds with individual case reports in sum emphasizing that *B. pseudomallei* can cause pyogenic or granulomatous lesions at virtually any site including prostate, spleen, liver, kidney, eyes, synovium, and heart (mycotic aneurysm). Melioidosis mycotic aneurism is usually fatal.

### 2.7.7. RELAPSE

Relapse in melioidosis, following various antimicrobial regimens, reflects the ability of *B. pseudomallei* to interfere with inducible nitric oxide synthase (iNOS) production—a factor in its ability to survive within phagocytic cells *(45)*, as well as its ability to produce glycocalyx and to form microcolonies in infected tissue *(46)*. β-Lactams do not penetrate intracellular sites and kill nonmultiplying bacteria; thus therapy with β-lactams may not prevent future relapse of melioidosis. The mean time to relapse is about 21 wk.

## *2.8. Diagnosis*

Prompt diagnosis, leading to early initiation of treatment, critically influences the prognosis. The patient's history, especially travel, occupational exposure to infected animals, or a history of intravenous drug use should alert the clinician to possible exposure to *B. pseudomallei*.

Melioidosis patients who present with acute pneumonia have symptoms that can resemble those of pneumonic plague, and stained organisms of *Y. pestis* resemble those of *Burkholderia*. Staining with methylene blue or Wright's stain shows a bipolar "safety pin" pattern very similar to that of *Y. pestis*. In addition to plague, inhalational melioidosis needs to be distinguished from inhalational anthrax and inhalational tularemia *(47)*. In patients who present during the nonspecific febrile prodrome, melioidosis should be considered along with anthrax, plague, smallpox, tularemia, brucellosis, Q fever, and viral hemorrhagic fevers *(46)*.

Depending on the stage of infection, radiographs may reveal miliary lesions, small multiple lung abscesses, or infiltrates involving upper lungs, with consolidation and cavitation. Patients who present with the diffuse, pustular eruption can be mistaken for victims of varicella or smallpox. Radiographs and sonograms can help demonstrate the extent of infection *(48)*.

Isolation and identification of *B. pseudomallei* is still the method of choice for definitive confirmatory diagnosis of melioidosis. Microbiologists should suspect *B. pseudomallei* when isolation in pure or predominantly pure culture reveals the presence of a small, oxidasc-positive motile, tiny Gram-negative rod from blood, pus, sputum, urine, other fluids, or skin from anyone who has ever spent time in an endemic area. Look for colonies with a pearly sheen, a sweet earthy smell, and a variably wrinkled colonial morphology (which can be confused with an aerobic spore-bearer). Culture needs no elaborate or expensive equipment but does requires experienced personnel, particularly in the interpretation of the results. Organisms grow in 5% sheep blood agar and in MacConkey agar at 35°C (in 24–48 h). They have a characteristic antibiogram (resistant to aminoglycosides, polymyxins, fluoroquinolones, and many β-lactams, but susceptibility to chloramphenicol, tetracyclines, and co-amoxiclav) *(49)*. Many commercial biochemical test kits reliably identify the organism to species level, but referral to a reference laboratory (level 3) for confirmation is recommended. The main drawback is that identification by culture takes at least 3–4 d to obtain the results and by that time it may be too late for successful management. An automatic BacT/Alert® nonradiomatric blood culture system reportedly detects about 62% of *B. pseudomallei*-positive cultures within 24 h of incubation and more than 90% within 48 h *(50)*.

The genome of *B. pseudomallei* has been almost unraveled *(51,52)*, and now, in addition to classical microbiological procedures (microscopy, culture and biochemical identification) polymerase chain reaction (PCR) techniques exist for detection and to distinguish different *Burkholderia (53)*. Detection using molecular studies (PCR) can be done but may require bacterial concentration steps *(54)*.

A number of serological tests for the detection of specific *B. pseudomallei* antibodies exist, all of which are in need of improvement; thus serodiagnosis of melioidosis abounds with problems *(55)*. It is possible to detect early acute cases of melioidosis serologically, but negative results do not exclude the illness. Enzyme-linked immunosorbent assay (ELISA) tests have variable sensitivities and specificities depending in part on the immunoglobulin or immunoglobulin subclass detected *(56)*. A fourfold increase in the titer for melioidosis is good presumptive laboratory test. Transporting a sample from a rural clinic and then carrying out the check can often mean a delay of more than 24 h—too long if, as often happens, melioidosis has already developed into full-blown septicemia. For many patients, death arrives before the test results.

## *2.9. Treatment*

Optimal antibiotic treatment for acute severe melioidosis remains enigmatic. Ideally, antimicrobial agents used in a regimen for melioidosis would have bactericidal effect, the ability to penetrate phagocytic cells, and the ability to destroy or inhibit the production of the glycocalyx. Currently, treatment, even for localized infection, is prolonged, often requiring up to 9 mo of antibiotic therapy *(57)*, and relapses are frequent. Morbidity and mortality of relapsed disease is similar to that of primary cases. The type of infection and the course of treatment determine the risk of long-term sequelae.

*Burkholderia pseudomallei* is usually susceptible in vitro to some third-generation cephalosporins (notably ceftazidime, but also cefotaxime and ceftriaxone), ureidopenicillins, carbapenems (such as imipenem and meropenem), amoxycillin with clavulanate [= co-amoxiclav (Augmentin®)], chloramphenicol, tetracyclines, trimethoprim-sulfamethoxazole (TMP-SXT; brand names Cotrimoxazole®, Apo-Sulfatrim®, Bactrim®, Novo-Trimel®, Protrin®, Roubac®, and Septra®) *(58)*, and fluoroquinolones *(59)*.

High-dose intravenous ceftazidime, with or without TMP-SXT, is currently the treatment of choice for severe melioidosis. Treatment is typically given in two phases, an acute parenteral phase for at least 10–14 d followed by an oral maintenance phase for an additional 18 wk. Oral maintenance therapy for 3–5 mo or longer may reduce the risk of relapse *(60)*. Cefoperazone with sulbactam plus TMP-SXT appears promising. A recent randomized study of 102 confirmed melioidosis patients that compared ceftazidime plus TMP-SXT with cefoperazone-sulbactam plus TMP-SXT demonstrated that both regimens resulted in similar in-hospital mortality and time to defervescence *(61)*. Comparative trials of other antibiotics are under way. The combination of meropenem with TMP-SXT, and to a lesser extent meropenem with other drugs *(62)*, looks promising and warrants study in properly conducted randomized studies. If sputum cultures remain positive for 6 mo, consider surgical removal of the lung abscess with lobectomy.

Patients with mild illness usually do well with oral antibiotics; however, they need prolonged therapy and must take antibiotics for 3–5 mo. All patients require life-long follow-up. The treatment of relapses is identical to that of primary cases.

In vitro, *B. pseudomallei* is resistant to penicillin, amino-penicillins, first- and second-generation cephalosporins, most aminoglycosides, most macrolides and rifampicin *(63,64)*. Studies from China indicate that *B. pseudomallei* produces a β-lactamase and is often resistant to penicillin and ampicillin, as well as to methicillin, oxacillin, gentamicin, carbenicillin, streptomycin, erythromycin, albomycin, oxytetracycline, chlortetracycline, polyxin B, and cefazolin *(65)*. A randomized, open-label study of 65 patients for maintenance treatment of melioidosis demonstrated culture-proven relapse of 22% using the unusual choice of a combination of ciprofloxacin and azithromycin for 12 wk, compared with a relapse rate of 3% when investigators used a combination of cotrimoxazole and doxycycline for 20 wk *(66)*.

## *2.10. Prognosis*

Currently, if there is a rapid correct diagnosis, and appropriate treatment is given early enough, mortality is approximately 40%. Overall in-hospital mortality, however, remains nearer 50%. The prognosis for recovery from mild infections is good. Studies from Australia and Papua Guinea show an overall mortality from melioidosis of 19–21%, with a mortality rate in septicemic cases of 39% and in nonsepticemic cases of 4% *(67)*.

## 2.11. Prevention

There is no human vaccine, but there extensive research is ongoing for the production of a vaccine *(68)*. Likewise, at this time, there is no pre-exposure or postexposure prophylactic medication. Prevention in endemic disease areas is complicated because contact with contaminated soil is quite common. Individuals should avoid exposure to water and soil from disturbed areas in periods of high rainfall, particularly in tropical areas. Prompt cleansing of scrapes, burns, or other open wounds in endemic areas and avoidance of needle sharing among drug addicts reduces the danger of infection. Persons at increased risk, such as diabetics with skin lesions, should avoid contact with contaminated soil. In health care settings, using common blood and body fluid precautions can prevent transmission. Hypochlorite solution, at 0.5%, effectively decontaminates the environment. Pasteurization will decontaminate milk. In tropical areas where people consume warm goat milk, farmers are urged to test the goat herd twice a year and cull any positive animals. Slaughterhouse workers should employ basic hygiene and protective clothing. Wearing boots during agricultural work can prevent infection through the feet and lower legs. Travelers returning from rural zones in endemic areas should disinfect shoes, clothing, and other potentially contaminated apparel and equipment.

# 3. GLANDERS

## 3.1. Definition

*Burkholderia mallei*, a Gram-negative bacterium, causes glanders, a disseminated disease, and farcy, a subcutaneous and lymphatic disease. This zoonosis primarily affects equids (horses, donkeys, and mules) but also Felidae, primates, and other species—particularly carnivorous animals. In humans, glanders is a painful and loathsome disease that can be pulmonary, septicemic, or chronic. *Burkholderia mallei* is a host-adapted pathogen that does not persist in nature outside a host.

## 3.2. Synonyms

Synonyms for the infection include glanders, farcy, and malleus. Older names for *B. mallei* include *Bacillus mallei*, *Pfeifferella mallei*, *Malleomyces mallei*, and *Pseudomonas mallei*.

## 3.3. History

Knowledge of the illness caused by *B. mallei* in equids dates back to antiquity, having been described in Greco-Roman times; this organism has caused heavy losses of horses down the centuries. The German bacteriologists Friedrich Löffler and Wilhelm Schütz isolated and identified the causal agent of farcy in 1882; they named it *Bacillus mallei (69)*. Soon thereafter Löffler provided a detailed microbiological description of the agent *(70)*.

## 3.4. Epidemiology and Transmision

The epidemiologic distribution of *B. mallei* is distinctly different than that of *B. pseudomallei*. *Burkholderia mallei* exists in nature only in infected susceptible hosts and, unlike *B. pseudomallei*, it is not found in water, soil, or plants. *Burkholderia mallei* is endemic in Africa, Asia (including China, Mongolia, India, Iraq, and Turkey), parts of Europe, and the Americas (Central and South).

Individuals with occupational exposure to infected animals (veterinarians, horse and donkey caretakers, and abattoir workers) and laboratory workers are at increased risk of infection. Despite this increased risk from occupational exposure, historically, humans have seldom acquired infection from infected animals despite frequent and often close contact. This may reflect the facts that strains virulent for equids are often less virulent for humans, or that the human exposure was to only low concentrations of bacteria from ill animals, or that other unidentified host factors were involved. *Burkholderia mallei* can enter the body by invading the nasal, oral, and conjunctival mucous membranes, by inhalation, and through abraded or lacerated skin. In the United States the most recent instance of endemic glanders happened in the spring of 2000, involving a 33-yr-old microbiologist with insulin-dependent diabetes mellitus. He worked in a Department of Defense laboratory with a number of pathogens including *Bacillus anthracis*, *B. mallei*, *B. pseudomallei*, *Y. pestis*, *Coxiella burnetii*, and *Borrelia* sp., and did not routinely wear latex gloves. He developed severe pulmonary glanders with respiratory failure, which had a great systemic impact including increasing difficulty with control of his diabetes. Prior to that event there had not been an endemic case of human glanders in the United States since 1945 *(71)*.

### 3.5. Role in Biological Warfare and Terrorism

*Burkholderia mallei* has a low potential for contagion, but it became a candidate for biological warfare because of the efficacy of aerosolized dissemination and the lethal nature of the disease.

In World War I, the Central Powers used *B. mallei* against equids on the Eastern Front *(72)*, in the United States, and in Romania *(73)*. The glanders outbreak among Russian horses and mules on the Eastern Front had an effect on troop and supply convoys as well as on artillery movement, which were dependent on horses and mules. Human cases in Russia increased with the infections during and after the disease in animals.

The Japanese reportedly infected horses, civilians, and prisoners of war with *B. mallei* during World War II. The Former Soviet Union tested *B. mallei* for use in biological warfare *(74)*. In May of 1947 the American Association of Scientific Workers, with the consent of the military, released a detailed study of the menace of germ warfare. The report warned that germ weapons rival the A-bomb as "one of the most important hazards to humanity which could result from the misuse of science." Drs. Theodore Rosebury and Elvin A. Kabat of Columbia University listed 33 bacteria and viruses that have the potential to spread mass pestilence and famine from planes. Included in their report were botulinum toxin, leptospira, anthrax, pneumonic plague, undulant fever (brucellosis), glanders, influenza, malaria, melioidosis, parrot fever (psittacosis), rabbit fever (tularemia), yellow fever, and several typhus-like diseases *(75)*. The report noted that in 1943–1944 the United States studied *B. mallei* for its biowarfare potential.

The Soviets weaponized anthrax and tested it at Vozrozdeniie Island in the Aral Sea *(76)*. Then, during their war in Afghanistan, the Soviets employed glanders to kill the animal transport used by the Afghan resistance *(77)*. More recently, Dr. Alibekov (now known as Dr. Alibek), who was first deputy director of Biopreparat in charge of the civilian branch of the former Soviet Union's Biowarfare program—and who continues to monitor the work of his old colleagues—has testified that Russian scientists have created genetically altered antibiotic-resistant strains of plague, anthrax, tularemia, and glanders *(78)*. According to Igor Domaradsky, former chairman of the Soviet Interagency Science and Technology Council on Molecular Biology and Genetics, Pokrov was one of the biggest of several Soviet facilities that altogether employed some 10,000 scientists to develop antiagricultural weapons. There have been several reports of theft or diversion of dangerous pathogens from these and other Soviet facilities; this clearly provides a potential source for terrorists desiring to acquire glanders or other biological agents for weaponization *(79)*. In addition, the Monterey Institute of International Studies states that it is probable that Egypt currently has glanders in its arsenal of agricultural biowarfare agents *(80)*.

### 3.6. Microbiological Characteristics

*Burkholderia mallei* are small (1–3 μm long × 0.5–1 μm wide), Gram-negative, non-motile, aerobic rods with a polysaccharide biopolymer capsule that adversely affects phagocytosis. The amotility of *B. mallei* contrasts with the motility of *B. pseudomallei*. Curiously, despite amotility, strains of *B. mallei* have the gene for the filament forming flagellin *(fliC) (81)*. These bacteria are catalase positive and grow on MacConkey media.

### 3.7. Clinicopathological Findings

Similar to melioidosis, those infected with glanders may be asymptomatic, or may manifest a wide range of symptoms. The use of *B. mallei* in a bioterrorism event would result in significant numbers of patients presenting with acute illness, which may herald primary pulmonary infection or fulminant sepsis. Necrosis of the tracheobronchial tree and pustular skin lesions characterize acute *B. mallei* infection. Patients typically have high fevers with pneumonia, mucositis, signs of sepsis, and multiple abscesses, predominantly involving the lungs, liver, and spleen.

Similar to melioidosis, the symptoms depend on the route of *B. mallei* infection. Under natural circumstances, patients may have localized, pus-filled cutaneous lesions, pulmonary damage, bloodstream infections, and chronic suppurative infections of the skin. Similar to melioidosis, glanders generally causes fever, rigors, muscle aches, chest pain, muscle tightness, headache, and malaise. In addition, many patients complain of excessive tearing of the eyes, photophobia, and diarrhea.

The pathological damage may be acute or chronic; it may be localized to the skin or lungs or may be systemic. Infections involving the mucous membrane, eyes, nose, and respiratory tract cause increased mucus production from the affected sites.

#### 3.7.1. Localized Infections

Local ulceration develops 1–5 d after contamination of broken skin. This is characteristically accompanied by swelling of regional lymph nodes.

#### 3.7.2. Pulmonary Infections

Pulmonary disease results either from inhalation or through hematogenous spread. In most of patients the incubation period for inhalational glanders is 10–14 d. Patients may have symptoms of septicemia in conjunction with pulmonary changes. Lung damage may manifest as pneumonia, pulmonary abscesses, and occasionally pleural effusions. Typically, chest radiographs reveal 0.5–1-cm miliary lesions and/or localized infection in the lobes of the lungs. There may be consolidation or cavitation. If the disease spreads systemically, patients may manifest cutaneous pustules.

#### 3.7.3. Bloodstream Infections

Untreated, septicemia is usually fatal within 7–10 d. Patients have high fever (39°C), rigors, headache, muscle pain, jaundice, photophobia, tachycardia, and diarrhea. The skin has a generalized redness (erythroderma) and often multiple cutaneous pustules, some of which become necrotizing lesions. Abscesses form throughout the body, especially the organs of the reticuloendothelial system. Cervical adenopathy and mild hepatomegaly or splenomegaly are common. There may be leukopenia or a mild shift to the left.

### 3.7.4. Mucous Membrane Infections

This form is fatal if untreated; it usually progresses rapidly into septicemic infection, and patients succumb to septic shock. Disease begins with nasal ulcers and nodules that secrete a bloody discharge. As it becomes systemic, patients manifest a papular and/or pustular rash that can resemble the rash of smallpox. Once again, abscesses form throughout the body, especially in the lungs and organs of the reticuloendothelial system.

### 3.7.5. Chronic Infections

Some patients develop necrotizing granulomas within the muscles of the arms and legs and in organs of the reticuloendothelial system including the spleen, liver, and lung.

Among Equidae, after an incubation of about 2 wk, clinical disease manifests as septicemia with high fever (up to 41°C) followed by a thick, mucopurulent nasal discharge and respiratory signs. Infection is frequently fatal. Cutaneous (farcy), nasal, and pulmonary forms can develop simultaneously. Acute disease is most common in donkeys and mules, whereas horses often have chronic infection. Chronic disease in horses manifests as a debilitating condition with nodular or ulcerative cutaneous and nasal lesions. Infected animals may live for years and may disseminate *B. mallei*. Recovered animals often fail to develop immunity *(82)*.

## 3.8. Diagnosis

Patients may have either mild leukocytosis with a left shift or leukopenia. Methylene blue stain of exudates may reveal scant, tiny, safety pin-shaped bacilli. Blood cultures are usually negative until the patient is moribund. Chest X-ray may show miliary lesions, small multiple lung abscesses, or bronchopneumonia. Similar to melioidosis, the serological tests can assist in the diagnosis, but a negative serology does not exclude the infection. Agglutination tests require 7–10 d for confirmation; high background titers in normal sera make the tests difficult to interpret, and results often come too late for the index case. Complement fixation tests with titers greater than 1:20 provide good evidence of infection. DNA-based testing is available but is currently not FDA approved. The mallein test is used to diagnosis *Burkholderia* infection in equids. The Soviets used the word "mallein" to describe the lipopolysaccharide (LPS) they derived from *B. mallei*. Dropping a few drops of mallein into one eye of a horse, using the other eye as a control, readily reveals whether a horse has been infected with glanders; however, the antigen crossreacts, horses infected with *B. pseudomallei* also have positive results.

## 3.9. Treatment

Treatment is empirical, but a reasonable choice is to treat systemic disease for a minimum of 2 wk of parenteral therapy, followed by 6 m of oral therapy. The suggested regimen for the parenteral treatment is ceftazidime 120 mg/kg/d iv in three divided doses and TMP-SMX (TMP 8 mg/kg/d; sulfa 50 mg/kg/d) iv in four divided doses. For localized disease, treatment alternatives are 2–5 mo of amoxicillin/clavulanate 60 mg/kg/d po in three divided doses, or tetracycline 40 mg/kg/d po in three divided doses, or TMP-SMX (TMP 4 mg/kg/d, sulfa 20 mg/kg/d) po in two divided doses. Others favor streptomycin in conjunction with tetracycline or imipenem, and some have suggested mono- or polytherapy with ceftazidime, sulfadizine, TMP-SMX, gentamicin, or imipenem. The most recent patient with glanders in the United States had a rapid improvement after 2 wk of parenteral treatment with imipenem and doxycycline, which was followed by 6 mo of oral therapy *(83)*.

### *3.10. Prevention*

There is no vaccine. Prevention and control depend on early detection, slaughter of infected animals, and proper cleaning and disinfection of the affected premises. This policy permitted the eradication of glanders from the United States, Great Britain, and Canada. Laboratory workers and researchers handling *Burkholderia* should pay close attention to biosafety precautions and should adhere to protocols. Researchers and laboratory workers should be aware of the signs and symptoms of the diseases caused by the organisms they handle and, if they are not disabled by disease, take responsibility for notifying their health care providers about their exposure. A worthy recommendation is the use of medical alert tags for those with occupational exposure *(84)*.

## REFERENCES

1. Yabuuchi E, Kosako Y, Oyaizu H, et al. Proposal of *Burkholderia* gen. nov. and transfer of seven species of the genus *Pseudomonas* homology group II to the new genus, with the type species *Burkholderia cepacia* (Palleroini and Holmes 1981) comb. nov. Microbiol Immunol 1992;36:1251–1275.
2. Anuntagool N, Sirisinha S. Antigenic relatedness between *Burkholderia pseudomallei* and *Burkholderia mallei*. Microbiol Immunol 2002;46:143–150.
3. Rogul M, Brendle JJ, Haapala DK, Alexander AD. Nucleic acid similarities among *Pseudomonas pseudomallei*, *Pseudomonas multivorans*, and *Actinobacillus mallei*. J Bacteriol 1970;101:827–835.
4. Khan SA, Levitt AM, Sage MJ, and the Centers for Disease Control and Prevention strategic Planning Working Group. Biological and chemical terrorism: strategic plan for preparedness and response. Recommendations of the CDC Strategic Planning Workgroup. MMWR 2000;49:1–14. Updated at: http://www.bt.cdc.gov/agent/agentlist.asp (Oct. 2002).
5. World Health Organization. International Statistical Classification of Diseases and Related Health Problems, 10th revision, vol. 1. WHO, Geneva, 1992.
6. Stanton AT, Fletcher W. Melioidosis. Studies from the Institute of Medical Research, Federated Malay States, vol 21. Bale and Danielson, Kuala Lumpur, Malaysia, 1932.
7. Huang CT. What is *Pseudomonas pseudomallei*? Elixir 1976;70–72.
8. Choy JL, Mayo M, Janmaat A, Currie BJ. Animal melioidosis in Australia. 2000;74:153–158.
9. Whitmore A, Krishnaswami CS. Account of the discovery of a hitherto undescribed infective disease occurring among the population of Rangoon. Indian Med Gaz 1912;47:262–267.
10. Whitmore A. An account of a glanders-like disease occurring in Rangoon. J Hyg 1913;XIII:1–34.
11. Stanton AT, Fletcher W. Melioidosis and its relation to glanders. J Hyg 1925;23:347–363.
12. Green R, Mankikar DS. A febrile case of melioidosis. BMJ 1945;1:308–311.
13. Chittivej C, Buspavanij S, Chaovanasai A. Melioidosis with case report in Thai. R Thai Army Med J 1955;8:11–18.
14. Weber DR, Douglas LE, Brundage WG, Stallkamp TC. Acute varieties of melioidosis occurring in U.S. soldiers in Vietnam. Am J Med 1969;46:234–244.
15. Suputtamongkol Y, Hall AJ, Dance DAB, Chaowagul W, Rajchanuvong A, Smith MD, White NJ. The epidemiology of melioidosis in Ubon Ratchatani, northeast Thailand. Int J Epidemiol 1994;23:1082–1090.
16. Dharakul T, Songsivilai S. Recent developments in the laboratory diagnosis of melioidosis. J Infect Dis Antimicrob Agents 1996;13:77–80.
17. Yang S. Melioidosis research in China. Acta Trop 2000;77:157–165.
18. Leelarasamee A. Melioidosis in Southeast Asia. Acta Trop 2000;74:129–132.
19. Dance, DAB. Melioidosis as an emerging global problem. Acta Trop 2000;74:115–119.

20. Heng BH, Goh KT, Yap EH, Loh H, Yeo M. Epidemiological surveillance of melioidosis in Singapore. Ann Acad Med Singapore 1998;27:478–484.
21. Dance DAB, King C, Aucken H, Knott CD, West PG, Pitt TL. An outbreak of melioidosis in imported primates in Britain. Vet Rec 1992;130:525–529.
22. Kibbler CC, Roberts CM, Ridgway GL, Spiro SG. Melioidosis in a patient from Bangladesh. Postgrad Med J 1991;67:764–766.
23. Dance DAB. Ecology of *Burkholderia pseudomallei* and the interactions between environmental *Burkholderia* spp. and human-animal hosts. Acta Trop 2000;74:159–168.
24. Brett PJ, DeShazer D, Woods DE. *Burkholderia thailandensis* sp. nov., a *Burkholderia pseudomallei*-like species. Int J Syst Bacteriol 1998;48:317–320.
25. Mollaret HH. 'L'affaire du Jardin des plantes' ou comment la mélioïdose fit son apparition en France. Med Mal Infect 1988;18:64–654
26. Suputtamongkol Y, Hall AJ, Dance DAB, et al. The epidemiology of melioidosis in Ubon Ratchatani, northeast Thailand. Int J Epidemiol 1994;23:1082–1090.
27. Torrens JK, McWhinney PHM, Tompkins DS. A deadly thorn: a case of imported melioidosis. Lancet 1999;353:1016.
28. Pruekprasert P, Jitsurong S. Septicemic melioidosis following near-drowning. Southeast Asian J Trop Med Public Health 1991;22:276–278.
29. Fournier J, Chambon L. La Mélioïdose et le Bacille de Whitmore. Éditions Médicales Flammarion, Paris, 1958.
30. Schlech WF, Turchik JB, Westlake RE, Klein GC, Band JD, Weaver RE. Laboratory-acquired infection with *Pseudomonas pseudomallei* (melioidosis). N Engl J Med 1981;305:113–1135.
31. Kunakorn M, Jayanetra P, Tanphaichitra D. Man-to-man transmission of melioidosis. Lancet 1991;33:1290–1291.
32. Dharakul T, Songsivilai S. The many facets of melioidosis. Trends Microbiol 1999;7:138–140.
33. Spillane PK, Fisher DA, Currie BJ. Neurological manifestations of kava intoxication. Med J Aust 1997;167:172–173.
34. Howe C, Sampath A, Spotnitz M. The pseudomallei group: a review. J Infect Dis 1971;124:598–606.
35. Jane's Chem-Bio Web. (2002) Features: Is it Safe to Drink the Water? The Chemical and Biological Threat to the U.S. Water Infrastructure. 02 July. Available to subscribers at: http://www4.janes.com (Accessed 22 November 2002).
36. Dodlin A. Antignes précipitait et antigens agglutinants de *Pseudomonas pseudomallei*. Ann De Limistitat Pasteur 1970;119:211–221.
37. Thepthai C, Dharakul T, Smithikarn S, Trakulsomboon S, Songsivilai S. Differentiation between non-virulent and virulent *Burkholderia pseudomallei* with monoclonal antibodies to the Ara+ or Ara− biotypes. Am J Trop Med Hyg 2001;65:10–12.
38. Lertpatanasuwan N, Sermsri K, Petkaseam Λ, Trakulsomboon S, Thamlikitkul, V, Suputtamongkol Y. Arabinose-positive *Burkholderia pseudomallei* infection in humans: case report. Clin Infect Dis 1999;28:927–928.
39. Li L, Chenyin S. Restricting property of *Pseudomonas pseudomallei* to the growth of other kinds of bacterial species. Chin J Zoonosis 1988;4:56–57.
40. Smith CJ, et al. Human melioidosis: an emerging medical problem. MIRCEN J 1987;3:343–366.
41. Mays EE, Ricketts EA. Melioidosis: recrudescence associated with bronchogenic carcinoma twenty-six years following initial geographic exposure. Chest 1975;68:261–263.
42. Everett ED, Nelson RA. Pulmonary melioidosis. Observations in thirty-nine cases. Am Rev Respir Dis 1975;112:331–340.
43. Rimington RA. Melioidosis in Northern Queensland. Med J Aust 1962;1:50–53.
44. Currie BJ, Fisher DA, Howard DM, Burrow JNC. Neurological melioidosis. Acta Trop 2000;74:145–151.
45. Utaisincharoen P, Tangthawornchaikul N, Kespichayawattana W, Chaisuriya P, Sirisinha S. *Burkholderia pseudomallei* interferes with inducible nitric oxide synthase (iNOS) production: a possible mechanism of evading macrophage killing. Microbiol Immunol 2001;45:307–313.
46. Vorachit M, Lam K, Jayanetra P, Costerton JW. Electron microscopy study of the mode of growth of *Pseudomonas pseudomallei* in vitro and in vivo. J Trop Med Hyg 1995;98:379–391.
47. Henretig FM, Cieslak TJ, Kortepeter MG, Fleisher GR. Medical management of the suspected victim of bioterrorism: an algorithmic approach to the undifferentiated patient. Emerg Med Clin North Am 2002;20:351–364.

48. Wibulpolprasert B, Dhiensiri T. Visceral organ abscesses in melioidosis: sonographic findings. J Clin Ultrasound 1999;27:29–34.
49. Dance DAB, Smith MD, Aucken HM, Pitt TL. Imported melioidosis in England and Wales. Lancet 1999;353:208.
50. Tiangpitayakor C, Songsivilai S, Piyasangthong N, Dharakul T. Speed of detection of *Burkholderia pseudomallei* in blood cultures and its correlation with the clinical outcome. Am J Trop Med Hyg 1997;57:96–99.
51. Songsivilai S, Dharakul T. Multiple replicons constitute the 6.5-megabase genome of *Burkholderia pseudomallei*. Acta Trop 2000;74:169–179.
52. Pitt TL, Trakulsomboon S, Dance DAB. Molecular phylogeny of *Burkholderia pseudomallei*. Acta Trop 2000;74:181–185.
53. Wongratanacheewin S, Komutrin K, Sermswan RW. Use of multiplex PCR patterns as genetic markers for *Burkholderia pseudomallei*. Acta Trop 2000;74:193–199.
54. Kunakorn M, Raksakait K, Sethaudom C, Sermswan RW, Dharakul T. Comparison of three PCR primer sets for diagnosis of septicemic melioidosis. Acta Trop 2000;74:247–251.
55. Sirisinha S, Anuntagool N, Dharakul T, et al. Recent developments in laboratory diagnosis of melioidosis. Acta Trop 2000;74:23–245.
56. Chenthamarakshan V, Kumutha MV, Vadivelu J, Puthucheary SD. Distribution of immunoglobulin classes and IgG subclasses against a culture filtrate antigen of *Burkholderia pseudomallei* in melioidosis patients J Med Microbiol 2001;50:55–61.
57. Tanphaichitra D, Srimuang S. Cellular immunity in tuberculosis, melioidosis, pasteurellosis, penicilliosis and role of levamisole and isoprinosine. Dev Biol Stand 1984;57:117–123.
58. Dance DAB, Wuthiekanun V, Chaowagul W, White NJ. The antimicrobial susceptibility of *Pseudomonas pseudomallei*. Emergence of resistance in-vitro and during treatment. J Antimicrob Chemother 1989;24:29–309.
59. Ashdown LR. In-vitro activities of the β-lactam and quinolone agents against *Pseudomonas pseudomallei*. J Antimicrob Agents Chemother 1988;32:1435.
60. Chaowagul W. Recent advances in the treatment of severe melioidosis. Acta Trop 2000;74:133–137.
61. Chetchotisakd P, Porramatikul S, Mootsikapun P, Anunnatsiri S, Thinkhamrop B. Randomized, double-blind, controlled study of cefoperazone-sulbactam plus cotrimoxazole versus ceftazidime plus cotrimoxazole for the treatment of severe melioidosis. Clin Infect Dis 2001;33:29–34.
62. Inglis TJ, Golledge CL, Clair A, Harvey J. Case report: recovery from persistent septicemic melioidosis. Am J Trop Med Hyg 2001;65:76–82.
63. Dance DAB, Wuthiekanun V, Chaowagul W, White NJ. The antimicrobial susceptibility of *Pseudomonas pseudomallei*. Emergence of resistance In-vitro and during treatment. J Antimicrob Chemother 1989;24:295–309.
64. Leelarasamee A, Bovornkitti S. Melioidosis: review and update. Rev Infect Dis 1989;11:413–425.
65. Li L, Zhenzi L, Ouer H, Yutu J. Investigation of endemic areas of melioidosis. Chin J Prev Med 1981;15:1–5.
66. Chetchotisakd P, Chaowagul W, Mootsikapun P, Budhsarawong D, Thinkamrop B. Maintenance therapy of melioidosis with ciprofloxacin plus azithromycin compared with cotrimoxazole plus doxycycline. Am J Trop Med Hyg 2001;64:24–27.
67. Currie BJ, Fisher DA, Howard DM, et al. The epidemiology of melioidosis in Australia and Papua New Guinea. Acta Trop 2000;74:121–127.
68. Iliukhin VI, Kislichkin NN, Merinova LK, et al. Perspektivy razrabotki zhivykh vaktsin dlia profilaktiki melioidoza. (Russian) (The outlook for the development of live vaccines for the prevention of melioidosis) Zh Mikrobiol Epidemiol Immunobiol 1999;3:52–55.
69. Boerner O. A preliminary report on work by the Imperial Health Care Office leading to discovery of the glanders bacillus. Dtsch Med Wochenschr (German) 1882;52:707–708.
70. Löffler F. Die Aetiologie der Rotzkrankheit. Arb Kais Gesundh Berlin 1886;1:141–198.
71. Howe C, Miller WR. Human glanders: report of six cases. Ann Intern Med 1947;26:93–115.
72. Lehavi O, Aizenstien O, Katz LH, Houvitz A. Glanders–a potential disease for biological warfare in humans and animals. Harefuah 2002;141(spec. no. 88–99):119.
73. Wheelis M. First shots fired in biological warfare. Nature 1998;395:213–213.
74. Housden T. Analysis: Threat from weapon stockpiles. BBC news. Tuesday, 30 October, 2001. http://news.bbc.co.uk/1/hi/world/europe/1628486.stm.
75. Arts and Science: Germ Warfare; Other Developments (May 18, 1947) World News Digest.

76. Jane's Chem-Bio Web. (2001) News, Special Report: Have Soviet-era Bio-weapons Infected Afghan Refugees? 14 November. Available to subscribers at: http://www4.janes.com (Accessed 22 November, 2002).
77. Margolis E. (1999) Biological Weaponry of Russia and China Poses Vicious Threat. Toronto Sun 20 May. Available at: http://www.rense.com/politics4/biowp.htm (Accessed 23 November, 2002).
78. Russia Reform Monitor, no. 422 March 31, 1998 American Foreign Policy Council, Washington, D.C. Available at http://www.afpc.org/rrm/rrm422.htm (Accessed 23 November, 2002).
79. Jane's Chem-Bio Web. (2002) News , Russian Biological Weapons Materials: The Price of Non-proliferation. 12 September. Available to subscribers at: http://www4.janes.com (Accessed 23 November, 2002).
80. Monterey Institute of International Studies. (2002) Chemical and Biological Weapons Resource Page. Agro-terrorism. Agricultural Biowarfare: State Programs to develop Offensive Capabilities. Available at http://cns.miis.edu/research/cbw/agprogs.htm (Accessed 23 November, 2002).
81. Sprague LD, Zysk G, Hagen RM, et al. A possible pitfall in the identification of *Burkholderia mallei* using molecular identification systems based on the sequence of the flagellin fliC gene. FEMS Immunol Med Microbiol 2002;34:231–236.
82. Aiello SE, Mays A, eds. The Merck Veterinary Manual, 8th ed. Merck & Co., Whitehouse Station, NJ, 1998.
83. Srinivasan A, Kraus CN, DeShazer D, et al. Glanders in a military research microbiologist. N Engl J Med 2001;345:256–258.
84. DeShazer D, Thomas D, Srinivasan A. Glanders in a military research microbiologist [Correspondence]. N Engl J Med 2001;345:1644.

# 11

## Botulinum Toxins

*Naomi E. Aronson, MD, FACP*

The opinions and assertions contained herein are those of the author and are not to be construed as official or as representing the position of the Department of the Army or the Department of Defense.

### CONTENTS

## 1. INTRODUCTION

Botulism, a clinical intoxication, was named from *botulus* (Latin for sausage) after a late 18th century German outbreak caused by blood sausage. Since World War I, outbreaks in the United States have been commonly associated with the home preservation of vegetables and fish. In Europe, home-cured ham and sausage are more frequent vehicles. *Clostridium botulinum* is an anaerobic organism that is widespread in soil and salt water and freshwater mud. It forms heat-resistant spores. Eight distinct protein toxins from germinating spores have been described; A, B, C1, C2, D, E, F, and G. Regional differences are noted, with type A predominating in the western United States, B in the eastern United States and Europe, and E in the Great Lakes, Alaska, and Southeast Asia areas.

Botulinum toxin is exceedingly potent: 0.1–1 μg of toxin is known to kill [0.001 μg/kg being the median lethal dose ($LD_{50}$)] *(1)*. Because of this deadly neurotoxicity, botulinum toxin has been considered a biological weapons agent. In 1935, Major Shiro Ishiri (head of Biowarfare Unit 731, Japan) fed botulinum toxin to prisoners in Manchuria with lethal results *(2)*. At Porton Down, UK, BTX toxins were developed, and some suggest that

From: *Physician's Guide to Terrorist Attack*
Edited by: M. J. Roy © Humana Press Inc., Totowa, NJ

botulinum toxin may have had a role in Reinhard Heydrich's assassination in 1942 *(3)*. Concern that Germany might have weaponized botulinum toxin led the Allies to prepare more than a million doses of botulinum vaccine for D-Day in Normandy *(2)*. The United States worked on the weaponization of botulinum toxin during World War II and through the 1960s, with microencapsulation techniques expanding the environmental persistence. Botulinum toxin was tested at the Soviet site Aralsk-7 on Vozrozhdeniye Island, and toxin gene splicing into other bacteria was reported *(2)*. In the 1980s, French police found a bathtub operation making botulinum toxin during a raid against a Red Army Faction in Paris *(4)*. Aum Shinrikyo, the cult responsible for the sarin gas attack on the Tokyo subway, unsuccessfully aerosolized anthrax and botulinum toxins in Tokyo several times between 1990 and 1995 *(5)*. Iraq produced 20,000 L (three times the amount needed to kill all humankind by inhalation) of botulinum toxin solution in 1989–1990, using 12,000 L in field tests or to fill warheads *(6)*. It is estimated that 8 kg of concentrated botulinum toxin, dispersed over 100 $km^2$, will deliver a median lethal dose to the entire unprotected population located there *(7)*.

Botulinum toxin is a category A (highest priority) biological agent in the CDC categories of risk. This category applies to organisms that spread easily, cause high death rates, can panic and disrupt society, and need special public health preparedness *(8)*. An aerosolized attack is the most likely scenario for the deliberate release of botulinum toxin, but the agent could also be used to sabotage food *(2)*. In an aerosolized attack, toxin particles would be 0.1–0.3 μm in size, and 1 g could kill up to 1.5 million persons *(9)*. Since botulinum toxin is quickly denatured in chlorine (84% inactivated at 20 min of 0.4% mg/L free available chlorine, similar to U.S. municipal water treatment) and by sunlight in 1–3 h, a water release was postulated to be of limited potency *(10)*.

## 2. THE TOXIN

Botulinum toxin is one of the most toxic substances (by weight) known *(1)*. The lethal inhalation dose is estimated at 0.7–0.9 ng *(2)*. Ingestion of toxin has greater efficacy than injection or entry through wounds or inhalation: the toxin does not penetrate intact skin. *C. botulinum* spores are highly heat resistant and may survive boiling for 3–4 h. Spores are killed by chlorine but are resistant to ultraviolet light, phenols, desiccation, and irradiation. In contrast, the toxin is heat labile and can be inactivated at more than 85°C for 5 min *(10)*. Besides *C. botulinum*, *C. baratii* (toxin F) and *C. butyricum* (toxin E) have been reported to cause human botulism. Limited cross-neutralization between the eight antigenically distinct toxin types has been found *(2)*.

Botulinum toxin is a dichain polypeptide, consisting of a heavy chain (100 kD) linked with a 50-kD light chain. The toxin light chain is a zinc-containing endopeptidase, which interferes with the synaptic vesicle's fusion with the terminal membrane of a motor neuron, functionally denervating it *(2)*. The endopeptidase cleaves specific sites on the synaptic fusion complex SNARE proteins (soluble *N*-ethylmaleimide-sensitive fusion factor attachment protein receptor). Recovery comes after the neuron grows new axons, which starts within 2 d of toxin exposure, but it may take months to complete. Botulinum toxin (Botox®, Myobloc®, Dysport®) is approved by the Food and Drug Administration (FDA) for therapeutic use. One vial has about 0.3% of a lethal inhalation dose, or 0.005% of a lethal oral dose *(2)*.

## 3. EPIDEMIOLOGY

A person can be exposed to botulinum toxin in several ways. Toxin can be ingested (foodborne botulism) or inhaled (bioterrorism) or can come from intestinal organisms that produce toxin locally (infant botulism); devitalized tissue with *C. botulinum* can produce toxin locally (wound botulism), or toxin can be injected (therapeutic botulism). Foodborne botulism requires that food ingested be contaminated by preformed botulinum toxin. Multiple factors are involved including contamination of food with *C. botulinum* spores and inadequate food preservation and reheating (78.5°C for at least 5 min). Permissive environments for the germination of spores and toxin production include temperatures in excess of 10°C, pH 4.6–4.8, anaerobic environment, and some water content.

In the United States, the geographic distribution of botulism was reported (1899–1996) to be 86% type A outbreaks west of the Mississippi River, 61% type B outbreaks east of the Mississippi River, and 84% type E outbreaks in Alaska. The median number of cases of foodborne botulism (1973–1996) annually reported to the Centers for Disease Control and Prevention (CDC) was 24, the mean number of outbreaks/year (1950–1996) was 9.4, and the mean number of persons/outbreak was 2.5 *(11)*. Worldwide, an average of 449 outbreaks are reported, with 930 cases annually *(12)*. Poland had the most cases, with 448 in 1984–1987 *(12)*. Of those worldwide cases for which a toxin is identified, 34% are type A, 52% type B, and 12% type E *(13)*. More than 90% of foodborne botulism worldwide is attributed to home-prepared or home-preserved foods, especially vegetables such as asparagus, green beans, beets, and corn. Many commercially produced, but not preserved, foods have been associated with outbreaks including salsa, sealed foil-baked potato, hazelnut yogurt, peanuts in jar, garlic in oil, sautéed onions, commercially made cheese sauce, traditionally prepared salted or fermented fish, restaurant canned jalapeño peppers, cream cheese, canned macrobiotic food, potato salad, commercial pot pie, and skordalia made with potato. A reported unusual vehicle was ceremonial peyote tea. Among Alaskan Natives, consumption of fermented meat and fish (stink heads, stink eggs) made when modern technology (e.g., plastic) intersects with traditional preparation, has led to many cases of type E botulism.

Wound botulism is much less common; *C. botulinum* can infect a wound and produce a toxin. The wounds themselves often appear uninfected. The median incubation period, if the wound was trauma-associated, has been 7 d. Wounds are usually avascular, often soil contaminated, and include deep puncture wounds, compound fractures, gunshot wounds, severe "road rash," or extensive crush injury. Other reported instances of wound botulism include associations with tooth abscess, sinusitis in a nasal cocaine abuser, and postoperative intestinal surgery *(14)*. The correlation of wound botulism with injectable drug use (especially black tar heroin from Mexico) through skin-popping and intravenous injection was noted more recently *(15)*. During 1986–1996 in the United States, 78 cases of wound botulism were reported to the CDC, mostly in injection drug users *(11)*.

Infant botulism is currently the leading form of botulism reported to the CDC. First recognized in 1976, 1442 cases were reported between 1976 and 1996. California (47% of cases), Utah, Delaware, and Hawaii had the highest incidence rates (range 5.7–9/100,000 live births) *(11)*. Infant botulism is caused when an infant (mean onset of age 13 wk, range 1–63 wk) ingests *C. botulinum* spores, which subsequently germinate and make toxin. The illness usually starts with constipation, a weak cry, poor suck/slowed feeding, and then hypotonia ("floppy baby"), weakness, neuromuscular paralysis, and ventilatory failure. Sources of spores are not usually known, but honey has been implicated *(16)*. Breast-feeding, constipation (chronically less than one bowel movement per day), and corn syrup are suggested as risk factors *(17)*. Cases of intestinal botulism in adults have occurred with a similar pathogenesis; most have been postoperatively, after antibiotics, or in the setting of inflammatory bowel disease *(18)*.

Inhalation of botulinum toxin suggests dispersion as a biological weapon. Aerosolized exposure of Rhesus monkeys to botulinum toxin A, at 5–10 times the $LD_{50}$, resulted in death in 2–4 d. Observed symptoms were muscular weakness, ptosis, and mouth breathing around 12–18 h before death, and then serous nasal discharge, salivation, rales, generalized weakness, and recumbency *(19)*. Another study showed that aerosol challenge of toxin serotypes C, D, and G are toxic to Rhesus macaques *(3)*. One accidental human botulinum toxin inhalation exposure has been reported from a German laboratory in 1962, among three lab workers. They were apparently exposed to botulinum toxin aerosolized from the coated fur of rabbits and guinea pigs. Symptoms occurred 3 d after exposure, and botulinum toxin was found in the sera of all who were exposed *(3)*.

Purified botulinum toxin [type A (Botox®, Allergen Inc.; Dysport®, Europe) and type B (Myobloc®, Elan Pharmaceutics)] has been approved by the FDA for therapy of blepharospasm, strabismus, cervical dystonia, and recently for the cosmesis of "frown lines" *(20–22)*. Off-label use has been extensive, for purposes such as laryngeal dystonia, cerebral palsy, migraine headaches, and facial twitches. Because of the low dose per vial, this commercially available form of botulinum toxin is not likely to be used as a weapon. It is estimated that at least 10 times a therapeutic dose would have to enter the circulation to give systemic symptoms. The new drug application cites an $LD_{50}$ for monkeys as approximately 40 U/kg by intramuscular injection *(21,22)*. The overall adverse event rates suggest that dry mouth and dysphagia are the most prominent and dose related. Transient ptosis was common (30%) in clinical trials for blepharospasm. Antibody formation was seen in 20%, increasing with repeat administration.

Having described the epidemiology of botulism recently, what features should raise concern for a bioterrorist release of botulinum toxin? These features include a simultaneous outbreak of large numbers of cases of afebrile, flaccid paralysis and cranial nerve palsies, unusual botulinum toxin types (C, D, F, G), a common geographic exposure but not a common dietary exposure, or several simultaneous outbreaks without a common source *(2)*. Botulism is not transmitted person to person. However, a microbe that was intentionally modified to make botulinum toxin might be contagious, so this must be considered in a deliberate release situation. Also, in an inhalational exposure, animals may also be affected. Animals are susceptible to botulism, and the clinical features are similar. Wild waterfowl (into the millions) have succumbed to type C botulism; this can sometimes be a problem in chickens (a condition known as *limberneck*) *(12)*.

## 4. CLINICAL PRESENTATION

### Case Vignette

A 47-year-old man presented to the emergency room (ER) complaining of double vision and dizziness developing over the past day. A close friend of his had recently been hospitalized in an intensive care unit because "he stopped breathing." He was assessed as having a normal physical examination and sent home with the discharge diagnosis of hysteria.

Two days later, a state health officer notified the individual that he had potentially been exposed to food implicated in his friend's illness (clinical botulism). The patient was then admitted to the hospital with approximately 3 days of symptoms, about 5 days after ingestion of normal-tasting home-canned jalapeño peppers during a meal shared with the friend who developed botulism. Since the ER visit, he had noted mild improvement in his dizzy feeling, but his vision was blurred and horizontally double. He denied headache, gastrointestinal symptoms, weakness, trouble talking, or swallowing. He had no prior significant medical history.

On physical examination he was cognitively intact and afebrile, with a supple neck. His examination showed normal-sized, reactive pupils, no ptosis, and paresis of the left medial rectus muscle. Sensory examination was intact, and deep tendon reflexes were 2+ bilaterally. No motor strength weakness was noted, and cerebellar function was normal. Initial laboratory testing was normal, including a complete blood count, serum electrolytes, magnesium, calcium, lactate dehydrogenase, and aminotransferase levels. A cranial computed tomography scan (with contrast) was normal. A lumbar puncture was performed, and cerebrospinal fluid showed 2 white blood cells/cmm, protein 28 mg/dL. Stool and serum were sent to the state health laboratory for mouse inoculation/botulinum toxin testing. Stool culture grew *Clostridium botulinum*. The stool was later found to contain type A botulinum toxin. Contents from the jar of jalapeños also demonstrated type A botulinum toxin.

After discussion with the Centers for Disease Control and Prevention and the state health department, a decision was made not to give the patient trivalent botulinum antitoxin, as his symptoms were mild and appeared to be improving. After 5 days of hospitalization, his ophthalmoplegia resolved, and he was discharged. He noted some fatigue on a 2-week follow-up but was otherwise back to baseline.

Testing for botulinum toxin will take days; therefore a clinical diagnosis is made on the basis of observed symptoms (Fig. 1). The characteristics of botulism include an afebrile, alert patient with an acute illness beginning with cranial nerve palsies followed by a symmetric, descending flaccid paralysis. Based on the level of toxin exposure, the interval from exposure to symptoms varies from 12 to 36 h (with a reported range of 6 h to 10 d) *(11)*. Foodborne, intestinal, wound, and inhalational exposures to botulinum toxin all present in a similar fashion, except that foodborne botulism may have more initial gastrointestinal symptoms such as nausea, vomiting, constipation, and/or diarrhea. Wound botulism may have a longer incubation period, up to 14 days *(14)*. Symptoms described in more than 50% of patients include dry mucous membranes (can see fissured tongue/pharyngeal pain), anticholinergic symptoms such as ileus, urinary retention, mydriasis, other ocular findings of blurred vision, diplopia, ptosis, dysphonia, dysphagia, dysarthria, dizziness, fatigue, neck or truncal weakness, or dyspnea *(23)*. Typical signs of accessory respiratory muscle use, restlessness, and gasping are unusual owing to weakened musculature, and precipitous respiratory deterioration can occur, so this should be followed by measurement of vital capacity *(24)*. In general, mental status changes, fever (unless aspiration pneumonitis is present), and paresthesias are unusual in botulism. Progressive paralysis descends, affecting first the cranial nerves, then the neck, the upper arms, the trunk, the diaphragm, the hands and legs, and last the fingers.

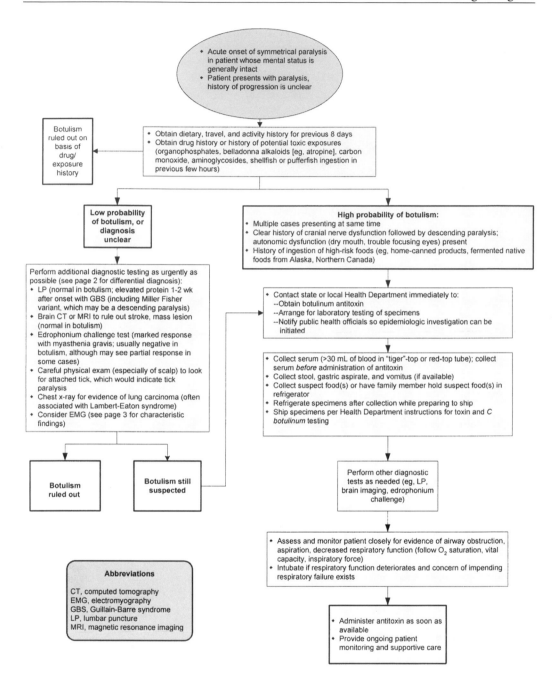

**Fig. 1.** Clinical pathway: botulism. Copyright 2002 Center for Infectious Disease Research & Policy, University of Minnesota (www.cidrap.umn.edu) and the Infectious Diseases Society of America (www.idsociety.org) . Reprinted by permission.

The physical examination generally shows absence of elevated temperature, intact mental status (although bulbar dysfunction can impair oral communication), and a normal sensory examination. Postural hypotension may be present. Frequent signs include skeletal muscle weakness (upper extremities > lower extremities), extraocular muscle palsies, decreased gag reflex, hypotonia, and ocular findings including ptosis, abnormal papillary response to light and/or accommodation, nystagmus, and mydriasis *(25)*. Deep tendon reflexes may be diminished in affected muscle groups but are often normal initially. Mucous membranes can be very dry, with crusting or fissures. Facial palsy, tongue weakness, and loss of head control (wobbly head) may be noted. Respiratory failure may occur precipitously, and death results from airway obstruction (upper airway muscle paralysis) and diaphragmatic/accessory respiratory muscle paralysis. With modern intensive care, case fatality rates vary from 5 to 10% for foodborne botulism to 15 to 44% for wound botulism *(9)*. The rate is higher in patients over 60 yr of age, those with rapid incubation periods, and index cases *(26)*. Very limited information exists on inhalational botulism in humans. Three laboratory workers, exposed to aerosol from animal fur, experienced symptoms within 3 d starting as a sensation of mucous plugging in the throat, trouble swallowing solids, and an upper respiratory infection sensation without fever. On d 4, mental numbness and slowed eye movement, mydriasis, and nystagmus were noted, speech was indistinct, gait uncertain, and weakness noted. Antitoxin given on d 4/5 resulted in reduced symptoms, with marked improvement by 2 wk *(3)*.

Laboratory findings in botulism include a normal complete blood count, serum chemistries, and central nervous system imaging with computed tomography/magnetic resonance imaging. Cerebrospinal fluid shows a normal glucose, protein, and cell count. Electrodiagnostic findings in botulism include normal sensory and motor conduction velocities, small M-wave amplitudes, increases in M-wave amplitude with repetitive nerve stimuli (20 or 50 Herz) or after exercise, short duration, low-amplitude motor unit action potential, increased jitter and blocking by single-fiber electromyography (EMG), and decreased compound muscle action potential after single-nerve stimuli. Multiple muscles should be tested since this varies *(27,28)*.

The course of botulism can be affected by the dose of ingested toxin, host characteristics, and the administration of botulinum antitoxin. There seem to be some toxin differences, with type E having a shorter incubation period, type B having the longest, and type A being associated with more severe illness (more likely to require intubation) *(9,26,29,30)*. Respiratory failure is one of the most severe complications. Duration of required ventilator support can be prolonged (usually 2–8 wk, up to months), and clinical recovery depends on the formation of new presynaptic endplates and neuromuscular junctions. In general, early botulism deaths occur from lack of recognition of the disease severity, and deaths occurring after 2 wk arise from complications of the intensive care unit (ICU) admission and long-term mechanical ventilation *(2)*. Aspiration pneumonia in patients with decreased gag reflex and respiratory failure constitutes a significant complication. Some have a persistent ileus, which can delay the onset of feeding. Residual symptoms with slow recovery have been recorded; autonomic and muscle symptoms (including exercise intolerance, dry eyes and mouth, difficulty swallowing, and weakness) persist in some for years *(30,31)*. Psychological sequelae can require specific intervention. Two studies have demonstrated that despite residual symptoms at 1–2 yr (fatigue, dyspnea), pulmonary function tests were fairly normal for most patients, with mean performances generally within normal limits *(32,33)*.

Table 1
Differential Diagnosis of Botulism

Guillain-Barré syndrome (Miller-Fisher variant)
Myasthenia gravis
Lambert-Eaton syndrome
Brain stem infarction or infection
Anticholinergic excess (atropine, jimson weed, belladonna, phenothiazine idiopathic reaction)
Diphtheria
Tick paralysis
Paralytic shellfish poisoning (saxitoxin)
Poliomyelitis
Organophosphate poisoning
Neurotoxic snake bite
Carcinomatosis of the cranial nerves
Acute intermittent porphyria
Hypermagnesemia
Psychiatric illness (conversion reaction)

## 5. DIFFERENTIAL DIAGNOSIS

Aside from an exposure history, botulism should be considered when evaluating a flaccid descending paralysis with cranial nerve palsies and a lack of sensory involvement. A cluster of cases should suggest this diagnosis *(34,35)*. A discussion of some of the more common similarly appearing illnesses follows (Table 1). Guillain-Barré syndrome (Miller-Fisher variant) may be differentiated by an elevated cerebrospinal fluid protein (although this may be normal initially), the presence of paresthesias, or EMG without facilitation after repetitive nerve stimulation. The presence of a reactive GQ1b ganglioside antibody would be more consistent with the Miller-Fisher variant. Myasthenia gravis may be differentiated by using an edrophonium chloride test (although this is occasionally positive in botulism) and EMG [decreasing muscle action potential (MAP) with repetitive stimulation]. Lambert-Eaton syndrome has EMG findings similar to those of botulism but greater augmentation; it usually spares cranial nerves and is associated with absent deep tendon reflexes and an abnormal chest radiograph. Chemical nerve agent poisoning would have associated convulsions, excessive salivation, miotic pupils, and paresthesias.

## 6. DIAGNOSIS

Botulism is primarily a clinical diagnosis. Laboratory confirmation is available in the United States through the CDC (Atlanta GA), some state and municipal public health laboratories, and the military reference toxin laboratory at the U.S. Army Medical Research Institute of Infectious Diseases (USAMRIID; Ft. Detrick, MD). Specimens of choice include serum, wound/tissue, stool, and food. Others that can be studied include sterile water enema fluid, nasal swab (if inhalation suspected, best within 24 h, up to 72 h after exposure), vomitus, and autopsy samples of intestinal fluids, liver, and spleen *(36)*. Toxin assays include a mouse bioassay (requires several days), an antigen capture enzyme-linked immunosorbent assay (ELISA; 5 h), and polymerase chain reaction (PCR; 2.5 h). Specific guidance for specimen handling can be reviewed at the CDC Laboratory

Specimen collection website *(37)*. The National Botulism Surveillance and Reference laboratory can be reached at 404-639-3867. Electrochemiluminescence assays have been described as the most sensitive immunoassay (as low as 10 fg/mL) for detection of botulinum toxins *(38,39)*. Given the potency of botulinum toxin, an immune response may not be detected *(3)*. Conversely, in those not treated with antitoxin, free toxin can be demonstrated in the serum for up to 28 d. Injection of sample by the intraperitoneal route into mice, observing for signs consistent with botulism, and then performing a toxin neutralization by adding type-specific and polyvalent antitoxin before injection are classic, but time-consuming, methods to detect botulinum toxin (can detect to up 0.03 mg botulinum toxin residues in 1–2 d) *(2,11)*. Samples can be cultured for *C. botulinum (40)*. In one foodborne outbreak, 53% of serum samples were toxin positive, 32% of stool samples were toxin positive, and in 79% *C. botulinum* was anaerobically cultured from the stool *(41)*. Serum samples for toxin should be obtained before antitoxin, which would interfere with the mouse bioassay. The sensitivity and diagnostic value of nasal swab culture is unknown, and, based on the recent anthrax experience, this may be more useful as part of an epidemiological investigation. PCR does not differentiate between living and dead organisms. A limitation of *C. botulinum* culture is that, in the absence of detectable toxin, it may not be causing disease, as the organism is ubiquitous in nature.

Laboratory biosafety recommendations are detailed by the FDA *(40)*. Sodium hypochlorite (0.1%) or sodium hydroxide (0.1 *N*) inactivates toxin, and these are recommended for spills or contaminated work spaces. Standard precautions are appropriate for collected samples, with shipping at 4°C.

## 7. MANAGEMENT

The most urgent clinical management is assessment of the respiratory reserve. Frequent vital capacity determinations are advised, and any significant decline should lead to endotracheal intubation/assisted ventilation. Supportive care can be life-saving; this includes nasogastric suctioning for ileus, bowel and bladder care, prevention of deep venous thromboses and decubitus ulcers, control of oropharyngeal secretions, and prevention of nosocomial pneumonia with reverse Trendelenberg 20–25° positioning with cervical vertebral support in nonventilated patients (helpful in infants but unstudied in adults) *(2)*. Cathartics, activated charcoal, and high colonic enemas can be used to encourage removal of retained toxin when ingestion is the likely route of intoxication, unless the patient is an infant or has an ileus. Magnesium-containing cathartics should be avoided, as they may potentiate the neuromuscular blockade.

Passive immunization with botulinum antitoxin is recommended in patients with neurological signs as soon as possible after clinical diagnosis. Antitoxin will not reverse the existing paralysis but should protect against subsequent nerve damage and has shown benefit in shortening the course of type A botulism when given within 24 h of symptom onset *(26)*. As botulinum toxin is rapidly and irreversibly bound at the neuromuscular junction, a beneficial effect is more likely realized if antitoxin is administered as soon as possible after exposure. Antitoxin can be withheld if the patient is improving without intervention. In animal experiments with aerosolized botulinum toxin, antitoxin is effective if given before the onset of clinical symptoms; after that, it does not protect against respiratory failure *(19)*. If the source of botulism is considered to be a wound, then it should be surgically debrided and antibiotics (penicillin or metronidazole) administered. Aminoglycosides and clindamycin should not be used, as they can potentiate the toxin-induced neuromuscular blockade. Theoretically, antibiotics could potentiate illness by increasing cell lysis and toxin release, as well as destroying competing intestinal flora, so they are not recommended in ingestion or inhalational botulism.

Several antitoxin preparations are available in the United States. The CDC and the state health departments (California and Alaska) control the release of this product; the CDC can be contacted 24 h/d at 404-639-2888. Antitoxin is stored at airports around the country (including New York, Chicago, Atlanta, Miami, Los Angeles, Seattle, San Francisco, and Honolulu) to facilitate rapid delivery. Previously the CDC Drug Service has distributed trivalent (ABE) botulinum toxin (Connaught Laboratories) in 10-mL multidose vials (each vial has 7500 IU of type A, 5500 IU of type B, and 8500 IU of type E), but the FDA has suspended the use of this product until further safety testing. Each IU neutralizes 1000 mouse $LD_{50}$ of toxin E or 10,000 mouse $LD_{50}$ of toxin A and B. Circulating equine antitoxin has a $t_{1/2}$ of 5–8 d (42). Currently the CDC is releasing equine botulinum antitoxin for types A/B (FDA approved) and another product, equine botulinum antitoxin, for type E [Investigational New Drug (IND)]. Since these standard products are horse-derived, potential complications include anaphylaxis, thermal reactions, and serum sickness hypersensitivity reactions. The vials should be diluted in 0.9% saline to a 1:10 dilution and infused slowly (minimum of 2 min per vial; the usual dose is 10 mL). Sensitivity skin testing is recommended on all patients before they receive antitoxin. A scratch test is outlined in the package insert. If the skin test is positive, then desensitization can be attempted by subcutaneous administration of 0.01–0.1 nL antitoxin, increasing the dose every 20 min until 2 mL can be sustained without much reaction. If a very large amount of botulinum toxin has been delivered (i.e., biological weapon), then serum can be tested for residual unbound toxin after treatment. Additional doses could be given 2–4 h after the initial dose. The CDC reports that from 1967 to 1977, 268 individuals received antitoxin; of them, 9% had an acute reaction, and 3.7% had a delayed hypersensitivity reaction (43). Receiving more than 40 mL serum was associated with an increased risk of serum sickness.

A "de-speciated" equine heptavalent antitoxin against all serotypes, derived by cleaving the allergenic Fc region leaving $F(ab)_2$ fragments, has been developed at USAMRIID and is available under IND status. Four percent horse antigens remain in this antitoxin, so there is some potential for an allergic response (44). The use of human-derived botulism immune globulin (BIG) could decrease these allergic reactions. This was studied in 1992 in a placebo-controlled trial for infant botulism that demonstrated efficacy and safety (45). Currently BIG is available as an orphan drug under open-label IND guidelines from the California Department of Health Services for the treatment of infant botulism. In general, horse-derived botulinum toxin is not used in infants owing to the side effects and potential for inapparent lifelong sensitization to horse serum products. The dose is given as a single intravenous 50-mg/kg infusion. A combination of several recombinant monoclonal antibodies has recently been found to potently neutralize botulinum toxin A. This technique could allow production of large amounts of nonallergenic antitoxin, free of the infectious diseases risks found in using plasma from horses and humans (46).

## 8. INFECTION CONTROL

An emergency response to a mass aerosolized exposure must include giving antitoxin to all ill persons and the mobilization of adequate supportive care resources, such as mechanical ventilators. Person-to-person transmission of botulinum does not occur, so standard precautions are adequate; isolation is not needed. Patients can be air-evacuated with careful attention to their respiratory sufficiency. Sodium hypochlorite 0.1% or sodium hydroxide 0.1 *N* are recommended in a laboratory setting to decontaminate work surfaces/clean up spills of cultures and/or toxin.

## 9. SPECIAL POPULATIONS

Children may be especially vulnerable to biological terrorism, because of their more permeable skin, smaller fluid reserve, rapid respiratory rate, high skin-to-mass ratio, and sometimes an inability to communicate symptoms *(47)*. The signs and symptoms of botulism are similar to those in adults (except for infant botulism) *(47)*. With limited information, there is no indication that more vulnerable populations such as children, immunocompromised hosts, and pregnant females should receive different treatment. Pregnant females and children have received the equine antitoxin without adverse effects.

## 10. PREVENTION

Botulinum toxin seems to be colorless, tasteless, and odorless. Germination of the *C. botulinum* spores can be prevented by refrigeration, freezing, drying, or salting, as well as through the use of food preservatives such as sodium nitrite. In home canning, spores can be destroyed when food is heated over 120°C for 30 min under pressure; pressure should be increased 0.5 pounds for every 1000 feet above sea level. Terminal heating during canning at 80°C for 20 min or boiling for more than 5 min assists in inactivating the neurotoxin *(27)*. For prevention of infant botulism, children younger than 12 mo should not be fed honey. For aerosolized botulinum toxin, clothing and skin should be washed immediately with soap and water and surfaces and objects cleaned with bleach. If the release of aerosolized botulinum toxin is anticipated, then covering the mucosal surfaces should confer some protection. A pentavalent toxoid (Michigan Department of Public Health) consisting of crude extracts of clostridial proteins (toxins A, B, C, D, and E) is available from the CDC under IND status. It is recommended for military personnel and laboratory workers with potential exposure to *C. botulinum* cultures or toxins. It has been administered to more than 10,000 persons between 1970 and the Gulf War and has induced serum antitoxin levels that corresponded to protective levels in animal studies *(48)*. Botulinum toxoid is given 0.5 mL subcutaneously at 0, 2, and 12 wk with a booster at 1 yr. This gives protective levels in 78% (toxin type B) to 91% (toxin type A) *(48)*.

Reactogenicity is reported as mild, with 2–4% getting local edema, induration, and erythema at 24–48 h at the injection site *(1)*. Local reactions increase with repeated doses. Up to 3% have systemic reactions of fever, myalgias, headache, and malaise. Postexposure prophylaxis with the heptavalent antitoxin has been effective in primate studies, but no human data have been published. A separate monovalent toxoid for type F has been produced by Porton Products (United Kingdom) and is more than 60% pure toxoid *(49)*. A recombinant vaccine is being developed using synthetic genes encoding for nontoxic, carboxyl-terminal fragments of *C. botulinum* neurotoxins. Studies have been completed in mice and nonhuman primates *(49)*.

## REFERENCES

1. Botulinum. In: Medical Management of Biological Casualties Handbook. USAMRIID, Ft. Detrick, MD, 2001, pp. 69–75 and Appendices. http://www.usamriid.army.mil/education/bluebook.html
2. Arnon SS, Schechter R, Inglesby TV, et al. Botulinum toxin as a biological weapon. JAMA 2001;285:1059–1070.

3. Middlebrooks JL, Franz DR. Botulinum toxins. In: Sidell FR, Takafuji ET, Franz DR, eds. Textbook of Military Medicine: Medical Aspects of Chemical and Biologic Warfare. Borden Institute, Washington, DC, 1997, pp. 643–653.

4. Compton JAF. Botulinum toxin. In: Military Chemical and Biological Agents: Chemical and Toxicological Properties. Telford Press, Caldwell, NJ, 1987, pp. 337–342.

5. Henderson DA. The looming threat of bioterrorism. Science 1999;283:1279–1282.

6. Zilinskas RA. Iraq's biologic weapons. JAMA 1997;278:418–424.

7. Franz DR. Defense against toxin weapons. In: Sidell FR, Takafuji ET, Franz DR, eds. Medical Aspects of Chemical and Biologic Warfare (Textbook of Military Medicine Part I). Borden Institute, Washington, DC, 1997, pp. 603–619.

8. CDC. Biologic and chemical terrorism: strategic plan for preparedness and response. MMWR 2000; 49:1–14.

9. Shapiro RL, Hatheway C, Swerdlow DL. Botulism in the United States: a clinical and epidemiologic review. Ann Intern Med 1998;129:221–228.

10. Siegel LS. Destruction of botulinum toxins in food and water. In: Hauschild AH, Dodds KL, eds. *Clostridium botulinum*: Ecology and Control in Foods. Marcel Dekker, New York, 1993, pp. 323–341.

11. CDC. Botulism in the United States, 1899–1996. In: Handbook for Epidemiologists, Clinicians, and Laboratory Workers. CDC/NCID, Atlanta, GA, 1998, 1–42.

12. Hathaway CL. Botulism: the present status of the disease. Curr Top Microbiol Immunol 1995; 195:55–75.

13. Hauschild AHW. Epidemiology of human foodborne botulism. In: Hauschild AHW, Dodds KL, eds. *Clostridium botulinum*: Ecology and Control in Foods. Marcel Dekker, New York, 1993, 69–104.

14. Werner SB, Passaro K, McGee J, et al. Wound botulism in California, 1951–1998: recent epidemic in heroin injectors. Clin Infect Dis 2000;31:1018–1024.

15. Passaro DS, Werner SB, McGee J, et al. Wound botulism associated with black tar heroin among injecting drug users. JAMA 1998;279:859–863.

16. Arnon SS, Midura TF, Damus K. Honey and other environmental risk factors for infant botulism. J Pediatr 1979;94:331–336.

17. Spika JS, Shaffer N, Nargett-Bean, et al. Risk factors for infant botulism in the U.S. Am J Dis Child 1989;143:828–832.

18. Chia JK, Clark JB, Ryan CA, Pollack M. Botulism in an adult associated with food-borne intestinal infection with *Clostridium botulinum*. N Engl J Med 1986;315:239–241.

19. Franz DR, Pitt LM, Clayton MA, Hanes MA, Ross KJ. Efficacy of prophylactic and therapeutic adminstration of antitoxin for inhalation botulism. In: Das-Gupta BR, ed. Botulinum and Tetanus Neurotoxins. Neurotransmission and Biomedical Aspects. Plenum Press, New York, 1993, pp. 473–476.

20. Jankovic J, Brin MF. Therapeutic uses of botulinum toxin. N Engl J Med 1991;324:1186–1194.

21. Botulinum Toxin Type A Purified Neurotoxin Complex. NDA/BLA 103000,5000. FDA Medical Officer review, 2002.

22. Botulinum Toxin Type B. NDA/BLA 98-1396. FDA Medical Officer review, 1999.

23. Hughes JM, Blumenthal JR, Merson MH, Lombard GL, Dowell VR, Gangarosa EJ. Clinical features of type A and B food-borne botulism. Ann Intern Med 1981;95:442–445.

24. Beller M, Gessner B, Wainwright R, Barrett D. Botulism in Alaska: A Guide for Physicians and Health Care Providers. Alaska Department of Health and Social Services, Anchorage, AK, 1994, pp. 1–28.

25. Caya JG. *Clostridium botulinum* and the ophthalmologist: a review of botulism; including biological warfare ramifications of botulinum toxin. Surv Ophthalmol 2001;46:25–34.

26. Tacket CO, Mann JM, Hargrett NT, Blake PA. Equine antitoxin use and other factors that predict outcome in type A foodborne botulism. Am J Med 1984;76:794–798.

27. Cherington M. Botulism: ten year experience. Arch Neurol 1974;30:432–437.

28. Pickett JB. AAEE Case Report #16: botulism. Muscle Nerve 1988;11:1201–1205.

29. Woodruff BA, Griffin PM, McCroskey LM, et al. Clinical and laboratory comparison of botulism from toxin types A, B, and E in the United States 1975–1988. J Infect Dis 1992;166:1281–1286.

30. Wainwright RB, Heyward WL, Middaugh JP, Hatheway CL, Harpster AP, Bender TR. Food-borne Botulism in Alaska, 1947–85: Epidemiology and clinical findings. J Infect Dis 1988;157:1158–1162.

31. Mann JM, Martin S, Hoffman R, Marazzo S. Patient recovery from type A botulism: morbidity assessment following a large outbreak. Am J Public Health 1981;71:266–269.

32. Wilcox P, Andolfatto G, Fairbarn MS, Pardy RL. Long-term follow-up of symptoms, pulmonary function, respiratory muscle strength and exercise performance after botulism. Am Rev Respir Dis 1989;139:157–163.

33. Schmidt-Nowara WW, Samet JM, Rosario PA. Early and late pulmonary complications of botulism. Arch Intern Med 1983;143:451–456.
34. Campbell WW, Swift TR. Differential diagnosis of acute weakness. South Med J 1981;74:1371–1375.
35. LoVecchio F, Jacobson S. Approach to generalized weakness and peripheral neuromuscular disease. Emerg Med Clin North Am 1997;3:605–623.
36. Miller JM. Agents of bioterrorism: preparing for bioterrorism at the community health care level. Infect Dis Clin North Am 2001;15:1132:1148–1150.
37. CDC website: http://www.bt.cdc.gov/Agent/Botulism (Laboratory Testing section).
38. Madsen JM. Toxins as weapons of mass destruction. Clin Lab Med 2001;21:593–605.
39. Henchal EA, Teska JD, Ludwig GV, Shoemaker DR, Ezzell JN. Current laboratory methods for biological threat agent identification. Clin Lab Med 2001;21:661–675.
40. Solomon HM, Lilly T. *Clostridium botulinum*. In: Jackson GH, Merker RI, Bandler R, eds. Bacteriological Analytical Manual Online (www.cfsan.fda.gov/~ebam/bam-toc.html). FDA Center for Food Safety and Applied Nutrition, Washington, DC, 2001.
41. Mann JM, Hatheway CL, Gardiner TM. Laboratory diagnosis in a large outbreak of type A botulism. Am J Epidemiol 1982;115:598–605.
42. Hatheway CH, Snyder JD, Seal JE, Edell TA, Lewis GE. Antitoxin levels in botulism patients treated with trivalent equine botulism antitoxin to toxin types A, B, and E. J Infect Dis 1984;150:407–412.
43. Black RE, Gunn RA. Hypersensitivity reactions associated with botulinal antitoxin. Am J Med 1980;69:567–570.
44. Hibbs RG, Weber JT, Corwin A, et al. Experience with the use of an investigational F(ab)$_2$ heptavalent botulism immune globulin of equine origin during an outbreak of type E botulism in Egypt. Clin Infect Dis 1996;23:337–340.
45. California Department of Health Services website. http://www.dhs.ca.gov/ps/dcdc/infantBot/openlbl.htm.
46. Nowakowski A, Wang C, Powers DB, et al. Potent neutralization of botulinum neurotoxin by recombinant oligoclonal antibody. Proc natl Acad Sic USA 2002;99:11,346–11,350.
47. American Academy of Pediatrics. Chemical-biologic terrorism and its impact on children: a subject review. Pediatrics 2000;105:662–670.
48. Siegel LS. Human immune response to botulinum pentavalent (ABCDE) toxoid determined by a neutralization test and by an enzyme-linked immunosorbent assay. J Clin Microbiol 1988;26:2351–2356.
49. Byrne M, Smith LA. Development of vaccines for prevention of botulism. Biochimie 2000;82:955–966.

# 12 Ricin Toxin

## Glenn Wortmann, *MD, FACP*

The opinions or assertions contained herein are the private views of the author and are not to be construed as official or as representing the position of the Department of the Army or the Department of Defense.

### CONTENTS

### Case Vignette

A 49-year-old man presented complaining of severe leg pain and general weakness for 1 day. The patient had been in his usual state of good health but had felt poorly since being jostled while waiting at a bus stop yesterday. The patient recalled feeling a blow to the back of his right thigh; he turned to see a man bending to pick up an umbrella. By the time the patient arrived at his office, he noted an "angry red spot, like a pimple" on the back of his thigh. After a night of feeling weak and feverish, the patient presented with exquisite leg pain and fever. Physical exam revealed a febrile, ill-appearing man who had a 6-cm-diameter area of induration and inflammation on his right thigh with significant inguinal adenopathy. The patient's white blood count (WBC) was 10,600/mm$^3$, and X-rays of the right thigh were read as normal. Over the next 12 hours, the patient developed hypotension, anuria, and hematemesis. A repeat WBC was 26,300/mm$^3$. The next day, the patient developed complete atrioventricular block and then cardiac arrest. A repeat WBC was 33,200/mm$^3$, and the patient expired soon thereafter. At autopsy, a small pellet with two holes forming a storage cavity was discovered embedded in the patient's thigh.

From: *Physician's Guide to Terrorist Attack*
Edited by: M. J. Roy © Humana Press Inc., Totowa, NJ

# 1. INTRODUCTION

The case vignette describes a true story of the assassination of the dissident Bulgarian broadcaster Georgi Markov, who was killed in 1978 *(1)*. The weapon used to slay Mr. Markov was an umbrella tipped with a platinum/iridium pellet loaded with ricin, and his attackers injected the toxin into his leg as he stood waiting at a London bus station. Mr. Markov was not the only dissident attacked with what is presumed to have been ricin during this time period. Vladimir Kostov, a Bulgarian State Radio and Television correspondent who had defected to Paris, was shot in the back with an identical pellet just 2 weeks before the attack on Markov. Mr. Kostov was in the hospital for 12 days before he eventually recovered *(1)*.

The bean of the castor plant, *Ricinus communis*, has been recognized since antiquity for its value and potential toxicity. In many parts of the world, castor beans are used for medicinal purposes. Ingestion of crushed decorticated raw beans as an emetic, roasted castor beans as a cathartic, peeled raw beans as a treatment for leprosy, and pulverized beans mixed with honey as a cure for syphilis have all been described *(2)*. Many countries use extracted castor oil as lubricating oil for machinery, and extraction of ricin toxin from the remaining castor meal is easily performed *(3)*. Although the intentional use of ricin as a weapon of biological warfare (with the exception of the two cases cited above) has not been described, more than 750 cases of intoxication have been reported *(4)*, and the agent was developed and tested (but never used in battle) by the United States and Britain during World War II *(5)*. More recently, Iraq admitted in 1995 that it had developed ricin as a biological warfare agent prior to the Gulf War, and the lay media has highlighted several cases of individuals possessing ricin for possible terrorist activities *(6)*. Unfortunately for the civilized world, the relatively high toxicity, low cost ($10,000–$20,000 for 800 g, which is an amount sufficient to inflict heavy casualties over 1 square mile), and ease of production make ricin an attractive agent for potential nefarious use *(7)*.

# 2. MECHANISM OF ACTION

Ricin toxin belongs to the A-B family of toxins, which also includes several bacterial toxins, such as diphtheria, pseudomonas, cholera, Shiga, and anthrax toxins *(8)*. Toxins in this group consist of an enzymatically active A-moiety and a receptor-binding B-moiety linked together by a disulfide bond *(9)*.

The B-chain portion of the molecule binds β-D-galactopyranoside moieties on glycoproteins and glycolipids, and thus there are millions of binding sites for ricin on an average cell *(9)*. Once bound to the cell surface, the toxin is internalized by endocytosis and routed to the cytosol. The A-chain is a glycosidase that removes an adenine residue from an exposed loop of the 28S ribosomal RNA. The toxin does not by itself break the RNA chain, but the depurinated RNA is susceptible to hydrolysis at alkaline pH. This loop is involved in the binding of elongation factors, and the modified ribosomes are unable to support protein synthesis. Inhibition of protein synthesis is therefore the mechanism by which ricin kills. The toxic A-chains are highly efficient, and one molecule inactivates a few thousand ribosomes per minute. A single A-chain can inactivate ribosomes faster than the cell can make new ones *(8)*, and one A-chain molecule can kill an animal cell *(10)*.

## 3. CLINICAL SIGNS AND SYMPTOMS

The signs and symptoms of ricin toxicity vary with the dose and route of exposure *(11)*. Oral ingestion has an estimated fatality rate of between 1.9% and 6% *(4)*, although this percentage depends on multiple factors. Variations in the composition of the beans (which vary in size and ricin content), the number of beans ingested, host factors, and the availability of supportive care all impact outcome. For symptomatic patients, the clinical course presents with the rapid onset of nausea, vomiting, and abdominal pain. Diarrhea, gastrointestinal bleeding, anuria, cramps, and vascular collapse can all occur. Most symptoms develop less than 6 h after ingestion, although the lag time from ingestion of the beans to onset of symptoms has ranged from 15 min to almost 10 h *(12)*. Mild hemolysis, abnormal liver or kidney function tests, and elevated creatine phosphokinase have been occasionally reported *(12)*. Progression to death occurs on the third day or later. The scant descriptions of autopsy findings report erosions and punctate hemorrhages in the stomach and small bowel *(4)*. Lymphoid necrosis in the mesenteric lymph nodes, gut-associated lymphoid tissue and spleen, liver necrosis, diffuse nephritis, and diffuse splenitis have also been described *(6)*.

The consequences of inhalation of ricin toxin on humans are not known, but animal studies have demonstrated acute marked to severe multifocal to coalescing fibrinopurulent pneumonia, mild to severe diffuse necrosis and acute inflammation of airways, and diffuse marked to severe alveolar flooding and peribronchovascular edema. Mild to moderate fibrinopurulent pleuritis, minimal to mild acute purulent tracheitis, and moderate to severe purulent mediastinal lymphadenitis were also described *(13)*. In experimental animals, time to death was dose-dependent and occurred 36–72 h post inhalation exposure *(14)*.

Parenteral ricin is considered to be about 700-fold more toxic than oral ricin *(15)*, and injection of ricin toxin leads to the clinical scenario described at the beginning of this chapter. In the case of Mr. Markov, severe local necrosis of muscle and regional lymph nodes, hemorrhagic necrosis of the small intestine, small hemorrhages throughout the heart, interstitial hemorrhages of the intestines, testicles, pancreas, and inguinal lymph nodes were noted *(1)*.

## 4. DIAGNOSIS

As with any unusual and uncommon disease, the recognition of ricin intoxication will most likely require a leading clinical history (e.g., the ingestion of castor beans) or the occurrence of multiple cases in a short period (suggesting a common-source etiology). In the setting of a biological warfare attack, ricin would most likely be used as an aerosol. Clinicians confronted with a large number of patients with acute lung injury should suspect exposure to a pulmonary irritant such as ricin. Other causes to consider would be staphylococcal enterotoxin B, Q fever, tularemia, plague, and some chemical warfare agents such as phosgene *(14)*. Factors discriminating ricin intoxication from other agents would be a clinical progression despite antibiotics (as opposed to infectious agents), the lack of mediastinitis (as is seen with pulmonary anthrax), a progressive decline in clinical status (patients exposed to staphylococcal enterotoxin B tend to stabilize), and a slower progression than patients exposed to phosgene *(14)*.

Laboratory confirmation of ricin toxin inhalation can be done through enzyme-linked immunosorbent assay (ELISA) analysis of a swab sample of the nasal mucosa (6). In addition, ELISA assays testing for the presence of ricin in blood or other bodily fluids might be useful (16). As ricin is highly immunogenic, acute as well as convalescent sera should be obtained from survivors for measurement of antibody response (14).

## 5. TREATMENT

There are no postexposure antidotes to ricin, and medical treatment is supportive. If oral ingestion is suspected, gastric decontamination with activated charcoal followed by cathartics such as magnesium citrate is recommended (14). Because ricin is not dialyzable (17), and little is excreted in the urine (18), hemodialysis or forced diuresis is not indicated. Most patients reportedly respond well to intravenous fluids and electrolyte replacement and recover without permanent sequelae (12).

The clinical experience with inhalational and parenteral intoxication is much more limited, and outcome data are not currently available. Ventilatory support, wound care, and careful attention to fluid and electrolyte replacements coupled with tincture of time are the only modalities currently available.

Fortunately, the risk to the health care provider treating ricin intoxication victims should be minimal, as secondary aerosolization is not believed to be a danger, and weak hypochlorite solutions (0.1% sodium hypochlorite) and/or soap and water can decontaminate skin surfaces (19). For the future, the identification of drugs which counter the toxicity of ricin (20) and the development of a protective vaccine are the most promising defenses against a biological warfare attack with this agent.

## REFERENCES

1. Crompton R, Gall D. Georgi Markov—death in a pellet. Med Leg J 1980;48:51–62.
2. Scarpa A, Guerci A. Various uses of the castor oil plant (Ricinus communis)—a review. J Ethnopharmacol 1982;5:117–137.
3. Wannemacher R, Hewetson J, Lemley P, et al. Comparison of detection of ricin in castor bean extracts by bioassays, immunoassays, and chemistry procedures. In: Gopalakrishnakone P, Tan C, eds, Recent Advances in Toxicology Research. National University of Singapore, Singapore, 1992, pp. 108–119.
4. Rauber A, Heard J. Castor bean toxicity re-examined: a new perspective. Vet Hum Toxicol 1995;27:490–502.
5. Cookson J, Nottingham J. A Survey of Chemical and Biological Warfare. Monthly Review Press, New York, 1969, p. 6.
6. Franz D, Jaax N. Ricin toxin. In: Sidell FR, Takafuji ET, Franz DR, eds. Textbook of Military Medicine: Medical Aspects of Chemical and Biologic Warfare. Borden Institute, Washington, DC, 1997, pp. 631–642.
7. Nelan BW. The price of fanaticism. Time. April 3, 1995:35–41.
8. Olsnes S, Wesche J, Falnes PO. Binding uptake, routing and translocation of toxins with intracellular sites of action. In: Alouf JE, Freer JH, eds, The Comprehensive Sourcebook of Bacterial Toxins. Academic Press, London, 1999, pp. 73–93.
9. Olsnes S, Koslov J. Ricin. Toxicon 2001;39:1723–1728.
10. Eiklid K, Olsnes S, Pihl A. Entry of lethal doses of abrin, ricin and modeccin into the cytosol of HeLa cells. Exp Cell Res 1980:126;321–326.
11. Olsnes S, Pihl A. Toxic lectins and related proteins. In: Cohen P, van Heyningen S, eds. Molecular Action of Toxins and Viruses. Elsevier Biomedical Press, Amsterdam, 1982, pp. 51–105.
12. Challoner KR, McCarron MM. Castor bean intoxication. Ann Emerg Med 1989;19:1177–1183.
13. Wilhelmsen C, Pitt M. Lesions of acute inhaled lethal ricin intoxication in rhesus monkeys. Vet Pathol 1993;30:482.
14. Eitzen E, Pavlin J, Cieslak T, Christopher G, Culpepper R. Ricin. In: Medical Management of Biological Casualties Handbook. U.S. Army Medical Research Institute of Infectious Diseases, Frederick, MD, 1998, pp. 101–106.

15. Hayes WJ. Pesticides Studies in Man. Williams & Wilkins, Baltimore, 1982, pp. 101–103.
16. Poli M, Rivera V, Hewetson J, Merrill G. Detection of ricin by colorimetric and chemiluminescence ELISA. Toxicon 1994;32:1371–1377.
17. Balint GA. Ricin: the toxic protein of castor oil seeds. Toxicology 1974;2:77–102.
18. Kopferschmitt J, Flesch F, Lughier A, et al. Acute voluntary intoxication by ricin. Hum Toxicol 1983;2:239–242.
19. Mackinnon P, Alderton M. An investigation of the degradation of the plant toxin, ricin, by sodium hypochlorite. Toxicon 2000;38:287–291.
20. Thompson W, Scovill J, Pace J. Drugs that show protective effects from ricin toxicity in in-vitro protein synthesis assays. Natural Toxins 1995;3:369–377.

# 13

## Staphylococcal Enterotoxin B

*David L. Blazes,* MD, MPH

**CONTENTS**

## 1. INTRODUCTION

Toxins are biologically derived substances that adversely affect living organisms. An astounding number of toxins produced by animals, plants, and bacteria are harmful to humans. Toxins cause food poisonings and envenomations, bleeding disorders, and neurological dysfunction. They act via many diverse mechanisms and produce some of the most dramatic illnesses in humans.

The most potent toxins known are those produced by bacteria. *Staphylococcus aureus* is a bacterium that is ubiquitous in nature and is a common cause of both infection and intoxication among humans. Because of its potency and ease of acquisition, one of the toxins produced by *S. aureus* [staphylococcal enterotoxin B (SEB)] has been considered a viable bioterror agent. In fact, some nations—including the United States in the 1960s— are known to have studied this toxin thoroughly for use as a biological weapon *(1)*. SEB is generally considered an incapacitating agent, but when exposure levels are high, SEB intoxication can certainly be lethal. The lethal dose $(LD_{50})$ for human inhalational exposure has been estimated to be approximately 0.02 µg/kg, whereas the effective dose

From: *Physician's Guide to Terrorist Attack*
Edited by: M. J. Roy © Humana Press Inc., Totowa, NJ

(ED$_{50}$) at which 50% of those exposed develop incapacitating symptoms is significantly lower, 0.0004 µg/kg *(2)*.

The following chapter discusses in detail what is known about the microbiology, immunology, clinical presentation, diagnosis, and treatment of intoxications with SEB. Because the most likely route of exposure to SEB in the purview of a bioterror event is inhalation, this presentation is emphasized.

---

**Case Vignette**

A 25-year-old graduate student was riding the Metro from class to his apartment in Washington, DC. At his Metro stop, he walked through a small cloud of dust that caused him to cough briefly. He noted that several city workers had been sweeping up a pile of grayish dust that had spilled out of a box in the trash. The student proceeded home and was well until 8 hours later that evening, when he noted the sudden onset of nausea. He had one episode of emesis and noted that he had a fever. He took some antiemetics, but he soon developed a headache as well as a dry cough with dyspnea and mild substernal chest pain. At this point, he presented to the local emergency department, where there were several other patients with similar complaints. All had ridden the Metro at approximately the same time that day and all noted in retrospect the dust clean-up effort. He had a temperature of 103°F, but his other vital signs were normal. He and the others were quarantined in a large treatment room, and laboratory and radiographic studies were obtained. The chest radiograph was normal, and laboratory examinations revealed normal serum chemistries and a leukocyte count of 10,000/ mm$^3$. Sputum Gram stain revealed no organisms. The student was admitted for observation, appropriate cultures of blood and sputum were obtained, and he was given acetaminophen for his headache and oxygen for the dyspnea. The following day, the headache and nausea had resolved, although he still had a low-grade fever. The fever persisted for the next 3 days, but he was otherwise asymptomatic. Cultures of blood and sputum remained negative, and he was discharged on the fifth day, having fully recovered. All the patients who presented with similar symptoms had similar courses and full recoveries. Residual dust samples from the Metro trashcan provided the diagnosis of staphylococcal enterotoxin B intoxication.

---

## 2. MICROBIOLOGY

The Gram-positive bacterium *S. aureus* produces at least 12 distinct exotoxins, A, B, C$_{1-3}$, D, E, G, H, I, J, and K. Most is known about SEB, which is a common cause of food poisoning in the United States. The exotoxins are secreted by bacteria and thus can exert their biological effects in the absence of viable bacteria. In addition, most of these toxins are stable to heat, desiccation and aerosolization, making them persistent in the environment *(1)*.

The staphylococcal enterotoxins are produced by the bacteria in the log phase of growth in batch culture, and the amount of toxin produced depends on the local physical and chemical environment *(1)*. The production of SEB is controlled at the transcriptional level by the accessory gene regulator (agr) locus *(3)*, although other genes are probably involved, owing to variable toxin production rates among agr+ isolates *(1,3)*.

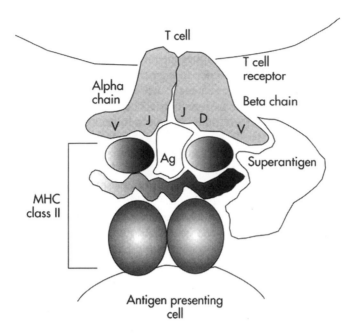

**Fig. 1.** A cross-sectional view of the interactions among a conventional peptide antigen, T-cell receptor (TCR), and MHC. The peptide sits within a groove in the MHC molecule formed by two α helices, bordered on the bottom by a β-pleated sheet. Superantigens are not processed to oligopeptides and therefore are not presented in the antigen groove. Instead, they bind to more conserved residues on the side of the MHC class II molecule and interact primarily with the Vβ region of the TCR. Reproduced from ref. *18*, copyright 1996 Mosby Inc., with permission from Elsevier Science.

SEB shares amino acid sequence homology with $SEC_{1-3}$ and streptococcal pyrogenic exotoxins A and C *(1,4)*. SEB additionally shares a similar three-dimensional structure with the toxin associated with staphylococcal toxic shock syndrome (TSST-1) and SEA *(5)*. The exact mechanisms by which SEB and related enterotoxins exert their effects have not been fully elucidated. However, these pyrogenic exotoxins as a group are very potent stimulators of the immune system, as covered in the immunology section below.

## 3. IMMUNOLOGY

The staphylococcal enterotoxins are classified as bacterial superantigens, which are some of the most potent known stimulators of the human immune system. A superantigen is a molecule that broadly binds to both the class II MHC of an antigen-presenting cell and the T-lymphocyte receptor (TCR), crosslinking these two molecules in a nontraditional fashion (Fig. 1). This novel method of binding bypasses the standard method of antigen presentation and allows unprocessed superantigen proteins to activate the cellular immune system. This independent binding is not MHC restricted and causes a massive stimulation of the immune system, activating up to 30% of the T-cell pool *(6)*. The particular superantigen will bind to the β-chain of the variable region of the MHC II molecule, and the magnitude of the immune response is dependent on the number of Vβ regions that are bound *(7)*. When these large numbers of T-cells are stimulated, a proinflammatory cytokine cascade is activated, leading to a Th1 predominant cellular immune response [interleukin-1 (IL-1), IL-2, tumor necrosis factor-α, and interferon-γ], and clinical signs of inflammation.

It appears that with increasing doses of superantigen, a faster and more vigorous immune response is produced. This dose-response relationship is conserved for many of the staphylococcal enterotoxins, including SEB *(7)*. In addition and opposite in effect, repeated exposures to the same superantigen can lead to immune tolerance through deletion or inactivation of various T-cell subsets *(7)*.

## 4. PATHOLOGY

There have been no pathological studies of SEB exposure in humans, but there are several reports documenting the pathology in non-human primates *(1,8)*. Pathological examination of rhesus monkeys exposed to lethal aerosolized doses of SEB showed abnormalities in the lungs, gastrointestinal tract, and vascular tissues. Grossly, the lungs from monkeys who died after SEB exposure were heavy and fluid filled, with atelectasis and many petechial hemorrhages *(1)*. Microscopically, there was extensive interstitial pulmonary edema with fibrin deposition and an inflammatory cell infiltrate *(1)*. In the gastrointestinal tract, there were petechial hemorrhages and mucosal ulcerations throughout the small and large intestines, as well as many small crypt abscesses in the colon. Vascular changes included generalized capillary leak resulting in tissue edema *(1)*.

## 5. CLINICAL SYNDROMES

SEB is a common cause of food poisoning, representing about 25% of cases yearly in the United States. The symptoms of exposure to SEB via the gastrointestinal tract are well described and include the rapid onset of nausea, emesis, and diarrhea in the absence of a systemic febrile response. Any clustering of such cases in today's threat climate should prompt an outbreak investigation. A respiratory exposure to SEB would be the more likely route in a bioterror event *(9)*, and the discussion here will focus on this presentation.

The aerosol route is the most efficient method to deliver an incapacitating or fatal dose of SEB to a large number of people. The mean incapacitating dose is many-fold less for an inhalation dose than for an enteric dose, and the clinical presentation is somewhat different as well.

Clinical symptoms have been documented for non-human primates in an experimental setting as well as in humans after an accidental exposure in a research laboratory *(1,8)*. Rhesus monkeys exposed to lethal doses of SEB via an aerosol route demonstrated a biphasic illness. They developed gastrointestinal signs within 24 h, including anorexia, emesis, and diarrhea, all of which were self-limited *(1)*. At 48 h, they rapidly developed a fatal systemic illness, which included lethargy, respiratory symptoms, and death or euthanasia *(1)*. There have been no controlled trials of human subjects exposed to SEB via aerosol, but an accidental exposure in a laboratory setting has given some insight into the incapacitating effects of SEB on humans.

Nine laboratory workers were accidentally exposed to SEB and developed various levels of incapacitation. The onset of illness was 3–4 h, and the duration was about 3–4 d. The severity of clinical illness ranged from mildly symptomatic to profoundly ill. None of the nine patients died *(1)*.

Similar to an enteral exposure to SEB, gastrointestinal symptoms were common among those exposed in the laboratory. Nausea, anorexia, and emesis were observed between 8 and 24 h, although none of the nine patients developed the diarrhea that is characteristic of food poisoning. There were no rashes documented among the nine patients, but myalgias were seen in a majority *(1)*.

Different from an enteral exposure to SEB, this aerosol exposure caused fever in all nine patients, with most experiencing rigors at the initiation of symptoms. Fevers were as high as 106°F. The mean time to the onset of fever was 12 h (range, 8–20 h), and the fevers lasted an average of 50 h (range, 12–76 h). In addition, eight of nine patients experienced varying degrees of headache, all of which resolved without neurological sequelae. The most prominent clinical features of inhalation of SEB were respiratory and included cough, dyspnea, and chest pain. The mean time to onset of respiratory symptoms was 10 h, and the duration ranged from 9 to 40 h. All patients reported a nonproductive cough. Five of the nine noted dyspnea and were found to have crackles on exam. Several patients were found to have pulmonary edema on chest radiograph, whereas others had either normal radiographs or peribronchial cuffing. Interestingly, seven of the nine patients noted substernal, pleuritic chest pain that was moderate in severity, occurred an average of 12 h after exposure, and lasted an average of 23 h (range, 4–84 h). All patients had normal electrocardiograms, all were normotensive, and none required intravenous fluid resuscitation *(1)*. All patients recovered with no known chronic sequelae.

## 6. DIAGNOSIS

Diagnosis of respiratory exposure to SEB requires a high index of suspicion and recognition of the above constellation of symptoms. If such a diagnosis is the result of a bioterror event, one might expect to see a cluster of similar cases from a common area. As some of the more lethal agents of bioterror may initially have a similar clinical presentation, it is important to identify the underlying etiology of the symptoms. This will allow appropriate treatment, prophylaxis, and reassurance to be dispensed. In general, SEB intoxication will present with the rapid onset of symptoms and then clinical stabilization. This is contrasted with inhalation anthrax, pneumonic plague, or tularemia pneumonia, all of which present less rapidly after exposure but progress clinically if untreated *(9)*.

Serological studies are of little value for the detection of acute exposure to SEB, as antibodies to staphylococcal toxins are common in the population and would not necessarily be found in the acute presentation. Direct detection of the toxin can be achieved in both clinical and environmental samples, often at picomolar or even femtomolar concentrations *(1,10,11)*. Environmental samples appropriate for testing include swabs from surfaces, dust, dirt, or other materials. Clinical samples include swabs from nasal passages taken within 12–24 h after exposure, urine, and serum. SEB antigen can be detected by polymerase chain reaction *(1)*, fluorometric capture enzyme-linked immunosorbent assay *(10)*, or surface plasmon resonance biosensor *(11)*, although the availability of these methods is currently limited to the research laboratory.

## 7. TREATMENT

Most patients with inhalational exposure to SEB will experience incapacitation rather than death. In general, treatment of inhalational exposure to SEB is supportive. Symptoms of nausea may be controlled with antiemetics. Fevers and myalgias may respond to antipyretics such as nonsteroidal anti-inflammatory drugs or acetaminophen. Respiratory status should be monitored closely, and severe cases of inhalational SEB exposure may require intensive care management.

There are several experimental therapies that may limit incapacitation or prevent death in severe SEB exposures. These have only been explored in animal models, but they have shown promise in reducing the deleterious effects of SEB intoxication. Chicken anti-SEB antibodies have conveyed passive protection from death for rhesus monkeys *(12)*. Another method of interfering with the superantigen effect of SEB is to block the TCR binding site, which has been accomplished with a peptide antagonist *(13)*. Finally, the drug perfenidone has been shown to downregulate the Th1 immune response, thus leading to decreased production of inflammatory cytokines and decreased incidence of death in mice exposed to lethal doses of SEB *(14)*.

## 8. PREVENTION

The best method of limiting the effect of inhalational exposure to SEB is to provide pre-exposure prophylaxis. Whether this is practical for the general population is unknown, although it is probably not cost effective owing to the low risk of intentional exposure and the low expected mortality rate. There have been several studies in animal models that demonstrate the protective efficacy of vaccines against SEB. A formalin-inactivated toxoid has shown efficacy in monkeys challenged with an inhalational exposure to SEB *(15)*. Other vaccines have been designed to protect against TSST-1, but they have shown cross-protection against several other staphylococcal toxins, including SEB. Some vaccine candidates have used adjuvants, such as the cholera toxin *(16)*, and others have used viruses (Venezuelan equine encephalitis) to import mutangenized SEB into the structural genes *(17)*. All have demonstrated some level of protective immunity in animal models but have yet to be explored in humans to date.

## 9. SUMMARY

SEB intoxication may occur via a gastrointestinal or respiratory exposure. The respiratory route of exposure would be expected in a bioterror event and results in an incapacitating illness characterized by fevers, respiratory symptoms, myalgias, and headaches. There is presently no specific therapy for SEB intoxication, although occasionally intensive care measures are required. The diagnosis requires a high index of suspicion and the timely laboratory evaluation of clinical and environmental samples. One important step in managing SEB intoxication is to exclude potentially life-threatening or contagious agents that initially may mimic SEB intoxication. Current research is demonstrating new methods for the detection, treatment, and prevention of SEB intoxication.

## REFERENCES

1. Ulrich RG, Sidell S, Taylor TT, et al. Staphylococcal enterotoxin B and related pyrogenic toxins. In: Sidell FR, Takafuji ET, Franz DR, eds. Textbook of Military Medicine: Medical Aspects of Chemical and Biologic Warfare. Borden Institute, Washington, DC, 1997, pp. 621–630.
2. Hursh S, McNally R, Fanzone J Jr, Mershon M. Staphylococcal enterotoxin B battlefield challenge modeling with medical and non-medical countermeasures. Technical Report MBDRP-95-2. Science Applications International, Joppa, MD, 1995.
3. Betley MJ, Borst DW, Regassa LB. Staphylococcal enterotoxins, toxic shock syndrome toxin, and streptococcal pyrogenic exotoxins: a comparative study of their molecular biology. Chem Immunol 1992;55:1–35.

4. Ulrich RG, Bavari S, Olson M. Bacterial superantigens in human diseases: structure, function, and diversity. Trends Microbiol 1995;3:463–468.
5. Prasad GS, Earhart CA, Murray DL, et al. Structure of the toxic shock toxin. Biochemistry 1993;32:13,761–13,766.
6. Drake CG, Kotzin BL. Superantigens: biology, immunology, and potential role in disease. J Clin Immunol 1992;12:149–162.
7. Reda KB, Rich RR. Superantigens. In: Rich RR, ed. Clinical Immunology: Principles and Practice. Mosby-Year Book, Chicago, 1996, pp. 132–148.
8. Mattix ME, Hunt RE, Wilhelmsen CL, et al. Aerosolized staphylococcal enterotoxin B-induced pulmonary lesions in rhesus monkeys (*Macaca mulatta*). Toxicol Pathol 1995;23:262–268.
9. Franz DR, Jahrling PB, Friedlander AM, et al. Clinical Recognition and management of patients exposed to biological warfare agents. JAMA 1997; 278:399–411.
10. Peruski AH, Johnson LH, Peruski LF. Rapid and sensitive detection of biological warfare agents using time resolved fluorescent assays. J Immunol Methods 2002;263:35–41.
11. Naimushin AN, Soelberg SD, Nguyen DK, et al. Detection of *Staphylococcus aureus* enterotoxin B at femtomolar levels with a miniature integrated two-channel surface plasmon resonance (SPR) sensor. Biosens Bioelectron 2002;17:573–584.
12. LeClaire RD, Hunt RE, Bavari S. Protection against bacterial superantigen staphylococcal enterotoxin B by passive vaccination. Infect Immun 2002;70:2278–2281.
13. Arad G, Hillman D, Levy R, Kaempfer R. Superantigen antagonist blocks Th1 cytokine gene induction and lethal shock. J Leukoc Biol 2001;69:921–927.
14. Hale ML, Margolin SB, Krakauer T, et al. Pirfenidone blocks the in vitro and in vivo effects of staphylococcal enterotoxin B. Infect Immun 2002;70:2989–2994.
15. Tseng J, Komisar JL, Trout RN, et al. Humoral immunity to aerosolized staphylococcal enterotoxin B (SEB), a superantigen, in monkeys vaccinated with SEB toxoid-containing microspheres. Infect Immun 1995;63:2880–2885.
16. Stiles BG, Garza AR, Ulrich RG, Boles JW. Mucosal vaccination with recombinantly attenuated staphylococcal enterotoxin B and protection in a murine model. Infect Immun 2001;69:2031–2036.
17. Lee JS, Dyas BK, Nystrom SS, et al. Immune protection against staphylococcal enterotoxin-induced toxic shock by vaccination with a Venezuelan equine encephalitis virus replicon. J Infect Dis 2002;185:1192–1196.
18. Rich RR. Clinical Immunology: Principles and Practice. St. Louis, MO, Mosby, 1996.

# 14 Mycotoxins

## Duane R. Hospenthal, *MD, PhD, FACP*

The opinions or assertions contained herein are the private views of the author and are not to be construed as official or as representing the position of the Department of the Army or the Department of Defense.

### CONTENTS

INTRODUCTION
CASE VIGNETTE
TRICHOTHECENE MYCOTOXINS
MECHANISMS OF TOXICITY
HISTORY OF NATURAL AND BIOLOGICAL WARFARE USE
CLINICAL PRESENTATION
DIAGNOSIS
TREATMENT/MANAGEMENT
PROPHYLAXIS/AVOIDANCE
REFERENCES

## 1. INTRODUCTION

Mycotoxins are a diverse group of fungal secondary metabolites that most commonly affect humans through their association with food and feed crops. Hundreds of mycotoxins have been identified throughout the world, and it is estimated that one-fourth of the world's food crops are contaminated with fungi that potentially produce mycotoxins *(1)*. This contamination may affect humans directly or indirectly through their economic effect on domesticated animals *(2–4)*. Some of the most important mycotoxins include the aflatoxins, ochratoxins, cyclopiazonic acid, zearalenone, fumonisins, and trichothecenes *(2,5–8)*. Of these substances, the trichothecene mycotoxins are the most likely agents to be used in biowarfare or bioterrorism, having been studied (and probably used) for this purpose in the past. The trichothecene mycotoxins, especially the one denoted T-2, pose a threat for potential use as bioweapons because of their ability to cause both lethal and nonlethal illness and their stability. These toxins may be harmful to humans by topical, inhalation, and oral routes and would probably be used in an aerosolized form. Topical exposure causes rapid skin discomfort and damage, a property that can help to rapidly distinguish T-2 exposure from that of other biological agents. Systemic disease may occur following skin, lung, or gastrointestinal absorption. Systemic illness may

From: *Physician's Guide to Terrorist Attack*
Edited by: M. J. Roy © Humana Press Inc., Totowa, NJ

include rapid lethality or a subacute syndrome similar to that seen in radiation exposure. Because of the stability of these toxins, small-scale poisoning of food or water supplies is a possible alternate delivery method.

### Case Vignette

A middle-aged man presents for medical attention with complaints of burning pain and redness of his forearms, face, and neck. Additionally, he reports mild blurring of his vision and increased tearing. His symptoms began shortly after he was sprayed with a yellowish, oily liquid, which appeared to be coming from a low-flying single-engine airplane. Other people who were also in the vicinity of this spray reported similar symptoms. In addition to skin and eye complaints, other exposed individuals also reported throat discomfort, dyspnea, and chest pain. On physical examination our patient has tender erythema of his exposed skin and scleral injection.

## 2. TRICHOTHECENE MYCOTOXINS

The trichothecene mycotoxins are a large group of compounds that have attracted interest as possible biowarfare/bioterrorism agents because of their unique chemical properties, ability to cause natural disease, and purported past use as bioweapons. Trichothecene mycotoxins are a group of over 150 low molecular weight compounds containing a trichothecene ring (6,9). Most commonly these are products of a few species of the genus *Fusarium*, although fungi from the genera *Cephalosporium*, *Cylindrocarpon*, *Myrothecium*, *Stachybotrys*, *Trichoderma*, *Trichothecium*, and *Verticimonosporium* can also produce them (10). Of the many trichothecenes, only the fusarial toxins deoxynivalenol (DON, vomitoxin), diacetoxyscirpenol (DAS), nivalenol (NIV), T-2, and HT-2 have been widely studied (11). T-2 toxin is commonly thought to be the most likely mycotoxin agent to be used for biological warfare or terrorism. This toxin is believed to be the cause of large outbreaks of alimentary toxic aleukia in the 1930s and 1940s and was the purported active ingredient in "yellow rain" in the 1970s and 1980s. T-2 toxin is a small (molecular weight 467), heat-stable molecule that is insoluble in water and resistant to heat and ultraviolet light inactivation (Fig. 1). This toxin is stable in open air and when exposed to sunlight. Neither boiling nor the temperatures achieved with routine autoclaving will inactivate the T-2 toxin (12). As mycotoxins are secondary fungal metabolites like many of our antibiotics, T-2 could be mass-produced with standard industrial or pharmaceutical fermentation equipment. Extraction of the toxin with organic solvents reportedly produces a yellow to brown oily liquid (13). Further purification can produce a yellow or white crystalline product.

## 3. MECHANISMS OF TOXICITY

T-2 toxin causes damage to mammalian cells chiefly through inhibition of protein synthesis (9,11). Toxin produces this effect by binding to the ribosome and interfering with this production (14). Direct effect on the eukaryotic cell membrane may also lead to compromise of this structure. Inhibition of RNA and DNA synthesis is currently believed to be a secondary effect of inhibition of protein synthesis. In mammals, these

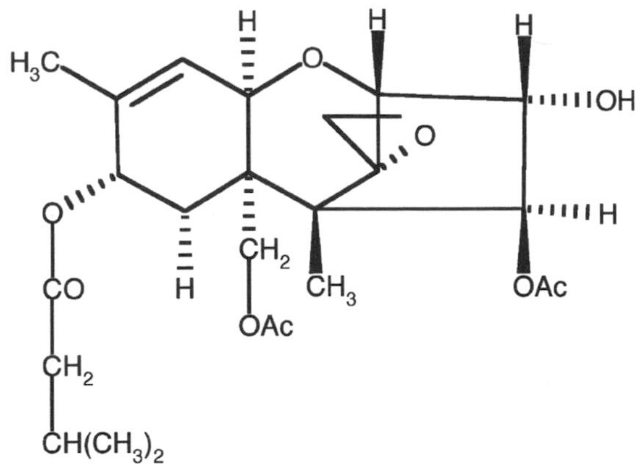

**Fig. 1.** Molecular structure of T-2 mycotoxin.

effects lead to cytotoxicity chiefly of rapidly dividing cells, thus accounting for their effect on the bone marrow and gastrointestinal tract.

Acute lethality has been studied in numerous animal models. Doses of T-2 required to produce death in 50% of challenged animals ($LD_{50}$) varies widely based on how the toxin is delivered and which species of animal is employed. $LD_{50}$ concentrations are generally in the single milligram range by nondermal routes. Although acute toxicity has been produced by oral, parenteral, and dermal challenges, delivery by the inhalational route is clearly the most lethal. The $LD_{50}$ of T-2 toxin in most animals is approximately 10–50 times smaller when given in an inhaled fashion *(13)*. In mice, inhalation of the toxin is 10 times more toxic than systemic administration and 20 times more toxic than oral ingestion *(15)*.

Toxin has been shown in animals to damage the immune system, including the production of apoptosis and DNA fragmentation in the thymus and spleen of rats and mice *(16,17)*. These immunosuppressive properties and decreased granulocyte production in the bone marrow explain the more chronic form of disease that mimics radiation exposure.

T-2 toxin is rapidly absorbed by the respiratory and gastrointestinal mucosa. Absorption through the skin is a slower process that can take hours. The trichothecene mycotoxins do not appear to require metabolic activation to produce their effects. Hepatic metabolism of these compounds rapidly leads to their excretion in the urine and stool. Animal models have not documented any accumulation of T-2 in the body with acute or chronic exposures *(11,18)*.

## 4. HISTORY OF NATURAL AND BIOLOGICAL WARFARE USE

In the late 1930s and 1940s, a large proportion of the population of the Orenburg district in Siberia became ill from eating contaminated breads, resulting in the death of an estimated 10% of the population *(14,19,20)*. This illness was given the name alimentary toxic aleukia (ATA) because of its effects on the gastrointestinal tract and suppression of the bone marrow. Studies linked ATA with the consumption of millet, wheat, and barley contaminated with fungi during overwintering. Four phases of disease have been described in this syndrome, occurring over a period of several months *(19)*. The first phase is typically an acute gastroenteritis that begins hours after ingestion of contaminated foodstuffs and usually lasts for 3–5 d. Symptoms described in this phase include burning sensation in the mouth, esophagus, and stomach, followed by nausea, vomiting, and diarrhea. This phase ends spontaneously as the subject passes into the second phase, which is usually asymptomatic (or clinically inapparent) and thus has been referred to as the latent period. This phase has also been called the leukopenic phase, as victims develop bone marrow suppression leading to leukopenia or even agranulocytosis during this period. Although phase two is said to be asymptomatic, some investigators have associated symptoms of weakness, easy fatigability, vertigo, headaches, palpitations, and even mild asthma with this phase.

The third phase of ATA is associated with severe bone marrow suppression, bleeding diatheses, and infectious complications of these. This stage, called the stage of evident sickness, appears 2–8 wk after ingestion of contaminated food, usually with the appearance of petechiae of the skin. Hemorrhagic syndromes and necrosis, especially of the structures of the mouth, were commonly noted in historic accounts. Fever and sepsis associated with severe leukopenia appears to be the major cause of mortality in ATA, and they are seen in this third phase. The fourth and final stage is the recovery phase. In patients who were supported through the third phase and survived, a period of up to 2 mo followed during which the bone marrow fully restored itself. Investigation of this syndrome identified toxin(s) produced by *Fusarium* as a probable etiology, and subsequent study in cats showed that an ATA-like syndrome could be produced using T-2 toxin produced from outbreak strains of *Fusarium (21)*. More recently, an epidemic of gastrointestinal disease was reported from the Kashmir Valley in India. In July through September of 1987, several thousand people became ill with symptoms including abdominal pain or fullness, throat irritation, and diarrhea. Epidemiological study of this outbreak identified bread prepared with wheat contaminated with *Fusarium* as a likely cause. Testing of food products found DON, nivalenol, and T-2 mycotoxins *(22)*.

The use of trichothecenes as biological warfare agents remains controversial. The strongest association of the use of mycotoxins as biological weapons comes from reports of their use in "yellow rain" attacks in Southeast Asia and Afghanistan from 1974 to 1981. Use of sprays containing a mixture of trichothecenes including T-2 has been reported in Laos, Cambodia, Afghanistan, and Iran *(23,24)*. The largest purported use was during the 1970s and 1980s in Laos, where around 6500 deaths have been attributed to "yellow rain" attacks *(25)*. Witnesses of these attacks described a yellowish oily substance, usually delivered by aerial spraying, that fell in large droplets, making a sound like rain on the roofs of buildings. Environmental samples and blood, urine, and tissue collected from attack areas and people exposed to these attacks have tested positive for mycotoxins, including T-2 *(26–28)*. Chiefly because of the remoteness of these attacks, the numbers of samples collected and tested were quite small. Skeptics introduced alternate explanations for the discovery of mycotoxins in these samples, including the possibility that toxins had been concentrated naturally in bee droppings, which themselves were concentrated in certain geographic areas by bee "cleansing flights" *(29–32)*. This explanation did not explain why polyethylene glycol, a man-made material, was found in some of these samples, or what toxin or chemical weapon explained the symptoms reported by those exposed to yellow rain, or the deaths of 10–20% of those exposed *(25,27–28)*. Another report of trichothecene mycotoxin use as a biological agent included the recovery of T-2 toxin from Iranian soldiers attacked by Iraqi weapons in the spring of 1984 *(24)*.

## 5. CLINICAL PRESENTATION

No well-described and documented study of the effect of T-2 or other trichothecene mycotoxins on humans exists. Clinical presentation and effects are extrapolated from animal studies, from anecdotal laboratory exposures, and from reports of natural or purported clandestine exposures. These latter two suffer additionally from retrospective collection of data and from the fact that mixtures of biological and/or chemical agents may have been involved in producing the reported symptoms and outcomes. Victims of attacks in Southeast Asia in the early 1980s believed to include mycotoxins reported a wide range of acute symptoms *(25,26,33)*. These always included eye and skin irritation along with gastrointestinal and respiratory distress. Specifically, eye irritation with pain, burning or tearing, eye redness, and blurring or other visual disturbances were described. Skin complaints included feelings of burning or itchiness, tenderness, redness, and sometimes development of small blisters in areas of exposed skin. Dryness of the mouth, bitter taste, prolonged vomiting and abdominal pain, diarrhea, and sometimes severe or fatal gastrointestinal hemorrhage occurred in those purportedly exposed to yellow rain. Hematemesis and hematochezia are reported to be the most characteristic presentation in exposures to yellow rain attack *(25)*. Dyspnea, shortness of breath, cough, wheezing, chest pain, nasal obstruction, rhinorrhea, nasal itchiness, epistaxis, and loss or change in voice was also reported. Other reported symptoms included headache, dizziness, ataxia, confusion, incoordination, collapse, paralysis, tachycardia, and muscle tremors or weakness. Death was described to occur both within minutes or hours of attack and for days afterward.

Clearly, the route or routes of exposure will affect the predicted clinical presentation. In an aerosolized attack, a combination of exposures including inhaled, ingested, or topical (dermal and ocular) may occur. As toxin can be absorbed systemically by any of these routes, systemic toxicity can occur acutely and chronically via any of them. Including animal data and probable historic exposures, the following symptoms are likely *(12,13)*.

> *Topical exposure* to unprotected skin and the eyes can result in symptoms within minutes to hours. Skin exposure to T-2 toxin can result in local erythema, pruritis, burning pain, and tenderness to touch. Blistering and progression to skin necrosis is possible. Ocular exposures will probably result in eye pain, excessive lacrimation, visual blurring and other disturbances in sight, and scleral injection.
>
> *Inhalational exposure* will probably produce nose and throat pain, nasal discharge or obstruction, nasal itching, sneezing, cough, dyspnea, chest pain, shortness of breath, hemoptysis, and voice change or loss.
>
> *Ingestional exposure* may cause mouth pain, esophageal pain, abdominal pain, diarrhea (often bloody and protracted), emesis, or hematemesis.
>
> *Systemic absorption* may lead to weakness, prostration, collapse, dizziness, incoordination, ataxia, tachycardia, hypotension, hypothermia, or death.
>
> *Late effects* of systemic absorption of subacute concentrations of T-2 toxin include bone marrow suppression leading to bleeding diatheses and infection.

## 6. DIAGNOSIS

Diagnosis is based on clinical presentation in conjunction with epidemiological and exposure data. Differential diagnosis includes exposure to other chemical agents and (in chronic forms) radiation. Smoke inhalation or exposure to industrial chemicals or pesticides could produce symptom complexes similar to acute exposure. Chemical weapons such as mustards and other blistering agents can produce acute eye and respiratory distress. In acute exposures, nasal or throat swabs should be obtained for analysis. Plasma and urine samples should be obtained from all persons who are believed to have been exposed to mycotoxin-containing agents. No rapid testing is available to detect the trichothecene mycotoxins. Testing is usually done with gas-liquid chromatography (GLC), combination GLC and mass spectrometry (MS), or high-performance liquid chromatography (HPLC). Immunoassays and bioassays have been evaluated for the detection of mycotoxins in food and feed crops and could potentially be used to study contaminated objects and areas.

## 7. TREATMENT/MANAGEMENT

No specific therapy exists for T-2 mycotoxin exposure. Removal of any unabsorbed toxin (decontamination) should occur as soon as possible. Outer clothing should be removed (and bagged) and exposed skin decontaminated with soap and water. Decontamination of skin may be effective in limiting absorption even if delayed for several hours. Persons with eye exposure should receive copious irrigation with normal saline. Persons with oral exposure should be given activated charcoal. Corticosteroids and colony-stimulating factors (CSFs) are potentially useful in the treatment of the more chronic effects of T-2 toxin exposures, although only limited animal research supports this use.

Virtually all treatment recommendations arise from controlled small animal study. Soap and water has been shown to be effective, and better than superactivated charcoal paste, in the treatment of dermal exposure in swine (34). Cleansing with detergent and water, even when delayed, appeared to be effective decontamination in rats (35). One study found removal with polyethylene glycol to be more effective than soap and water when large doses of T-2 were applied to rats (36). A topical skin protectant (cream containing perfluoroalkylpolyether and polytetrafluoroethylene) being developed by the military, has been shown to protect rabbits from dermal toxicity (37). This agent is not currently available for general use. Oral administration of activated charcoal following oral challenge with T-2 has been shown to be protective in female rat models (38,39). Orally administered activated charcoal improved survival in mice challenged orally, as well as parenterally with T-2 toxin (40). Superactivated charcoal enhanced rat survival when given within 3 h of T-2 toxin exposure (41). Swine were protected from acute toxicity by activated charcoal and magnesium sulfate (42). Corticosteroids, specifically dexamethasone and prednisolone, have been shown to decrease acute lethality in a murine model of toxin exposure (43,44). Dexamethasone has also been shown to decrease lethality in rats (45,46). Administration of methylthiazolidine-4-carboxylate improved survival in mice, apparently by maintaining the hepatic glutathione levels (47). Human recombinant granulocyte-CSF (rhG-CSF) produced decreased lethality and protected mice from leukopenia in at least one study of T-2 intoxication (48).

## 8 PROPHYLAXIS/AVOIDANCE

No specific prophylactic medications or immunizations exist. Prevention is chiefly by avoiding exposure to the toxin. Appropriate protective clothing and masks should prevent skin or inhalational exposure. Removal of toxin that contacts the skin with soap and water cleansing should limit absorption and may prevent systemic toxicity. Proper decontamination of contaminated areas and objects should decrease exposure to others. The toxin can be inactivated on contaminated surfaces with a 3–5% solution of sodium hypochlorite *(13)* or by a 1% hypochlorite solution that contains 0.1 *M* sodium hydroxide (NaOH) *(12)*. A 1-h contact time is suggested with the use of the latter product.

# REFERENCES

1.  Fink-Gremmels J. Mycotoxins: their implications for human and animal health. Vet Q 1999;21:115–120.
2.  Hollinger K, Ekperigin HE. Mycotoxicosis in food producing animals. Vet Clin North Am Food Anim Pract 1999;15:133–165.
3.  Hussein HS, Brasel JM. Toxicity, metabolism, and impact of mycotoxins on humans and animals. Toxicology 2001;167:101–134.
4.  Peraica M, Radic B, Lucic A, Pavlovic M. Toxic effects of mycotoxins in humans. Bull WHO 1999;77:754–766.
5.  Abarca ML, Accensi F, Bragulat MR, Cabanes FJ. Current importance of ochratoxin A-producing *Aspergillus* spp. J Food Prot 2001;64:903–906.
6.  Coulombe RA. Biological actions of mycotoxins. J Dairy Sci 1999;376:880–891.
7.  Osweiler GD. Mycotoxins. Contemporary issues of food animal health and productivity. Vet Clin North Am Food Anim Pract 2000;16:511–530.
8.  Pitt JI. Toxigenic fungi: which are important? Med Mycol 2000;38(suppl 1):17–22.
9.  Yagen B, Bialer M. Metabolism and pharmacokinetics of T-2 toxin and related trichothecenes. Drug Metab Rev 1993;25:281–323.
10. Sweeney MJ, Dobson ADW. Mycotoxin production by *Aspergillus*, *Fusarium* and *Penicillium* species. Int J Food Microbiol 1998;43:141–158.
11. Buck WB, Cote L. Trichothecene mycotoxins. In: Keeler RF, Tu AT, cds. Handbook of Natural Toxins. Vol. 6. Toxicology of Plant and Fungal Compounds Marcel Dekker, New York, 1991, pp. 523–555.
12. Kortepeter M, ed. T-2 mycotoxins. In: USAMRIID's Medical Management of Biologic Casualties Handbook, 4th ed. U.S. Army Medical Research Institute of Infectious Diseases, Fort Detrick, MD, 2001, pp. 146–153. (available online at www.usamriid.army.mil/education/bluebook.html).
13. Wannemacher RW, Wiener SL. Trichothecene mycotoxins. In: Sidell FR, Takafuji ET, Franz DR, eds, Textbook of Military Medicine: Medical Aspects of Chemical and Biologic Warfare. Borden Institute, Washington, DC, 1997, pp. 655–676.
14. Ueno Y. Mode of action of trichothecenes. Ann Nutr Aliment 1977;31:885–900.
15. Creasia DA, Thurman JD, Jones LJ, et al. Acute inhalational toxicity of T-2 mycotoxin in mice. Fund Appl Toxicol 1987;8:230–235.
16. Ihara T, Sugamata M, Sekijima M, Okumura H, Yoshino N, Ueno Y. Apoptotic cellular damage in mice after 1-2 toxin-induced acute toxicosis. Nat Toxins 1997;5:141–145.
17. Sugamata M, Hattori T, Ihara T, Okumura H, Yoshino N, Ueno Y. Fine structural changes and apoptotic cell death by T-2 mycotoxin. J Toxicol Sci 1998;23(suppl II):148–154.
18. Naseem SM, Pace JG, Wannemacher RW. A high-performance liquid chromatographic method for determining ($^3$H)T-2 and its metabolites in biological fluids of the cynomolgus monkey. J Anal Toxicol 1995;19:151–156.
19. Mayer CF. Endemic panmyelotoxicosis in the Russian grain belt. Part one: The clinical aspects of alimentary toxic aleukia (ATA). A comprehensive review. Mil Surg 1953;113:173–189.
20. Mayer CF. Endemic panmyelotoxicosis in the Russian grain belt. Part two: The botany, phytopathology, and toxicology of Russian cereal food. Mil Surg 1953;113:295–315.
21. Lutsky I, Mor N, Yagen B, Joffe AZ. The role of T-2 toxin in experimental alimentary toxic aleukia: a toxicity study in cats. Toxicol Appl Pharmacol 1978;43:111–124.
22. Bhat RV, Beedu SR, Ramakrishna Y, Munshi KL. Outbreak of trichothecene mycotoxicosis associated with consumption of mould-damaged wheat products in Kashmir Valley, India. Lancet 1989;1:35–37.
23. Haig AM. Chemical Warfare in Southeast Asia and Afghanistan. March 22, 1982 Report to Congress. US Government Printing Office, Washington, DC, 1982.
24. Heyndricks A, Sookvanichsilp N, van den Heede M. Detection of trichothecene mycotoxins (yellow rain) in blood, urine and faeces of Iranian soldiers treated as victims of a gas attack. Arch Belges 1984;(suppl):143–146.

25. Watson SA, Mirocha CJ, Hayes AW. Analysis of trichothecenes in samples from Southeast Asia associated with "yellow rain." Fund Appl Toxicol 1984;4:700–717.
26. Mirocha CJ, Pawlosky RA, Chatterjee K, Watson S, Hayes W. Analysis for *Fusarium* toxins in various samples implicated in biological warfare in Southeast Asia. J Assoc Off Anal Chem 1983;66:1485–1499.
27. Rosen JD. Presence of mycotoxins and a made-made material in a "yellow rain" sample. Arch Belges 1984;(suppl):173–176.
28. RosenRT, Rosen JD. Presence of four *Fusarium* mycotoxins and synthetic material in 'yellow rain.' Evidence for the use of chemical weapons in Laos. Biomed Mass Spectrom 1982;9:443–450.
29. Ashton PS, Meselson M, Robinson JPP, Seeley TD. Origin of yellow rain. Science 1983;222:366–368.
30. Dashek WV, Mayfield JE, Llewellyn GC, O'Rear CE, Bata A. Trichothecenes and yellow rain: possible biological warfare agents. Bioessays 1986;4:27–30.
31. Marshall E. Yellow rain evidence slowly whittled away. Science 1986;233:18–19.
32. Nowicke JW, Meselson M. Yellow rain—a palynological analysis. Nature 1984;309:205–206.
33. Stahl C J, Green CC, Farnum JB. The incident at Tuol Chrey: pathologic and toxicologic examinations of a casualty after chemical attack. J Forensic Sci 1985;30:317–337.
34. Biehl ML, Lambert RJ, Haschek WM, Buck WB, Schaeffer DJ. Evaluation of a superactivated charcoal paste and detergent and water in prevention of T-2 toxin-induced local cutaneous effects in topically exposed swine. Fundam Appl Toxicol 1989;13:523–532.
35. Bunner BL, Wannemacher RW, Dinterman RE, Broski FH. Cutaneous absorption and decontamination of ($^3$H)T-2 toxin in the rat model. J Toxicol Environ Health 1989;26:413–423.
36. Fairhurst S, Maxwell SA, Scawin JW, Swanston DW. Skin effects of trichothecenes and their amelioration by decontamination. Toxicology 1987;46:307–319.
37. Liu DK, Wannemacher RW, Snider TH, Hayes TL. Efficacy of the topical skin protectant in advanced development. J Appl Toxicol 1999;19:S41–S45.
38. Bratich PM, Buck WB, Haschek WM. Prevention of T-2 toxin-induced morphologic effects in the rat by highly activated charcoal. Arch Toxicol 1990;64:251–253.
39. Buck WB, Bratich PM. Activated charcoal: preventing unnecessary death by poisoning. Vet Med 1986;86:73–77.
40. Fricke RF, Jorge J. Assessment of efficacy of activated charcoal for treatment of acute T-2 toxin poisoning. Clin Toxicol 1990;28:421–431.
41. Galey FD, Lambert RJ, Busse M, Buck WB. Therapeutic efficacy of superactive charcoal in rats exposed to oral lethal doses of T-2 toxin. Toxicon 1987;25:493–499.
42. Poppenga RH, Lundeen GR, Beasley VR, Buck WB. Assessment of a general therapeutic protocol for the treatment of acute T-2 toxicosis in swine. Vet Hum Toxicol 1987;29:237–239.
43. Ryu J, Shiraki N, Ueno Y. Effects of drugs and metabolic inhibitors on the acute toxicity of T-2 toxin in mice. Toxicon 1987;25:743–750.
44. Fricke RF, Jorge J. Beneficial effect of dexamethasone in decreasing the lethality of acute T-2 toxicosis. Gen Pharmacol 1991;22:1087–1091.
45. Shohami E, Wisotsky B, Kempski O, Feuerstein G. Therapeutic effect of dexamethasone in T-2 toxicosis. Pharm Res 1987;4:527–530.
46. Tremel H, Strugala G, Forth W, Fichtl B. Dexamethasone decreases lethality of rats in acute poisoning with T-2 toxin. Arch Toxicol 1985;57:74–75.
47. Fricke RF, Jorge J. Methylthiazolidine-4-carboxylate for treatment of acute T-2 toxin exposure. J Appl Toxicol 1991;11:135–140.
48. Ohtani K, Nanya T, Aoyama Y, et al. Recombinant human granulocyte colony-stimulating factor accelerates regeneration after T-2 toxin-induced hemopoietic injury and lessens lethality in mice. J Toxicol Sci 1993;18:155–166.

# 15 | Smallpox

## James V. Lawler, MD, and Timothy H. Burgess, MD, MPH

The opinions or assertions contained herein are the private views of the authors and are not to be construed as official or as representing the position of the Department of the Navy or the Department of Defense.

### CONTENTS

## 1. INTRODUCTION

Smallpox is a febrile exanthematous illness caused by the variola virus, a member of the *Poxviridae* family. Smallpox was endemic in developing regions and periodically epidemic worldwide until the late 1970s. It is thought to have had among the greatest impacts on humanity of any infectious disease. The origin of the disease is unknown, but evidence of potential infection dates well back into ancient history. Several Egyptian mummies, including that of Ramses V from the 18th Egyptian Dynasty (16th–14th centuries BC), bear scars suggestive of smallpox *(1,2)*. Smallpox has been proposed as the source of several ancient epidemics, including the Plague of Athens in 430 BC described by Thucydides. Chinese writings from the 4th century AD and Indian writings from some 300 years later confirm the presence of the disease in these regions, although there are suggestions of its presence centuries earlier *(1)*. Smallpox reached its peak in the crowded

From: *Physician's Guide to Terrorist Attack*
Edited by: M. J. Roy © Humana Press Inc., Totowa, NJ

cities of 18th century Europe, taking 400,000 lives per year and killing five reigning European monarchs *(2,3)*. During this period, 10% of Swedish infants died of smallpox each year, and 10% of all deaths in London were attributable to the disease *(2)*.

At the height of the epidemics of the 1700s, Europeans were introduced to variolation, inoculating the skin of healthy individuals with lesions from smallpox patients. This technique had been practiced in India and East Asia for centuries, as it was recognized that cutaneous inoculation resulted in a less severe disease with much lower mortality while providing long-lasting immunity to recurrent smallpox infection *(1)*. Acceptance of variolation varied significantly between European countries, and although the practice spread slowly, it appeared to diminish the rate of disease in Europe and the American colonies. At the end of the 18th century, Edward Jenner performed his famous experiments inoculating people with material from cowpox lesions. In 1798, he published his treatise, *An Inquiry into the Causes and Effects of the Variolae Vaccinae, a Disease Discovered in some of the Western Counties of England Particularly Gloucestershire, and Known by the Name of Cow Pox*, at his own expense after his original reports of vaccination success were met with significant criticism *(2,3)*. Jenner's method of *vaccination* was much safer than variolation, which was still associated with the risk of severe disease and death, and his method provided lasting immunity *(1)*. Vaccination spread rapidly throughout Europe and America, and by the early 20th century smallpox was rarely seen in Western nations *(3)*.

Smallpox continued to be an endemic disease of tropical, underdeveloped countries until the late 20th century. The last naturally acquired case of smallpox occurred in Somalia in 1977, and the last recorded cases occurred in laboratory workers in Birmingham, England in 1978 *(1)*. Smallpox was declared eradicated by the World Health Organization (WHO) in May 1980. Global eradication was the result of a monumental coordinated vaccination effort by the WHO that began in 1959 and culminated in the Intensified Smallpox Eradication Program launched in 1967. Unfortunately, the threat of a recurrent epidemic remains, despite the official eradication of smallpox, because of its production as an agent of biological warfare. The former Soviet Union is known to have had a large smallpox weaponization program, producing large quantities of the variola virus for that purpose *(4)*. The WHO had recognized variola samples held at the U.S. Centers for Disease Control and Prevention (CDC) in Atlanta and the Research Institute of Viral Preparations in Moscow (later moved to the Vektor Institute in Novosibirsk, Russia) as the only repositories of the virus left in the world as of 1984. However, the U. S. Central Intelligence Agency reportedly surmised that at least four nations possessed samples of variola as late as 2002 *(5)*.

The fact that vaccination has not been practiced for 30 years in most Western counties has left a large population with little or no immunity, and the effects of an intentional release of smallpox into such a population are potentially devastating. The possible magnitude may be appreciated by considering the effects of smallpox on early Native American populations, which were naïve to smallpox prior to the arrival of European conquistadors. In the 2 years after the arrival of Hernan Cortez, 3.5 million Aztecs died of diseases, of which smallpox is thought to be the most prominent. In 1837, a whole Mandan Indian village on the Missouri river was decimated by smallpox brought in by a riverboat. In 2 weeks, smallpox reduced the population of the village from 2000 to less than 40 *(6)*.

As a result of the threat of biological warfare and terrorism, smallpox remains a disease of significant importance. Few practicing clinicians have ever seen the disease, so its recognition may be difficult. Because of the importance of early recognition and aggressive vaccination in the prevention of disease spread, a thorough understanding of the disease is necessary in preparation for what was previously an unthinkable event, the intentional reintroduction of smallpox. A comprehensive description of the disease can be found in the volume *Smallpox and Its Eradication*, by Fenner et al., published by the WHO after the success of the eradication campaign *(1)* and recently made available via the internet (www.who.int/emc/diseases/smallpox/Smallpoxeradication.html). The clinical features of smallpox have been recently reviewed *(7,8)*, and guidelines for prevention and management have been published by the CDC *(9)*. This chapter reviews and summarizes information on the clinical presentation, epidemiology, pathogenesis, prevention, and therapy of the disease.

## 2. CLINICAL MANIFESTATIONS AND PRESENTATION

Smallpox is a severe febrile illness, its most prominent feature being a rash appearing 2–4 d after a febrile prodrome and following a recognizable progression over the next 2–3 wk. Two distinct forms of smallpox are recognized. The prototypical disease, variola major, was seen mostly in Asia and Africa and had a 30% fatality rate in unvaccinated individuals. Variola minor, also known as alastrim, was recognized in Europe, parts of Africa, and South America after the late 19th century *(1)*. It was marked by a less severe course and had a 1% mortality in unvaccinated individuals. Initially distinguished on epidemiological grounds, viruses isolated from outbreaks of variola major and minor have been shown by restriction fragment length polymorphism (RFLP) analysis to have unique genomic properties and thus represent distinct entities *(10,11)*.

## 3. VARIOLA MAJOR

The clinical course of smallpox has been well described *(1,7,8)*. The incubation period was commonly reported to last from 7 to 17 d, although epidemiological data reviewed in the WHO publication suggest that the extreme of the incubation period could be 19 d or possibly longer. The incubation period for the vast majority of cases appears to have been 10–12 d in the pre-eradication era. Illness began with 2–3 d of high fever (38.5–40.5°C), prostration, headache, backache, and chills. Nausea, vomiting, and abdominal pain were sometimes seen, as well as altered mental status. The fact that fever preceded the rash was an important point in distinguishing smallpox from other febrile exanthems. The rash appeared first in the mucosa of the mouth and on the face, hands, and forearms. The lesions are initially macular but quickly became papular. Over the next few days, the lesions spread centrally, becoming most abundant on the face and extremities. The lesions progressed from papules to pustular vesicles. Lesions in a particular part of the body progressed in regional synchrony. For instance, at a given point in the course of the illness, lesions on the face may have progressed to vesicles, whereas lesions on the palms lagged a day behind and were still papular, but all facial lesions would be vesicular and all palmar lesions papular. Finally, the lesions have been described as "deep," not superficial (in contrast to the vesicles of chickenpox), and were typically loculated and umbilicated. Vesicles crusted by d 8–9 and formed scabs. Scabs usually separated around d 14, leaving

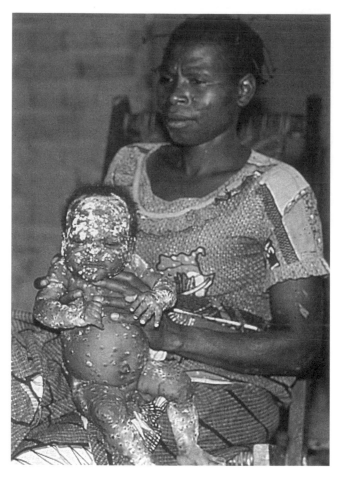

**Fig. 1.** Clinical smallpox. Photograph by Daniel H. Connor, M.D.Taken at Oicha, Eastern Zaire (Democratic Republic of the Congo), August, 1968.

a permanent hypopigmented scar, after which patients were considered no longer infectious (Figs. 1 and 2).

The mortality rate for ordinary-type smallpox was around 30%, although variations were noted ranging from 20 to 50% depending on circumstances. Death was ascribed to toxemia with attendant hypotension and shock, although the exact pathogenic mechanisms are probably unknown. Variola virus was disseminated systemically, and complications can arise involving most organ systems.

### 3.1. Hemorrhagic and Flat-Type Variants

A minority of patients with variola major in the pre-eradication era had an atypical, malignant course of the illness *(1,7,8)*. Hemorrhagic smallpox was seen in less than 3% of cases but was marked by extensive mucosal hemorrhage and petechiae, high viremia, and almost universal mortality. Flat-type smallpox, also known as hemorrhagic type II, had a slow evolution of soft, flat lesions with a hemorrhagic base. It appeared in 2–5% of patients and had a mortality of 95% in unvaccinated individuals. The cause of hem-

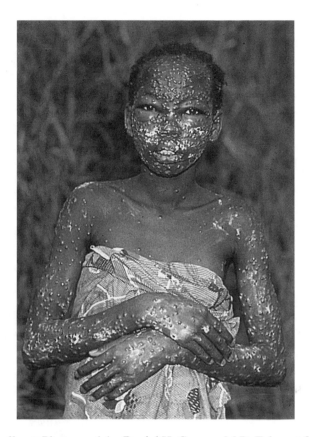

**Fig. 2.** Clinical smallpox. Photograph by Daniel H. Connor, M.D. Taken at Oicha, Eastern Zaire (Democratic Republic of the Congo), August, 1968.

orrhagic-type smallpox is unclear. Rao demonstrated that contacts of patients with hemorrhagic-type smallpox in his series did not have a higher incidence of this type of infection. This led experts to attribute its pathogenesis to host immune factors rather than a particularly virulent strain of virus *(1)*. A recent report describing a 1971 outbreak in Aralsk, Kazhakstan that had an unusually high rate of hemorrhagic-type smallpox has caused some to speculate that particular strain virulence factors (possibly engineered) could contribute to hemorrhagic disease *(12)*.

### 3.2. Smallpox in Vaccinated Individuals

The most significant and desired effect of vaccination is the prevention of any manifestation of clinical smallpox. However, some vaccinated persons did develop smallpox, and in those persons, a history of vaccination within 10 years (or possibly longer) resulted in a less severe course of illness *(1,13–15)*. A possible exception to this rule was hemorrhagic smallpox, which may not have been affected by prior vaccination *(1)*. Vaccination was associated with most, if not all, of the cases of modified-type smallpox, a much milder illness resembling variola minor. This was characterized by a much more rapid progression through the stages of eruption, decreased density of lesions, absence of fever after the pre-eruptive stage, rare toxemia, and very low mortality *(1)*. Even when vaccinated patients had an illness more consistent with ordinary-type smallpox, the exanthem was often less severe with fewer lesions. These lesions tended to be more superficial and progressed rapidly, in sometimes half the time of normal cases. Prior vaccination was almost always present in patients with *variola sine eruptione*, a brief febrile illness without rash that could be confirmed as smallpox only through serological testing *(1)*.

The varied presentations of vaccine-modified smallpox may pose a difficult challenge to clinicians in the event of a future outbreak. Such cases frequently presented without classical manifestations of smallpox. The rash could be rapidly progressing, superficial, and nonpustular and could progress in varying stages. It could be mistaken for other febrile illness with vesicular eruption such as chickenpox (varicella).

## 4. VARIOLA MINOR

Any future epidemic of smallpox will probably be caused by the intentional release of smallpox as a biological weapon, and one would therefore assume that variola major would be the virus introduced. Variola minor is of historical interest, however, and may be useful in understanding the pathogenesis of smallpox infection.

As was previously mentioned, variola minor was found primarily in Europe, North and South America, and certain parts of Africa and was not recognized as a separate entity until the late 19th century *(1)*. The illness went by the names "amaas" in South Africa and "alastrim" in South America *(3)*. Clinically, it was impossible to differentiate variola minor from modified-type or mild, discrete ordinary-type smallpox on a case-by-case basis. The distinction could only be made through epidemiological study during an outbreak or in the laboratory through virological testing *(1,3)*. In general, the pre-eruptive stage was milder and the skin lesions were smaller, more discrete, and more rapidly progressing. Fever during the eruptive stage was rare, as was significant toxemia. Flat-type smallpox was not associated with variola minor, and only a few cases of hemorrhagic-type smallpox were reported. Overall, the mortality of variola minor infection was around 1% in unvaccinated persons *(1)*.

## 5. LABORATORY FINDINGS

Accounts of clinical observation of smallpox cases are relatively abundant, but fewer data exist regarding abnormalities of hematological or biochemical parameters. This is in part because most cases were encountered in countries with little or no medical infrastructure and a paucity of laboratory capabilities. Hospitalization was associated with worse outcome in some countries, so a large proportion of patients remained at home *(1)*. Regardless of the availability, most laboratory and radiographic tests were of little use in diagnosis. Ordinary-type smallpox was often accompanied by neutropenia and relative leukocytosis in the early eruptive stage. Mild thrombocytopenia and hypoalbuminemia were also encountered. These findings tended to correlate with severity of disease. As would be expected, patients with hemorrhagic-type smallpox had significant thrombocytopenia and coagulopathy as demonstrated by abnormal bleeding time and prothrombin time *(1)*.

## 6. VIROLOGY AND PATHOGENESIS

Variola virus is a member of the *Poxviridae* family, a large group of viruses that infect both vertebrates and invertebrates. Molluscum contagiosum virus and variola virus are the only members that are found strictly in humans *(16)*. Poxviruses are the largest of all viruses, with a genome consisting of a single molecule of double-stranded DNA, ranging in size from 130 to over 300 kb *(16)*. The physical properties of the poxviruses are similar. They are described as brick-shaped or ovoid and are 200–400 nm in length *(1)*. They consist of a core that contains DNA, lateral bodies (the function of which is unknown), and an outer membrane. Extracellular viruses sometimes possess an envelope that is acquired from a host cell prior to virion budding *(16)*. Poxviruses replicate and assemble in the cytoplasm. They can pass directly from cell to cell, be released from a lysed cell, or bud off a living host cell to infect other cells *(16)*.

Infection with poxviruses appears to have a profound effect on host cells and immune responses. Infection of tissue culture cells results in abrupt cessation of host cell protein synthesis, changes in membrane permeability, and cytopathic changes *(16)*. Poxviruses possess several defense mechanisms against host immune response including proteins that inhibit the complement cascade and proteins that mimic or bind cytokines, as well as proteins that inhibit apoptosis in infected cells *(17)*. Manipulating the genes that express these proteins can alter the virulence of poxviruses *(16)*.

The genus *Orthopoxvirus* contains a group of closely related poxviruses of vertebrates; among these are variola, vaccinia, cowpox, and monkeypox. These viruses are distinguished from other genuses of poxviruses by their crossreactivity in hemagglutinin inhibition, gel precipitation, crossneutralization, and several other serological assays *(1)*. By RFLP analysis, genomes of these viruses have a very well-preserved central region, allowing classification within the genus, whereas heterology in the terminal regions can be used to differentiate species *(1,10,11)*. The close relation of these viruses and serological crossreactivity helps to explain why infection with one species can protect against subsequent infection with a different species, as is the case with vaccinia and variola.

Variola viruses consist of a number of distinct strains. Although strain differences are difficult to differentiate antigenically or serologically, they are demonstrated functionally by the wide variation in mortality from epidemics in different areas *(3)*. These differences did not appear to be related to host factors and persisted when particular strains were transported to different regions *(1)*. The clearest distinction was between strains of the virus that caused outbreaks with a mortality of 5–40% and strains associated with a mortality of 0.1–2%. This led to the classifications of variola major and minor *(1)*. The genetic differences between strains have been analyzed by RFLP mapping *(10,11)*. These studies found that strains of variola minor were similar but differed from strains of variola major. Although subtle differences between strains of variola major were found, none could be found to correlate with severity of disease.

Strain-associated differences in pathogenicity among the orthopoxviruses are not unique to variola. Of particular interest are variations among different strains of vaccinia used in vaccination efforts. These differences were shown to correlate with adverse events from vaccination and the potentially protective effect of vaccination *(1)*.

Studies with various models of *Orthopoxvirus* infections have suggested a basic sequence of events that probably reflects the course of variola infection in humans *(1,18)*. From the initial site of inoculation, usually the mucosa of the oropharynx or upper respiratory system in naturally acquired smallpox, the virus was transported to regional lymph nodes, where significant replication first occurred. From regional lymph nodes, the virus was spread to large lymphoid organs such as the spleen and deep lymph node chains. This probably occurred through a low-level primary viremia. After further replication in the lymphoid organs, a secondary viremia occurred, resulting in generalized dissemination to most organs, including the skin. This generalized dissemination and replication of the virus in end organs probably coincided with the onset of clinical illness. Viremia with variola virus is thought to be primarily cell-associated and of low magnitude. It was a rare occurrence for researchers to detect any viremia in patients, especially after the onset of clinical disease. The exception to this was in hemorrhagic-type smallpox, in which high titers of virus were detected up to the point of death.

Except for the readily apparent enanthem and exanthem, the pathological effects of systemic infection and replication of variola virus were not remarkable *(1,4,18)*. Pathological examination of various organs failed to demonstrate any consistent findings associated with infection, other than those associated with the skin and mucous membranes. Specific organ injury resulting in death was rarely discernable. Studies of lethal monkeypox infections in monkeys have demonstrated a precipitous drop in blood pressure prior to death that is associated with a rapid rise in interleukin-6 (IL-6), IL-10, and tumor necrosis factor (TNF)-$\alpha$ and -$\beta$ *(19)*. This "cytokine storm" may underlie the toxemia and eventual death seen in severe cases of ordinary-type or flat-type smallpox.

## 7. EPIDEMIOLOGY AND TRANSMISSION

In endemic countries, transmission of smallpox occurred year round *(1)*. As with most infectious diseases, there was significant variation with the seasons, cases being most prevalent in the winter and spring *(1,15,20)*. There was also variation over 3–8-yr cycles, probably related to population susceptibility and exposure and potentially climate *(15)*.

Invasion of smallpox virus occurred primarily through the oropharynx and respiratory route *(1,3)*. Entry could also be gained through nonintact skin, but a cutaneous route of infection was usually the result of intentional inoculation. Variola virus was shed in large amounts from infected cases in oropharyngeal secretions starting on d 3–4 of illness *(1,21)*, probably because the mucosal enanthem lesions were first to appear and were rapidly ulcerating. Shedding continued up to the 14th day of illness but tended to be shorter and of less magnitude in less severe cases *(1)*. Although some investigators were able to demonstrate virus in oropharyngeal swabs in the incubation period, this was not thought to translate into infectivity during this stage of the illness *(1,3,22)*. Virions were probably passed to uninfected people by direct contact or large droplets and were introduced into the mucous membranes (oropharynx and nasopharynx) where infection was established. Viral titers in vesicular fluid, pustular fluid, and scabs were also high; however, this did not appear to be very important as a route of transmission *(1,23)*. Epidemiological evidence clearly demonstrated that susceptible contacts were at much higher risk of infection from contact with smallpox patients during the first week of the rash rather than later in the illness, when large amounts of virus were being shed in separating scabs. Virus in scabs, although viable, is thought to be tightly bound in the fibrin matrix and thus much less infectious *(1,3)*.

Variola virus is relatively hardy in the environment. It is susceptible to high temperatures and high humidity, but viable virus could be recovered from old scabs after years of storage in temperate climates *(1)*. High titers of virus were isolated from the bedding and clothes of smallpox patients, most likely from contamination with oropharyngeal secretions *(23)*. The virus is viable for at least a short time in droplets and aerosols. Fortunately, most uncomplicated cases of smallpox did not involve frequent coughing or sneezing to generate small-particle aerosols. When these symptoms did occur, however, distant transmission was a risk *(1)*.

Although the highest risk of transmission of smallpox is from direct patient contact, indirect transmission is possible. Transmission through fomites was clearly, albeit infrequently, documented, especially in laundry workers or other handlers of contaminated clothes or linens *(3)*. Airborne transmission was thought to be relatively rare. Proximity to active cases on trains and buses in India was frequent, but infection was not commonly linked to such exposures *(1)*. Evidence of distant aerosol transmission was clearly documented, however. The most famous such study examined the spread of smallpox introduced to a German hospital by a single returning traveler in 1970 *(20)*. The index case was hospitalized for 3 d before a diagnosis of smallpox was made. Despite an aggressive immunization program, 19 people at the hospital developed smallpox, and many of them were 1 or 2 floors above the index case. The distribution of subsequent cases in the hospital closely mirrored the distribution of smoke that was released as a test from the index case's room. One man who developed smallpox was a visitor who spent only 15 min in the hospital, on the same floor as the index case but in a section several rooms away from any patient care area.

It is important to note that some contacts of smallpox patients (10% in one study) who never manifested clinical illness still had detectable viral shedding from oropharyngeal secretions *(22)*. These apparent subclinical infections usually occurred in previously vaccinated individuals. Although it was difficult to trace significant transmission from such asymptomatic carriers, they may have played a minor role in perpetuating the spread of smallpox *(1)*.

Overall, smallpox was relatively efficient in its transmission from infected patient to susceptible host, although it did not appear to achieve the level of infectivity of measles or chickenpox. A review of studies from endemic countries found an average secondary attack rate of 58.4% among unvaccinated household contacts *(1)*. Rates among unvaccinated hospital workers in nonendemic countries may have been higher, perhaps because of the absence of prior immunity or because of the high level of exposure *(14)*. The vast majority of secondary cases were the result of intimate household contacts *(13,20,24,25)*. Transmission outside the home was lower. Because patients were ill for days before the onset of the enanthem and subsequent infectivity, they generally quarantined themselves by staying home in bed, thus reducing contact with other potential hosts *(1,26)*.

In predicting the ramifications of a future outbreak, one of the most pertinent studies is Thomas Mack's review of the effects of 49 importations of smallpox into Western countries during the period 1950–1971 *(14)*. Such countries had not seen endemic smallpox for decades and did not have the population benefits of repeated exposures or subclinical infections. As a result, any immunity was probably the result of vaccination. The population in this review differed from the present-day population, however, because vaccination was still standard among developed countries. The difficulty of diagnosis in these cases is evidenced by the fact that only 21 of the 41 identified importing travelers were placed in isolation within 2 d of the onset of illness, and only 27 cases were in isolation within 10 d. This was in an era prior to the eradication of the disease, with patients apparently providing a history of travel to endemic countries. Remarkably, the diagnosis was made by the index case himself in 29 of 41 cases. In the Mack review, 936 cases of smallpox resulted from these importations. Variola major probably accounted for 44 outbreaks with 680 cases. Thirteen importations resulted in no subsequent transmission. Importations in which a diagnosis was made only after at least one transmission resulted in an average of four additional cases. More than half of the generated cases of variola major were transmitted in the hospital, with health care professionals and families of health care professionals accounting for 146/211 of in-hospital transmission. The vast majority of cases outside of the hospital occurred in family members or intimate contacts of the patient.

With variola major, age and vaccination status appeared to have a profound effect on mortality among hospital worker cases, hospital-acquired cases, and community-acquired cases. Overall mortality rates, regardless of vaccination status, for ages 0–9, 10–49, and 50+ yr were 20, 12, and 29%, respectively. For those never vaccinated, mortality rates rose to 40, 49, and 91%, respectively. Even young adult hospital workers had a surprisingly high mortality rate without pre-exposure vaccination, with 14 of 20 (70%) cases resulting in death. Only 12 of these persons received postexposure vaccination, with 7 deaths in this group. Mack's review reveals several germane points about smallpox outbreaks in nonendemic countries. Errors and delays in diagnosis of smallpox in the absence of a known outbreak were common *(1)*. The spread of the disease was relatively slow, since at least 10 d is required between generations, and most outbreaks were halted within two generations of transmission *(20)*. Persons at high risk for acquisition of infection could be predicted, as transmission almost always occurred to very close contacts. Hospital workers and inpatient contacts appear to be at especially high risk of infection. Finally, mortality rates in unvaccinated individuals from nonendemic areas may be much higher than rates commonly reported for variola major infection.

## 8. DIFFERENTIAL DIAGNOSIS

The differentiation of smallpox from other illnesses was sometimes challenging to even the most experienced clinicians. The present paucity of first-hand knowledge of smallpox among health care workers will probably make timely diagnosis even more difficult. During the pre-eruptive stage, the disease has no truly distinguishing characteristics, and without the benefit of prior knowledge of exposure or an ongoing epidemic, a diagnosis of smallpox would probably never be entertained. Only after the appearance of the rash is one able to look for characteristic features of the disease.

The differential diagnosis of fever and macular or maculopapular rash is a long list indeed. Early in the eruptive stage, smallpox can mimic any classic exanthemous illnesses of childhood (such as measles, rubella, roseola, erythema infectiosum), viral illnesses such as enterovirus or adenovirus, rickettsial spotted fevers, leptospirosis, syphilis, or other bacterial infections. It is helpful that in smallpox, the patient has a prodromal febrile illness for days prior to the onset of rash, as opposed to many of these illnesses, in which fever and rash have an onset with close temporal relationship. In addition, patients with smallpox tend to be more ill than patients with more typical viral diseases.

The progression of smallpox lesions and their appearance in the more advanced stages serves to differentiate smallpox from most other diseases. Illnesses that may be confused with smallpox in later stages of the eruption are those that have a prominent vesicular or pustular rash, especially chickenpox. Other diseases commonly manifesting such a rash are disseminated herpes simplex (including eczema herpeticum), coxsackievirus, rickettsialpox (*Rickettsia akari*), mycoplasma, *Vibrio vulnificus*, and (rarely) bacteremia with bacteria such as *Moraxella*. Noninfectious diseases can also sometimes present with fever and vesicular rash, especially erythema multiforme, drug eruption, or (rarely) Behçet's syndrome *(1,7,27)*. Several features usually differentiated smallpox from these other illnesses. The rash was preceded by an enanthem (mucous membrane eruption) and was first seen on the face, upper trunk, or (rarely) forearms, with spread to the eventual centrifugal pattern. Fever usually abated with the appearance of the rash and recurred a few days later. Lesions in the same region progressed in synchrony (unlike chickenpox, in which adjacent lesions may be in different stages). Lesions were deep and firm. One suggested test to differentiate smallpox and chickenpox is the "thumbnail test": the examiner firmly rubs his or her (preferably gloved) thumbnail over the lesion *(28)*. A vesicle that ruptures is likely to be from varicella, whereas the deep nature of smallpox lesions will generally prevent the lesion from rupturing.

Hemorrhagic-type smallpox may be difficult to diagnose clinically, since patients die before the rash progresses to a vesicular or pustular form *(1)*. Hemorrhagic smallpox was frequently misdiagnosed as acute leukemia or meningococcemia *(4)*. In a patient residing in or traveling to countries with endemic viral hemorrhagic fevers, it may be impossible to make a definitive clinical diagnosis early in the course. Dengue virus is ubiquitous throughout the tropics, and the incidence of dengue hemorrhagic fever is on the rise *(29)*. However, the cutaneous findings in this disease are much less prominent than with smallpox, and mortality is significantly less. In fact, any patient who survives an apparent hemorrhagic fever is unlikely to have had smallpox. Some of the more severe hemorrhagic fevers such as filovirus infections (Ebola, Marburg) may be difficult to distinguish from hemorrhagic-type smallpox strictly on clinical grounds. Fortunately, these diseases are geographically restricted. A severe hemorrhagic fever in any patient in North America or Europe without recent travel to Africa or Asia should suggest smallpox.

Diagnostic difficulty was greatest in the setting of a previously vaccinated patient. In this instance, modified-type smallpox or a less severe form of ordinary-type smallpox was the common presentation *(1,3)*. As was noted earlier, skin findings in these forms of smallpox frequently did not appear prototypical. They tended to be less dense, to have less frequent classical distribution, to progress much faster, and to appear more superficial. Patients were typically less ill, and fever often did not recur after the pre-eruptive stage ended. Vaccine-modified smallpox would most likely be confused with chickenpox. The lack of a prodromal fever preceding the eruption, the wide variation of lesion stages, the more superficial nature of lesions, and the characteristic "centripetal" distribution of lesions (more dense on the trunk than on the face or extremities) should assist in the diagnosis of chickenpox as opposed to smallpox.

The most difficult disease to distinguish from smallpox on clinical grounds alone would be human monkeypox infection. This is a rare disease encountered in Central and Western Africa, obtained primarily through a zoonotic cycle, although person-to-person transmission has occurred *(30)*. It is generally less severe than variola major and has the frequent finding of lymphadenopathy, a feature not found in smallpox. However, it is practically impossible for even the most experienced clinician to differentiate the two infections without laboratory confirmation. Since this is a rare disease that has been considered for use as a biological weapon, even a confirmed case of monkeypox should alert medical staff to the likelihood of biological attack.

## 9. DIAGNOSIS

Research and development of easy-to-use rapid diagnostic tests for smallpox is ongoing, but no such tests are commercially available at the time of this writing. The initial diagnosis of smallpox remains a clinical one, and physicians or other health care providers should not await laboratory confirmation prior to instituting appropriate infection control and public health measures. However, confirmation of alternative diagnoses, particularly chickenpox, can be rapidly accomplished by means of techniques such as direct fluorescent antibody (DFA) staining. Such alternative diagnoses should be expeditiously pursued in the appropriate settings, since confirmation would avert unnecessary public health measures. Laboratory diagnosis of variola requires the handling of potentially infectious samples and should be done only in reference laboratories under biosafety level 4 (BL-4) safety containment (4).

The most rapid diagnostic tools available are light and electron microscopy. Scrapings of the vesicular or pustular lesions or scabs can be examined for characteristic findings. An experienced microscopist may be able to discern Guanieri bodies using Giemsa or Gispen's modified silver stains under light microscopy (31). Guanieri bodies are aggregates of virions within the cytoplasm of infected cells. Electron microscopy using a negative staining technique is a much more sensitive test. Recognition of the large, brick-shaped virions is diagnostic of a poxvirus, although the particular species may not be identified. This technique can easily differentiate poxviruses from other viruses (such as herpesviruses) and was used extensively in the Intensified Smallpox Eradication Program (1).

Antigen detection methods and serological tests for antibodies to variola can also be used for diagnosis. The most widely used method for antigen detection was gel precipitation, which detected the presence of viral antigen in vesicular or pustular fluid by using vaccinia hyperimmune serum (1). This test was rapid and did not require a microscope. However, it requires the supply of vaccinia hyperimmune serum and a laboratory and technicians capable of performing such a test. In addition, this test cannot differentiate between the different species of Orthopoxvirus (smallpox, vaccinia, cowpox, monkeypox.) Serological testing can be done by a variety of means, such as enzyme-liked immunosorbent assay (ELISA), Western blot, or virus neutralization assay, but this is most useful in retrospective diagnosis (18).

Historically, the definitive identification of variola virus has been made from live virus culture with a variety of biological tests. Poxviruses grow on a variety of cell lines, but the most useful medium has been the chorioallantoic membrane of the chick. All orthopoxviruses that infect humans produce unique pockmarks on the chick chorioallantoic membrane that allow their identification (1).

Nucleic acid techniques have been used for specific virus identification. Endonuclease digestion and RFLP is an established technique that can provide unequivocal identification (10,11), Nucleic acid amplification tests such as polymerase chain reaction (PCR) are available in specialized laboratories and may provide rapid diagnosis (4).

## 10. VACCINATION

Vaccination against smallpox has a long history and was the genesis of modern vaccine study and immunology. Vaccination was the key component in the WHO's successful eradication program, a crowning achievement in the field of public health. Vaccination will remain the cornerstone of any response to a future outbreak, and clinicians should have a solid understanding of the principles underlying smallpox vaccination. Conditions associated rarely with vaccinia complications (see Subheading 10.2.) represent contraindications to pre-exposure vaccination. However, many experts suggest that there are no contraindications to vaccinia administration for persons exposed to confirmed smallpox cases.

## *10.1. Vaccinia*

Sometime between the end of the 18th century, when Jenner's work launched massive vaccination efforts, and the early 20th century, the virus used for vaccination against smallpox changed from cowpox to vaccinia *(18)*. Vaccinia is a closely related member of the genus *Orthopoxvirus*, and its origins are still a source of debate. Similar to cowpox, inoculation of vaccinia into the skin of naïve hosts results in a self-limited infection that imparts immunity to subsequent smallpox infection *(1)*.

The general principles of production of vaccinia vaccine remained relatively unchanged throughout the 20th century. Stocks of vaccinia or "seed" were maintained through repeated passages in a pool of animals. Vaccinia was inoculated into the skin of an animal host or "vaccinifer," usually into the shaved skin of the abdomen of a cow or calf. A pox lesion developed at the site, which was then scraped to supply a raw pulp. The pulp was then ground, purified, and mixed with a stabilizing and antibiotic solution. This liquid vaccine was effective but did not store or travel well *(1)*. The discovery of freeze drying techniques in the middle of the 20th century allowed for long-term storage and transport of vaccine *(32)*, one of the keys to the success of the WHO eradication campaign.

For most of the 20th century, smallpox vaccines were produced in a large number of individual production facilities using different animal vaccinifers, different vaccinia strains, and different purification techniques. The potency and purity of vaccines varied significantly, especially those from production facilities in underdeveloped countries *(1)*. In the 1960s, the WHO implemented guidelines requiring a "seed lot" system for vaccine production *(32)*. This attempt to standardize vaccines encouraged use of only a limited number of known strains for production. The most commonly used strains in Europe and the United States, respectively, were the Lister strain and the New York City Board of Health (NYCBH) strain (the source strain for the Dryvax® vaccine) *(1,32)*. As a result, vaccines used during the Intensified Eradication Program were much more potent and much more reliable than many of the vaccines used before.

The U.S. stockpile of smallpox vaccine as of late 2002 was produced using growth on calf skin (Dryvax, Wyeth Laboratories). This vaccine has been maintained in storage, as production ceased over 20 yr ago. The harvested calf lymph was processed with polymyxin B sulfate, dihydrostreptomycin sulfate, chlortetracycline hydrochloride, and neomycin sulfate and was then dried by lyophilization. The vaccine is reconstituted with a diluent containing 50% glycerine and 0.25% phenol in sterile water *(33)*. Supplies of this vaccine are limited, as only 15.4 million doses were stockpiled *(34)*. Studies have recently shown that the vaccine can be diluted up to fivefold without significantly reducing efficacy, thus expanding the available supply of vaccine *(35,36)*. To boost future availability of smallpox vaccine, the U.S. Department of Health and Human Services awarded contracts in 2000 and in 2001 for the production of new smallpox vaccines to total over 200 million doses *(37)*. These vaccines will use the NYCBH strain but will be grown in tissue culture rather than live animals. As of late 2002, phase I trials of the first of these vaccines showed 100% efficacy in take *(38)*.

To ensure adequate vaccination, the WHO set specific guidelines for vaccine administration and follow-up. The vaccine is administered with a standardized bifurcated needle dipped into the reconstituted vaccine and used to puncture the superficial skin. The WHO Smallpox Eradication unit suggested a universal 15 strokes with the needle regardless of prior vaccination status *(1)*. Vaccinees should be examined 6–8 d after vaccination to determine "take." The WHO Expert Committee on Smallpox classified vaccine response into two types: (1) major reaction and (2) equivocal reaction *(1,32)*. A major reaction consists of a vesicular or pustular lesion or an ulcerated or crusted lesion surrounded by palpable induration and is considered evidence of adequate vaccination. An equivocal reaction is any vaccination site that does not possess these qualities. It may be the result of prior immunity or a defective lot of vaccine that does not produce adequate immune response. An equivocal reaction is evidence of vaccine failure and should not be considered to impart protection. Such patients should be revaccinated.

Most vaccines produced later in the campaign against smallpox (such as the Dryvax) were so potent that even recently vaccinated individuals with presumably high levels of immunity had a classic Jennerian response (major reaction) elicited by revaccination *(1)*. The response follows a stereotypical course, beginning with erythema, pruritis, and a papular lesion 3–4 d after vaccination. A vesicle forms, which becomes umbilicated and then pustular by the 9th d. The pustule crusts over and scabs by the 14th d, and the scab finally separates between the 17th and 21st d, leaving a characteristic scar. Fever and mild constitutional symptoms may be present in association with the pustular phase, and swelling and tenderness of draining lymph nodes is not uncommon *(1,39)*. Viremia and virus isolation from tonsillar swabs were demonstrated in modest numbers of vaccinees with European strain. Existence of systemic infection with NYCBH strain (i.e., Dryvax) has not been demonstrated in the absence of adverse reactions and remains controversial *(32)*.

## 10.2. Complications of Vaccination

Adverse reactions to smallpox vaccination were historically relatively uncommon with the standard vaccine preparations used in Western countries. The most common complication was accidental inoculation, either of a remote part of the vaccinee's body or of another unvaccinated person *(32)*. The most common areas of autoinoculation were the eyelid, vulva, and perineum. The vast majority of these episodes were benign. Three more severe types of adverse skin reactions were reported after vaccination. In order of frequency, they are generalized vaccinia, eczema vaccinatum, and vaccinia necrosum (also known as progressive vaccinia). In addition, encephalitis rarely (and unpredictably) follows vaccinia administration *(1,32,39)*.

### 10.2.1. GENERALIZED VACCINIA

This condition represents an exaggerated manifestation of the systemic vaccinia infection usually induced by vaccination. Few to many vaccinial lesions develop between the 6th and 9th d after vaccination. Patients may experience high fevers and constitutional symptoms along with the diffuse eruption. The lesions vary in size but usually follow the same course as primary vaccination lesions. This reaction usually occurs in otherwise healthy individuals and is associated with full recovery *(1)*.

### 10.2.2. ECZEMA VACCINATUM

For unknown reasons, patients with eczema or atopic dermatitis can experience an unusual and severe course of vaccinia infection. Hypothesized mechanisms involve immunological abnormalities in the skin of patients with atopic dermatitis. These include tissue-specific cytokine imbalance between interferon-γ (low) and IL-4 (high) favoring a Th2 cellular immune response, and deficiencies in innate responses manifested by abnormal natural killer cell function, paucity of neutrophil infiltration, and diminished endogenous antimicrobial peptides *(40)*. This complication occurs in both vaccinated patients and unvaccinated contacts who have either active eczema or a history of eczema.

Eczematous skin or areas previously affected by eczema develop an eruption relatively concurrent with the lesion at the site of vaccination (or after a 5-d incubation period in contacts of vaccinees) that becomes inflamed and can later spread to normal skin. Patients may experience severe constitutional symptoms, lymphadenopathy, and high fevers. Infants with large areas of involved skin have a significant mortality. Treatment with vaccinia immune globulin (VIG) appears to reduce mortality (1).

### 10.2.3. Progressive Vaccinia (Vaccinia Necrosum)

Patients with an immune deficiency disorder can have a persistent vaccinia infection at the site of inoculation or sometimes at remote sites. These lesions gradually spread over the course of weeks to months. Mortality was high, 4 of 11 patients in the 1968 nationwide survey (41). Treatment with methisazone appeared to have some beneficial effect, and agents such as cidofovir may be useful today (1). VIG probably does not offer much in these cases, as the defect appears to be one of cell-mediated immunity. Fortunately, this complication was rare in the 1960s. Our present population has a much higher incidence of deficiencies in cell-mediated immunity, with the greatly increased frequency of transplant or chemotherapy recipients and the advent of a significant proportion of people with HIV infection. It has therefore been postulated that the rate of progressive vaccinia may be higher today than during the pre-eradication era (7,42).

## 10.3. Central Nervous System Complications

The most feared complication for people without contraindication to vaccination is postvaccinial encephalitis. This complication was more common with vaccinia strains used in Europe, although it was certainly seen in the United States as well (32). A number of somewhat distinct pathological disorders are lumped into this term, and "postvaccinial central-nervous-system disease" is technically more accurate (1,41). When this complication was seen in the era of large-scale vaccination, children under 2 yr generally manifested an encephalopathy with the onset of fevers and seizures occurring 6–10 d after vaccination. Focal neurological signs were common, and recovery was frequently incomplete. The more common presentation, in persons older than 2 yr, was a classic viral encephalitis. Patients had the onset of fever, headache, and malaise 11–15 d after vaccination and went on to develop altered mental status, sometimes progressing to seizures or coma or death (1,32). Mortality ranged from 10 to 35%, with one-fourth of patients dying in the 1968 nationwide survey (32,41).

## 10.4. Other Complications

Other complications of vaccination were rare. Erythema multiforme occurred in 118 postvaccine patients in the 1968 10-state survey (out of an estimated 1.6 million vaccinees) (43). Fetal infection was rarely documented and was of unknown significance. Skin tumor at the site of previous vaccination was documented on occasion, as was vaccinial osteomyelitis. Bacterial infection was sometimes seen at the site of vaccination, but this was less common in modern vaccine preparations that contained a much lower bacterial load (1).

## 10.5. Incidence of Complications

Rates of adverse outcomes varied with immune status of the vaccinee, purity of the vaccine (absence of bacterial contamination), and the strain of vaccinia used in the vaccine (1). The most complete studies of complications in the United States come from two CDC surveys conducted in the 1968 *(41,43)*. The 10-state survey involved a more aggressive effort to find complications and may reflect a more accurate estimate of rates *(1)*. Almost all vaccinations in the United States at this time used the NYCBH strain *(32)*. The nationwide survey found 572 total complications out of over 14 million vaccinations, whereas the 10-state survey found 968 complications out of over 1.6 million vaccinations. The significantly higher rate in the second study was attributed to the increased capture of less severe presentations of complications *(43)*. In both studies, complications were much less common with revaccination as opposed to primary vaccination, by an order of magnitude. Adverse reactions were somewhat less common in individuals from 5 to 19 yr of age, with higher rates for younger and older recipients. One striking figure was the rate of postvaccinial encephalitis in children under 1 yr old (6.5 per million in the nationwide study and 42.3 per million in the 10-state study), which was several times higher than the rates for other age groups. Mortality in the nationwide study was 1 per million.

## *10.6. Protective Efficacy*

The protection afforded by vaccination is not exactly known. As was noted earlier, production techniques prior to 1968 yielded vaccines of varying potency. Vaccination techniques were also frequently suboptimal *(1)*. Most efficacy studies were performed in developing nations with endemic smallpox; subclinical variola infection in vaccinated individuals probably had some effect in boosting immunity *(44)*. Classification of a person as "vaccinated" usually relied on the presence of a classic scar. Given the techniques and quality of vaccines used in these countries in the early and mid-20th century, however, many of these scars could have been caused by bacterial infection or immune reaction to impurities in the vaccine rather than a true immune response to vaccinia *(1)*. Studies from the Indian subcontinent in the 1960s and early 1970s reported a rate of protection over 95% *(13,15)*. Considering the factors mentioned above and the fact that the time between vaccination and contact with infectious cases was unknown in these studies, they probably underestimated the true protective effect *(32)*.

In addition to protecting against the development of clinical disease, vaccination was shown to greatly modify the severity of smallpox in persons who did manifest disease. One study found that 25% of previously vaccinated individuals had the milder modified-type smallpox. Even in those who developed ordinary-type smallpox, the majority (83.5%) had the discrete form that carried a much lower mortality. Flat-type smallpox was much less common in vaccinated patients as well *(32)*. Mack's study of imported smallpox outbreaks in Europe between 1950 and 1971 found that mortality of clinical smallpox in patients vaccinated within the past 10 yr was 1 of 72, compared with 41 of 79 in patients who were never vaccinated *(14)*.

## *10.7. Postexposure Prophylaxis*

Postexposure vaccination was one of the most important techniques for containing spread in the Intensified Eradication Program and is likely to remain so in the event of a future smallpox release. Protection afforded by postexposure vaccination is because disease following cutaneous inoculation with vaccinia (or variola for that matter) follows a more rapid course than does naturally transmitted smallpox, allowing the immune system to mount a response prior to the onset of clinical smallpox *(1)*. This accelerated course is exaggerated further in previously vaccinated persons. There is relatively good evidence from contact studies that postexposure vaccination reduces the incidence of clinical disease, and there is excellent evidence that it has a profound effect on the severity of disease *(1,13–15,20,24,25)*. In Mack's study, postexposure vaccination in persons never before vaccinated cut mortality almost in half.

### *10.8. Duration of Protection*

For the same reasons that the primary protective effect of vaccination is not precisely known, the durability of protection afforded by vaccination is also difficult to quantify *(1,3)*. Neutralizing antibodies have been detected in serum up to 40 yr after vaccination, although they do not necessarily correlate with protection *(45)*. Cellular immune responses have been elicited from patients' lymphocytes decades after vaccination *(46–48)*. Studies from the Indian subcontinent seemed to demonstrate protection from infection for at least 5 yr *(1)*. Most impressive is the low mortality in of smallpox patients vaccinated more than 20 yr earlier presented in Mack's study. The 11% mortality seen in these patients was significantly lower than the mortality in unvaccinated patients and in patients receiving postexposure vaccination *(14)*.

Because of the uncertain duration of protection and data from studies that support waning immunity with the passage of years, current recommendations are for periodic revaccination in individuals deemed at risk for infection. Laboratory workers occupationally exposed to orthopoxviruses are generally vaccinated every 3 yr. In the event of a smallpox release, there may be potential benefit even in those vaccinated more recently. It is probably prudent, therefore, to vaccinate all contacts, even those "up to date" on their vaccination status. There are probably no contraindications to vaccinia administration for persons exposed to confirmed smallpox cases, since those at risk for complications from vaccinia are presumably at commensurately increased risk for complications from variola infection.

## 11. TREATMENT

Through the last human case of smallpox infection in 1978, standard treatment for smallpox patients remained primarily supportive, and this is the case today. No specific antiviral therapy with demonstrated benefit in human smallpox is currently available, although evaluation of potentially useful agents has been identified as an important priority by the Institute of Medicine *(7)*. Almost all data regarding clinical outcome have been garnered from studies of patients in underdeveloped countries before the advent of modern medical practice. The effect of modern supportive care upon outcome in smallpox cases is unknown. Of particular importance would presumably be careful attention to fluid and electrolyte balance, pain management, and control of secondary infections (particularly impetigo complicating skin lesions and bacterial pneumonia), as well as management of specific complications such as hemorrhage.

### *11.1. Antiviral Drugs*

Some studies of the efficacy of early antiviral drugs were performed when smallpox was endemic, and a few showed some evidence of benefit, although minor *(1)*. The thiosemicarbazones, in particular methisazone (Marboran®) and the related agent M & B 7714, had excellent activity in mouse models of vaccinia and variola. However, randomized, placebo-controlled human trials for post-exposure prophylaxis of smallpox infection yielded disappointing results *(1,49)*. A small decrease in mortality was seen in vaccinated individuals, but no difference was detected in unvaccinated subjects. In addition, side effects of nausea and vomiting were sometimes severe *(1,50)*. Vaccination was clearly superior in effectiveness and ease of administration, and the chemotherapeutic agents were never used significantly for prophylaxis or treatment.

Since the eradication of smallpox, a variety of antiviral compounds has become available, and some have shown in vitro activity against orthopoxviruses. These include inosine monophosphate (IMP) dehydrogenase inhibitors, s-adenosylhomocysteine hydrolase inhibitors, orotidine monophosphate decarboxylase inhibitors, cytosine triphosphate synthetase inhibitors, thymidylate synthetase inhibitors, nucleoside analogs, thiosemicarbazones, and acyclic nucleoside phosphonates *(19,50)*. Most of this work has been performed with orthopoxviruses other than variola, but some drugs have demonstrated in vitro activity specifically against variola virus. Of the current commercially available drugs, HPMPC (cidofovir), bis-POM PMEA (adefovir dipivoxil), and ribavirin have been shown to have an $IC_{50}$ in tissue culture assays below levels associated with cytotoxicity *(19)*. The in vitro and limited animal data available for these three agents will be reviewed here.

### 11.1.1. CIDOFOVIR

Cidofovir is a nucleotide analog with activity against DNA viruses, including members of the adenovirus, papillomavirus, and herpesvirus families *(51)*. It has been approved for use in cytomegalovirus (CMV) retinitis in AIDS patients. It has a very long intracellular half-life and thus requires dosing only every other week. It has been associated with severe nephrotoxicity in some instances, which has been ameliorated with aggressive hydration and concomitant administration of probenicid. Iritis and uveitis have been seen with relative frequency in postmarketing studies *(52,53)*. Cidifovir has been tested in a variety of in vitro and in vivo models. In vitro culture assays, it is effective against a spectrum of poxvirus infections, including vaccinia and variola *(50)*. It has been shown to be effective in preventing tail lesion formation in mice after vaccinia infection and was effective in preventing end-organ replication of vaccinia and mortality in vaccinia-infected SCID mice *(54)*.

Cidofovir has been studied in mice infected with cowpox by respiratory inoculation. In one study, mice were exposed to aerosolized cowpox virus and were treated with cidofovir or placebo *(55)*. All control mice died, whereas in mice given a subcutaneous injection of 100 mg/kg cidofovir anywhere from 4 d prior to 3 d after infection, survival was 80–100%. In another study, intranasal cidofovir from 2.5 to 40 mg/kg given in a single dose was shown to be effective in reducing mortality in mice given an intranasal inoculation of cowpox virus *(56)*. Protection was dose- and time-dependent: of mice treated 1 d after infection with 10–40 mg/kg of cidofovir, survival was 29/30 compared with 0/10 in controls; mice treated 3 d after infection with 40 mg/kg of cidofovir experienced a 60% survival rate, compared with 100% mortality in controls. Bray et al. *(57)* found that aerosolized cidofovir was as efficacious as subcutaneous cidofovir at much lower doses (0.5–5 mg/kg) if given early in the course of murine cowpox infection, on d 0 or 1 *(57)*. However, later administration of aerosolized cidofovir appeared to be less protective than subcutaneous administration.

Obviously, no human data exist concerning cidofovir in the treatment of smallpox, but case reports have documented successes against other poxvirus infections. Topical and parenteral cidofovir has effectively treated patients with severe immunodeficiency disorders (AIDS and Wiskott-Aldrich syndrome) and disfiguring molluscum contagiosum *(58,59)*. Topical cidofovir has also been associated with complete resolution of human orf (ecthyma contagiosum), another poxvirus infection *(49)*.

### 11.1.2. Adefovir

Adefovir dipivoxil is the orally bioavailable form of adefovir, a cytidine analog originally developed as an antiretroviral drug for use against HIV. Trials of adefovir dipivoxil for HIV were stopped because of nephrotoxicity and other side effects encountered with doses (usually 60 mg/d or greater) required for reverse-transcriptase inhibition. However, adefovir has been used at lower doses (10–30 mg/d) against hepatitis B infection without significant adverse effects *(60–62)*. It has recently been approved by the Food and Drug Administration (FDA) for use against hepatitis B. Adefovir dipivoxil has shown in vitro activity against cowpox, monkeypox, camelpox, and variola viruses at noncytotoxic concentrations but did not show efficacy against vaccinia *(19)*. To date, no published study has examined adefovir's efficacy in a live animal model.

### 11.1.3. Ribavirin

Ribavirin is an IMP dehydrogenase inhibitor that has been studied for several decades. It has clinical utility against respiratory syncitial virus and hepatitis C, influenza A and B, Lassa fever, measles, Hantaan virus, Junin virus, and other viral infections. Ribavirin is associated with bone marrow suppression that can be dose-limiting, a particular concern in the setting of potential hemorrhagic complications. It is also potentially teratogenic and cannot be used in pregnancy *(63)*. Studies have found varying activity against orthopoxviruses in vitro *(50,64)*. However, ribavirin inhibited variola infection in Vero and BSC cell cultures *(19)*. In live animal models, topical ribavirin was effective in treating vaccinia keratitis in rabbits and in preventing tail lesions in vaccinia infected mice *(65,66)*. Ribavirin alone has been shown to delay or prevent death in studies of intranasal, lethal cowpox infection in mice, depending on inoculation dose of virus and dose of drug *(64,67)*. Subcutaneous injections of ribavirin, 100 mg/kg/d for 5 d, followed by one dose of cidofovir (75 mg/kg on d 6) improved survival over placebo or either of the drugs used individually on the same schedule *(67)*. There are no published data regarding the use of ribavirin in human orthopoxvirus infections.

In summary, *no definitive antiviral treatment exists* for human variola infection. Although some antiviral drugs have shown promise in experimental studies, none is labeled for use in any human orthopoxvirus infection. Excepting a deliberate release of smallpox, data regarding treatment will be confined to animal models or anecdotal cases of human infection with related orthopoxviruses. The validity of extrapolating animal data to treatment of human smallpox is obviously unknown. Of the clinically available drugs, cidofovir has the most promising animal data and has been effective in the treatment of human orthopoxvirus infections other than smallpox. At present, no recommendation can be made for the use of any antiviral agent for treatment of smallpox outside the setting of an investigational new drug (IND) clinical trial.

## 12. INFECTION CONTROL AND PRECAUTIONS

An outbreak of smallpox will constitute an infection control and public health emergency of the highest magnitude. Containment will require the coordinated efforts of first responders, physicians, hospital staff, public health and infection control personnel, and (in the civilian setting) civic leaders and media. In a military operational environment, medical personnel must work closely with the chain of command to ensure open communication and rapid action. At the time of this writing, the Department of Defense (DoD) has initiated vaccination of selected "first-line" health care workers, and similar plans are being formulated in the civilian sector. Plans and policies are still being revised, and the subsequent section does not constitute official DoD policy.

The containment of a smallpox outbreak must start with the individual infected patient. There is no substitute for early diagnosis (in particular, early confirmation of alternative diagnoses to rule out smallpox) and rapid implementation of infection control measures. Physicians, nurses, and ancillary health care workers should maintain an appropriate index of suspicion, and possible cases of smallpox should be immediately isolated. Potential cases of smallpox should be promptly reported to the local or state health department (9). Although an appropriate index of suspicion and vigilance are critical at all times, it must be remembered that, barring reintroduction of variola, all cases potentially suspicious for smallpox will by definition represent other disease entities (most often adult varicella). Thus, prudent consideration of the differential diagnosis and early involvement of infectious disease consultants are critical.

Probably by orders of magnitude, the highest risk of smallpox transmission occurs in people who have close and sustained contact with an infected patient (13,14,20,24,25). Transmission is much more likely in a hospital setting rather than in the community, since patients are probably most infectious when they reach the hospital and are in closer proximity to more potential contacts (1). An exception to this may be the close billeting often encountered in garrison or among deployed military units, especially if a case is unrecognized and the patient is sent back to rest in quarters. Initial containment efforts should concentrate on such close contacts.

Once a diagnosis of smallpox is entertained, however unlikely, the patient should be placed in strict contact and airborne precautions. The possibility of aerosolized nosocomial transmission, although rare, clearly exists, even several floors removed from the infected patient. Patients should be contained in a negative pressure isolation room with high-efficiency particulate air filtration (4). In a deployed setting, where field or commandeered hospitals may not have such isolation facilities, it is essential to find a room as far removed from the rest of the patient care facility as possible that has a completely separate air flow. Transport through hallways should be avoided when possible. In situations in which this is unavoidable, a surgical mask or small-particle mask should be placed on the patient. Strict contact precautions are probably the most effective measure in preventing transmission. Gowns, gloves, and meticulous handwashing are essential in interrupting the most common route of transmission (9).

The remainder of the discussion assumes the possibility that smallpox may be reintroduced. Vaccination provides the best protection against infection. For a treatment facility admitting smallpox patients, the most prudent course of action is to vaccinate the entire hospital staff and all patients (4,9). Any patient admitted with a presumed diagnosis of smallpox should be vaccinated to prevent subsequent infection in an originally misdiagnosed patient. If possible, health care professionals who also have a history of past vaccination should be used for direct care of smallpox patients, since they are likely to have a brisker immune response to revaccination. Previous expert recommendations suggested that VIG (0.3 mL/kg) should be coadministered with vaccine to patients and staff who have contraindications to vaccination *(4)*. However, current recommendations do not include an indication for VIG in this setting. VIG supply is limited at the time of this writing, and its use is indicated only for treatment of severe complications of vaccination (*eczema vaccinatum*, progressive vaccinia). Until vaccine take has been assessed in health care providers, aerosol-protective masks should be worn within the patient care area *(9)*.

Risk management must also extend to ancillary staff. The virus can survive on fomites and is present in especially high titers in clothing and bedding of patients *(23)*. Items coming in contact with the patient should be considered biohazards and dealt with appropriately. All laundry and linens should be placed in biohazard bags and incinerated or autoclaved if they are to be relaundered. Blood, bodily fluids, and other clinical samples pose a risk to laboratory workers, especially with centrifuging or other manipulations likely to cause aerosolization *(4)*. Any laboratory work with smallpox must be done under maximal (BL-4) containment by experienced technicians. The CDC can give instructions on packaging and transport of clinical specimens *(9)*. Ill patients with smallpox will probably require body fluid chemistries and hematological profiles. Often there may be no time to wait for transport of samples to a BL-4 laboratory or establishment of such a laboratory on site. Without specific guidance in these instances, common sense dictates that these specimens should only be handled by vaccinated laboratory workers in a laboratory area or building completely separated (including ventilation) from the rest of the facility and under the highest biosafety level available. Mortuary workers should also be vaccinated and must take precautions, as transmission has been associated with corpses, especially in patients who died of hemorrhagic-type smallpox *(1)*.

Any intentional release of smallpox is likely to infect a number of patients, and cases may quickly overwhelm even the largest of medical treatment facilities. In such instances, some current plans call for establishment of separate facilities to isolate cases from noninfected patients and providers. Facilities should be segregated from the general population to achieve the largest buffer possible. Contingency plans for smallpox outbreaks should establish locations, personnel, and equipment designation for these facilities, as *de novo* assembly of this type of operation would be difficult under the strain of an existing epidemic. Specific guidelines for the establishment of such facilities can be found in the CDC Smallpox Response Plan and Guidelines *(9)*.

Control of the spread of disease among a population will be a challenge, but this effort will be helped by the fact that the disease spreads somewhat slowly. Vaccination is the cornerstone of any public health effort. General strategies include mass vaccination of whole communities or populations and "ring vaccination," in which vaccination focuses on the contacts of known cases. Patients with the disease become infectious only after the onset of illness, allowing time to initiate isolation and vaccination of close contacts if a known outbreak exists. Models of civilian smallpox attack have predicted that ring vaccination will be effective in controlling disease spread as long as there is some residual immunity in the community from childhood vaccinations *(68,69)*. Vaccination within the first 4 d after contact with an infectious case provides protection against infection and significant protection against severe disease *(1)*. Contacts of cases should be vaccinated and observed daily with a daily recording of temperature. Any symptoms of illness or a temperature greater than 38°C should instigate immediate isolation *(4,9)*. Problems may potentially arise in the instance of asymptomatic shedders, generally vaccinated individuals with subclinical infection *(22)*. Close contacts of health care workers may be at risk for infection through this mechanism, and vaccination for them may be warranted. Chemoprophylaxis with cidofovir could have a role in contacts for whom vaccine is contraindicated and VIG is unavailable, although, as discussed, this would be an unlabeled use and can only be recommended in the setting of an IND trial.

Few data exist on decontamination of persons or surfaces in close contact with infected patients. Extrapolating from experimental data with vaccinia, aerosolized smallpox is probably rapidly inactivated by UV light. In the absence of UV light and under ideal conditions of low temperature and humidity, the virus may persist for 24–48 h *(1)*. Virus may persist in droplets on surfaces as well. Standard hospital hypochlorite or quaternary ammonium solution disinfectants should be adequate for cleaning contaminated surfaces *(4)*. As long as disposable gowns, gloves, masks, and other contact precautions are taken, personnel should be at low risk for body surface contamination.

# REFERENCES

1. Fenner F, Henderson DA, Arita I, Jezek Z, Ladayi ID. Smallpox and Its Eradication. World Health Organization, Geneva, 1988.
2. Radetsky M. Smallpox: a history of its rise and fall. Pediatr Infect Dis J 1999;18:85–93.
3. Dixon CW. Smallpox. J & A Churchill, London, 1962.
4. Henderson DA, Inglesby TV, Bartlett JG, et al. Smallpox as a biological weapon: medical and public health management. Working Group on Civilian Biodefense. JAMA 1999;281:2127–2137.
5. Gellman B. 4 nations thought to possess smallpox. Washington Post, Washington, DC, November 5, 2002:A01.
6. Diamond J. Guns, Germs, and Steel: The Fates of Human Societies. WW Norton, New York, 1999.
7. Breman JG, Henderson DA. Diagnosis and management of smallpox. N Engl J Med 2002;346: 1300–1308.
8. Henderson DA. Smallpox: clinical and epidemiologic features. Emerg Infect Dis 1999;5:537–539.
9. Anonymous. CDC Smallpox Response Plan and Guidelines. Draft 3.0. U. S. Centers for Disease Control and Prevention, Atlanta, GA, 2002.
10. Esposito JJ, Obijeski JF, Nakano JH. Orthopoxvirus DNA: strain differentiation by electrophoresis of restriction endonuclease fragmented virion DNA. Virology 1978;89:53–66.
11. Esposito JJ, Knight JC. Orthopoxvirus DNA: a comparison of restriction profiles and maps. Virology 1985;143:230–251.
12. Enserink M. Biowarfare. Did bioweapons test cause a deadly smallpox outbreak? Science 2002;296: 2116–2117.
13. Heiner GG, Fatima N, McCrumb FR Jr. A study of intrafamilial transmission of smallpox. Am J Epidemiol 1971;94:316–326.
14. Mack TM. Smallpox in Europe, 1950-1971. J Infect Dis 1972;125:161–169.
15. Thomas DB, McCormack WM, Arita I, Khan MM, Islam S, Mack TM. Endemic smallpox in rural East Pakistan. I. Methodology, clinical and epidemiologic characteristics of cases, and intervillage transmission. Am J Epidemiol 1971;93:361–372.
16. Moss B. Poxviridae: the viruses and their replication. In: Knipe DM, Howley PM, eds. Fields Virology. Lippincot Williams & Wilkins, Philadelphia, 2001, pp. 2849–2883.
17. Alcami A, Koszinowski UH. Viral mechanisms of immune evasion. Trends Microbiol 2000;8:410–418.
18. Esposito JJ, Fenner F. Poxviruses. In: Knipe DM, Howley PM, eds. Fields Virology. Lippincott Williams & Wilkins, Philadelphia, 2001, pp. 2885–2921.
19. Jahrling PB, Zaucha GM, Huggins JW. Contermeasures to the reemergence of smallpox virus as an agent of bioterrorism. In: Scheld WM, Craig WA, Hughes JM, eds. Emerging Infections 4. ASM Press, Washington, DC, 2000.
20. Wehrle PF, Posch J, Richter KH, Henderson DA. An airborne outbreak of smallpox in a German hospital and its significance with respect to other recent outbreaks in Europe. Bull WHO 1970;43:669–679.
21. Downie AW, Saint Vincent L, Meiklejohn M, et al. Studies on the virus content of mouth washings in the acute phase of smallpox. Bull WHO 1961;25:49–53.

22. Sarkar JK, Mitra AC, Mukherjee MK, De SK. Virus excretion in smallpox. 2. Excretion in the throats of household contacts. Bull WHO 1973;48:523–527.
23. Downie AW, Meiklejohn M, St Vincent L, Rao AR, Sundara Babu BV, Kempe CH. The recovery of smallpox virus from patients and their environment in a smallpox hospital. Bull WHO 1965;33: 615–622.
24. Henderson RH, Yekpe M. Smallpox transmission in Southern Dahomey. A study of a village outbreak. Am J Epidemiol 1969;90:423–428.
25. Thomas DB, Arita I, McCormack WM, Khan MM, Islam S, Mack TM. Endemic smallpox in rural East Pakistan. II. Intervillage transmission and infectiousness. Am J Epidemiol 1971;93:373–383.
26. Mack T. A different view of smallpox and vaccination. N Engl J Med 2003;348:460–463.
27. Weber DJ, Cohen MS, Fine J. The acutely ill patient with fever and rash. In: Mandell GL, Bennett JE, Dolin R, eds. Principles and Practice of Infectious Diseases. Churchill Livingstone, Philadelphia, 2000, pp. 633–650.
28. Damon I. Smallpox false alarms: lessons for the clinician. Bioterrorism Symposium Presentation, 40th Annual Meeting of the Infectious Diseases Society of America, 2002.
29. Gubler DJ. Dengue and dengue hemorrhagic fever. Clin Microbiol Rev 1998; 11:480–496.
30. Jezek Z, Szczeniowski M, Paluku KM, Mutombo M. Human monkeypox: clinical features of 282 patients. J Infect Dis 1987;156:293–298.
31. McClain DJ. Smallpox. In: Sidell FR, Takafuji ET, Franz DR, eds. Part I: Medical Aspects of Chemical and Biological Warfare. Office of the Surgeon General, U.S. Department of the Army, Washington, DC, 1997, pp. 539–559.
32. Henderson DA, Moss B. Smallpox and vaccinia. In: Plotkin SA, Orenstein WA, Zorab R, eds. Vaccines. WB Saunders, Philadelphia, 1999.
33. Anonymous. Dryvax (Smallpox Vaccine, Dried, Calf Lymph Type) Package Insert, vol 2002. Wyeth Laboratories, 2002.
34. LeDuc JW, Jahrling PB. Strengthening national preparedness for smallpox: an update. Emerg Infect Dis 2001;7:155–157.
35. Frey SE, Couch RB, Tacket CO, et al. Clinical responses to undiluted and diluted smallpox vaccine. N Engl J Med 2002; 346:1265–1274.
36. Frey SE, Newman FK, Cruz J, et al. Dose-related effects of smallpox vaccine. N Engl J Med 2002; 346:1275–1280.
37. Anonymous. HHS awards $428 million contract to produce smallpox vaccine. United States Department of Health and Human Services, Washington, DC, accessed at http://www.hhs.gov/news/press/2001pres/20011128.html, 2001, p. 2.
38. Anonymous. Acambis reports successfull phase I trial of cell-culture-grown smallpox vaccine. Center for Infectious Disease Research & Policy, Minneapolis, accessed at http://www1.umn.edu/cidrap/content/bt/smallpox.news.acam.html, 2002, p. 1.
39. Anonymous. Vaccinia (smallpox) vaccine: recommendations of the Advisory Committee on Immunization Practices (ACIP), 2001. MMWR 2001;50:1–25.
40. Engler RJM, Kenner J, Leung DYM. Smallpox vaccination: risk considerations for patients with atopic dermatitis. J Allergy Clin Immunol 2002;110:357–365.
41. Lane JM, Ruben FL, Neff JM, Millar JD. Complications of smallpox vaccination, 1968. N Engl J Med 1969;281:1201–1208.
42. Bartlett JG. Smallpox vaccination and patients with human immunodeficiency virus infection or acquired immunodeficiency syndrome. Clin Infect Dis 2003;36:468–471.
43. Lane JM, Ruben FL, Neff JM, Millar JD. Complications of smallpox vaccination, 1968: results of ten statewide surveys. J Infect Dis 1970;122:303–309.
44. Heiner GG, Fatima N, Daniel RW, Cole JL, Anthony RL, McCrumb FR Jr. A study of inapparent infection in smallpox. Am J Epidemiol 1971;94:252–268.
45. McCarthy K, Downie AW, Bradley WH. The antibody response in man following infection with viruses of the pox group. II. Antibody response following vaccination. J Hygi 1958;56:466–478.
46. Moller-Larsen A, Haahr S. Humoral and cell-mediated immune responses in humans before and after revaccination with vaccinia virus. Infect Immun 1978;19:34–39.
47. Perrin LH, Reynolds D, Zinkernagel R, Oldstone MBA. Generation of virus-specific cytolytic activity in human peripheral lymphocytes after vaccination with vaccinia virus and measles virus. Med Microbiol Immunol 1978;166:71–79.

48. Demkowicz WE, Littaua RA, Wang J, Ennis FA. Human cytotoxic T-cell memory. long-lived responses to vaccinia virus. J Virol 1996;70:2627–2631.

49. Geerinck K, Lukito G, Snoeck R, et al. A case of human orf in an immunocompromised patient treated successfully with cidofovir cream. J Med Virol 2001;64:543–549.

50. De Clercq E. Vaccinia virus inhibitors as a paradigm for the chemotherapy of poxvirus infections. Clin Microbiol Rev 2001;14:382–397.

51. Naesens L, Snoeck R, Andrei G, Balzarini J, Neyts J, De Clercq E. HPMC (cidofovir), PMEA (adefovir) and related acyclic nucleoside phosphonate analogues: a review of their pharmacology and clinical potential in the treatment of viral infections. Antiviral Chem Chemother 1997;8:1–23.

52. Plosker GL, Noble S. Cidofovir: a review of its use in cytomegalovirus retinitis in patients with AIDS. Drugs 1999;58:325–345.

53. Wachsman M, Petty BG, Cundy KC, et al. Pharmacokinetics, safety and bioavailability of HPMPC (cidofovir) in human immunodeficiency virus-infected subjects. Antiviral Res 1996;29:153–161.

54. Neyts J, De Clercq E. Efficacy of (S)-1-(3-hydroxy-2-phosphonylmethoxypropyl)cytosine for the treatment of lethal vaccinia virus infections in severe combined immune deficiency (SCID) mice. J Med Virol 1993;41:242–246.

55. Bray M, Martinez M, Smee DF, Kefauver D, Thompson E, Huggins JW. Cidofovir protects mice against lethal aerosol or intranasal cowpox virus challenge. J Infect Dis 2000;181:10–19.

56. Smee DF, Bailey KW, Wong M, Sidwell RW. Intranasal treatment of cowpox virus respiratory infections in mice with cidofovir. Antiviral Res 2000;47:171–177.

57. Bray M, Martinez M, Kefauver D, West M, Roy C. Treatment of aerosolized cowpox virus infection in mice with aerosolized cidofovir. Antiviral Res 2002;54:129–142.

58. Davies EG, Thrasher A, Lacey K, Harper J. Topical cidofovir for severe molluscum contagiosum. Lancet 1999;353:2042.

59. Meadows KP, Tyring SK, Pavia AT, Rallis TM. Resolution of recalcitrant molluscum contagiosum virus lesions in human immunodeficiency virus-infected patients treated with cidofovir. Arch Dermatol 1997;133:987–990.

60. Perrillo R, Schiff E, Yoshida E, et al. Adefovir dipivoxil for the treatment of lamivudine-resistant hepatitis B mutants. Hepatology 2000;32:129–134.

61. Benhamou Y, Bochet M, Thibault V, et al. Safety and efficacy of adefovir dipivoxil in patients co-infected with HIV-1 and lamivudine-resistant hepatitis B virus: an open-label pilot study. Lancet 2001;358:718–723.

62. Noble S, Goa KL. Adefovir dipivoxil. Drugs 1999;58:479–487; discussion 488–489.

63. Kucers A, Crowe SM, Grayson ML, Hoy JF. The Use of Antibiotics. Butterworth Heineman, Oxford, 1997.

64. Smee DF, Huggins JW. Potential of the IMP dehydrogenase inhibitors for intiviral therapies of poxvirus infections. International Society for Antiviral Research. Eleventh International Conference on Antiviral Research, San Diego, CA, 1998.

65. De Clercq E, Luczak M, Shugar D, Torrence PF, Waters JA, Witkop B. Effect of cytosine arabinoside, iododeoxyuridine, ethyldeoxyuridine, thiocyanatodeoxyuridine, and ribavirin on tail lesion formation in mice infected with vaccinia virus. Proc Soc Exp Biol Med 1976;151:487–490.

66. Sidwell RW, Allen LB, Khare GP, et al. Effect of 1-b-D-ribofuranosyl-1,2,4-triazole-3-carboxamide (Virazole, ICN 129) on herpes and vaccinia keratitis and encephalitis in laboratory animals. Antimicrob Agents Chemother 1973;3:242–246.

67. Smee DF, Bailey KW, Sidwell RW. Treatment of cowpox virus respiratory infections in mice with ribavirin as a single agent or followed sequentially by cidofovir. Antivir Chem Chemother 2000;11:303–309.

68. Halloran ME, Longini IM Jr, Nizam A, Yang Y. Containing bioterrorist smallpox. Science 2002;298:1428–1432.

69. Bozzette SA, Boer R, Bhatnagar V, et al. A model for a smallpox-vaccination policy. N Engl J Med 2003;348:416–425.

# 16 Viral Hemorrhagic Fevers

*Thomas W. Geisbert, PhD, Aileen M. Marty, MD, FACP, and Peter B. Jahrling, PhD*

The views, opinions, and findings contained herein are those of the authors and should not be construed as an official Department of the Army, Department of the Navy, or Department of Defense position, policy, or decision unless so designated by other documentation.

## CONTENTS

---

### Case Vignette

A 15-year-old European boy, who had been in Kenya for 1 month, was admitted to the hospital with a 3-day history of headache, malaise, anorexia, fever, and vomiting. Throughout the course of the illness, he developed copious bloody diarrhea, hypotension, leukocytosis, thrombocytopenia, and prolonged prothrombin and partial thromboplastin times consistent with disseminated intravascular coagulation (DIC). Despite intensive supportive therapy, which included antibiotics, steroids, heparin, fresh plasma, and blood transfusions, his condition steadily deteriorated, and he died on the 11th day of illness. Based on the characteristic clinical picture, provisional diagnoses were either viral hemorrhagic fever or, less likely, typhoid fever with "extreme toxicity." An autopsy was performed soon after death. Postmortem examination showed extensive petechial and purpuric hemorrhage in the skin, conjunctiva, and gastrointestinal mucosa. Blood-tinged pleural, pericardial, and peritoneal effusions were copious, and retroperitoneal edema was striking. The lungs and tracheobronchial tree were

---

From: *Physician's Guide to Terrorist Attack*
Edited by: M. J. Roy © Humana Press Inc., Totowa, NJ

hemorrhagic. Multiple petechial hemorrhages were observed on the epicardium, renal cortex and pelvis, and urinary bladder. Marburg virus was isolated from fluids and tissues and was identified in tissues by immunohistochemistry, electron microscopy, and immunoelectron microscopy *(1)*.

## 1. INTRODUCTION

Viral hemorrhagic fever (VHF) is an acute febrile syndrome characterized by systemic involvement, which in severe infection includes generalized bleeding. Patients with VHF manifest combinations of malaise, prostration, generalized signs of increased vascular permeability, and coagulation abnormalities *(2)*. Although the more severely ill patients manifest bleeding, this does not result in a life-threatening loss of blood volume, rather, it indicates damage to the vascular endothelium and is an index of how severe the disease is in specific target organs.

The viral agents responsible for VHFs are taxonomically diverse. They are all single-stranded ribonucleic acid (ssRNA) viruses that can infect humans through contact with contaminated animal reservoirs or arthropod vectors. Under natural conditions they all cause significant infectious diseases, although their geographical ranges may be tightly circumscribed. The relatively recent advent of jet travel, coupled with human demographics, increases the opportunity for humans to contract these infections, and from time to time sporadic cases of VHFs are exported from endemic areas to new areas. Clinical and epidemiological data on the VHFs are sparse; outbreaks are sporadic and unexpected and typically develop in geographical areas where cultural mores and logistical barriers hamper systematic investigations.

VHFs, many of which spread easily in hospitals to patients and staff alike, causing high morbidity and mortality, gained public notoriety in the last decade largely as a result of the enormous interest and alarm generated by the news media. Ebola virus has received the overwhelming majority of this notoriety primarily as a consequence of the highly publicized isolation of a new Ebola virus species in a suburb of Washington, DC, in 1989 *(3)*, coupled with its high case-fatality rate (nearly 90% in some outbreaks), unusual and striking morphology, and dramatic clinical presentation and lack of effective specific treatment. Progress in understanding the origins of the pathophysiological changes that make Ebola and other VHF infections of humans so devastating has been slow, primarily because most of these viruses require special containment for safe research.

Many of the VHF agents are highly infectious via the aerosol route, and most are quite stable as respirable aerosols. This means that they satisfy at least one criterion for weaponization, and some clearly have potential as biological terrorism and warfare threats. Most of these agents replicate in cell culture to concentrations sufficiently high to produce a small terrorist weapon, one suitable for introducing lethal doses of virus into the air intake of an airplane or office building. Some replicate to even higher concentrations, with obvious potential ramifications. Since the VHF agents cause serious diseases with high morbidity and mortality, their existence as endemic disease threats, and as potential biological warfare weapons, suggests a formidable potential impact on public health.

## 2. POTENTIAL ROLE IN BIOLOGICAL WARFARE AND TERRORISM

Public concern regarding the dangers posed by VHFs reflects the potential for high morbidity and mortality from these infections, coupled with the potential for their spread agents as a result of increased international commerce and jet travel, as well as the heightened awareness of bioterrorism advanced by the events surrounding September 11, 2001. The Centers for Disease Control and Prevention (CDC) recently classified VHF viruses as category A bioweapon agents *(4)*. This classification undertakes the task of identifying agents that require special action for public health preparedness. Such agents are associated with high mortality rates, ease of dissemination or transmission from person to person, and potential for major public panic and social disruption.

The Japanese studied VHF for use in warfare during their activities with Unit 731; specifically, they studied hantaviruses and noted that rodents served as reservoirs *(5)*. The former Soviet Union, Russia, and the United States weaponized several VHF viruses *(6– 8)*, and both the former Soviet Union and Russia produced large quantities of Ebola, Marburg, Lassa, Junin, and Machupo viruses until 1992 *(6,8)*. In fact, Soviet researchers determined that only a few virions of Marburg virus administered aerogenically can produce a lethal infection in monkeys *(9)*. Likewise, Soviet researchers showed that very small doses of Ebola virus produced lethal infection in monkeys when administered in aerosol form *(10)*. A number of studies reveal that aerosol preparations of Ebola *(10,11)*, Marburg *(9,12)*, Lassa *(13)*, and Junin *(14)* viruses can produce lethal infection of non-human primates. Some argue that these viruses are too dangerous to develop as weapons since there are no effective vaccines or therapies; however, this view contradicts historical facts. In October of 1992, the Japanese cult Aum Shinrikyo unsuccessfully sent a "medical mission to Zaire" in an attempt to obtain Ebola virus as part of an effort to develop biological weapons *(15)*.

There is evidence suggesting that North Korea weaponized yellow fever virus *(7,16)*. Moreover, the U.S. offensive biological weapons program developed yellow fever and Rift Valley fever viruses as weapons before terminating its program 1969 *(7)*. An aerosol attack using 50 kg of aerosolized Marburg, Machupo, or Rift valley fever viruses on a city of 500,000 residents would reach an estimated downwind distance of 1 km and cause 35,000 casualties, with mortality rates of 25, 35, and 0.5%, respectively.

The Working Group on Civilian Biodefense recently excluded the viruses causing dengue hemorrhagic fever, Crimean-Congo hemorrhagic fever (CCHF), and the agents of hemorrhagic fever with renal syndrome (HFRS) as potential biological weapons *(17)*. They excluded dengue virus by reasoning that it is not transmissible by small-particle aerosol *(18)*. Exclusion of CCHF and the agents of HFRS for bioterrorism purposes is based primarily on technical problems, the principle barrier being that these agents do not readily replicate to high concentrations in cell culture, which is a necessity for weaponization of an infectious organism *(17)*.

## 3. HISTORY, EPIDEMIOLOGY, AND TRANSMISSION

Under natural conditions, members of the Arenaviridae, Bunyaviridae, Filoviridae, and Flaviviridae families (Table 1) that cause VHF have a specific geographical distribution and diverse modes of transmission. Although the natural reservoir for Filoviridae

Table 1
Viral Hemorrhagic Fevers of Humans

| Virus family and genus | Virus | Disease | Natural distribution | Source | Incubation (d) |
|---|---|---|---|---|---|
| Arenaviridae | | | | | |
| Arenavirus | Lassa | Lassa fever | West Africa | Rodent | 5–16 |
| | Junin | Argentine HF | South America | Rodent | 7–14 |
| | Machupo | Bolivian HF | South America | Rodent | 9–15 |
| | Sabia | Brazilian HF | South America | Rodent | 7–14 |
| | Guanarito | Venezuelan HF | South America | Rodent | 7–14 |
| | Whitewater Arroyo | Unnamed HF | North America | Rodent | Unknown |
| Bunyaviridae | | | | | |
| Nairovirus | Crimean-Congo HF | Crimean-Congo HF | Africa, Central Asia, Eastern Europe, Middle East | Tick | 3–12 |
| Phlebovirus | Rift Valley fever | Rift Valley fever | Africa, Saudi Arabia, Yemen | Mosquito | 2–6 |
| Hantavirus | Agents of HFRS | HFRS | Asia, Balkans, Europe[a] | Rodent | 9–35 |
| Filoviridae | | | | | |
| Ebolavirus[b] | Ebola | Ebola HF | Africa | Unknown | 2–21 |
| Marburgvirus | Marburg | Marburg HF | Africa | Unknown | 2–14 |
| Flaviviridae | | | | | |
| Flavivirus | Dengue | Dengue HF | Asia, Africa, Pacific, Americas | Mosquito | Unknown |
| | Yellow fever | Yellow fever | Africa, Tropical Americas | Mosquito | 3–6 |
| | Omsk HF | Omsk HF | Central Asia | Tick | 2–9 |
| | Kyasanur Forest disease | Kyasanur Forest disease | India | Tick | 2–9 |

Abbreviations: HF, hemorrhagic fever; HFRS, hemorrhagic fever with renal syndrome.
[a]The agents of hantavirus pulmonary syndrome have been isolated in North America.
[b]There are four species of Ebola: Zaire, Sudan, Reston, and Ivory Coast.

remains unknown, as a group, the VHF viruses are linked to the ecology of their vectors or reservoirs, whether rodents or arthropods. Not only do these characteristics have great significance in the natural transmission cycle for arenaviruses and bunyaviruses (rodents to humans) and for flaviviruses (arthropods), but they also make nosocomial transmission a concern. In this regard, most reservoirs tend to be rural, and a patient's history of being in a rural locale is an important factor to consider when reaching a diagnosis. Human-to-human spread is possible for all VHF viruses, but pandemics are unlikely.

### 3.1. The Arenaviridae

Arenaviruses take their name from their sand-like appearance under the electron microscope. There are two complexes of arenaviruses, the Old World (e.g., Lassa virus) and New World groups (South American and North American Hemorrhagic fever viruses) (2). Arenaviruses survive in nature by a life-long association with specific rodent reservoirs. Rodents spread the virus to humans, and outbreaks can usually be related to some perturbation in the ecosystem that brings humans in contact with rodents or material contaminated by rodent products. Arenaviruses initiate infection in the nasopharyngeal mucosa.

Lassa fever made a dramatic appearance in 1969 when an American nurse working at a modest mission station in Lassa, a small town in northeastern Nigeria, became ill and started a chain of nosocomial infections that extended from health care workers in Africa to laboratory workers in the United States. Lassa virus produces Lassa fever, a major febrile disease of West Africa that causes 10–15% of adult febrile admissions to the hospital and perhaps 40% of nonsurgical deaths (19). Lassa virus infects 100,000–300,000 people annually in West Africa, killing 5000–10000, and leaving approximately 30,000 deaf (19,20). Lassa fever causes high mortality in pregnant women and is also a pediatric disease. Most Lassa virus infections are traceable to contact with the carrier rodent, the rat *Mastomys natalensis*, but nosocomial transmission is also possible. Lassa fever has periodically been imported to the Europe, the United States, Japan, and Canada by travelers from West Africa (21), and in 2000, there were at least four such fatal cases in the United Kingdom, Germany, and the Netherlands (22).

Argentine hemorrhagic fever (AHF) was described in 1943, and Junin virus was first isolated from one of its victims in 1958. Junin virus is carried by field voles such as *Calomys musculinus* and *Calomys laucha* and is associated with agricultural activities in the pampas of Argentina, where there have been 300–600 cases per year since 1955 (23). Transmission is airborne from fomites, from contaminated food or water, or through damaged skin. Direct person-to-person transmission is rare.

In 1959, physicians in the Beni department of Bolivia noted a sporadic hemorrhagic illness in patients from rural areas; it soon became known as Bolivian hemorrhagic fever (BHF). In 1963, MacKenzie and colleagues isolated Machupo virus from patients with BHF and soon thereafter, he (together with Johnson and others) identified the voles *Calomys callous* as the rodent reservoir (24). Machupo virus produced several outbreaks of disease in the 1960s, but more recently BHF has manifested only sporadically; there was a cluster of cases in 1994. Transmission is through contaminated food and water and direct contact through skin abrasions; there is only rare documentation of human-to-human transmission.

In 1989 an outbreak of VHF involving several hundred patients in the municipality of Guanarito, Portuguesa State, Venezuela, led to the isolation of Guanarito virus and identification of its probable animal reservoir: the cotton rat *Sigmodon alstoin (25)*. Sabia virus caused a fatal VHF infection in Brazil in 1990, followed by a severe laboratory infection in Brazil in 1992 and another laboratory infection in the United States in 1994 *(26)*. The most recently recognized arenavirus linked to VHF is Whitewater Arroyo, which apparently caused three fatal cases of hemorrhagic fever in California in 1990–2000 *(27)*.

### 3.2. The Bunyaviridae

Included among the Bunyaviridae are members of the genus *Phlebovirus* (e.g., Rift Valley fever virus); *Nairovirus* (e.g., Crimean-Congo hemorrhagic fever virus); and *Hantavirus* (e.g., Sin Nombre virus). Transmission of Bunyaviridae ranges from arthropod transmission (largely by mosquitoes, ticks, and phlebotomine flies), or, as is the case for hantaviruses, by contact with rodents or rodent products. Transmission by aerosol is also documented.

The *Phlebovirus* Rift Valley fever (RVF) virus, which causes Rift Valley fever, is a significant human pathogen. Outbreaks of this major African disease often reflect unusual increases in mosquito populations *(28)*. RVF virus primarily affects domestic livestock and can cause epizootic disease in domestic animals. Daubne and colleagues *(29)* first described RVF in 1931 as an enzootic hepatitis among sheep, cattle, and humans in Kenya. In 1950–1951, an epizootic of RVF in Kenya resulted in the death of an estimated 100,000 sheep. An RVF epizootic can lead to an epidemic among humans who are exposed to diseased animals. Risk factors for human infection include contact with infected blood, especially in slaughterhouses, and handling of contaminated meat during food preparation. Exposure to aerosols of RVF virus is a potential source of infection for laboratory workers. In 2000, Rift Valley fever spread for the first time beyond the African continent to Saudi Arabia and Yemen, affecting both livestock and humans *(30)*.

Crimean-Congo hemorrhagic fever (CCHF) is a zoonotic disease transmitted not only through the bite of at least 29 species of ticks, of which *Hyalomma marginatum* is the most important, but also by exposure to infected animals or their carcasses, by contact with blood and bodily secretions of infected persons, and by aerosol. The agent of CCHF is a *Nairovirus*. Although descriptions of this illness can be traced to antiquity, its first recognition was in 1944–1945, when there was a large outbreak in the Steppe region of the western Crimea among Soviet troops and peasants helping with the harvest. In 1956, a similar illness was identified in a febrile child from what was then the Belgian Congo (now the Democratic Republic of the Congo), but it was not until 1969 that researchers realized that the pathogen causing Crimean hemorrhagic fever was the same as that responsible for the illness in the Congo. The linkage of the two place names resulted in the current name for the disease and the virus. CCHF is endemic in many countries in Africa, Europe, and Asia; it causes sporadic, yet particularly severe, VHF in endemic areas *(31)*. CCHF has frequently caused small, hospital-centered outbreaks, owing to the copious hemorrhage and highly infective nature of this virus via the aerosol route. An outbreak of a hemorrhagic fever in the Pakistani-Afghan border during the 2001–2002 U.S. campaign against terrorists is suspected to be CCHF, although the closely related Hazara virus has not been excluded.

Hantaviruses, unlike the other bunyaviruses, are not transmitted via infected arthropods, rather, contact with infected rodents and their excreta leads to human infections. Researchers have documented transmission by aerosol *(32)*. Of the 17 types of hantaviruses known, at least 8 (Hantaan, Seoul, Puumala, Dobrava, Sin Nombre, New York, Black Canal Creek, and Bayou) can cause significant clinical illness. Each has its own rodent vector, geographical distribution, and clinicopathological expression. The poor hygienic conditions of combat promote exposure to rodents, and a review of illness during the U.S. Civil War, and the First and Second World Wars suggests that there were outbreaks of hantaviral infections among troops. Hantaviral disease was described in Manchuria along the Amur River, and later among United Nations troops during the Korean War, where it became known as Korean hemorrhagic fever *(33)*. The prototype virus from this group, Hantaan, which causes Korean hemorrhagic fever with renal syndrome (HFRS), was isolated in 1977. Hantaan virus is borne in nature by the striped field mouse *Apodemus agrarious*.

Hantaan virus is still active in Korea, Japan, and China. Seoul virus causes a milder form of HFRS and may be distributed worldwide. Other hantaviruses associated with HFRS include the Puumala virus, which is associated with bank voles (*Clethrionomys glareolus*). An epidemic in 1993 in the Four Corners region of the United States led to the identification of a new hantavirus (Sin Nombre virus) and eventually to identification of several related viruses (Black Canal Creek, New York, and Bayou); all of these have been associated with the hantavirus pulmonary syndrome (HPS) *(34,35)*. The classical features of the syndrome of acute febrile illness associated with prominent cardiorespiratory compromise has been extended to include clinical variants, including disease with frank hemorrhage *(35)*.

### 3.3. The Filoviridae

The Filoviridae include the causative agents of Ebola and Marburg hemorrhagic fevers. Under electron microscopy, these filoviruses have an exotic, thread-like appearance. Marburg virus was first recognized in 1967 when there were three simultaneous outbreaks of a lethal epidemic of VHF at Marburg, Frankfurt, and Belgrade among laboratory workers exposed to the blood and tissues of African green monkeys (*Ceropithecus aethiops*) imported from Uganda. Secondary transmission to medical personnel and family members was also documented *(36)*. G.A. Martini *(36)* recognized the initial outbreak from his clinical practice in Marburg, Germany. In all, 31 patients became infected, 7 of whom died. The 23% human mortality and bizarre morphology of the virions had a great psychological impact and led to new quarantine procedures for imported animals. During the next two decades, Marburg virus was associated with sporadic, isolated, usually fatal cases among residents and travelers in southeast Africa. In 1998–2000, there was an outbreak of Marburg hemorrhagic fever in Durba, Democratic Republic of the Congo, linked to individuals working in a gold mine *(37)*.

Ebola viruses, taxonomically related to Marburg viruses, were first recognized during near-simultaneous explosive outbreaks in 1976 in small communities in the former Zaire (now the Democratic Republic of the Congo) *(38)* and Sudan *(39)*. There was significant secondary transmission through reuse of unsterilized needles and syringes and nosocomial contacts. These independent outbreaks involved serologically distinct viral species. The Ebola-Zaire outbreak involved 318 cases and 280 deaths (88% mortality), and the Ebola-Sudan outbreak involved 280 cases and 148 deaths (53% mortality). Since 1976, Ebola virus has appeared sporadically in Africa, causing several small- to mid-size outbreaks between 1976 and 1979. In 1995, there was a large epidemic of Ebola-Zaire hemorrhagic fever involving 315 cases, with an 81% case fatality rate, in Kikwit, a community in the former Zaire *(40)*. Meanwhile, between 1994 and 1996, there were smaller outbreaks caused by the Ebola-Zaire virus in Gabon *(41)*. More recently, in 2000, Gulu, Uganda suffered a large epidemic of VHF attributed to the Sudan species of Ebola virus *(42)*. In 1989, a third species of Ebola virus appeared in Reston, Virginia, in association with an outbreak of VHF among cynomolgus monkeys (*Macaca fascicularis*) imported to the United States from the Philippines *(3)*. Hundreds of monkeys were infected (with high mortality) in this episode, but no human cases occurred, although four animal caretakers seroconverted without overt disease. Epizootics in cynomolgus monkeys recurred at other facilities in the United States and Europe through 1992, and again in 1996. A fourth species of Ebola virus, Ivory Coast, was identified in Côte d'Ivoire in 1994; this species was associated with chimpanzees, and only one nonfatal human infection was identified *(43)*.

Very little is known about the natural history of filoviruses. Animal reservoirs and arthropod vectors have been aggressively sought without success.

### 3.4. The Flaviviridae

Viruses responsible for VHF of the family Flaviviridae (type species Yellow fever virus) are members of the genus *Flavivirus*. These include the viruses of yellow fever, dengue, Kyasanur Forest disease, and Omsk. Mosquitoes transmit yellow fever, found throughout Africa and South America, and dengue, found throughout the Americas, Asia, and Africa *(44)*. Yellow fever was probably transported from Africa to the Americas during the slave trade. Probable early accounts of yellow fever in the Americas date to a 1648 outbreak in the Yucatan Peninsula. Carlos Finlay, a Cuban physician, identified *Aedes aegypti* as a likely vector and promulgated the theory of mosquito transmission. Dr. Finlay provided the Walter Reed commission with the mosquito and facilitated the U.S. experiments demonstrating that an extrinsic incubation period in the mosquito was needed prior to transmission. Benjamin Rush described classic dengue as "breakbone fever" in 1789. In 1954, dengue hemorrhagic fever/dengue shock syndrome (DHF/DSS) was described in the Philippines, and for a while it was known as Philippine hemorrhagic fever. There are four dengue virus serotypes, 1, 2, 3, and 4. DHF/DSS manifests in infants less than 1 year of age, born to dengue-immune mothers, and to persons older than 1 year of age with prior immunity to one serotype of dengue virus, undergoing infection with a second serotype. Humans are the reservoir of dengue virus, but a jungle cycle involving forest mosquitoes and monkeys, similar to that associated with yellow fever, is recognized. In 1981, Cuba reported the first serologically confirmed instance of DHF/DSS outside of Asia. Both yellow fever and dengue have had a major impact on military campaigns and military medicine.

The tick-borne flaviviruses include the agents of Kyasanur Forest disease of India *(45)* and Omsk hemorrhagic fever, seen mainly in Siberia *(46)*. Kyasanur forest disease, also called "monkey disease," was first described in 1957 in the Kyasanur forest of Mysore, India. Both diseases have a biphasic course; the initial phase includes a prominent pulmonary component, followed by a neurological phase with central nervous system manifestations.

## 4. VIROLOGICAL CHARACTERISTICS AND PATHOGENESIS

Despite the diversity of the four families of viruses (Arenaviridae, Bunyaviridae, Filoviridae, and Flaviviridae) that contribute pathogens to the group of VHF agents

(Table 1), all these viruses share common characteristics. They are all relatively simple RNA viruses, and they all have lipid envelopes. This renders them relatively susceptible to detergents, as well as to low-pH environments and household bleach. Conversely, they are quite stable at neutral pH, especially when protein is present. Thus, these viruses are stable in blood for long periods and can be isolated from a patient's blood after weeks of storage at refrigerator or even ambient temperatures.

Except for dengue viruses, they are all biosafety level 3 (BSL-3) or BSL-4 agents because they tend to be stable and highly infectious as fine-particle aerosols, and they produce very serious disease.

VHF viruses can all cause thrombocytopenia. Patients with Ebola, Lassa, and Junin virus infections can manifest platelet dysfunction. Coagulation factor levels drop, reflecting hepatic damage, cytokine interactions, and/or disseminated intravascular coagulopathy. Evidence suggests that inflammatory mediators from macrophages and other cells of the immune system may trigger many of the pathological manifestations seen in filoviruses and arenaviruses.

## 5. CLINICOPATHOLOGIC FINDINGS

There is a wide spectrum of clinical manifestations with varying degrees of severity in patients infected with these viruses, and not all patients develop classic VHF syndrome. The exact nature of the disease depends on the viral virulence and strain characteristics, routes of exposure, dose, and host factors. For example, DHF/DSS typically develops only in patients previously exposed to heterologous dengue serotypes *(47)*. The target organ in VHF syndrome is the vascular bed; correspondingly, the dominant clinical features are usually a consequence of microvascular damage and changes in vascular permeability *(48)*. Common presenting complaints are fever, myalgia, and prostration; clinical examination may reveal only conjunctival injection, mild hypotension, flushing, and petechial hemorrhages. Full-blown VHF typically evolves to shock and generalized bleeding from the mucous membranes and is often accompanied by evidence of neurological, hematopoietic, or pulmonary involvement. Hepatic involvement is common, but only a small percentage of patients with Rift Valley fever, CCHF, Marburg hemorrhagic fever, Ebola hemorrhagic fever, and yellow fever manifest a clinical picture dominated by jaundice and other evidence of hepatic failure. Renal failure is proportional to cardiovascular compromise, except for patients with HFRS caused by hantaviruses, in which renal failure is an integral part of the disease process, and oliguria is a prominent feature of the acutely ill patient *(33)*. VHF mortality may be substantial, ranging from 5 to 20% or higher in recognized cases. Ebola outbreaks in Africa have had particularly high case fatality rates, from 50% up to 90% *(38–40)*.

The overall incubation period for VHF ranges from 2 to 35 days. There is a prodrome period that may include a high fever, headache, malaise, myalgias, arthralgia, abdominal pain, nausea, and diarrhea, which usually lasts less than a week. The clinical characteristics vary with the viral agent involved. Filoviruses, flaviviruses, and Rift Valley fever tend to have an abrupt onset, whereas arenaviruses have more insidious onset. For Lassa fever patients, hemorrhagic manifestations are not pronounced, and neurological complications are infrequent, develop late, and manifest only in the most severely ill group. Deafness is a frequent sequela of severe Lassa fever. For the South American arenaviruses (Argentine and Bolivian hemorrhagic fevers), neurological and hemorrhagic manifestations are much more prominent. RVF virus is primarily hepatotropic, and hemorrhagic disease is infrequent. In recent outbreaks in Egypt, retinitis was a frequently reported component of Rift Valley fever *(49)*.

Unlike Rift Valley fever, in which hemorrhage is not prominent, CCHF infection is usually associated with profound disseminated intravascular coagulation (DIC) (Fig. 1A). Patients with CCHF may bleed profusely, and since this occurs during the acute, viremic phase, contact with blood of an infected patient is a special concern; a number of nosocomial outbreaks have been associated with CCHF virus.

The picture for diseases caused by hantaviruses is evolving, especially now in the context of HPS syndrome. The pathogenesis of HFRS may be somewhat different; immunopathological events seem to be a major factor. When patients present with HFRS, they are typically oliguric. Surprisingly, the oliguria commences while the patient's viremia is resolving and patients are mounting a demonstrable antibody response. This has practical significance in that renal dialysis can be started with relative safety.

Clinical data from human outbreaks caused by filoviruses are sparse. Although mortality is high, outbreaks are rare and sporadic. Marburg and Ebola viruses produce prominent maculopapular rashes in both human and nonhuman primates (Fig. 1B), and DIC is a major factor in their pathogenesis. Therefore, treatment of the DIC should be considered, if practicable, for these patients.

Among the flaviviruses, yellow fever virus is, of course, hepatotropic; black vomit caused by hematemesis has been associated with this disease. Patients with yellow fever develop clinical jaundice and die with something comparable to hepatorenal syndrome. Dengue hemorrhagic fever and shock are uncommon, life-threatening complications of dengue and are thought (especially in children) to result from an immunopathological mechanism triggered by sequential infections with different dengue viral serotypes *(47)*. Although this is the general epidemiological pattern, dengue virus may also rarely cause hemorrhagic fevers in adults and in primary infections *(50)*.

Laboratory findings for VHFs may include thrombocytopenia (or abnormal platelet function), leukopenia (except for Lassa fever, in which there is leukocytosis). Some patients have anemia and others have hemoconcentration; most have elevated liver enzymes. Bilirubin is elevated in RVF and yellow fever. Prothrombin time, activated partial thromboplastin time, and bleeding time are often prolonged. Patients in DIC will have elevated fibrin degradation products and decreased fibrinogen. Urine tests may reveal proteinuria and hematuria; those with renal failure may have oliguria or azotemia. Blood, occult or overt, may be present in stools.

## 6. DIAGNOSIS

In the event of a covert bioterrorist attack, a high degree of suspicion would be required to have any realistic chance of diagnosing VHF rapidly. Thus, it is unclear whether clinicians would initially recognize VHF, but a cluster of such cases would probably alert clinicians to this possibility. Under natural conditions these viruses have a geographically restricted distribution linked to the ecology of the reservoir species and vectors; thus, a detailed travel history is critical in making the diagnosis of VHF. Patients with arenaviral or hantaviral infections often recall seeing rodents during the presumed incubation period, but, since the viruses spread to humans by aerosolized excreta or environmental contamination, actual contact with the reservoir is not necessary. Large mosquito populations are common during the seasons when RVF virus and the flaviviruses are transmitted, but a history of mosquito bite is sufficiently common to be of little assistance in making a

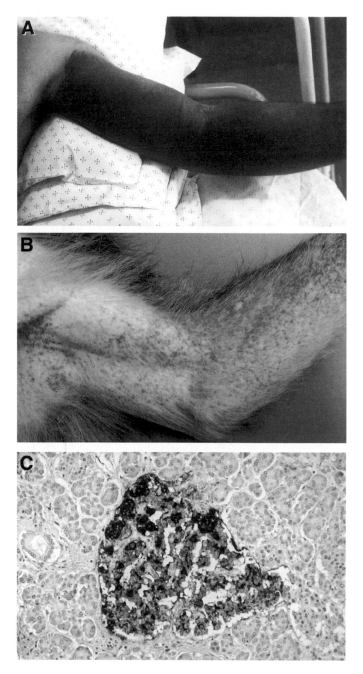

**Fig. 1. (A)** Massive cutaneous ecchymosis associated with late-stage Crimean-Congo hemorrhagic fever virus infection, 7–10 d after clinical onset. Ecchymosis indicates multiple abnormalities in the coagulation system, coupled with loss of vascular integrity. The cause of the sharply demarcated proximal border on this patient's lesion is unknown. (Courtesy of Robert Swanepoel, PhD, DTVM, MRCVS, National Institute of Virology, Sanderingham, South Africa.) **(B)** Characteristic petechial rash of the left arm of a cynomolgus macaque resulting from Ebola virus (Zaire) infection. **(C)** Immunohistochemical stain from the pancreas of a fatal human case of Marburg hemorrhagic fever. Note that Marburg virus-positive staining (red) is limited to the pancreatic islet, with multifocal distribution within the islet. Steptavidin-alkaline phosphatase method; section counterstained with hematoxylin. Original magnification 20×.

diagnosis, whereas tick bites or nosocomial exposures are of some significance when CCHF is suspected. History of exposure to animals in slaughterhouses should raise suspicions of Rift Valley fever and CCHF in a patient with VHF.

The variable clinical presentation of these diseases presents a major diagnostic challenge. VHF should be suspected in any patient presenting with a severe febrile illness and evidence of vascular involvement (subnormal blood pressure, postural hypotension, petechiae, hemorrhagic diathesis, flushing of the face and chest, nondependent edema), who has traveled to an endemic area, or where intelligence suggests a biological warfare or biological terrorist threat. Signs and symptoms suggesting additional organ system involvement are common (headache, photophobia, pharyngitis, cough, nausea or vomiting, diarrhea, constipation, abdominal pain, hyperesthesia, dizziness, confusion, and tremor), but they rarely dominate the picture. The macular eruption characteristic of Marburg and Ebola hemorrhagic fevers has considerable clinical importance.

As previously noted, laboratory findings can be helpful, although they vary from disease to disease, and summarization is difficult. Leukopenia may be suggestive, but in some patients, white blood cell counts may be normal or even elevated. Thrombocytopenia is a component of most VHF diseases, but to a varying extent. In some, platelet counts may be near normal, and platelet function tests are required to explain the bleeding diathesis. A positive tourniquet test has been particularly useful in diagnosing dengue hemorrhagic fever, but this sign may be associated with other hemorrhagic fevers as well. Proteinuria or hematuria or both are common in VHF, and their absence virtually rules out Argentine hemorrhagic fever, Bolivian hemorrhagic fever, and HFRS. Hematocrits are usually normal, and if there is sufficient loss of vascular integrity, perhaps mixed with dehydration, hematocrits may be increased. Soluble cytosolic liver-associated enzymes such as aspartate aminotransferase (AST) are frequently elevated. VHF viruses are not primarily hepatotropic, but the liver is involved, and an elevated AST may help to distinguish VHF from a simple febrile disease.

For much of the world, the major differential diagnosis is malaria. It must be borne in mind that parasitemia in patients partially immune to malaria does not prove that malaria is responsible for symptoms. Typhoid fever and rickettsial and leptospiral diseases are major confounding infections; nontyphoidal salmonellosis, shigellosis, relapsing fever, fulminant hepatitis, and meningococcemia are some of the other important diagnoses to exclude. Ascertaining the cause of DIC is usually surrounded by confusion. Many conditions that cause DIC, such as acute leukemia, lupus erythematosus, idiopathic or thrombotic thrombocytopenic purpura, and hemolytic uremic syndrome, could be mistaken for VHF.

Definitive diagnosis in an individual case rests on specific virological diagnosis. Most patients have readily detectable viremia at presentation (the exception is those with hantaviral infections). Infectious virus and viral antigens can be detected and identified by a number of assays using fresh or frozen serum or plasma samples. Likewise, early immunoglobulin (Ig) M antibody responses to the VHF-causing agents can be detected by enzyme-linked immunosorbent assays (ELISAs), often during the acute illness. Diagnosis by viral cultivation and identification requires 3–10 days for most (longer for the hantaviruses); with the exception of dengue, specialized microbiological containment is required for safe handling of these viruses (51). Appropriate precautions should be observed in collection, handling, shipping, and processing of diagnostic samples (*see* "Packaging Protocols for Biological Agents/Diseases" at http://www.bt.cdc.gov/agent/

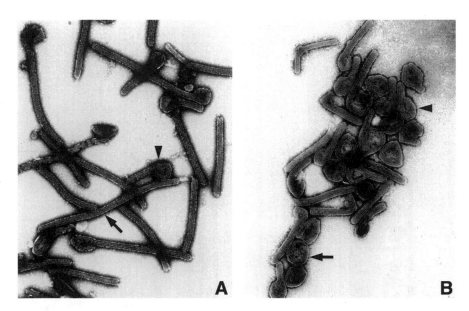

**Fig. 2. (A)** Negatively contrasted Ebola viral particles recovered from fluid of infected African green monkey kidney cells. Note high proportion of filamentous forms (arrow) compared with true "6"-shaped forms (arrowhead) and no circular forms. **(B)** Negatively contrasted Marburg viral particles recovered from fluid of infected African green monkey kidney cells. Note high proportion of circular (arrow) and "6"-shaped forms (arrowhead) compared with filamentous virions. Viral particles in both panels are 80 nm in diameter; Ebola virions from unpurified cell cultures average approximately 1200 nm in length, and Marburg virions average approximately 870 nm in length *(58)*.

vhf/index.asp). Both the CDC and the U.S. Army Medical Research Institute of Infectious Diseases (USAMRIID; Fort Detrick, MD) have diagnostic laboratories operating at the maximum BSL-4. Viral isolation should not be attempted without BSL-4 containment.

In contrast, most antigen-capture and antibody-detection ELISAs for these agents can be performed with samples that have been inactivated by treatment with β-propiolactone *(52)*. Likewise, diagnostic tests based on reverse transcriptase polymerase chain reaction (RT-PCR) technology are safely performed on samples following RNA extraction using chloroform and methanol. RT-PCR has been successfully applied to the real-time diagnosis of most of the VHF agents *(53–56)*. When isolation of the infectious virus is difficult or impractical, RT-PCR has proven to be extremely valuable, for example, with HPS: Sin Nombre virus was recognized by PCR months before it was finally isolated in culture *(34)*.

When the identity of a VHF agent is totally unknown, isolation in cell culture and direct visualization by electron microscopy (Fig. 2), followed by immunological identification by immunohistochemical techniques are often successful *(3,57)*. Filoviruses and arenaviruses induce intracytoplasmic inclusions that are morphologically unique to each viral family (Fig. 3). Moreover, Ebola and Marburg viruses can be distinguished from each other by their distinctive inclusion material *(58)*; trained microscopists can distinguish these filoviral genera by virion size and shape *(58)*.

Immunohistochemical stains (IHS) can detect VHF viruses in tissue sections. The application of IHS to skin snips can provide a relatively rapid diagnosis. Immunohis-

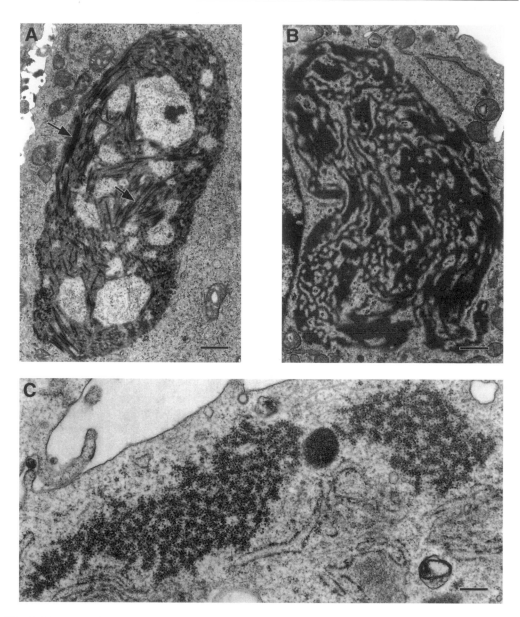

**Fig. 3.** Transmission electron micrographs of thin sections through African green monkey kidney cells showing intracytoplasmic viral inclusions. (**A**) Ebola viral inclusion composed of an amorphous matrix containing preformed nucleocapsids (arrows) that are easily distinguished from the less electron-dense matrix. Scale bar = 770 nm. (**B**) Marburg viral inclusion composed of electron-dense amorphous material. Note the absence of preformed nucleocapsids seen in Ebola inclusions. Scale bar = 640 nm. (**C**) Lassa viral inclusion composed of a moderately electron-dense matrix, with aggregates of dense, 20–25-nm granules. Scale bar = 270 nm.

tochemical techniques are also useful for retrospective diagnosis using formalin-fixed tissues, in which viral antigens can be detected and identified using batteries of specific immune sera and monoclonal antibodies (Fig. 1C).

Although intensive efforts are being directed toward the development of simple, qualitative tests for rapid diagnosis in the field, definitive diagnosis for these diseases today requires, at a minimum, an ELISA capability coupled with specialized immunological reagents, supplemented with an RT-PCR capability.

# 7. MEDICAL MANAGEMENT

Patients with VHF syndrome will require close supervision, and some require intensive care. Since the pathogenesis of VHF is not entirely understood and availability of antiviral drugs is limited, treatment is largely supportive. The care is essentially the same as the conventional care provided to patients with other causes of multisystem failure. The challenge is to provide this support while minimizing the risk of infection to other patients and medical personnel.

## 7.1. Supportive Care

Patients with VHF syndrome generally benefit from rapid, nontraumatic hospitalization to prevent unnecessary damage to the fragile capillary bed. Transportation of these patients, especially by air, is usually contraindicated because of the effects of drastic changes in ambient pressure on lung water balance. Frequently patients manifest restlessness, confusion, myalgia, and hyoperesthesia; this should be managed by reassurance and other supportive measures, including the judicious use of sedatives and pain relief and amnestic medications.

Secondary infections are common and should be sought and aggressively treated. Concomitant malaria should be treated aggressively with a regimen known to be effective against the geographical strain of the parasite; however, the presence of malaria, particularly in immune individuals, should not preclude management of the patient for VHF syndrome if such is clinically indicated.

Intravenous lines, catheters, and other invasive techniques should be avoided unless they are clearly indicated for appropriate management of the patient. Attention should be given to pulmonary toilet, the usual measures to prevent superinfection, and the provision of supplemental oxygen. Immunosuppression with steroids or other agents has no empirical and little theoretical basis and is contraindicated except possibly for HFRS.

The diffuse nature of the vascular pathological process may lead to a requirement for support of several organ systems. Myocardial lesions detected at autopsy reflect cardiac insufficiency ante mortem. Pulmonary insufficiency may develop, and, particularly with yellow fever, hepatorenal syndrome is prominent (44).

## 7.2. Treatment of Bleeding

The management of bleeding is controversial. Uncontrolled clinical observations support vigorous administration of fresh frozen plasma, clotting factor concentrates, and platelets, as well as early use of heparin for prophylaxis of DIC. In the absence of definitive evidence, mild bleeding manifestations should not be treated at all. More severe hemorrhage requires appropriate replacement therapy. When there is definitive laboratory evidence of DIC, consider the use of heparin therapy if appropriate laboratory support is available.

## 7.3. Treatment of Hypotension and Shock

Management of hypotension and shock is difficult. Patients are often modestly dehydrated from heat, fever, anorexia, vomiting, and diarrhea, in any combination. There are covert losses of intravascular volume through hemorrhage and increased vascular permeability *(59)*. Nevertheless, these patients often respond poorly to fluid infusions and readily develop pulmonary edema, possibly from myocardial impairment and increased pulmonary vascular permeability. Asanguineous fluids (either colloid or crystalloid solutions) should be given, but cautiously. Although it has never been evaluated critically for VHFs, dopamine might be the agent of choice for patients with shock who are unresponsive to fluid replacement. α-Adrenergic vasoconstricting agents have not been clinically helpful except when emergent intervention to treat profound hypotension is necessary. Vasodilators have never been systematically evaluated. Pharmacological doses of corticosteroids (e.g., methylprednisolone 30 mg/kg) provide another possible, but untested, therapeutic modality in treating shock.

## *7.4. Isolation and Containment*

Patients with VHF syndrome generally have significant quantities of virus in their blood, and perhaps in other secretions as well (with the exception of dengue and classical hantavirus disease). Secondary infections among contacts and medical personnel not parenterally exposed are well documented. Thus, caution is needed in evaluating and treating patients with suspected VHF syndrome. Over-reaction on the part of medical personnel is inappropriate and detrimental to both patient and staff, but it is prudent to provide isolation measures as rigorous as feasible *(60)*. At a minimum, isolation measures should include the following:

• Stringent barrier nursing
• Mask, gown, glove, and needle precautions
• Hazard labeling of specimens submitted to the clinical laboratory
• Restricted access to the patient
• Autoclaving or liberal disinfection of contaminated materials, using hypochlorite or phenolic disinfectants.

For more intensive care, however, increased precautions are advisable. Members of the patient care team should be limited to a small number of selected, trained individuals, and special care should be directed toward eliminating all parenteral exposures. Use of endoscopy, respirators, arterial catheters, routine blood sampling, and extensive laboratory analysis increase opportunities for aerosol dissemination of infectious blood and body fluids. For medical personnel, the wearing of flexible plastic hoods equipped with battery-powered blowers provides excellent protection of the mucous membranes and airways.

## *7.5. Specific Antiviral Therapy*

Currently, there are no antiviral drugs approved by U.S. Food and Drug Administration (FDA) for treatment of the VHFs. Ribavirin is a nonimmunosuppressive nucleoside analog with broad antiviral properties *(61)* and is of proven value for some of the VHF agents. Ribavirin was shown to reduce mortality from Lassa fever in high-risk patients *(62)*, and it presumably decreases morbidity in all patients with Lassa fever, for whom current recommendations are to treat initially with ribavirin 30 mg/kg, administered intravenously, followed by 15 mg/kg every 6 h for 4 d, and then 7.5 mg/kg every 8 h for an additional 6 d *(60)*. Treatment is most effective if begun within 7 d of onset; lower intravenous doses or oral administration of 2 g followed by 1 g/d for 10 d may also be useful. Although oral ribavirin is FDA-approved, in combination with interferon-α, for treatment of chronic hepatitis C virus infection, intravenous ribavirin is of limited availability in the United States. It is manufactured by ICN Pharmaceuticals (Costa Mesa, CA) for compassionate use under an investigational new drug (IND) application.

The primary adverse effects caused by ribavirin have been anemia and hyperbilirubinemia related to a mild hemolysis and reversible block of erythropoiesis. The anemia did not require transfusions or cessation of therapy in the published Sierra Leone study *(62)* or in subsequent unpublished limited trials in West Africa. Ribavirin is contraindicated in pregnant women and is classified as a pregnancy category X drug *(63)*. However, in cases of VHF of unknown etiology or secondary to an arenavirus or Rift Valley fever, the benefits of treatment are likely to outweigh any fetal risk. Safety of oral or intravenous ribavirin in infants and children has not been established; aerosolized ribavirin has been approved by the FDA to treat respiratory syncytial virus infection in children.

A similar dose of ribavirin initiated within 4 d of disease is efficacious in patients with HFRS *(64)*. In Argentina, ribavirin has been shown to reduce virological parameters of Junin virus infection (i.e., Argentine hemorrhagic fever) and is now used routinely as an adjunct to immune plasma. Unfortunately, ribavirin does not penetrate the brain and is expected to protect only against the visceral, not the neurological phase of Junin infection *(64,65)*.

Small studies investigating the use of ribavirin in the treatment of Bolivian hemorrhagic fever and CCHF have been promising, as have preclinical studies for Rift Valley fever *(64)*. Conversely, ribavirin is ineffective against both the filoviruses and the flaviviruses. No other antiviral compounds are currently available for VHF agents.

Interferon-$\alpha$ has no role in therapy, with the possible exception of Rift Valley fever *(66)*, in which fatal hemorrhagic fever has been associated with low interferon responses in experimental animals. Exogenous interferon-$\gamma$, does, however, hold promise in treatment of arenaviral infections when used as an adjunct to ribavirin.

### 7.6. Immunoprophylaxis and Immunotherapy

Passive immunization has been attempted for treatment of the diseases caused by VHFs. This approach has often been taken in desperation, owing to the limited availability of effective antiviral drugs. Studies and case reports describing successes and clinical utility *(67–75)* are frequently tempered by more systematic studies in which efficacy is less obvious and/or of no benefit *(62,76,77)*. In the case of dengue virus, passive immunization has been associated with enhanced viral replication in experimentally infected animals *(78)*. For all VHF viruses, the benefit of passive immunization seems to be correlated with the concentration of neutralizing antibodies, which are readily induced by some, but not all, of these viruses.

Argentine hemorrhagic fever responds to antibody therapy with two or more units of convalescent plasma that contain adequate amounts of neutralizing antibody (or an equivalent amount of immune globulin), provided that treatment is initiated within 8 d of onset *(68)*. Antibody therapy is also beneficial in the treatment of Bolivian hemorrhagic fever. Efficacy of immune plasma in treatment of Lassa fever *(79)* and CCHF *(80)* is limited by low neutralizing antibody titers and the consequent need for careful donor selection.

In the future, passive immunization strategies using recombinant human monoclonal antibodies may have utility against the VHF agents, given the potential benefit of passive immunization described in a number of studies *(68,72,74,75,81)*. In HFRS, a passive immunization approach is contraindicated for treatment, since an active immune response is usually already evolving in most patients when they are first recognized, although plasma containing neutralizing antibodies has been used empirically in prophylaxis of high-risk exposures.

## 7.7. Active Immunization

The only established and licensed virus-specific vaccine available against any of the hemorrhagic fever viruses is the yellow fever live attenuated 17D vaccine, which is mandatory for travelers to endemic areas of Africa and South America *(82)*. For prophylaxis against Argentine hemorrhagic fever virus, a live attenuated Junin vaccine strain (Candid #1) was developed at USAMRIID *(83)* as part of an international cooperative project (USAMRIID-Pan American Health Organization) and is available as an IND. Candid #1 was proved to be effective in phase III studies in Argentina *(84)*, and plans are proceeding to obtain a New Drug license. Candid #1 elicits high levels of protective antibodies of 9 years' duration in approximately 90% of the people vaccinated with a single dose. This vaccine also provides protection against Bolivian hemorrhagic fever in experimentally infected primates. Two IND vaccines were developed at USAMRIID against Rift Valley fever; a formalin-inactivated vaccine that requires three boosters, which has been in use for 20 years, and a live-attenuated RVF virus strain (MP-12). The inactivated vaccine has been administered to laboratory workers and appears to be safe and efficacious, but the ability to produce this vaccine in the United States no longer exists *(85)*.

For Hantaan virus, a formalin-inactivated rodent brain vaccine is available in Korea but is not generally considered acceptable by U.S. standards. Another USAMRIID product, a genetically engineered vaccinia construct, expressing hantaviral structural proteins, is in phase II safety testing in U.S. volunteers. A formalin-inactivated Kyasanur Forest disease vaccine was shown to be protective in field trials in India *(86)*. For dengue, a number of live attenuated strains of all four serotypes are entering phase II efficacy testing. However, none of these vaccines in phase I or II IND status will be available as licensed products in the near term. For the remaining VHF agents, the availability of effective vaccines is more distant. Several promising vaccines are in development including platforms that have shown efficacy in nonhuman primate models of Ebola hemorrhagic fever *(87)* and Lassa fever *(88)*. Development of an Ebola vaccine, conducted jointly by The Vaccine Research Center at the National Institutes of Allergy and Infectious Diseases and USAMRIID, is the most advanced effort among these remaining VHF agents.

## REFERENCES

1. Geisbert TW, Jaax NK. Marburg hemorrhagic fever: report of a case studied by immunohistochemistry and electron microscopy. Ultrastruct Pathol 1998;22:3–17.
2. Jahrling PB. Viral hemorrhagic fevers. In: Sidell FR, Takafuji ET, Franz DR, eds. Textbook of Military Medicine: Medical Aspects of Chemical and Biologic Warfare. Borden Institute, Washington, DC, 1997, pp. 591–603.
3. Jahrling PB, Geisbert TW, Dalgard DW, et al. Preliminary report: isolation of Ebola virus from monkeys imported to the USA. Lancet 1990;335:502–505.
4. Centers for Disease Control and Prevention. Category A agents. Available at: http://www.bt.cdc.gov/Agent/agentlist.asp (accessed November 18, 2002).
5. Williams P, Wallace D. Unit 731, Japan's Secret Biological Warfare in World War II. Free Press, New York, 1989, pp. 38–40.

6. Alibek K, Handelman S. Biohazard: The Chilling True Story of the Largest Covert Biological Weapons Program in the World. Told from the Inside by the Man Who Ran It. Random House, New York, 1999.
7. Center for Nonproliferation Studies. Chemical and biological weapons: possession and programs past and present. November 2000. Available at: http://cns.miis.edu/research/cbw/possess.htm (accessed November 18, 2002).
8. Miller J, Engelberg S, Broad WJ. Germs: Biological Weapons and America's Secret War. Simon & Schuster, Waterville, ME, 2001.
9. Bazhutin NB, Belanov EF, Spiridonov VA, et al. Vliianie sposobov eksperimental'nogo zarazheniia virusom Marburg naosobennosti protekaniia bolezni u zelenykh martyshek (Russian) [The effect of the methods for producing an experimental Marburg virus infection on the characteristics of the course of the disease in green monkeys.] Vopr Virusol 1992;37:153–156.
10. P'yankov OV, Sergeev AN, P'yankova OG, Chepurnov AA. Eksperimental'naia likhoradka ebola u makak rezusov (Russian) [Experimental Ebola fever in macaca rhesus.] Vopr Virusol 1995;40:113–115.
11. Johnson E, Jaax N, White J, Jahrling P. Lethal experimental infections of rhesus monkeys by aerosolized Ebola virus. Int J Exp Pathol 1995;76:227–236.
12. Lub MI, Sergeev AN, P'iankov OV, P'iankova OG, Petrishchenko VA, Kotlyarov LA. Nekotorye patogeneticheskie kharakteristiki zabolevaniia obez'ian, aerogenno infitsirovannykh virusom Marburg. (Russian) [Certain pathogenetic characteristics of a disease in monkeys infected with the Marburg virus by an airborne route.] Vopr Virusol 1995;40:158–161.
13. Stephenson EH, Larsen EW, Dominik JW. Effect of environmental factors on aerosol-induced Lassa virus infection. J Med Virol 1984;14:295–303.
14. Kenyon RH, McKee KT, Zack PM, et al. Aerosol infection of rhesus macaques with Junin virus. Intervirology 1992;33:23–31.
15. Global Proliferation of Weapons of Mass Destruction: Hearings Before the Permanent Subcommittee on Investigations of the Committee on Governmental Affairs, United States Senate, 104th Congress, 1st-2nd Session (1996). Available at http://www.fas.org/irp/congress/1995_rpt/aum/part0.5.htm (accessed on November 19, 2002).
16. Federation of American Scientists. Chemical and Biological Arms Control Program. Weapons of Mass Destruction Around the World. Report on North Korea. Biological Systems. Available at http://www.fas.org/nuke/guide/dprk/bw/index.html (accessed November 20, 2002).
17. Borio L, Inglesby T, Peters CJ, et al., and The Working Group on Civilian Biodefense. Hemorrhagic fever viruses as biological weapons. JAMA 2002;287:2391–2405. Available at http://jama.ama-assn.org/issues/v287n18/ffull/jst20006.html (accessed November 20, 2002).
18. Peters CJ, Jahrling PB, Khan AS. Patients infected with high-hazard viruses. Arch Virol 1996; 11(suppl):141–168.
19. McCormick JB, Webb PA, Krebbs JW, Johnson KM, Smith E. A prospective study of epidemiology and ecology of Lassa fever. J Infect Dis 1987;155:437–444.
20. Birmingham K Kenyon G. Lassa fever is unheralded problem in West Africa. Nat Med 2001;7:878.
21. Freedman DO, Woodall J. Emerging infectious diseases and risk to the traveler. Med Clin North Am 1999;83:865–883.
22. Schmitz H, Kohler B, Laue T, et al. Monitoring of clinical and laboratory data in two cases of imported Lassa fever. Microbes Infect 2002;4:43–50.
23. Maiztegui J, Feuillade M, Briggiler A. Progessive extension of the endemic area and changing incidence of Argentine hemorrhagic fever. Med Microbiol Immunol 1986;175:149–152.
24. Johnson KM, Wiebenga NH, Mackenzie RB, et al. Virus isolations from human cases of hemorrhagic fever in Bolivia. Proc Soc Exp Biol Med 1965;118:113–118.
25. Salas R, de Manzione N, Tesh RB, et al. Venezuelan haemorrhagic fever. Lancet 1991;338:1033–1036.
26. Lisieux T, Coimbra M, Nassar ES, et al. New arenavirus isolated in Brazil. Lancet 1994;343:391–392.
27. Centers for Disease Control and Prevention. Fatal illness associated with a new world arenavirus—California. MMWR 2000;49:709–711. Available at: http://www.cdc.gov/mmwr/preview/mmwrhtml/mm4931a1.htm (accessed 19 November 2002).
28. Easterday BC. Rift Valley fever. Adv Vet Sci 1965;10:65–127.
29. Daubney R, Hudson JR, Garnham PC. Enzootic hepatitis or Rift Valley fever. An undescribed virus disease of sheep, cattle and man from East Africa. J Pathol Bacteriol 1931;34:545–579.
30. Shawky S. Rift Valley fever. Saudi Med J 2000;21:1109–1115.
31. van Eeden PJ, van Eeden, SF, Joubert JR, King JB, van de Wal BW, Michell WL. A nosocomial outbreak of Crimean-Congo haemorrhagic fever at Tygerberg Hospital, II: Management of patients. S Afr Med J 1985;68:718–721.

32. Nuzum EO, Rossi CA, Stephenson EH, LeDuc JW. Aerosol transmission of Hantaan and related viruses to laboratory rats. Am J Trop Med Hyg 1988;38:636.

33. Lee HW. Hemorrhagic fever with renal syndrome in Korea. Rev Infect Dis 1989;11(suppl 4):S864–S876.

34. Butler CJ, Peters CJ. Hantaviruses and hantavirus pulmonary syndrome. Clin Infect Dis 1994;19:387–395.

35. Peters CJ, Khan AS. Hantavirus pulmonary syndrome: the new American hemorrhagic fever. Clin Infect Dis 2002;34:1224–1231.

36. Martini GA, Siegert R. Marburg Virus Disease. Springer-Verlag, Berlin, 1971.

37. Zeller H. Les leçons de l'épidémie a virus Marburg a Durba, République Démocratique du Congo (1998–2000). (French) [Lessons from the Marburg virus epidemic in Durba, Democratic Republic of the Congo (1998–2000)]. Med Trop (Mars) 2000;60(suppl): 23–26.

38. World Health Organization International Study Team. Ebola haemorrhagic fever in Zaire, 1976. Bull WHO 1978;56:271–293.

39. World Health Organization International Study Team. Ebola haemorrhagic fever in Sudan, 1976. Bull WHO 1978;56:247–270.

40. Khan AS, Tshioko FK, Heymann DL, et al. The reemergence of Ebola hemorrhagic fever, Democratic Republic of the Congo, 1995. J Infect Dis 1995;179(suppl 1):S76–S86.

41. Georges-Courbot MC, Sanchez A, Lu CY, et al. Isolation and phylogenetic characterization of Ebola viruses causing different outbreaks in Gabon. Emerg Infect Dis 1997;3:59–62.

42. Centers for Disease Control and Prevention. Outbreak of Ebola hemorrhagic fever Uganda, August 2000–January 2001. MMWR 2001;50:73–77. Available at: http://www.cdc.gov/mmwr/preview/mmwrhtml/mm5005a1.htm (accessed on 19 November 2002).

43. Le Guenno B, Formenty P, Wyers M, Gounon P, Walker F, Boesch C. Isolation and partial characterization of a new strain of Ebola virus. Lancet 1995;345:1271–1274.

44. Monath TP. Yellow fever: Victor Victoria? Conqueror, conquest? Epidemics and research in the last forty years and prospects for the future. Am J Trop Med Hyg 1991;45:1–43.

45. Pavri K. Clinical, clinicopathological, and hematologic features of Kyasanur Forest disease. Rev Infect Dis 1989;11(suppl 4):S854–S859.

46. Chumakov MP. Studies of virus hemorrhagic fevers. J Hyg Epidemiol Microbiol Immunol 1959; 7:125–135.

47. Halstead SB. Antibody, macrophages, dengue virus infection, shock, and hemorrhage: a pathogenetic cascade. Rev Infect Dis 1989;11(suppl 4):S830–S839.

48. McKay DG, Margaretten W. Disseminated intravascular coagulation in virus diseases. Arch Intern Med 1967;120:129–152.

49. WHO Collaborating Centre for Research and Training in Veterinary Epidemiology and Management. Report of the WHO/IZSTE Consultation on Recent Developments in Rift Valley Fever (RVF) (With the Participation of FAO and OIE). 1993;128:1–23. Civitella del Tronto, Italy, 14–15 September, 1993. WHO/CDS/VPH/93.123.

50. Rosen L. Disease exacerbation caused by sequential dengue infections: myth or reality? Rev Infect Dis 1989;11(suppl 4):S840–S842.

51. Centers for Disease Control and Prevention, National Institutes of Health. Biosafety in Microbiology and Biomedical Laboratories. Government Printing Office, Washington, DC, 1993. HHS Publication (CDC) 93-8395. Also available at: http://www.orcbs.msu.edu/biological/BMBL/BMBL-1.htm. (accessed November 18, 2002).

52. van der Groen G, Elliot LH. Use of betapropiolactone inactivated Ebola, Marburg and Lassa intracellular antigens in immunofluorescent antibody assay. Ann Soc Belg Med Trop 1982;62:49–54.

53. Trappier SG, Contay AL, Farrar BB, Auperin DD, McCormick JB, Fisher-Hoch SP. Evaluation for the polymerase chain reaction for diagnosis of Lassa virus infection. Am J Trop Med Hyg 1993;49:214–221.

54. Ksiazek TG, Rollin PE, Jahrling PB, Dalgard DW, Peters CJ. Enzyme immunosorbent assay for Ebola virus antigens in tissues of infected primates. J Clin Microbiol 1992;30:947–950.

55. Leroy EM, Baize S, Lu CY, et al. Diagnosis of Ebola hemorrhagic fever by RT-PCR in an epidemic setting. J Med Virol 2000;60:463–467.

56. Drosten C, Gottig S, Schilling S, et al. Rapid detection and quantification of RNA of Ebola and Marburg viruses, Lassa virus, Crimean-Congo hemorrhagic fever virus, Rift Valley fever virus, dengue virus, and yellow fever virus by real-time reverse transcription-PCR. J Clin Microbiol 2002;40:2323–2330. Available to members at: http://jcm.asm.org/cgi/content/full/40/7/2323?view=full&pmid=12089242 (accessed 19 November, 2002).

57. Geisbert TW, Rhoderick JB, Jahrling PB. Rapid identification of Ebola and related filoviruses in fluid specimens by indirect immunoelectron microscopy. J Clin Pathol 1991;44:521–522.

58. Geisbert TW, Jahrling PB. Differentiation of filoviruses by electron microscopy. Virus Res 1995; 39:129–150.

59. Fisher-Hoch SP. Arenavirus pathophysiology. In Salvato MS, ed. The Arenaviridae. Plenum Press, New York, 1993, pp. 299–323.

60. Centers for Disease Control. Management of patients with suspected viral hemorrhagic fever. MMWR 1988;37(suppl 3):1–16. Available at http://www.cdc.gov/mmwr/preview/mmwrhtml/00037085.htm (accessed November 19, 2002), and Update available at: http://www.bt.cdc.gov/agent/vhf/index.asp (accessed November 18, 2002).

61. Canonico PG, Kende M, Luscri BJ, Huggins JW. In-vivo activity of antivirals against exotic RNA viral infections. J Antimicrob Chemother 1984;14(suppl A):27–41.

62. McCormick JB, King IJ, Webb PA, et al. Lassa fever. Effective therapy with ribavirin. N Engl J Med 1986;314:20–26.

63. Rebetol product information. Available at: http://www.rebetol.com/index.html (and http://www.spfiles.com/pirebetol.pdf) (accessed November 19, 2002).

64. Huggins JW. Prospects for treatment of viral hemorrhagic fevers with ribavirin, a broad-spectrum antiviral drug. Rev Infect Dis 1989;11(suppl 4):S750–S761.

65. Kilgore PE, Ksiazek TG, Rollin PE, et al. Treatment of Bolivian hemorrhagic fever with intravenous ribavirin. Clin Infect Dis 1997;24:718–722.

66. Morrill JC, Jennings GB, Cosgriff TM, Gibbs PH, Peters CJ. Prevention of Rift Valley fever in rhesus monkeys with interferon-α. Rev Infect Dis 1989;11(suppl 4):S815–S825.

67. Emond RT, Evans B, Bowen ET, Lloyd G. A case of Ebola virus infection. BMJ 1977;2:541–544.

68. Enria DA, Fernandez NJ, Briggiler AM, Lewis SC, Maiztegui JI. Importance of neutralizing antibodies in treatment of Argentine hemorrhagic fever with immune plasma. Lancet 1984;4:255–256.

69. Peters CJ, Jones D, Trotter R, et al. Experimental Rift Valley fever in rhesus macaques. Arch Virol 1988;99:31–44.

70. Monath TP, Maher M, Casals J, Kissling RE, Cacciapuoti A. Lassa fever in the Eastern Province of Sierra Leone, 1970–1972, II: Clinical observations and virological studies on selected hospital cases. Am J Trop Med Hyg 1974;23:1140–1149.

71. Mupapa K, Massamba M, Kibadi K, et al. Treatment of Ebola hemorrhagic fever with blood transfusions from convalescent patients. J Infect Dis 1999;179(suppl 1):S18–S23.

72. Stille W, Bohle E, Helm E, van Rey W, Siede W. Uber eine durch *Cercopithecus aethiops* ubertragene Infektionskrankheit. ("Grune-Meerkatzen-Krankheit", "Green Monkey Disease") (German) [On an infectious disease transmitted by *Cercopithecus aethiops* ("Green monkey disease")]. Dtsch Med Wochenschr 1968;93:572–582.

73. Leifer E, Gocke DJ, Bourne H. Lassa fever, a new virus disease in man from West Africa, II: report of a laboratory-acquired infection treated with plasma from a person recently recovered from the disease. Am J Trop Med Hyg 1970;19:677–679.

74. Frame JD, Verbrugge GP, Gill RG, Pinneo L. The use of Lassa fever convalescent plasma in Nigeria. Trans R Soc Trop Med Hyg 1984;78:319–324.

75. Maiztegui JI, Fernandez NJ, de Damilano AJ. Efficacy of immune plasma in treatment of Argentine haemorrhagic fever and association between treatment and a late neurological syndrome. Lancet 1979;2:1216–1217.

76. White HA. Lassa fever: a study of 23 hospital cases. Trans R Soc Trop Med Hyg 1972;66:390–401.

77. Clayton AJ. Lassa immune serum. Bull WHO 1977;55:435–439.

78. Halstead SB. In vivo enhancement of dengue virus infection in rhesus monkeys by passively transferred antibody. J Infect Dis 1979;140:527–533.

79. Jahrling PB, Frame JD, Rhoderick JB, Monson MH. Endemic Lassa fever in Liberia, IV: selection of optimally effective plasma for treatment by passive immunization. Trans R Soc Trop Med Hyg 1985;79:380–384.

80. Shepherd AJ, Swanepoel R, Leman PA. Antibody response in Crimean-Congo hemorrhagic fever. Rev Infect Dis 1989;11(suppl 4):S801–S806.

81. Parren PW, Geisbert TW, Maruyama T, Jahrling PB, Burton DR. Pre- and post-exposure prophylaxis of Ebola virus infection in an animal model by passive transfer of a neutralizing human antibody. J Virol 2002;76:6408–6412. Available to members at http://jvi.asm.org/cgi/content/full/76/12/6408?view=full&pmid=12021376 (accessed November 19, 2002).

82. Monath TP. Yellow fever: an update. Lancet Infect Dis 2001;1:11–20.

83. McKee KT, Oro JG, Kuehne AI, Spisso JA, Mahlandt BG. Candid No. 1 Argentine hemorrhagic fever vaccine protects against lethal Junin virus challenge in rhesus macaques. Intervirology 1992;34:154–163.

84. Maiztegui JI, McKee KT, Barrera Oro JG, et al. Protective efficacy of a live attenuated vaccine against Argentine hemorrhagic fever. J Infect Dis 1998;177:277–283.

85. Pittman PR, Liu CT, Cannon TL, et al. Immunogenicity of an inactivated Rift Valley fever vaccine in humans. Vaccine 1999;18:181–189.

86. Dandawate CN, Desai GB, Achar TR, Banerjee K. Field evaluation of formalin inactivated Kyasanur Forest disease virus tissue culture vaccine in 3 districts of Karnataka state. Indian J Med Res 1994;99: 152–158.

87. Sullivan NJ, Sanchez A, Rollin PE, Yang ZY, Nabel GJ. Development of a preventative vaccine for Ebola virus infection in primates. Nature 2000;408:605–609. Available at http://www.nature.com/cgi-taf/ DynaPage.taf?file=/nature/journal/v408/n6812/full/408605a0_fs.html (accessed November 19, 2002).

88. Fisher-Hoch SP, Hutwagner L, Brown B, McCormick JB. Effective vaccine for Lassa fever. J Virol 2000;74:6777–6783.

# 17  Viral Encephalitides

## Niranjan Kanesa-thasan, MD, MTMH

The views expressed in this chapter are those of the author and do not reflect the official policy or position of the Department of the Army, the Department of Defense, or the U.S. government.

### CONTENTS

## 1. INTRODUCTION

Biological agents that cause viral encephalitis (inflammation of the brain and its meninges) are arthropod-borne viruses (arboviruses) that normally infect an arthropod vector or an intermediate host to disseminate infection. However, these viruses are also capable of transmission through man-made aerosols, as occurs in laboratory-associated infection or potentially during suspected a biological warfare attack *(1)*. Both mosquito-borne and aerosol routes of transmission may result in epidemic numbers of casualties or disability from viral encephalitis. In the past, biological warfare programs of the United States and the former Soviet Union pursued development and aerosol weaponization of viral encephalitis agents *(2)*. The following discussion will focus on viral biological warfare agents of encephalitis, their clinical features, diagnosis, treatment, and prevention.

The principal biological warfare agents of viral encephalitis are the alphaviruses (genus *Alphavirus*, family Togaviridae), which are small enveloped arboviruses containing single-stranded RNA genomes *(3)*. The three major agents in this group are Venezuelan equine encephalitis (VEE), eastern equine encephalitis (EEE), and western equine encephalitis (WEE). The alphaviruses are incapacitating, highly infectious, but rarely lethal viruses. They are considered potential biological warfare agents because large viral

From: *Physician's Guide to Terrorist Attack*
Edited by: M. J. Roy © Humana Press Inc., Totowa, NJ

concentrations are readily cultivated in vitro, remain stable during laboratory and weaponization procedures, and induce reproducible infections after short incubation periods when delivered by aerosol *(4)*. In addition, alphaviruses are genetically variable (three related viruses with multiple genotypes of each) and amenable to genetic manipulation *(5)*. This latter property has been used to generate candidate vaccines against the viruses but potentially may be used to nefarious purpose. Vaccination has proved effective against alphavirus encephalitis *(6)*, and new approaches promise enhanced prophylaxis against the disease.

## 2. EPIDEMIOLOGY

The alphaviruses are genetically distinct viruses maintained by distinct mosquito-vertebrate cycles in nature. These viruses occur naturally throughout the Western hemisphere and result in febrile illness and sporadic cases of meningo-encephalitis in humans *(7)*. VEE is also associated with epidemic disease in susceptible human populations during an epizootic (an epidemic in animals that are the natural hosts for the virus) of equine encephalitis. Birds (WEE, EEE), horses (epizootic VEE), and other animals (e.g., rodents in enzootic VEE) play prominent roles as natural reservoirs for these pathogens, whereas humans are considered accidental or "dead-end" hosts *(8)*.

Epidemiological clues are critical for distinguishing a natural outbreak of alphavirus encephalitis in susceptible individuals from a potential biological warfare attack *(9)*. Simultaneous and synchronous onset of cases of alphavirus encephalitis in the absence of a preceding epizootic is an important feature of biological warfare use *(10)*. Clustering or grouping of cases in military personnel while classically susceptible populations (children or elderly adults) are spared may be associated with a biological warfare attack. Laboratory identification of these viruses outside naturally endemic (EEE, WEE) or enzootic (VEE) areas would strongly suggest a biological warfare attack, as originally suspected in the recent unexpected appearance of West Nile virus associated with encephalitis cases in the Northern hemisphere *(11)*. Finally, alphavirus diseases are associated with seasonal foci of mosquito abundance, typically warm, wet, swampy areas. In the United States, cases of encephalitis usually peak in the late summer/early fall *(12)*. Appearance of these viruses outside periods of seasonal variation, for example, VEE during the winter in temperate climates, could indicate human manipulation of the agent.

## 3. PATHOGENESIS AND CLINICAL FEATURES

The alphaviruses may enter the body through the bloodstream, after the bite of an infected mosquito, or through the nasal and airway mucosa after aerosol exposure. Subsequent dissemination by Langerhans cells to the draining peripheral lymphoid tissues is followed by viremia *(13)*. Invasion of the brain parenchyma occurs through viral penetration of the brain vasculature or through axonal transport from the olfactory lobes. The latter route has been implicated as a major mechanism for central nervous system involvement after aerosol exposure *(14)*; however, disease pathogenesis after aerosol exposure of humans is essentially unknown *(15)*. The pathology of fatal encephalitis includes vasculitis with perivascular cuffing within the parenchyma, and neuronal destruction and gliosis in the cortex and thalamus with sparing of the cerebellum and spinal cord *(16)*. The alphaviruses do not persist in the human host after the acute disease.

After either subcutaneous or aerosol exposure, alphavirus infections may induce no symptoms or an undifferentiated acute febrile illness with or without systemic symptoms. The exception is VEE, in which each infection may result in apparent disease *(17,18)*. Typically, less than 1% of naturally acquired febrile alphavirus illnesses will progress to neurological disease *(19)*, and many hundreds of infections occur for each clinical case of encephalitis. However, experience with laboratory-acquired infections suggests that more rapid onset of illness and perhaps increased severity of disease, including encephalitis, may result from aerosol exposure *(20,21)*. Appearance of antibodies, particularly neutralizing antibodies, after infection or vaccination with alphaviruses correlates with protection against subcutaneous and possibly aerosol virus exposure *(22)*.

There are few characteristic clinical features to distinguish alphavirus encephalitides; summary descriptions of each agent and a Case Vignette follow. Typically, sudden fever, headache, vomiting, and dizziness may rapidly lead to frank mental status changes, including disorientation, obtundation, seizures, paresis, focal neurological signs, stupor, and coma. Frank encephalitis is followed by complete recovery, residual neurological sequelae, or death. Case fatality rates from alphavirus encephalitis range from less than 10% (VEE, WEE) to 60% (EEE). Children, especially those younger than 1 yr, are at risk for severe disease with death or neurological sequelae with WEE and EEE, whereas adults older than 55 are at greater risk with EEE viruses *(7)*.

### 3.1. VEE

After an incubation period of 2–6 d, VEE infection typically presents with abrupt onset of chills, fever, headache, and myalgias *(17)*. Many cases develop flu-like illness with prominent drowsiness, pharyngitis, myalgias, and/or arthralgias. Gastrointestinal symptoms of anorexia, nausea, vomiting, or diarrhea are also common *(8)*. Physical findings include fever (temperature >38.0°C), conjunctival injection, erythematous pharynx without exudate, and muscle tenderness. Illness resolves in most adults after a few days of nonspecific febrile illness, yet convalescence may be prolonged (1–2 wk).

A minority of adults (typically <1%) may proceed to neurological illness; this figure may be higher (4–5%) in children *(19)*. Most of these demonstrate mild central nervous system (CNS) involvement with lethargy, somnolence, or confusion that may be accompanied by nuchal rigidity *(23)*. Rarely, more severe illness results in a variety of neurological presentations, including seizures, ataxia, paralysis, or coma. Encephalitis, if present, is associated with a case fatality rate of less than 10–20% in adults and higher in children *(24)*. Recovery after encephalitis is often complete *(25)*. Laboratory findings include leukopenia and lymphopenia, with elevated serum aspartate transaminase and lactate dehydrogenase levels. VEE has been implicated in cases of congenital infection with encephalitis *(26)*.

### 3.2. EEE

In EEE, the prodromal illness is followed by the abrupt onset of fever, chills, malaise, myalgia, and arthralgia. Encephalitis may follow, with high fevers to 41.3°C, headache, malaise, irritability, drowsiness, anorexia, vomiting, diarrhea, seizures, and coma *(27)*. Clinical signs include nuchal rigidity, tremors and muscular twitching; edema in children is associated with paralysis *(7)*. Death occurs in 50–75% of cases, which makes EEE the most severe arboviral encephalitis *(28)*. Those who recover are left with severe sequelae (persistence of intellectual dysfunction, seizures, paralysis), and in many cases, increased mortality *(29)*.

### *3.3. WEE*

Onset of illness in WEE follows a prolonged incubation period of 5–15 d, which may be shorter in children or after aerosol exposure. Naturally acquired WEE infection is symptomatic in only 1:1150 infected adults and induces the mildest disease *(30)*. Illness presents with abrupt fever, malaise, and headache and progresses to nausea or vomiting *(31)*. Early CNS involvement occurs, with somnolence, delirium, and progresses to coma. Examination reveals nuchal rigidity, impaired sensorium, or upper motor neuron deficits with abnormal reflexes *(15)*. Death occurs in 10% of encephalitis cases, with higher rates in more severely affected individuals; survivors recover completely but slowly *(32)*. Congenital infections have been documented with coincident encephalitis and sequelae in affected infants *(33)*.

## 4. DIAGNOSIS

### Case Vignette

A 35-year-old male physician was accidentally exposed to VEE by aerosol while working in the laboratory. Within 48 hours after exposure to contaminated dust from cages housing VEE-infected mice, he experienced abrupt onset of general malaise and headache. The next day, while at work, he developed fever to 39.4°C accompanied by severe frontal headache as well as back and muscle aches. He also had a slight sore throat. Soon afterwards, he went home for bed rest and took aspirin without relief of symptoms. During the next 2 days, he sustained fever, chills, dizziness, nausea, and fatigue so profound that "every movement demanded considerable effort." By day 4, he had to rest frequently and was unable to do any active work. Eventually, he went to bed and "slept soundly for 22 hours." Upon arising, he felt better, with decreased fever, headache, and myalgias. He improved over the next 2 days but was still anorexic, weak, and fatigued quickly. However, on day 8, he had an abrupt relapse in symptoms of headache, myalgias, and chills with a recrudescence of fever to 39.7°C. He was irritable, vomited once, and then became somnolent for 5 days during which he "slept almost continuously day and night" but was easily aroused. The febrile illness resolved on day 12; during his illness, the patient experienced a 5-kg weight loss. He was only able to resume work 2 weeks after onset of illness, while continuing to note easy fatigability. The patient noted sequelae of insomnia and minor tremors, which persisted for over 4 months after his illness.

(Adapted from ref. *40*.)

Diagnosis of alphavirus encephalitis is often aided by a travel or occupational history, which indicates risk for mosquito-borne infection in an endemic area within the past several weeks before disease onset. VEE, EEE, and WEE must be considered if there were concurrent or preceding recent outbreaks of animal diseases in areas visited, particularly epidemics of equine encephalitis. In personnel at risk for exposure to biological warfare agents, queries would refer to characteristic abrupt onset of fever or neurological symptoms, presence of similar and coincident disease in colleagues, and cases of encephalitis within the same locale. Completion of vaccination against these agents (*see* Subheading 6., Prevention, below), particularly VEE, may significantly decrease the possibility of neurological disease.

Other entities that may be considered with multiple cases of meningo-encephalitis are biological warfare agents such as *Brucella* species, *Yersinia pestis*, and *Coxsiella burnetti* (covered elsewhere in this volume). Sporadic cases of encephalitis may require extensive evaluation to rule out potential causes of disease (*34*). Relatively common and treatable causes of viral encephalitis, such as herpesviruses or human immunodeficiency virus, should always be considered. Other viral causes of encephalitis include the flaviviruses and bunyaviruses, arboviral pathogens often found worldwide in the same biomes as the alphaviruses (*15*). In addition, nonviral and noninfectious causes of encephalomyelitis must be considered in the differential diagnosis, such as tuberculosis, partially treated meningitis, or subdural hematoma.

Definitive diagnosis may require lumbar puncture, computed tomography (CT), electroencephalogram (EEG), or other advanced testing. Cerebrospinal fluid (CSF) in VEE reveals aseptic meningitis, with up to 500 mononuclear cells/μL. Elevated CSF pressure is typical in EEE, along with an increased inflammatory reaction (up to 2000 cells/μL) that may reveal neutrophil predominance (*7*). The CSF in WEE resembles that of VEE, with a lymphocytic pleocytosis of 10–400 cells/μL.

An alphavirus infection is confirmed in the laboratory by either virus isolation or antibody determination. Virus may be recovered from serum or pharyngeal washes in VEE and WEE patients during the first days of their febrile illness but is rarely present upon clinical presentation with encephalitis. Antibodies may be detectable several days after onset of illness and should be present in either the serum or CSF of encephalitis cases. Specific IgM antibodies may be measured by enzyme immunoassay (*35*), but the diagnosis is usually confirmed by demonstration of a fourfold rise in specific IgG antibodies by another serological assay such as neutralization or hemagglutination inhibition antibody assays.

## 5. MANAGEMENT AND TREATMENT

Cases with neurological symptoms should be monitored for fever and respiratory insufficiency. Periodic neurological examination should be conducted for muscle weakness, diminished sensorium, hyperactive deep tendon reflexes, sensory disturbances, limb paralysis, paresis of the shoulder girdle or arms, tremors, abnormal movements, and cranial nerve abnormalities (gaze paralysis, speech disorders). Nuchal rigidity may be present and should prompt evaluation of the CSF. In obtunded patients, the Glasgow coma scale can be used to track progression of mental status changes and gauge the need for medical evacuation or consultation.

There is no specific drug treatment for alphavirus encephalitis. Patients are managed with supportive care, including fluids, analgesics, antipyretics, and anticonvulsants as needed. Arboviruses are not directly transmitted from person to person; thus universal precautions are sufficient for caregivers. Obtunded patients should be closely monitored for seizures or aspiration; decreasing Glasgow coma scale score or onset of seizures or focal neurological symptoms indicate disease progression and a requirement for specialized neurological evaluation. Onset of coma or respiratory failure necessitates intensive care for airway management and possible assisted ventilation.

# 6. PREVENTION

In endemic regions, protection against alphavirus encephalitis is primarily achieved by limiting exposure to mosquito vectors by using insect repellents and other personal protective measures. In biological warfare arenas, attempts may be made to control or eliminate reservoirs of infection, either by mosquito abatement or by reduction of potential vertebrate hosts. However, the principal means of prevention may be vaccination using several alphavirus vaccines. One investigational vaccine for VEE, TC-83, is a live attenuated virus that is used to induce active immunity in over 80% of recipients *(36)*. This vaccine, although effective against homologous VEE strains, also causes fever and systemic symptoms in over 20% of vaccinees and fails to produce antibodies in another 20% *(37)*. An experimental inactivated VEE vaccine, C-84, is used to boost these individuals successfully. Similar experimental inactivated vaccines for WEE and EEE exist; although these are well tolerated, they are only moderately immunogenic *(38)*. New, improved vaccines for the alphaviruses have shown efficacy in animal models and are proceeding toward clinical trials *(39)*. Availability of effective vaccines will be an essential component of protection against these potential biological warfare agents.

# REFERENCES

1. Hanson RP, Sulkin SE, Beuscher EL, Hammon WM, McKinney RW, Work TH. Arbovirus infections of laboratory workers. Science 1967;158:1283–1286.
2. Leitenberg M. Biological weapons in the twentieth century: a review and analysis. Crit Rev Microbiol 2001;27:267–320.
3. Strauss JH, Strauss EG. The alphaviruses: gene expression, replication, and evolution. Microbiol. Rev. 1994;58:491–562.
4. Huxsoll DL, Patrick WC, Parrott CD. Veterinary services in biological disasters. J Am Vet Med Assoc 1987;190:714–722.
5. Davis NL, Powell N, Greenwald GF, et al. Attenuating mutations in the E2 glycoprotein gene of Venezuelan equine encephalitis virus: construction of single and multiple mutants in a full-length cDNA clone. Virology 1991;183:20–31.
6. McKinney RW. Inactivated and live VEE vaccines—a review. In: Venezuelan Encephalitis: Proceedings of the Workshop-Symposium on Venezuelan Encephalitis Virus, 14–17 September, 1971. Pan American Health Organization, Washington, DC, 1972, pp. 369–377.
7. Calisher CH. Medically important arboviruses of the United States and Canada. Clin Microbiol Rev 1994;7:89–116.
8. Walton TE, Grayson MA. Venezuelan equine encephalitis. In: Monath TP, ed. The Arboviruses: Epidemiology and Ecology, vol 5. CRC Press, Boca Raton, FL, 1988, pp. 203–231.
9. Pavlin JA. Epidemiology of bioterrorism. Emerg Infect Dis 1999;5:528–530.
10. Franz DR, Jahrling PB, Friedlander AM, et al. Clinical recognition and management of patients exposed to biological warfare agents. JAMA 1997;278:399–411.
11. Fine A, Layton M. Lessons from the West Nile viral encephalitis outbreak in New York, 1999: implications for bioterrorism preparedness. Clin Infect Dis 2001;32:277–282.
12. Tsai TF. Arboviral infections in the United States. Infect Dis Clin North Am 1991;5:73–102.
13. MacDonald GH, Johnston RE. Role of dendritic cell targeting in Venezuelan equine encephalitis virus pathogenesis. J Virol 2000;74:914–922.
14. Ryzhikov AB, Tkacheva NV, Sergeev AN, Ryabchikova EI. Venezuelan equine encephalitis virus propagation in the olfactory tract of normal and immunized mice. Biomed Sci 1991;2:607–614.
15. Smith JF, Davis K, Hart MK, et al. Viral encephalitides. In: Sidell FR, Takafuji ET, Franz DR, eds. Textbook of Military Medicine: Medical Aspects of Chemical and Biologic Warfare. Borden Institute, Washington, DC, 1997, pp. 561–589.
16. de la Monte S, Castro F, Bonilla NJ, Gaskin de Urdaneta A, Hutchins GM. The systemic pathology of Venezuelan equine encephalitis virus infection in humans. Am J Trop Med Hyg 1985;34:194–202.
17. Franck PT, Johnson KM. An outbreak of Venezuelan equine encephalitis in man in the Panama Canal Zone. Am J Trop Med Hyg 1970;19:860–863.

18. Sanchez JL, Takafuji ET, Lednar WM, et al. Venezuelan equine encephalomyelitis: report of an outbreak associated with jungle exposure. Mil Med 1984;149:618–621.
19. Martin DH, Eddy GA, Sudia WD, Reeves WC, Newhouse VF, Johnson KM. An epidemiologic study of Venezuelan equine encephalomyelitis in Costa Rica, 1970. Am J Epidemiol 1972;95:2565–2578.
20. Slepushkin AN. An epidemiological study of laboratory infections with Venezuelan equine encephalomyelitis. Vopr Virusol 1959;3:311–314.
21. Anonymous. Treatment of Biological Warfare Casualties (Field Manual). Headquarters, Departments of the Army, the Navy, and the Air Force, and Commandant, Marine Corps, Washington, DC, 2000.
22. Jahrling PB, Stephenson EH. Protective efficacies of live attenuated and formaldehyde-inactivated Venezuelan equine encephalitis virus vaccines against aerosol challenge in hamsters. J Clin Microbiol 1984;19:429–431.
23. Sanmartin C. Diseased hosts: man. In: Venezuelan Encephalitis: Proceedings of the Workshop-Symposium on Venezuelan Encephalitis Virus, 14–17 September, 1971. Pan American Health Organization, Washington, DC, 1972, pp. 186–188.
24. Bowen GS, Fashinell TR, Dean PB, Gregg MB. Clinical aspects of human Venezuelan equine encephalitis in Texas. Bull Pan Am Health Organ 1976;10:46–57.
25. Leon CA. Sequelae of Venezuelan equine encephalitis in humans: a four year follow-up. Int J Epidemiol 1975;4:131–140.
26. Parsonson IM, Della-Porta AJ, Snowdon WA. Developmental disorders of the fetus in some arthropod-borne virus infections. Am J Trop Med Hyg 1981;30:660–673.
27. Deresiewicz RL, Thaler SJ, Hsu L, Zamani AA. Clinical and neuroradiographic manifestations of Eastern equine encephalitis. N Engl J Med 1997;336:1867–1874.
28. Feemster RF. Equine encephalitis in Massachusetts. N Engl J Med 1958;257:107–113.
29. Ayres JC, Feemster RF. The sequelae of eastern equine encephalomyelitis. N Engl J Med 1949;240: 960–962.
30. Reeves WC, Hammon WM. Epidemiology of the arthropod-borne viral encephalitides in Kern County, California, 1943–52. Univ Calif Public Health 1962;4:257.
31. Sciple GW, Ray CG, Holden P, La Motte LC, Irons JV, Chin TDY. Encephalitis in the high plains of Texas. Am J Epidemiol 1968;87:87–98.
32. Earnest MP, Goolishian HA, Calverly JR, Hayes RO, Hill HR. Neurologic, intellectual, and psychologic sequelae following western encephalitis. Neurology 1971;21:969–974.
33. Shinefield HR, Townsend TE. Transplacental transmission of western equine encephalomyelitis. J Ped 1953;43:21–25.
34. Whitley RJ, Gnann JW. Viral encephalitis: familiar infections and emerging pathogens. Lancet 2002;359:507–513.
35. Calisher CH, El-Kafrawi AO, Al-Deen Mahmud MI, et al. Complex-specific immunoglobulin M antibody patterns in humans infected with alphaviruses. J Clin Microbiol 1986;23:155–159.
36. McKinney RW, Berge TO, Sawyer WD, Tigertt WD, Crozier D. Use of an attenuated strain of Venezuelan equine encephalomyelitis virus for immunization in man. Am J Trop Med Hyg 1963;12:597–603.
37. Pittman PR, Makuch RS, Mangiafico JA, Cannon TL, Gibbs PH, Peters CJ. Long-term duration of detectable neutralizing antibodies after administration of live-attenuated VEE vaccine and following booster vaccination with inactivated VEE vaccine. Vaccine 1996;14:337–343.
38. Cieslak TJ, Christopher GW, Kortepeter MG, et al. Immunization against potential biological warfare agents. Clin Infect Dis 2000;30:843–850.
39. Hart MK, Caswell-Stephan K, Bakken R, et al. Improved mucosal protection against Venezuelan equine encephalitis virus is induced by the molecularly defined, live-attenuated V3526 vaccine candidate. Vaccine 2000;18:3067–3075.
40. Lennette EH, Koprowski H. Human infection with Venezuelan equine encephalomyelitis virus. JAMA 1943;123:1088–1095.

# III CHEMICAL AGENTS

# 18

## Pulmonary Toxic Agents

*Rafael E. Padilla,* MD

## 1. INTRODUCTION

The world changed at 0846 on September 11, 2001, when a group of terrorists used a coordinated attack of civilian aircraft loaded with jet fuel to wreak havoc on the World Trade Center. This incident served as a warning to industrial, military, and political leaders that common chemicals used in the manufacture of household products could possibly be used to inflict massive casualties within a community *(1,2)*. Pulmonary toxic agents are prevalent throughout the world because of the worldwide demands placed on industry for dyestuffs, textiles, metals, pharmaceuticals, plastics, and pesticides. These chemicals are often warehoused and transported via container barge, on interstate highway, and on railways. The industrial mishap in Bhopal, India underscores the importance of safeguarding these chemicals so that they may not be used for military or political gain. Some of these chemicals are well known in the annals of military history and evoke a great fear that some day they may be used once again in war, declared or otherwise. In World War I, approximately 1.2 million troops suffered a chemical gas exposure, resulting in 100,000 deaths *(3)*.

The human body requires the exchange of carbon dioxide and the replenishment of oxygen in order to survive. The pulmonary system therefore provides a potential portal of entry for toxic biological and chemical agents. Exposure to toxic pulmonary agents can present a myriad of challenging clinical scenarios to physicians treating these patients.

From: *Physician's Guide to Terrorist Attack*
Edited by: M. J. Roy © Humana Press Inc., Totowa, NJ

The history of the exposed patient is often difficult to obtain, and the symptoms may represent a wide array of pathology. This chapter will discuss a variety of toxic agents that enter the human body via the bronchopulmonary system. We will focus primarily on the diagnosis and treatment of the respiratory manifestations, although patients can develop multisystem organ failure from inhaled toxins. Toxic pulmonary agents can cause physiological embarrassment by many mechanisms, including topical damage, asphyxiation, and allergic reactions. The amount of damage is further complicated by the physiochemical properties of the agent, relative concentration of the agent, activity level of the victim at the time of exposure, and duration of exposure *(4)*.

### Case Vignette

A 27-year-old man welding in a closed space began coughing and experienced tearing after a few minutes. He left the area, walked outside, and noted some improvement in his symptoms. The supervisor noted an odd smell in the area but took no action other than to send the welder home. The welder did well for 8 hours after the exposure but then was brought to the emergency department by his wife because of difficulty breathing. He was hospitalized with hypotension, cyanosis, tachycardia, and pulmonary edema. Oxygen therapy was begun, but his condition continued to deteriorate, and he was intubated. He was given a course of steroid therapy and required dopamine for pressure support. Invasive monitoring confirmed the diagnosis of noncardiogenic pulmonary edema. Antibiotic therapy was instituted, but he continued to deteriorate, with the development of bilateral pneumothoraces, elevated white blood cells, and subcutaneous emphysema. Autopsy demonstrated pulmonary edema with severe bronchiolar necrosis.

## 2. CHLORINE GAS

Chlorine gas is used throughout the world in metal refinement and the production of agricultural chemicals, plastics, solvents, and their intermediates. As a result, chlorine is readily available in many industrial settings. It has also been used as a weapon of mass destruction. The first time it was used in this manner was in 1915 in Ypres, Belgium. The Germans released approximately 150 tons of chlorine gas along a 7000-m battlefront within a 10-min period, resulting in numerous injuries and deaths.

Currently, chlorine gas is transported in a pressurized liquid form but, when released, rapidly converts to a gaseous form. It forms a greenish yellowish cloud characterized by a dense, acrid, pungent smell. It tends to settle in low-lying areas and is readily detectable on first exposure. However, tolerance to its smell builds up rapidly, and therefore odor is not reliable as a monitor, especially for people who work within industrial and chemical complexes. The most common initial symptoms include shortness of breath, nausea, and vomiting, and patients' emesis may smell of chlorine *(5)*. Other frequent presenting symptoms include substernal tightness and rigorous coughing, often accompanied by hemoptysis. Chlorine gas can cause severe burning of the eyes, nose, and throat. It can also burn the larynx, which has been reported to induce fatal laryngospasm. Therefore, the initial assessment of victims should include a check for stridor, and if airway compromise is suspected, intubation should be performed immediately. The severity of the injury to the pulmonary tissues is related to the concentration of gas, duration of exposure, and water content of the tissue. The chemical reaction occurs when chlorine reacts with water to form hypochlorite and hydrochloric acid, which are caustic to the bronchioles and alveoli. Nebulized sodium bicarbonate has been used in uncontrolled case series to neutralize the hydrochloric acid produced by a chlorine gas exposure.

## 3. PHOSGENE

Phosgene is a ubiquitous chemical used in the manufacture of dyes, pharmaceuticals, and pesticides. It also is formed as a byproduct of welding around chlorinated solvents. Combustion of degreasing compounds, chlorinated solvents, and polyurethane has been shown to create phosgene. The estimated annual worldwide production is over 5 billion pounds *(6)*. At room temperature and normal pressure phosgene is colorless.

Phosgene was the most lethal offensive weapon used by the Germans in World War I. It has been estimated that 80% of all World War I deaths related to an inhaled pulmonary toxin were the result of a phosgene attack *(3,6,7)*. Troops exposed to phosgene gas reported observing a white cloud over the battlefield, whose density varied with the ambient humidity. They also described a characteristic smell of newly mown hay but found it to be unreliable as a protective indicator *(8,9)*. Smell did not correlate directly with higher concentrations *(6)*. The odor was also noted to be acrid and pungent, but tolerance builds rapidly and therefore odor detection will not adequately prevent harmful exposures. Phosgene settles in low-lying areas because of its increased density relative to air; however, because of its volatile nature, it is not persistent in the area of exposure. Its persistence will increase during cold weather, and it may condense to form liquid contaminating skin and ophthalmic areas.

Phosgene rapidly hydrolyzes to hydrochloric acid and carbon dioxide, damaging the cells lining the upper respiratory tract. Interestingly, the release of hydrochloric acid causes inflammation and localized damage, but the major effect is from acetylation within the tissue. The acetylation of amino, sulfhydryl, and hydroxyl groups leads to a disruption of enzymatic processes and disrupts the blood-to-air interface *(9,10)*. It is believed that phosgene also alters the level of pulmonary surfactants.

After limited exposure, a mild cough, chest discomfort, and/or slight dyspnea may be reported within 30 min. Moderate exposure typically results in prominent lacrimation and an objectionable taste. More severe exposure is manifest by a persistent cough with frothy sputum and marked dyspnea that can progress to pulmonary edema within the first 2–6 h. Hydrolysis of phosgene in the upper airway may release hydrochloric acid, causing a caustic burn and inducing laryngospasm, which may be fatal. As with exposure to chlorine, patients should be kept at rest since exertion may hasten pulmonary edema. Vigilant monitoring is especially critical in the first 24 h after exposure, owing to the risk for rapid progression of pulmonary edema. Pretreatment with hexamethamine tetramine has been used to minimize the effects of an anticipated phosgene gas exposure *(5,8,10)*. The long-term effects of a phosgene gas exposure have also been studied. Increased rates of cancer or respiratory diseases were not seen in cohort studies.

## 4. DIPHOSGENE

Diphosgene was developed by the Germans because it could destroy the conventional gas filters used during World War I, which had provided effective protection against chlorine and phosgene gas attacks *(11)*. Diphosgene is a compound that must be transported in glass vessels to prevent vaporization into its components of phosgene and chloroform. Soldiers exposed to diphosgene attacks described it as colorless but sharing with phosgene the smell of newly mown hay. Because of its increased density relative to air, like phosgene and chlorine gas, it settles in low-lying areas. The clinical sequelae likewise mimic those of phosgene gas exposure. Diphosgene can accumulate in the body because humans have no biological mechanism for detoxification.

## 5. CHLOROPICRIN

Chloropicrin is a colorless, slightly oily, heavy liquid at room temperature; it is used by the military as a chemical warning agent because it has an irritating tear gas odor. It also causes irritation of the skin and upper respiratory tract *(12)*. Chloropicrin is used commercially as a warning agent, primarily in conjunction with methyl bromide, in the use of high-value crops like the strawberry industry. Chloropicrin has been used as an insecticide and soil fumigant for over 80 yr. It is still most widely used for soil fumigation, as well as to control nematodes, bacteria, insects, and weeds, allowing the use of a lesser amount of methyl bromide. Chloropicrin is also used to treat wood posts as a preservative and as a warning agent for sulfuryl fluoride. Sulfuryl fluoride is used as a structural fumigant in warehouses storing cereal and grains.

Chloropicrin is gradually hydrolyzed in the presence of sunlight and microbes, with the primary byproduct of carbon dioxide. In the air, the half-life may be up to 20 d, with decomposition to many compounds including phosgene, which in turn hydrolyzes to carbon dioxide and hydrochloric acid *(13)*.

Patients exposed to chloropicrin generally present with tearing and eye irritation that improves with the termination of exposure. Continued exposure can cause irritation of the airway manifest by dyspnea. The median and small bronchi are affected the most. Alveolar damage can cause pulmonary edema, coma, and death. Chloropicrin can react with the hydroxyl groups within hemoglobin to interfere with oxygen transport. Smokers, who have a higher level of carboxyhemoglobin, may have more difficulty with oxygenation because chloropicrin reacts with the sulfhydryl group on the hemoglobin molecule. Accompanying symptoms may include vertigo, fatigue, gastrointestinal spasms, and diarrhea. The presence of pleuritic chest pain and elevated creatinine kinase levels may be a direct toxic effect of chloropicrin on skeletal muscle *(12)*.

## 6. ZINC OXIDE

Zinc oxide has historically been employed by military forces for use in grenades, candles, and firepots, as well as more recently with artillery shells and bombs, where it usually includes a combination of aluminum and zinc chloride. Zinc chloride is a respiratory irritant and a corrosive agent. As it burns it absorbs moisture from the air, creating a grayish white smoke that provides camouflage for movement of troops and materials.

After exposure, patients can present with an array of symptoms including myalgias, chills, headache, fever, malaise, and cough, often referred to as metal fume fever *(4,14)*. The pulmonary inflammatory response fatigues with repeated exposures to zinc oxide *(15)*. Symptoms usually begin within 6 h and resolve within 12 h after the person leaves the area of exposure, but it is important to observe patients for approximately 48 h after heavy exposure. Mild exposure is typically heralded by nausea and nose and throat irritation. More severe exposure is often characterized by nausea, retching, sore throat, hoarseness, and substernal chest tightness that may quickly progress to pulmonary edema. Toxicity from this chemical agent is generally thought to be a result of the topical effects of zinc chloride. Other products of combustion, such as carbon monoxide and phosgene gas, also can cause respiratory effects. Exposure to high doses of zinc oxide has been known to cause sudden collapse and death. The mechanism is thought to be upper airway obstruction. High-level exposures to zinc oxide have been treated in the past with serum chelating agents such as calcium ethylenediaminetetraacetic acid (EDTA) and British anti-Lewisite (BAL, or dimercaprol) to reduce serum zinc levels *(5,16,17)*. Survivors of major exposure have also been shown to have a persistent decrease in pulmonary function for months after exposure.

## 7. METHYL ISOCYANATE

Methyl isocyanate achieved international notoriety in 1984, when it was released in an industrial accident at a Union Carbide plant in Bhopal, India. This resulted in the death of approximately 3000 people and adverse health effects estimated for another 170,000 survivors *(1,7)*. Methyl isocyanate is a highly flammable intermediate used in the insecticide, herbicide, and chemical industries. Interaction with water results in a powerful exothermic reaction, producing a rapid buildup of carbon dioxide and pressure. The vapor is characterized by a sharp odor, an ability to travel long distances, and a propensity to accumulate in low-lying areas. The liquid form is colorless.

Pulmonary edema is the predominant cause of death in those victims exposed to methyl isocyanate; however, secondary respiratory infections from bronchitis and bronchial pneumonia may result following an exposure. Additional secondary effects seen after the Bhopal disaster include an increase in stillbirths, spontaneous miscarriages, pelvic inflammatory disease, increased menstrual bleeding, and decreased ability to lactate. Other short-term effects from methyl isocyanate included irritation of the eyes, nausea, gastritis, fever, and liver and kidney dysfunction.

## 8. PERFLUOROISOBUTYLENE

Perfluoroisobutylene (PFIB) is often a byproduct of high-temperature fires, especially those occurring in closed office spaces. The gas form that is produced is both colorless and odorless, resulting from incinerated organo-fluorines. Organo-fluorines are used in industrial and military applications such as tanks, aircrafts, and elevators because of their lubricant properties and chemical inertia. However, the release of byproducts such as PFIB from high-temperature fires can cause a condition known as polymer fume fever *(4,5,16)*. Teflon (which is polytetrafluoroethylene) is one of the more common organofluoride polymers. Teflon generally begins to burn at temperatures greater than 450°C. A febrile, influenza-like illness appears typically within 1–2 h after exposure. The fever may be as high as 104°F, accompanied by chills, malaise, sore throat, diaphoresis, and chest tightness. These symptoms usually subside over the next 24–48 h without long-term sequelae. A severe exposure to PFIB can result in the rapid onset of pulmonary edema within 2–4 h. However, even in such cases it is usually self-limited, rarely requiring treatment beyond supplemental oxygen, and clearing within 48 h.

# 9. TREATMENT

The treatment of patients who are exposed to pulmonary toxic agents is typically very similar, regardless of the particular agent. Victims should be immediately removed from low-lying areas; they should be moved uphill and/or upwind to triage areas. Decontamination should begin simultaneously with treating victims by removing their clothing in an open-air environment *(1,18)*. This should decrease the risk to emergency and rescue personnel from any residual vapors trapped in their clothing. Ideally, this should be done as close to the site of exposure as possible and prior to transporting the victim. It is important to try to avoid converting rescuers into victims. During the decontamination process, victims should be kept from overexertion. Exertion following any exposure to a pulmonary toxic agent has been shown to intensify the damage resulting from the agent *(5)*.

Airway, breathing, and circulation (the ABCs) should be rapidly assessed, with consideration of intubation if the airway appears to be compromised. Patients with suspected toxic pulmonary agents must initially have a rapid and careful assessment and, if necessary, surgical establishment of the victim's airway using a cricothyrotomy for life-threatening laryngospasm. If the eyes, nose, and oropharynx are badly burned, then concomitant chemical laryngitis should also be considered, and the patient should be observed for hoarseness and stridor. The intubation of victims may be extremely difficult because the caustic properties of the chemicals result in an increase in secretions and inflammation of the tissues. In the presence of obvious facial cutaneous burns, a clinician may decide to intubate the victim electively or monitor the patient in the intensive care unit. If an eye injury is suspected, contact lenses should be removed and irrigated with a balanced salt solution.

Victims of an inhalational attack may also suffer from blunt and penetrating trauma following the possible explosion that often follows the release of these volatile agents *(19)*. Once the ABCs have been established, then a history should be obtained as quickly as possible to facilitate appropriate care of the patient and development of a strategic plan with various other agencies involved in responding to the disaster.

Most of the toxic pulmonary agents have characteristic properties that can be elicited from victims. They include the color and smell of the agent and the inherent physical properties of a gas (e.g., density; Table 1) Descriptions should also be elicited from first responders, since an agent may linger at the scene and may be colorless and/or odorless (for example, PFIB gas created by pyrolysis of common fabrics, paints, and fluids used in office buildings). Treating physicians should in turn communicate pertinent data to appropriate military and or civilian authorities to incorporate in triage decisions as well as to protect rescue personnel treating the initial victims *(18,20–22)*.

After obtaining the history of present illness, a pertinent past medical history should be elicited. This should include previous medical and surgical interventions, current use of tobacco products, current medications, allergies to any medications, and general state of physical fitness. It is also important to verify the activity level of a victim at the time of exposure. A victim who was engaged in active exertion such as running will have had greater minute ventilation and as a result, potentially greater exposure to the affording toxic agents. For similar reasons, it is important to ensure that exposed individuals remain at rest after an initial evaluation. Transport from the affected areas should be rapid, while minimizing exertion on the part of those individuals not wearing protective breathing apparatus.

**Table 1**
**Characteristics of Pulmonary Toxic Gases**

| Feature | Chlorine | Phosgene | Diphosgene | Chloropicrin | Zinc oxide | Methyl isocyanate | PFIB |
|---|---|---|---|---|---|---|---|
| Color of cloud | Greenish yellow | Colorless to white | Colorless | Colorless | Gray/white smoke | Colorless | Colorless |
| Smell | Dense/acrid pungent | Newly mown hay | Newly mown hay | Tear gas | Sweet/Acrid | Sharp | Odorless |

If the airway has been shown to be patent and ventilation is adequate, then oxygenation can be monitored by either cannulation of an arterial line for obtaining arterial blood gases or noninvasively by monitoring oxygen saturation level. Oxygen is the mainstay of therapy, with the goal of keeping the $PaO_2$ above 60 torr. This may require endotracheal intubation, mechanical ventilation, and invasive monitoring to guide fluid therapy. The use of extracorporeal membrane oxygenation may be a consideration in those severe cases in which patients have become refactory to conventional ventilatory support.

The upper airways humidify and filter inspired air; as a result, different toxins may have different patterns of distribution within the lungs. For example, soluble toxic agents, like chlorine, tend to affect the areas of the upper airway, and the less soluble gases tend to produce affects in the peripheral airways and alveoli. Airways less than 2 mm are generally those most affected by insoluble gases, because airflow at that level occurs primarily by diffusion. Similarly, the size of the incoming particle will affect the distribution of damage done by a particular agent. Large particles (>10 μm) tend to be deposited in the upper airway, medium-sized particles (2.5–6 μm) tend be deposited in the lower airways, and very small particles (2.5 μm) tend to reach the most distal airways and alveoli. Substances reaching the alveoli in particular cause an enormous amount of damage due to the more limited air movement at that level of the lung.

After exposure to an inhaled pulmonary toxic agent, noncardiogenic pulmonary edema may be a lethal complication, with the highest risk period at 2–4 h; a latency of as much as 24 h is possible. It is therefore important to have a high level of vigilance both for relatively early as well as for delayed complications. Treatment sites should be equipped to establish intravenous access and to provide bronchodilators and humidified oxygen. If bronchospasm is severe, epinephrine or another $B_2$ agonist may be used to treat the injured victim. Humidified air decreases the degree of damage to the tissues of the upper airway resulting from a direct caustic exposure.

The chest radiographs of patients exposed to toxic pulmonary gases are most often normal immediately after exposure, while patients have limited or no symptoms *(4)*. When signs and symptoms develop, the chest X-ray most often shows diffuse pulmonary infiltrates without cardiomegaly. There is also often an increase in hilar markings and ill-defined shadows in the perihilar regions. Auscultation of the chest should be done at regular intervals and whenever new symptoms appear. The presence of wheezing in an otherwise healthy individual early after an exposure suggests that the exposure was severe. Patients often develop latent hypoxemia, dyspnea, and bronchospasm as a result of noncardiogenic pulmonary edema.

Diuretics should be avoided despite the presence of pulmonary edema, since the pathogenesis is via damage to alveolar and capillary membranes, not fluid overload. Failure to improve after the first 48 h should lead to consideration of bacterial superinfections. In this instance, sputum Gram stain and cultures, as well as blood cultures, can be helpful in directing antibiotic therapy. Most people are able to survive a chemical gas attack without lingering sequelae. Death within the first 24 h is usually the result of either laryngospasm or acute respiratory failure. After 24–48 h, bacterial superinfection leading to pneumonia may cause further pulmonary complications, and multisystem organ failure poses the greatest mortality risk. Bronchospasm is not common, but when it does occur, bronchodilators and steroid therapy are helpful as adjunctive therapy. The administration of corticosteroids early after exposure may decrease the degree of pulmonary edema. Rarely, aminophylline may be needed for severe bronchospastic crises.

# REFERENCES

1. Brennan RJ, Waeckerle JF, Sharp TW, Lillibridge SR. Chemical warfare agents: emergency medical and public health issues. Ann Emerg Med 1999;343:191–204.
2. Biological and chemical terrorism: strategic plan for preparedness and response. Recommendations of the CDC Strategic Planning Workgroup. MMWR 2000;49:RR–4.
3. Williams J. CBRNE—Lung-damaging agents, chloropicrin. Med J 2003 (accessed February 9, 2003 at http//www.emedicine.com/emerg/topic907.htm).
4. Balmes JR. Occupational and respiratory diseases. Review. Prim Care 2000;27:1009–1038.
5. Urbanetti, JS. Toxic inhalation injury. In: Sidell FR, Takafuji ET, Franz DR, eds. Textbook of Military Medicine: Medical Aspects of Chemical and Biologic Warfare. Borden Institute, Washington, DC, 1997, pp. 247–270.
6. Borak J, Diller WF. Phosgene exposure: mechanisms of injury and treatment strategies. J Occup Environ Med 2001;l43:110–119.
7. Harrison RJ. Chemicals and gases. Review. Prim Care 2000;27:917–982.
8. International Programme on Chemical Safety. Health and Safety Guide No.106. Phosgene. Health and Safety Guide. World Health Organization, Geneva, 1998 (accessed February 13, 2002 at http://www.inchem.org /documents/hsq/hsq/hsq106.htm).
9. United Nations Environment Programme, International Labour Organization, World Health Organization. International Programme on Chemical Safety. Environmental Health Criteria 193.Phosgene. World Health Organization, Geneva, 1997 (accessed February 13, 2002 at http://www.inchem.org/documents/ehc/ehc/ehc193.htm).
10. Environmental Protection Agency. Proposed Acute Exposure Guideline Levels. Oak Ridge National Laboratory, 2000 (accessed February 13, 2002 at http://www.epa.gov/fedrgstr/EPA-TOX/2000/December/Day-13/4862.htm).
11. Mowatt-Larssen E, Rega PP, Vollmer T. CBRNE—Lung-damaging agents, diphosgene. Med J 2001;3:10 (accessed February 13, 2002 at http//emedicine.com/emerg/topic906.htm).
12. Prudhomme JC, Bhatia R, Nutik JM, Shusterman DJ. Chest wall pain and possible rhabdomyolysis after choloropicrin exposure—a case series. J Occup Environ Med 2000;41:17–22.
13. Noltkamper D, Burgher S. Toxicity, phosgene. eMed J 2000 (accessed February 13, 2002 at http//www.emedicine.com/emerg/topic849.htm).
14. Frank AL. Approach to the patient with an occupational or environmental illness. Prim Care 2000;27:877–894.
15. Fine JM, Gordon T, Chen LC, et al. Characterization of clinical tolerance to inhaled zinc oxide in naïve subjects and sheet metal workers. J Occup Environ Med 2000;42:1085–1091.
16. Smith DT, Du Pont AM, Cullen NM. CBRNE—Lung-damaging agents, toxic smokes: Nox, Hc, Rp, Fs, Fm, Sgf2, Teflon. Med J 2001;2:10 (accessed February 13, 2002 at http://www.emedicine.com/emerg/topic908.htm)
17. Hu H. Occupational and environmental medicine: exposure to metals. Prim Care 2000,27.983–996.
18. Burgess JL, Kirk M, Borron SW,Cisek J. Emergency department hazardous materials protocol for contaminated patients. Ann Emerg Med 1999;34:205–212.
19. Wightman JM, Gladish SL. Explosions and blast injuries. Ann Emerg Med 2001;37:664–678.
20. Treat KN, Williams JM , Furbee PM, Manley WG, Russell FK, Stamper CD. Hospital preparedness for weapons of mass destruction incident: an initial assessment. Ann Emerg Med 2001;38:562–565.
21. Kvetan V. Critical care medicine, terrorism and disasters: are we ready? Crit Care Med 1999;27:873–874.
22. Tur-Kaspa I, Lev EI, Hendler I, Siebner R, Shapira Y, Shemer J. Preparing hospitals for toxiological mass casualties events. Crit Care Med ;1999;27:1004–1008.

# 19 Cyanide

*Steven I. Baskin,* PharmD, PhD, FCP, FACC, DABT, *FATS, Jonathan S. Kurche,* BS, *and Beverly I. Maliner,* DO, MPH, FABFP

The opinion or assertions contained in this paper are the private views of the authors and are not to be construed as official or as a reflection of the views of the Army or Department of Defense.

## CONTENTS

## 1. INTRODUCTION

Cyanide in its various forms ($CN^-$, HCN, NaCN, KCN, $CaCN_2$, CNCl, CNBr, $FeCN_2$, cyanogenic glycosides) is a rapidly acting lethal agent that is capable of incapacitating humans at doses of 10 mg/L within 10–18 s (1). Cyanide or plant materials containing cyanide have been utilized as poisons since antiquity (2). Cyanide-containing extracts from numerous plants were used over the years before chemical cyanide was isolated by the Swedish pharmacist and chemist Scheele from the dye Prussian blue in 1782 (3). Scheele also reportedly demonstrated the lethal toxicity of HCN gas when he died after breaking a vial of it in his laboratory shortly thereafter (4).

Cyanogenic glycosides are found abundantly in the Roseacea family (e.g., cherry, almond, apricot, peach, cassava) as well as in many other species (5). Consumption of inappropriately processed plants still containing cyanogenic glycosides or other chemical forms of cyanide have contributed to toxicity or death, particularly in migrant or nomadic peoples. Inappropriate use of apricot pits and bitter almonds have also been reported to cause toxicity or death from cyanide (6).

From: *Physician's Guide to Terrorist Attack*
Edited by: M. J. Roy © Humana Press Inc., Totowa, NJ

Industrial or commercial contact with cyanide is known to contribute to poisoning in the workplace. Electroplating, plastics processing, mining and ore extraction, fumigation, and steel manufacture as well as decomposition of synthetic fibers (i.e., nylon) by fire could also be a cause of cyanide release (7–9). In general, combustion of synthetic products that contain carbon and nitrogen will release cyanide. There are higher concentrations of blood cyanide levels among smokers (0.17 µg/mL) than among nonsmokers (0.06 mg/mL) (10).

## 2. CYANIDE AS A CHEMICAL WARFARE AGENT AND AS AN AGENT OF TERRORISM

Cyanides are well recognized as military and terror weapon agents. Nero used cherry laurel water, which contains cyanide, to kill those who opposed his rule, including members of his family (11). The use of cyanide as an offensive chemical agent was proposed during the Crimean and Franco-Prussian wars, but it was not until World War I that the French first utilized cyanide as HCN under the name Forestite (12). HCN, however, has a high volatility, is lighter than air, and is consequently easy to disperse. Cyanide offensive weapons remained ineffective until late in the war (1916), when cyanogen chloride was introduced by the French. Cyanogen chloride is heavier and less volatile than HCN, has a cumulative effect on its victims, and is a potent lachrymator at low concentrations (12). At high concentrations cyanogen chloride rapidly paralyzes the respiratory system's nerve center (13).

In World War II, a hydrogen cyanide formulation known as Zyklon (e.g., Zyklon B, HCN adsorbed onto a dispersible pharmaceutical base) was utilized by the Germans to exterminate over 2 million soldiers and civilians. Poison gas was also used to kill Yugoslavian partisans at the beginning of the war (14,15). More recently, cyanide's use has been reported in Hama, Syria, where over 10,000 individuals were killed in the 1980s (16), and in Halabja, Iraq, in the 1990s (17). In the United States, sensational incidents, such as the mass suicide of the Jonestown cult by cyanide in 1978 and the placing of cyanide in over-the-counter Tylenol pain relief tablets with the intent to kill consumers, have gained a place for cyanide in the minds of Americans (18).

Terrorist organizations, such as the Aum Shinrikyo in Japan, attempted to disperse and release multiple threat agents, including cyanide (19). Multiple reports of cyanide's attempted use as a poison by terrorist groups such as Al-Qaeda and the PLO Martyrs Brigade have proliferated in the press in recent years. Based on recent news accounts, including arrests made to foil a recent suspected terrorist cyanide attack against the London underground (20), cyanide remains a viable and concerning threat chemical throughout the industrialized world. Even in countries where industrial accidents involving cyanide are rare, cyanide is a weapon of convenience and is considered to be among the most likely chemicals to be used by terrorists.

## 3. THE BIOCHEMICAL AND PHYSIOLOGICAL BASIS FOR CYANIDE TOXICITY

Cyanide is known to bind and inactivate many cellular targets; it is thought to induce histotoxic anoxia by inhibiting the oxidized iron in the enzyme cytochrome c oxidase, the terminal electron transporter in the metabolic electron transport chain in mitochondria. Cytochrome c oxidase oxidizes cytochrome c and reduces $O_2$ to form $H_2O$. After an initial effect on excitable tissue, binding of cyanide to cytochrome oxidase effectively inhibits aerobic cell metabolism (21,22). The binding can occur between 30 s and several minutes; the lower the pH and the greater the cyanide concentration, the more rapidly the reaction takes place. Cyanide exposure brings about rapid onset of lactic acidosis as the metabolic machinery of the cell switches from aerobic to anaerobic metabolism (23), which may concomitantly enhance toxicity.

Other enzymes that are inhibited by cyanide include met- (oxidized) myoglobin and methemoglobin, which forms the basis of one of the methods of cyanide therapy, as well as myeloperoxidase, succinic dehydrogenase, superoxide dismutase, and carbonic anhydrase (4,24). Sun et al. (25) also reported that cyanide may interact with disulfide groups on the $N$-methyl-D-aspartate (NMDA) receptor regulatory sites to enhance receptor function, and Arden et al. (26) noted that cyanide may have a differential effect on different types of NMDA receptors. Combined with the understanding that minute quantities of cyanide are endogenous (27), this has prompted some to hypothesize that cyanide may act as a neuromodulator (28). Cyanide has also been shown to be produced by myeloperoxidase in activated neutrophils (3).

One might imagine that with cyanide-containing compounds present in the environment and at low levels in the body, intrinsic biochemical pathways for cyanide detoxification would have evolved. The most pharmacologically significant route of cyanide metabolism is excretion in the urine as thiocyanate (SCN$^-$) (3). Thiocyanate is markedly less toxic than cyanide, and its formation is essentially irreversible. Production of thiocyanate proceeds primarily by the transfer of sulfane sulfur—divalent sulfur attached to another sulfur—to cyanide by the enzyme rhodanese; however, other pathways exist for formation of thiocyanate. Deamination of cysteine, which is aided by the presence of $\alpha$-keto acids, leads to production of 3-mercaptopyruvate, a substrate for the enzyme 3-mercaptopyruvate sulfur transferase, which catalyzes the transfer of sulfur from 3-mercaptopyruvate to cyanide-forming thiocyanate and pyruvate. Other enzymes, such as vitamin B$_6$-dependent $\gamma$-cystathionase, contribute to the pool of sulfane sulfurs by cleaving cysteine-cysteine bonds (cystine) to form a cysteine persulfide and alanine or pyruvate and ammonium. These reactions occur mainly in the mitochondria of the liver and kidneys, although they can be found elsewhere. Many of these pathways now appear to also serve the purpose of mobilizing sulfur for construction of iron-sulfur cluster proteins.

Westley and coworkers (29), who contributed the most to the current understanding of sulfane sulfur metabolism, also noted the possible existence of a "thiosulfate reductase" among the other enzymes identified for mobilization of sulfane sulfur. They were not, however, able to isolate it. Recent studies in *E. coli* bacteria have revealed two enzymes involved in the formation of iron-sulfur proteins, IscS and IscU. IscS is a vitamin B$_6$-dependent cystiene desulfurase capable of sequestering inorganic sulfur and has been found, in the presence of reducing agents, to yield sulfide (S$^{2-}$), which is transferred to IscU (30). IscU is an iron-sulfur cluster scaffold protein. Both IscS and IscU homologs have been found in yeast and higher eukaryotes, including humans. The human IscU isoform has been sequenced and is known to be trafficked to the cytosol and to the mitochondria (31). Understanding these enzymes may give greater insight into pathways of sulfur metabolism and lead to new ideas about cyanide detoxification.

To review, the enzymes that appear to be responsible for cyanide's conversion to thiocyanate are primarily rhodanase and 3-mercaptopyruvate sulfur transferase, although albumin has been shown to have some detoxifying activity as well. The enzymatic routes of thiocyanate production are efficient, but they lack sufficient pools of substrate to deal with the amount of cyanide present in poisonings. They can be exploited by administration of sulfur donors, such as thiosulfate. They account for about 53% of cyanide metabolism *(32)*.

Another pathway of cyanide metabolism includes combination with cystine (the dithiol conjugation of two cystiene amino acids) to form 2-iminothiazolidine-4-carboxylic acid (2-ICA), which usually accounts for about 23% of cyanide metabolism. This assumes that the pH of the body is unchanged. However, if one is poisoned with cyanide, onset of lactic acidosis favors formation of 2-ICA rather than thiocyanate, as rhodanese activity falls off rapidly at low pH. 2-ICA has been found to have its own intrinsic neurotoxicity and is a convulsant *(33)*.

Other paths of cyanide metabolism include enzymatic and nonenzymatic production of cyanate ($CNO^-$), which accounts for 5–20% of detoxification, formation of cyanohydrin (approximately 2%), cyanide (1–2%), and other products.

In the average human, the combined metabolic routes detoxify approximately 0.017 mg of cyanide/kg body weight/min. Cyanide does not follow Haber's rule, which assumes that the effect of exposure to a toxin is cumulative over time and that the constant product of concentration and time ($C \times t$) will have a constant effect. With cyanide the $LCt_{50}$ (the vapor or aerosol exposure with respect to time that is lethal for 50% of the exposure population) for a short exposure to a high concentration is different from a long exposure to a low concentration. In other words, whereas exposure to 1000 mg m$^{-3}$ of cyanide for 1 min ($C \times t = 1000$ mg min m$^{-3}$) may be lethal for 50% of a given population, exposure to 67 mg m$^{-3}$ for 15 min ($C \times t = 1005$ mg min m$^{-3}$) will not be *(34)*. Although this property of cyanide pharmacology may challenge intuition, it is somewhat simpler to understand when viewed in conjunction with what has been covered regarding cyanide metabolism. A modification of Haber's rule to account for metabolic elimination of toxin, so that ($C - e$) $\times t$ determines the effect of cyanide, can resolve the discrepancy. Taking cyanide metabolism into account can explain the variation between the effects of long- and short-term cyanide exposure, and it is important to keep in mind when assessing symptoms. Furthermore, the dependence of cyanide mortality on metabolic processes of detoxification underscores the need to maintain the thiosulfate pool.

## 4. TOXICITY

Cyanides appear to be orders of magnitude less toxic compared with other lethal chemical warfare agents. In World War I, cyanide was delivered by a pulmonary route, with the $LCt_{50}$ 2500–5000 mg min m$^{-3}$. This is approximately the same as for phosgene but about 20 times that for nerve agents and 2–3 times that for sulfur mustard. However, because cyanide readily diffuses through epithelium and is also lethal if administered orally, rectally, ocularly, or vaginally or to intact or abraided skin and because comparatively large amounts are readily delivered to the target population, lethality from a cyanide event may be high.

Effects from cyanide toxicity are those of progressive histotoxic tissue hypoxia. They include vascular, visual, pulmonary, central nervous system (CNS), cardiac, autonomic, endocrine, and metabolic actions (Table 1). Usually the first effect observed is a transient respiratory gasp. This is generally believed to be owing to the effect of cyanide on chemoreceptor bodies in the aortic arch. Historically, this phenomena was used to mea-

Table 1
Systemic Effects of Cyanide Poisoning[a]

| System | Effect |
| --- | --- |
| Vascular | Initial transient increase, followed by a decrease in cardiac output; falling blood pressure owing to decrease in cardiac inotropic effect and vasodilation |
| Cardiac | Initial increase in heart rate followed by a decrease, both accompanied by arrhythmias and negative inotropy |
| Pulmonary | Respiratory gasp caused by stimulation of chemoreceptor bodies near aortic bifurcation followed by hyperventilation; over time, frequency of breath and breathing diminish |
| Visual | Decrease in capacity to focus, late-onset mydriasis secondary to hypoxia |
| Central nervous system (CNS) | Initially manifest as diminished awareness and increased release of enkephalins followed by loss of consciousness with progression to convulsions and/or late-appearing indications of CNS depression including fixed and dilated pupils or coma |
| Autonomic nervous system | Route- and dose-dependent; can include an increase in spleen contraction, emesis, defecation, urination, and salivation |
| Endocrine | Histamine and epinephrine release |
| Metabolic | Decrease in energy by inhibition of cytochrome oxidase, lactic acidosis, reduction in phosphocreatine, reduction in ATP |

[a]Many effects are dose- and route-dependent.
From Baskin SI, Brewer TG. Cyanide poisoning. In: Sidell FR, Takafuji ET, Franz DR, spc. eds. and Davis LB, Mathews Quick C, eds. Textbook on Military Medicine: Medical Aspects of Chemical and Biological Warfare. TMM Publications, Borden Institute, Walter Reed Army Medical Center, Washington, DC, 1997.

sure circulation time clinically. However, William Osler found the procedure had an unacceptable rate of morbidity, and it was discontinued.

Early signs and symptoms can include dyspnea, headache, and findings of CNS excitement, including anxiety, personality changes, and agitation progressing to seizures *(35)*. Diaphoresis, flushing, weakness, and vertigo may also be present. Because cyanide impairs tissue utilization of oxygen, an increase in oxyhemoglobin is observed rapidly. The "cherry red" skin color is caused by to the increased venous blood oxygenation. However, skin color changes are not always seen. The odor of bitter almonds has been used to identify cyanide, but because the odor is only detectable in 40–60% of cases, it cannot be considered reliable.

Late-appearing indications of CNS depression, such as coma and dilated, unresponsive pupils, are compatible with, but not specific for, cyanide poisoning *(35–37)*.

Nonlethal chronic exposure to cyanide has been shown to lead to neurological problems, and some neurodegenerative diseases have been linked to chronic low-dose administration, including parkinsonian symptoms *(38,39)*, tropical ataxic neuropathy, and the upper motor neuron disease "Konzo" *(40,41)*, as well as tobacco amblyopia, Leber's optic atrophy, and amyotrophic lateral sclerosis *(41)*.

Table 2
Cyanide Blood Concentrations and Associated Clinical Effects[a]

| Cyanide Concentration (μg/mL) | Signs & symptoms |
| --- | --- |
| 0.2-0.5 | None |
| 0.5–1.0 | Tachycardia, flushing |
| 1.0–2.5 | Obtunded |
| 2.5–3.0 | Coma |
| >3.0 | Death |

[a]Many effects are dose- and route-dependent.

From Baskin SI, Brewer TG. Cyanide poisoning. In: Sidell FR, Takafuji ET, Franz DR, spc. eds. and Davis LB, Mathews Quick C, eds. Textbook on Military Medicine: Medical Aspects of Chemical and Biological Warfare. TMM Publications, Borden Institute, Walter Reed Army Medical Center, Washington, DC, 1997.

## 5. LABORATORY FINDINGS

Laboratory observations include a decrease in the arteriovenous difference of the partial pressure of oxygen ($pO_2$) in the blood with progression to lactic acidosis. Timely measurement of blood and urine concentrations could provide useful guidelines. However, direct analysis of cyanide in body fluid can be difficult (42), particularly given the short half-life of cyanide. Time of sampling and methods of sample storage are important considerations. Cyanide concentrations in tissue in liver, heart, lung, or spleen may be more accurate indicators of exposure to cyanide (43). (For details on measuring cyanide concentrations in body fluids and tissues, see ref. 44.) Table 2 should provide a guideline for cyanide blood concentrations and associated effects.

## 6. PRINCIPLES OF THERAPY

Many different approaches to the treatment of cyanide intoxication have been explored, including the administration of drugs that directly bind cyanide and remove it from the bloodstream, those that induce changes in components of the bloodstream to cause them to bind cyanide directly such as methemoglobin-formers, and sulfur donors for the rhodanese reaction (45). Current methods for the treatment of cyanide intoxication generally call for administration of both methemoglobin-formers and sulfur donors, the result of which is theorized to be the combined removal of cyanide from the patient's system and reversal of cyanide binding to the metabolic enzyme cytochrome oxidase.

The therapeutic value of methemoglobin induction is that there is enough of a surplus of hemoglobin to generate relatively high methemoglobin levels without interfering significantly in oxygen transport (46). Traditional thinking regarding the use of methemoglobin-formers has followed from the fact that oxidized (met-) hemoglobin has a higher affinity for cyanide than does cytochrome oxidase (47) and that induction of methemoglobinemia can create an affinity gradient to pull cyanide off this critical enzyme. Although alternative therapeutic mechanisms have been suggested for administration of methemoglobin-formers—such as the possibility that met-myoglobin, which also has a higher affinity for cyanide than cytochrome oxidase and is more locally available in cells, may play a more direct role in cyanide detoxification than hemoglobin (48)—there remains a strong correlation between levels of induction of methemoglobin and recovery.

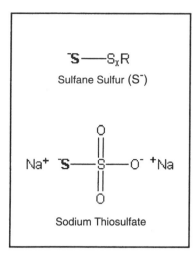

**Fig. 1.** Structure of sulfane sulfur (S⁻), where R is any conjugate attached to sulfur $S_x$, which is attached to the divalent sulfane sulfur. Sodium thiosulfate, a cyanide antidote, has structural sulfane sulfur.

Administration of thiosulfate provides substrate for the rhodanese cyanide detoxification reaction. As described previously, rhodanese catalyzes the transfer of sulfane sulfur (Fig. 1) to cyanide to form thiocyanate, which is excreted. Thiosulfate is an effective cyanide antagonist by itself *(49)*; however, it exhibits limited distribution to the brain, the organ most sensitive to cyanide *(50)*. Studies have shown, however, that cyanide increases the ability of thiosulfate to enter cardiac cells in isolated guinea pig hearts *(51)*.

Regardless of the specific method of cyanide antagonism, therapy for cyanide follows a few important principles. These are elimination of exposure, establishment of supportive therapy such as respiratory and cardiac support measures, and specific antidotal therapy. Each of these is addressed below to provide suitable instruction for physician reference, and individual advertisements and cautions are given to allow thoughtful supportive therapy.

### 6.1. Pediatric Considerations

There is little literature distinguishing the presentation and care of pediatric cyanide intoxications from adult cases. One might presume that, because of their smaller size and relatively higher metabolic rates and faster respiratory rates, children might be more likely to become severely intoxicated from a given exposure. Because the levels of activity of methemoglobin reductase, the enzyme that converts methemoglobin back to oxyhemoglobin, vary widely, and tend to be lower in children, and because children tend to be less tolerant of methemoglobinemia, there is greater concern for methemoglobin toxicity in pediatric patients. Therefore, antidotal dosage is calculated by body weight (discussed in Subheading 6.4., Antidotal Therapy, below). In the presence of anemia it may be prudent to give somewhat less antidote so that excessive methemoglobin is not generated. Nonanemic children weighing greater than 25 kg might receive the full adult dose of nitrite *(52)*. Methemoglobin levels bear monitoring in order that they not exceed safe levels, although the most important indicator of treatment effectiveness is clinical response.

## 6.2. Elimination of Exposure

The most basic, immediate treatment for cyanide intoxication is removal of the victim from any potential source of exposure. This includes isolation from the environment containing cyanide, removal of all contaminated clothing, rinsing the skin with soap and water, and lavage with activated charcoal for cyanide ingestion. Following these steps can significantly reduce the amount of cyanide to be detoxified in the body (53). Of course, cyanide intoxication progresses rapidly from initial onset to cardiac arrhythmias and convulsions, so the need to eliminate exposure must also be balanced by the need to administer treatment.

## 6.3. Supportive Therapy

Supportive therapies can positively affect patient outcome without risk from specific antidotes (54). The patient should be kept warm. For conscious patients, treatment should include supplemental oxygen, which by itself has not conclusively been shown to be an effective cyanide treatment but in connection with specific antidotes has been shown to potentiate the antidotal effect (55,56). Oxygen has also been shown to be effective prophylactically. Hyperbaric oxygen treatment, however, does not appear to be any more beneficial than oxygen at atmospheric pressure (57).

For unconscious, seizing, hypopneic, or hypotensive patients, more aggressive therapies should be considered. It is critical to maintain an open airway and ensure an adequate cardiac output. Cyanide casualties may require artificial resuscitation (58), antiarrhythmic drugs, and control of seizures through the use of benzodiazapine anticonvulsants (59). Treatment may also include control of lactic acidosis by intravenous administration of sodium bicarbonate.

Only those intoxications characterized by seizures, loss of consciousness, impaired respiration, hypotension, or severe metabolic acidosis require antidotal therapy, discussed in the next section. Some patients might require specific cardiovascular support, such as the use of vasopressors, until adequate blood pressure is restored.

## 6.4. Antidotal Therapy

In conjunction with symptomatic supportive therapies, administration of amyl nitrite and sodium nitrite, followed by administration of sodium thiosulfate, is the recommended treatment for cyanide intoxication. Antidotal therapy should be reserved for unconscious and severely intoxicated patients. Use of these compounds requires specific precautions and careful observation of the patient; when employed, they should provide a positive outcome.

### 6.4.1. NITRITES

Amyl nitrite and sodium nitrite, with or without sodium thiosulfate, are used as antidotes for cyanide (57). Nitrites are used inhalationally in the form of amyl nitrite ampules and intravenously in the form of sodium nitrite. Both accomplish the same purpose, which is to induce a relative methemoglobinemia. The nitrites work very rapidly, within seconds. Clinical response is typically seen in less than 5 min. Because nitrites tend to cause profound hypotension, therapy may need to be administered intermittently to allow for recovery of blood pressure. Resulting headaches can be managed with acetaminophen or nonsteroidal anti-inflammatories (NSAIDs). The rapid recovery expected with nitrites is noted in the cases given below.

The antidotal action of amyl nitrite was first noted as early as 1888 *(60)*. The easy availability of an inhalational antidote makes amyl nitrite appropriate for some casualties. However, marked vasodilation with orthostatic hypotension, dizziness, and headache, in addition to the unpredictable levels of methemoglobin formed *(61)*, limits its utility. Typically amyl nitrite inhalant, USP, is contained in a breakable glass ampule, wrapped in gauze. Amyl nitrite is usually used for the initial induction of methemoglobinemia. Simultaneous with the administration of oxygen, the broken amyl nitrite ampule should be held in front of the patient's mouth or placed within the mask or air-supply system for 15–30 s at 2- to 3-min intervals *(62)*.

Sodium nitrite, USP (30 mg/mL), should be given to an adult intravenously over 5–15 min, with careful monitoring of blood pressure. A single dose is sufficient to raise the methemoglobin level to 20% in an adult *(63)*, and a second dose, up to half as large as the initial one, can be given. Each sodium nitrite USP ampule contains 300 mg in 10 mL sterile water. Recommended dosage is 300 mg at the given rate, no more than 2 mL/min. The solution may be diluted in 50–100 mL intravenous fluid and infused slowly with careful monitoring of blood pressure *(64)*. The recommended dose for children is 0.33 mL of the 10% solution per kilogram of body weight *(52)*, or 0.2 mL/kg body weight for a 3% solution, not to exceed 10 mL, and adjusted for hemoglobin.

It is important to emphasize that treatment endpoints are primarily driven by patient response, not methemoglobin levels. Rapid reversal of histotoxic anoxia is desired, and so nitrites are given quite rapidly. The oft-cited goal of 25–30% methemoglobin is, however, more a ceiling than a floor. Above that range, oxygen-carrying deficits are caused by methemoglobin itself *(65)*. Case reports indicate that successful treatment with either amyl or sodium nitrite frequently results in much lower methemoglobin levels.

In cases of excessive methemoglobinemia, the blood will appear chocolate brown or otherwise atypical in color and will not redden with exposure to air *(66)*. Symptoms of excessive methemoglobinemia can include cyanosis, vomiting, shock, and coma. If excessive methemoglobinemia is induced, administer 1% methylene blue solution intravenously. A total dose of 1–2 mg/kg body weight should be administered over 5–10 min and should be repeated in 1 h if necessary to alleviate symptoms.

The provider should remember that oxygen saturation is not measured accurately by conventional pulse oximetry in the presence of methemoglobinemia *(66)*. In addition, methemoglobin measurements do not fully reflect levels of hemoglobin available for oxygen transport, as some proportion of the remaining hemoglobin is in the form of cyanomethemoglobin, nitrosohemoglobin, and other species that are not effective transporters of oxygen. Either oxyhemoglobin measurement or co-oximetry are possibly better tools to assess residual oxygen-carrying capacity *(67)*.

Methemoglobin-inducing substances should probably not be given to fire victims, even if cyanide intoxication is suspected, because neither methemoglobin nor carboxyhemoglobin (formed by carbon monoxide) transport oxygen. Alternative therapy in this situation consists of administering oxygen, thiosulfate, and other standard supportive measures.

### 6.4.2. THIOSULFATE

The second antidote is sodium thiosulfate. Its purpose is to provide a substrate sulfur donor for the rhodanase enzyme in order that the cyanide be biotransformed into the excretable form, thiocyanate. Sodium thiosulfate is essentially a nontoxic drug; however, nausea and vomiting have been associated with rapid intravenous administration to volunteers *(68)*. Thiosulfate is considered safe for use even in patients who might already have reduced oxygen-carrying capacity for other reasons such as fire/smoke inhalation and might therefore be intolerant of induced methemoglobinemia. In such persons, it is reasonable to consider using thiosulfate alone. Unfortunately, sodium thiosulfate acts more slowly than nitrites and should therefore be used in conjunction with nitrites in severely intoxicated persons whenever possible.

Sodium thiosulfate, USP, is supplied as a sterile, nonpyrogenic solution of sodium thiosulfate in water for injection. The standard dose of sodium thiosulfate, which is supplied in 50-mL ampules, is 50 mL of the 250 mg/mL (12.5 g), given intravenously over a 20-min period *(64)*. A second treatment with half of the initial dose may be given. The pediatric dose is 1.65 mL per kilogram of body weight, not to exceed 12.5 g *(52)*.

### 6.4.3. OTHER ANTIDOTAL COMPOUNDS

In other countries, most notably France, the primary cyanide antidote is hydroxo-cobalamin ($B_{12}$). The cobalt ion in this drug rapidly attracts the cyanide off the mitochondria, resulting in rapid reversal of histotoxic hypoxia and recovery of critical life-sustaining functions. It is used in conjunction with thiosulfate as described above and is considered quite safe, particularly in fire victims. Unfortunately, because hydroxocobalamin acts stochiometrically, binding in a 1:1 fashion with cyanide, and because the formulation available in the United States is not designed for this purpose, the volume required to achieve a therapeutic effect is prohibitive.

The chelating agent cobalt EDTA has also been used extensively for treating cyanide poisoning. However, because of its adverse cardiovascular side effects and because it is often poorly tolerated, this drug is better reserved as a second-line therapy in confirmed cyanide intoxications *(69)*.

Many case histories support the efficacy of early intervention using respiratory support combined with nitrite therapy and thiosulfates. Patients poisoned with multiple $LD_{50}$s of cyanide frequently recover if therapy is given in a timely manner. Even the most aggressive therapy may fail, however, if begun after obvious encephalopathy is present. Recovery is also more uncertain if cyanide intoxication is complicated by other intoxications such as ethanol *(70,71)*.

Regardless of the antidote selected, early evidence of benefit is reversal of hypotension, restoration of spontaneous respirations, and recovery from metabolic acidosis. Return to full consciousness and mental alertness may take longer and will depend on the degree of anoxic injury sustained. Patients will benefit from a period of observation of up to 48 h so that retreatment might be instituted should their clinical condition relapse.

### Case Vignettes

Case 1 *(71)*

A male industrial worker received an inhalational exposure to industrial hydrogen cyanide. His collapse was witnessed by another trained employee. He was noted to become unconscious approximately 30 seconds after exposure. He was evaluated, treated with an amyl nitrite ampule, and forced ventilation began within 3 minutes. When he reached the plant treatment center (at about 5 minutes) he was unconscious and without spontaneous ventilation. His blood pressure was 130/84 and his pulse 100. His emergency treatment consisted of forced oxygen and amyl nitrite until he rejected the amyl nitrite. This patient responded to therapy within 5 minutes. He was fully recovered at 6 hours except for a slight headache that responded to aspirin. He returned to work that same day. This is one of several similar cases treated at the same plant over many years. They demonstrate that prompt measures to offset tissue anoxia can reverse the effect of cyanide exposure. The inhalational cyanide response protocol in this plant did not include the routine use of sodium thiocyanate or even intravenous support, even for lethal exposures. Induction of methemoglobinemia with adjunctive use of oxygen and cardiopulmonary resuscitation (CPR) as necessary were usually all that was needed, presumably because a portion of cellular respiration was restored nearly immediately as cyanide transferred from the cytochrome oxidase to methemoglobin. It is likely that methemoglobin levels did not reach the recommended 25–30% using only amyl nitrite. In addition, once methemoglobin has bound cyanide, the circulating cyanomethemoglobin will not be detected; desired clinical effects are still achieved and actual oxygen-carrying capacity will still be reduced. The data suggest that relatively low measured levels of methemoglobin may be sufficient to reverse low-level intoxication (73). Indeed, patient status is the only measure of need for additional treatment. Neither measured cyanide levels nor measured methemoglobin levels substitute.

### Case 2

This gentleman, a colleague of Case 1, sustained an unwitnessed exposure to cyanide when he violated plant safety standards. He was found approximately 20 minutes after his inhalational and dermal exposure. When he was found, his pupils were dilated and fixed, and he was without heartbeat or respirations. He failed to respond to intravenous sodium nitrate, sodium thiosulfate, CPR, adrenalin, and forced oxygenation. He was pronounced dead after 1 hour. It is entirely possible that—had he been observed and received immediate antidotal therapy—he would have survived. Yen et al. (70) also discuss the futility of initiating treatment of persons who already display evidence of anoxic encephalopathy with signs such as deep coma or dilated and nonreactive pupils.

### Case 3 (73,74; compiled from two case reports)

A 31-year-old man who had been found comatose in bed with seizures was brought to the emergency department of a Japanese hospital. On admission, he was deeply comatose, with a blood pressure of 100/70 mmHg, heart rate of 54 beats/min, and respiratory rate of 15 breaths/min. His face was slightly flushed. Because his respiratory rate soon decreased to 6 breaths/min, he was intubated to receive controlled mechanical ventilation. The axillary temperature was 36°C. Analysis of arterial blood gas on admission showed severe metabolic acidosis: pH, 7.049; $PaCO_2$, 28 torr; $PaO_2$ 329 torr (normal); base excess, −20.7 mEq/L; and $H2CO_3-$, 7.8 mEq/L. Because drug intoxication was suspected, gastric lavage and activated charcoal with cathartics were administered. Thirty minutes after admission, emergency department staff were informed that the patient might have taken potassium cyanide, which was found in the bathroom. They immediately administered antidotes for cyanide poisoning. The patient revived in 30 minutes. Because sodium nitrite is not available in Japan, antidotes used were amyl nitrite ampules and sodium thiosulfate *(74)*. The severe metabolic acidosis improved rapidly, reaching a normal value 2 hours after treatment. His recovery chemistries were notable for elevated CPK MM, indicating destruction of skeletal muscle. He was discharged to psychiatry after apparently recovering fully. Approximately 4 months later, he was evaluated for stiffness and weakness of all four limbs along with a lack of clarity in speech. Symptom onset was approximately 1 month after his suicide attempt. Symptom severity was gradually progressive for about 2 months and then stabilized to its current level. On examination, the dominating feature was hemiplegic dystonia with bilateral involvement characterized by flexed upper limbs, extended lower limbs, and normal deep tendon reflexes. He required ambulatory support owing to his dystonic gait. Routine chemistries and testing for Wilson's disease were normal. CT and MRI showed bilateral putamen lesions. His condition improved with levodopa and carbidopa therapy but not with anticholinergics. This patient demonstrates cyanide's tendency to preferentially injure the basal ganglia *(76,77)*, resulting in delayed onset of extrapyramidal signs. Nonetheless, this is an uncommon consequence of severe cyanide intoxication, perhaps because few who sustain acute central nervous system anoxic injury survive to experience the delayed effects.

# REFERENCES

1. Magnum GH, Skipper HE. Hydrocyanic acid: the toxicity and speed of action on man. Edgewood Arsenal Memorandum Report (Project A 3.5-1), Aberdeen Proving Ground, MD, (T.D.M.R. 471), 1942.
2. Sykes AH. Early studies on the toxicology of cyanide. In: Vennesland B, Conn EE, Knowles CJ, Westley J, Wissing F, eds. Cyanide in Biology. Academic Press, New York, 1981, pp. 1–9.
3. Vinnesland B, Castric PA, Conn EE, Solomonson LP, Volini M, Westley J. Cyanide Metabolism. Fed Proc 1982;41:2639–2648.
4. Ballantyne B. Toxicology of cyanides. In: Ballantyne B, Marrs TC, eds. Clinical and Experimental Toxicology of Cyanides. Wright, Bristol, England, 1987, pp. 41–126.
5. Seigler DS. Cyanogenic glucosides and lipids. In: Vennesland B, Conn EE, Knowles CJ, Westley J, Wissing F, eds. Cyanide in Biology. Academic Press, New York, 1981, pp. 133–143.
6. Hall AH, Rumack BH, Schaffer MI, Linden CH. Clinical toxicology of cyanide: North American clinical experiences. In: Ballantyne B, Marrs TC, eds. Clinical and Experimental Toxicology of Cyanides. Wright, Bristol, England, 1987, pp. 313–314.
7. Bryson DB. Acute industrial cyanide intoxication and its treatment. In: Ballantyne B, Marrs TC, eds. Clinical and Experimental Toxicology of Cyanides. Wright, Bristol, England, 1987, pp. 348–358.
8. Anderson RA, Harland WA. Fire deaths in the Glasgow area, III: The role of hydrogen cyanide. Med Sci Law 1982;22:35–40.
9. Baud FJ, Barriot P, Toffis V, et al. Elevated blood cyanide concentrations in victims of smoke inhalation. N Engl J Med 1991;325:1761–1766.
10. Clark CJ, Campbell D, Reid WH. Blood carboxyhaemoglobin and cyanide levels in fire survivors. Lancet. 1981;i:1332–1335. Quoted in: Hall AH, Rumack BH, Schaffer MI, Linden CH. Clinical toxicology of cyanide: North American clinical experiences. In: Ballantyne B, Marrs TC, eds. Clinical and Experimental Toxicology of Cyanides. Wright, Bristol, England, 1987, pp. 321–333.

11. Sollman T. A Manual of Pharmacology and Its Applications to Therapeutics and Toxicology, 7th ed., WB Saunders, Philadelphia, 1948.
12. Jacobs MB. War Gases: Their Identification and Decontamination, Interscience Publishers, New York, 1942.
13. Prentiss AM. Chemicals in War: A Treatise on Chemical War. McGraw-Hill, New York, 1937, pp. 171–175.
14. Robinson JP. The problem of chemical and biological warfare, vol 1. In: Robinson JP, ed. The Rise of CB Weapons: A Study of the Historical, Technical, Military, Legal and Political Aspects of CBW, and Possible Disarmament Measures. Humanities Press, New York, 1971:155–156.
15. Baskin SI. Zyklon. In: La Cleur W, ed. Encyclopedia of the Holocaust. Yale University Press, New Haven, CT, 1998.
16. Lang JS, Mullin D, Fenyvesi C, Rosenberg R, Barnes J. Is the "protector of lions" losing his touch? US News & World Report. November, 1986;10:29.
17. Heylin M, ed. US decries apparent chemical arms attack. Chem Eng News 1988;66:23.
18. Wolnick KA, Fricke FL, Bonnin E, Gaston CM, Satzger RD. The Tylenol tampering incident—tracing the source. Anal Chem 1984;56:466A–470A, 474A.
19. Sidell FR. Chemical Casualty Consultant, Bel Air, MD. Personal communication, August, 1996.
20. Jaber H, Rufford N. MI5 foils poison gas attack on the tube. London Times, Nov. 17, 2002:1.
21. Warburg O. Inhibition of the action of prussic acid in living cells. Hoppe-Seylers Z Physiol Chem 1911;76:331–346.
22. Keilin D. Cytochrome and respiratory enzymes. Proc R Soc Lond B Biol Sci 1929;104:206–251.
23. Katsumata Y, Sato K, Yada S, Suzuki O, Yoshino M. Kinetic analysis of anaerobic metabolism in rats during acute cyanide poisoning. Life Sci 1983;33:151–155.
24. Solomonson LP. Cyanide as a metabolic inhibitor. In: Vennesland B, Conn EE, Knowles CJ, Westley J, Wissing F, eds. Cyanide in Biology. Academic Press, New York, 1981, pp. 11–28.
25. Sun PW, Rane SG, Gunasekar PG, Borowitz JL, Isom GE. Cyanide interaction with redox modulatory sites enhances NMDA receptor responses. J Biochem Mol Toxicol 1999;13:253-259.
26. Arden SR, Sinor JD, Potthoff WK, Aizenman E. Subunit-specific interactions of cyanide with the N-methyl-D-aspartate receptor. J Biol Chem 1998;273:21,505–21,511.
27. Lundquist P, Rosling H, Sorbo B. The origin of hydrogen CN in breath. Arch Toxicol 1988;61:270–274
28. Borowitz J, Gunasekar P, Isom G. Hydrogen cyanide generation by mu opiate receptor activation: possible neuromodulatory role of endogenous cyanide. Brain Res 1997;768:294–300.
29. Westley J. Cyanide and sulfane sulfur. In: Vennesland B, Conn EE, Knowles CJ, Westley J, Wissing F, eds. Cyanide in Biology. Academic Press, New York, 1981, pp. 61–76.
30. Urbina HD, Silberg JJ, Hoff KG, Vickery LE. Transfer of sulfur from IscS to IscU during Fe/S cluster assembly. J Biol Chem 2001;276:44,521–44,526.
31. Tong WH, Rouault T. Distinct iron-sulfur cluster assembly complexes exist in the cytosol and mitochondria of human cells. EMBO J 2000;19:5692–5700.
32. Wood JL, Cooley SL. Detoxication of cyanide by cystine. J Biol Chem 1956;218:449–457.
33. Bitner RS, Yim GW, Isom GE. 2-Iminothiazolidine-4-carboxylic acid produces hippocampal CA1 lesions independent of seizure excitation and glutamate receptor activation. Neurotoxicology 1997;18:191–200.
34. Marrs TC, Maynard RL, Sidell FR. Physiochemical and general toxicology of chemical warfare agents. In: Chemical Warfare Agents: Toxicology and Treatment. John Wiley & Sons, Chichester, England, 1996, pp. 27–81.
35. Hall AH, Rumack BH. Clinical toxicology of cyanide. Ann Emerg Med 1986;15:1067–1074.
36. Egekeze JO, Oehme FW. Cyanides and their toxicity: a literature review. Vet Q 1980;2:104–114.
37. Izraeli S, Israeli A, Danon Y. Pharmacological treatment of cyanide poisoning. Harefuah 1988;114: 338–342.
38. Kanthasamy AG, Borowitz JL, Pavlakovic G, Isom GE. Dopaminergic neurotoxicity of CN: neurochemical, histological, and behavioral characterization. Toxicol Appl Pharmacol 1994;126:156–163.
39. Uitti RJ, Rajput AH, Ashenhurst EM, Rozdilsky B. Cyanide-induced parkinsonism: a clinicopathologic report. Neurology 1985;35:921–925.
40. Isom GE, Gunasekar PG, Borowitz JL. Cyanide and neurodegenerative disease. In: Bondy S, ed. Chemical and Neurodegenerative Disease Prominent Press, Scottsdale, AZ, 1999, p. 101–129.
41. Baskin SI, Rockwood GA. Neurotoxicological effects of cyanide and its potential therapies. Mil Psychol 2002;14:159–177.

42. Groff WA Sr, Stemler FW, Kaminskis A, Froehlich HL, Johnson RP. Plasma free cyanide and blood total cyanide: a rapid completely automated microdistillation assay. Clin Toxicol 1985;23:133–163.

43. Sunshine I, Finkle B. The necessity for tissue studies in fatal cyanide poisoning. Int Arch Gewerbepathol Gewerbehyg 1964;20:558–561.

44. Department of the US Army. Assay Techniques for Detection of Exposure to Sulfur Mustard, Cholinesterase Inhibitors, Sarin, Soman, GF, and Cyanide. Technical Bulletin Medical 296. Headquarters, DA, Washington, DC, 22 May, 1996..

45. Way JL, Leung P, Cannon E, et al. The mechanism of cyanide intoxication and its antagonism. In: Cyanide Compounds in Biology. John Wiley & Sons, New York, 1988, pp. 232–243.

46. Babior BM, Stossel TP. Hemoglobin and oxygen transport: disorders of oxygen binding. In: Babior BM, Stossel TP. Hematology: A Pathophysiological Approach, 3rd ed. Churchill Livingstone, New York, 1994, pp. 27–42.

47. Viana C, Cagnoli H, Cendan J. L'action du nitrite de sodium dans l'intoxication par les cyanures. Soc Biol Montevideo 1933;9:1649–1651.

48. Steinhaus RK, Baskin, SI, Clark JH, Kirby SD. Formation of methemoglobin and metmyoglobin using 8-aminoquinoline derivatives or sodium nitrite and subsequent reaction with cyanide. J Appl Toxicol 1990;10:345–351.

49. Gallo D. Antidotal actions of sodium thiosulfate in hydrocyanic acid poisoning. CR Soc Biol 1932;111:84–87.

50. Isom GE, Way JL. Lethality of cyanide in the absence of inhibition of liver cytochrome oxidase. Biochem Pharmacol 1976;25:605–608.

51. Baskin SI, Froehlich HL, Groff WA. The disassociation of reversal of cyanide (CN) toxicity and methemoglobin (MH) formation by nitrite (N) on the isolated heart. Fed Proc 1986;45:196.

52. Berlin CM. The treatment of cyanide poisoning in children. Pediatrics 1970;6:793–796.

53. Lambert RJ, Kindler BL, Schaeffer DJ. The efficacy of superactivated charcoal in treating rats exposed to a lethal oral dose of potassium cyanide. Ann Emerg Med 1988;17:595–598.

54. Graham DL, Laman D, Theodore J, Robin ED. Acute cyanide poisoning complicated by lactic acidosis and pulmonary edema. Arch Intern Med 1977;137:1051–1055.

55. Takano T, Miyazaki Y, Nashimoto I. Effect of hyperbaric oxygen on cyanide intoxication: in situ changes in intracellular oxidation reduction. Undersea Biomed Res 1980;7:191–197.

56. Way JL, Gibbon SL, Sheehy M. Effect of oxygen on cyanide intoxication: 1. Prophylactic protection. J Pharmacol Exp Ther 1966;153:381–385.

57. Way JL, Sylvester D, Morgan RL, et al. Recent perspectives on the toxicodynamic basis of cyanide antagonism. Fundam Appl Toxicol 1984;4:S231–S239.

58. Blake J. Observations and experiments on the mode in which various poisonous agents act on the animal body. Edinb Med Surg 1840;53:35–49.

59. Brivet F, Delfraissy JF, Bertrand P, Dormont J. Acute cyanide poisoning: recovery with non-specific supportive therapy. Intensive Care Med 1983;9:33–35.

60. Pedigo LG. Antagonism between amyl nitrite and prussic acid. Trans Med Soc Virginia 1888;19:124–131.

61. Way JL. Cyanide intoxication and its mechanism of antagonism. Annu Rev Pharmacol Toxicol 1984;24:451–481.

62. Eli Lilly and Company. Cyanide antidote package: instructions for the treatment of cyanide poisoning. Indianapolis, IN, 46285, 1987.

63. Chen KK, Rose CL. Nitrite and thiosulfate therapy in cyanide poisoning. JAMA 1952;149:113–119.

64. Baskin SI, Horowitz AM, Neally EW. The antidotal action of sodium nitrite and sodium thiosulfate against cyanide poisoning. J Clin Pharmacol 1992;32:368–375.

65. Bunn HF. Disorders of hemoglobin. In: Braunwald E, Wilson JD, Martin JB, Fauci AS. Harrison's Principles of Internal Medicine, 11th ed. McGraw-Hill, New York, 1987, pp. 1518–1527.

66. CDC. Methemoglobin formation following unintentional ingestion of sodium nitrite—New York, 2002. MMWR 2002;51;639–642.

67. Wright RO, Lewander, WJ, Woolf, AD. Methemoglobinemia: etiology, pharmacology, and clinical management. Ann Emerg Med 1999;34:646–656.

68. Ikankovich AD, Braverman B, Stephens TS, Shulman M, Heyman HJ. Sodium thiosulfate disposition in humans: relation to sodium nitroprusside toxicity. Anesthesiology 1983;58:11–17.

69. Dicobalt edetate. In: Reynolds JEF, Parfitt K, Parsons AV, Sweetman SC, eds. Martindale: The Extra Pharmacopoeia, 29th ed. Pharmaceutical Press, London, 1989, p. 839.

70. Yen D, Tsai J, Wang LM, et al. The clinical experience of acute cyanide poisoning. Am J Emerg Med 1995;13:524–528.
71. Wurzburg H. Treatment of cyanide poisoning in an industrial setting. Vet Hum Toxicol 1996; 38:44–47.
72. Borron SW, Baud FJ. Acute cyanide poisoning: clinical spectrum, diagnosis, and treatment. Arh Hig Rada Toksikol 1996;47:307–322.
73. Nakatani T, Kosugi Y, Mori A, Tajimi K, Kobayashi K. Changes in the parameters of oxygen metabolism in a clinical course recovering from potassium cyanide. Am J Emerg Med 1993;11:213–217.
74. Borgohain R. Delayed onset generalized dystonia after cyanide poisoning. Clin Neurol Neurosurg 1995;97:213–215.
75. Kasamo K, Okuhata Y, Satoh R, et al. Chronological changes of MRI findings on striatal damage after acute cyanide intoxication: pathogenesis of the damage and its selectivity, and prevention for neurological sequelae: a case report. Eur Arch Psychiatry Clin Neurosci 1993;243:71–74.
76. Patel MN, Yim G, Isom G. N-methyl-D-aspartate receptors mediate cyanide-induced cytotoxicity in hippocampal cultures. Neurotoxicology 1993;14:35–40.

# 20    Vesicants

## Edward Lucci, MD, FACP

The opinions or assertions contained herein are the private views of the author and are not to be construed as official or as representing the position of the Department of the Army or the Department of Defense.

### CONTENTS

---

### Case Vignette

Three patients presented to the Emergency Department with similar complaints of smoke inhalation after being exposed to a gray-blue cloud of smoke and mist generated by an explosion in the Washington Metro subway system. One patient noted droplets of liquid on her skin and reported a distinct pungent smell of garlic. Shortly after the smoke exposure, all three patients began experiencing a burning sensation in their eyes and throat, as well as difficulty breathing. Over the next 4 hours all three patients reported a similar progression of symptoms, noting a worsening burning in the throat, severe eye pain, and photophobia. On exam, each patient had evidence of diffuse conjunctivitis. In addition, all three patients reported the onset of skin erythema and itching in the regions of skin exposed to the smoke and mist, particularly on the face and neck. The areas of skin erythema gradually developed painful burning sensation and small vesicles.

The charge nurse informs you that other patients are arriving in the Emergency Room triage area with similar complaints including painful skin blisters.

## 1. SULFUR MUSTARD

### 1.1. Background

Concern over the recurrence of the threat of sulfur mustard continues to grow. Sulfur mustard, often referred to as "mustard" or "mustard gas" has created more battlefield

From: *Physician's Guide to Terrorist Attack*
Edited by: M. J. Roy © Humana Press Inc., Totowa, NJ

casualties than all other chemical agents combined since it was first introduced on the battlefield at Ypres, Belgium in 1917. There have been at least 12 reported uses since that time, most recently in the Middle East in the 1980s, when it was used against both military and civilian populations *(1)*. Today, at least a dozen countries have sulfur mustard in their arsenals *(2)*.

Sulfur mustard [NATO designations: H, HD, HT; chemical name: bis (2-chloroethyl) sulfide] is generally regarded as one of the two most important chemical agents in existence, the other being nerve agent. Under comparable conditions of exposure, however, sulfur mustard is much less potent than nerve agent. It has been referred to as the king of battlefield war gases and the "weapon of choice" in modern tactical warfare *(3)*. The term "mustard gas" is a misnomer because the chemical is a liquid at normal environmental temperatures. U.S. stockpiles consist of H (Levinstein mustard: 70% sulfur mustard and 30% sulfur impurities), HD (distilled purified sulfur mustard), and HT (a mixture of HD and agent T) *(4)*. Agent T is added to HD to improve its stability, primarily by lowering its freezing point *(2,4,5)*. The toxicities of HT and L are not as well characterized as sulfur mustard, but it is clear that both agents possess similar vesicant properties *(4)*. Nitrogen mustard has never been used on the battlefield and is not felt to be an important military threat agent *(2)*.

Potential sources of exposure to chemical agents for civilian populations include acts of terrorism, industrial accidents, inadvertent release from chemical weapons stockpiles, and military attack *(6)*. Most of the U.S. military stockpile is stored at eight separate locations in the continental United States. Destruction by high-temperature incineration is being carried out on Johnston Island in the South Pacific with a scheduled completion date of 2004 *(4,5)*.

As a result of the dual-use nature of chemical weapons technology, any country (regardless of size or industrial capacity) capable of producing petrochemicals, pesticides, or detergents has the potential to produce a variety of chemical warfare agents, with sulfur mustard being the most feasible *(2,7)*. In a recent report to Congress, the Central Intelligence Agency revealed that there is considerable activity in manufacturing and stockpiling chemical weapons, including vesicants (blister agents), in Iran, Iraq, Sudan, Syria, Libya, and North Korea, and many of these countries continue to seek dual-use materials, equipment, and expertise from abroad *(8)*. Iraq has rebuilt key portions of its chemical production infrastructure since the Gulf War *(8)*. Additionally, China and Russia have substantial weapons of mass destruction programs and, in many cases, have failed to enforce export controls on these items.

Iranian casualties from sulfur mustard during the Iran-Iraq war included many women and children living near the war front *(9)*. Iraq attacked its own Kurdish population with mustard during the 1980s *(2,4)*. In 1988, Osama Bin Laden stated that he considered acquiring weapons of mass destruction a religious duty. A Bin Laden associate on trial in Egypt in 1999 claimed his group had chemical weapons, raising the specter of mustard use in a terrorist scenario *(8)*. As yet, there have been no terrorist events using sulfur mustard; however, a number of non-battlefield exposures to sulfur mustard have occurred, including those among Danish fisherman, school children, an American souvenir collector, and workers in a munitions stockpile *(7,10–14)*.

The most recent U.S. military experience with significant mustard casualties occurred in 1943 during World War II when a U.S. warship in the Italian harbor of Bari, Italy was sunk. The ship released mustard liquid and vapor into the oil slick that resulted from the destruction of 16 ships and thousands of tons of high explosives in the harbor. There were 617 U.S. casualties from mustard exposure, with 83 deaths, along with an unknown number of Italian civilian casualties. It was an alert medical officer with previous chemical warfare training who first recognized that these casualties were dying from sulfur mustard poisoning, and not immersion shock or blast injury, when they demonstrated unusual skin blistering *(2,15)*.

## 1.2. Properties of Sulfur Mustard

Sulfur mustard is a stable, oily liquid with a distinct mustard or garlic odor (detectable at 1–2 mg/m$^3$). It is barely soluble in water, but dissolves well in various other materials including oils and organic solvents, such as petroleum distillates and alcohols. It is easily absorbed by paint and readily permeates rubber, which will remain contaminated for long periods *(4,7)*.

Mustard's toxicity is greatly dependent on environmental conditions. It is of low volatility, with little vapor produced in cool weather, but at high temperatures, it becomes a significant vapor hazard. The vapor of sulfur mustard is 5.4 times heavier than air, and its vapor clouds will hug the ground and sink into trenches; thus standing may provide a degree of protection as the concentration of agent nearer to the ground may be significantly higher. Mustard's freezing point is 57°F. It is often mixed with other agents in colder climates to lower its freezing point *(2,16)*.

Sulfur mustard is considered a persistent chemical agent because it will remain present in the environment for more than 24 hours when dispersed. It has enough volatility at ordinary temperatures to produce mustard vapor hazard in the air immediately surrounding liquid mustard droplets. Droplets released from an explosion could deposit on numerous surfaces and slowly evaporate, thus posing a risk from dermal contact and vapor inhalation. During the Iran-Iraq war, air samples from bomb craters detected mustard vapor concentrations for as long as 14 days after dispersion *(4)*.

## 1.3. Sulfur Mustard Toxicity

Although more toxic chemical warfare agents exist, sulfur mustard has retained its military usefulness because of its unique characteristics: it is inexpensive, persistent, easily manufactured, highly toxic, and difficult to protect against and to treat *(7)*.

Sulfur mustard is a highly reactive simple sulfur compound and a strong alkylating agent that readily reacts with cellular components of DNA, RNA, and proteins *(7)*. It is considered poisonous to cells and is particularly toxic to mitotic cells *(4)*. Multiple hypotheses for the basis of its biochemical mechanism of action have been proposed. The special properties that give sulfur mustard its tremendous chemical reactivity include the presence of a sulfur atom with an unsaturated valence and the chloroethyl side chains, which when ionized acquire the capacity to insert into other molecules or form addition compounds *(7,17)*. The basis for its skin toxicity is its ability to form a highly reactive moiety that readily interacts with biological molecules in tissue, including enzymes, proteins, glutathione, and DNA. Alkylation of DNA by sulfur mustard results in intrastrand crosslinks, strand breaks, and inhibition of DNA synthesis. This triggers the activation of a repair enzyme cascade that may explain the cleavage of the basal epidermal cell layer to the basement membrane and the resulting blister formation *(2,18)*. Within minutes in the "biological milieu" *(16)*, the reactive sulfur mustard molecule attaches to another molecule and is no longer reactive *(2)*. The clinical relevance of this reactivity and quick transformation is that within minutes of exposure sulfur mustard has started to cause tissue damage. It is no longer present as intact mustard in either tissue or blister fluid; however, clothing, hair, and skin surfaces can remain contaminated for hours *(2)*.

The exact biochemical mechanism of action of sulfur mustard is still uncertain. No one theory alone explains all the phenomena seen after sulfur mustard exposure *(2,16,18,19)*.

## *1.4. Clinical Manifestations of Mustard Toxicity*

Sulfur mustard exposure does not cause any immediately noticeable effects. There is an asymptomatic latency period. As a result, victims generally experience multiple sites of injury. The primary impediment to successful early management of mustard casualties continues to be the latency of onset of effects after exposure. During the latency period before the casualty or health care worker is aware of exposure, there continues to be the risk of spreading the agent until effective decontamination is accomplished. Early removal of the protective mask in a contaminated environment has caused many mustard injuries.

Factors that shorten the duration of the latency period include increased temperature and humidity, intensity and site of exposure, and variation in individual susceptibility. Latency periods have ranged from 1 hour to over 24 hours *(19)*. Tissues that come into direct contact with either vapor or liquid droplets are at risk, i.e., exposed skin surfaces, eyes, nose, throat, trachea, bronchial airways, and the upper gastrointestinal tract. The moist surfaces of perspiring skin, conjunctiva of the eye, airway mucosa, and mucous membranes preferentially absorb sulfur mustard. The most vulnerable areas are moist body parts in general *(9)*.

The main target organs in sulfur mustard exposures remain the skin, the eyes, and the respiratory tract, the organs with which it is most likely to come in direct contact. Systemic toxic effects occur, tend to be dose dependent, and affect primarily tissues with a rapid cell turnover rate, such as lymphoid cells, bone marrow, and gastrointestinal mucosa (Table 1).

### 1.4.1. SKIN INJURY

Skin lesions are common with mustard exposure (Table 2). In an Iranian study of 535 mustard casualties, more than 90% had skin lesions. Approximately 20% of sulfur mustard that contacts the skin is absorbed *(2,7,20)*. The remainder disappears rapidly in the circulation or evaporates *(7)*. Exposure leads to dose-related skin injury, ranging from erythema (resembling sunburn) and edema to vesication and necrosis *(2,7,9)*.

Liquid droplets produce deeper and more severe blistering than vapor exposure on the skin. Vapor skin injury usually results in a first- or second-degree burn, whereas liquid mustard may produce third-degree burns *(2)*. Thinner skin areas are also more easily affected, and moisture on the skin promotes absorption. For liquid mustard, a 10-μg droplet will produce vesication. A lethal dose of liquid sulfur mustard is a relatively small amount, roughly the equivalent of 1 teaspoon (7.0 g) *(2)*. Vapor exposure is measured as a product of the concentration and time of exposure: $Ct = mg \times min/m^3$ *(2)*. The threshold for skin damage from vapor exposure is dependent on multiple factors including skin site, sweating, and temperature and is approximately $200 mg \times min/m^3$ *(2)*. Higher temperatures and increased moisture potentiate mustard effects *(18)*. Large individual differences in sensitivity to sulfur mustard exist.

Table 1
Clinical Effects of Mustard Exposure

| Organ | Severity | Effects | Onset of first effect (h) |
|---|---|---|---|
| Eyes | Mild | Tearing | 4–12 |
| | Moderate | Above effect, plus reddening, lid edema, moderate pain | 3–6 |
| | Severe | Marked lid edema | 1–2 |
| | | Possible corneal damage | |
| | | Severe pain | |
| Airways | Mild | Rhinorrhea | 6–24 |
| | | Sneezing | |
| | | Epistaxis | |
| | | Hoarseness | |
| | | Hacking cough | |
| | Severe | Above effects, plus productive cough, mild to severe dyspnea | 2–6 |
| Skin | Mild | Erythema | 2–24 |
| | Severe | Vesication | |

Reprinted from Sidell FR, Urbanetti JS, Smith WJ, et al. Vesicants. In: Zajtchuk R, Bellamy RF, Jenkins DP, eds. Textbook of Military Medicine, Part I: Medical Aspects of Chemical and Biological Warfare. Borden Institute, Washington DC, 1997, pp. 197–228.

Table 2
Typical Development of Mustard Skin Lesion

| Effect | Time after vapor exposure (h) |
|---|---|
| Earliest appearance of erythema | 1 |
| Definite erythema | 2–3 |
| Raised erythema (edema) | 8–12 |
| Pinhead vesication | 13–22 |
| Vesicles coalescing into blisters or necrosis | 16–48 |
| Maximum blisters or necrosis | 42–72 |
| Complete skin surface denudation | 6–9 d |
| Removal of scab | 20–28 d |
| Complete healing | 22–29 d |

Reprinted from Smith WJ, Dunn MA. Medical defense against blistering chemical warfare agents. Arch Dermatol 1991;127:1207–1213. Copyrighted 1991 American Medical Association.

Vesication (blisters) develops after a variable period of erythema and itching. The typical blister is superficial, thin-walled, filled with translucent yellowish fluid, and surrounded by erythema (Fig. 1) (2,18,21). Blister formation is a complicated pathological phenomenon, and the progression of histological changes has been well documented

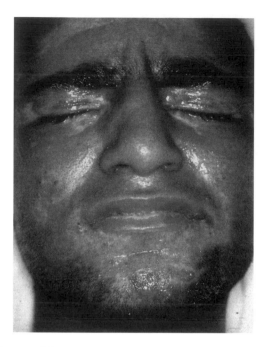

**Fig. 1.** Mild facial erythema with some mucosal involvement in a mustard casualty. (Reprinted from Bennion SD, David-Bajar K. Cutaneous reactions to nuclear, biological, and chemical warfare. In: Zajtchuk R, Bellamy RF, Jenkins DP, eds. Textbook of Military Medicine, Part III: Military Dermatology. Office of the Surgeon General, Department of the Army, Falls Church, VA, 1994, pp. 96–97.)

*(22).* Research efforts have focused on alkylation of DNA as a key intracellular event leading to blister formation *(19).* Once fixed in the skin (in 2–4 min), mustard cannot be extracted, and its effects become irreversible. The key cellular target of the skin is the basal epidermal cell, which when damaged attenuates the healing process. Basal cells of the epidermis are rapidly killed by mustard *(4).* Although fixation of mustard to the tissues occurs in minutes, histological changes within the dermis require 30–60 min to become evident and are not completely manifested until 2–3 d after exposure *(9,21).* Over the course of 12–16 h, separation occurs at the dermal-epidermal junction, promoting blister formation *(19,21).* Clinically, mustard blisters appear similar to other thermal or chemical burns *(21).* Blister fluid is nontoxic *(2,19,21).* The base of the neck, the axillae, and inguinal areas are often intensely involved (Figs. 2 and 3) *(9).* Large areas of darkened skin, exfoliation, and occasionally deep ulceration may occur without passing through a blistering stage *(9,19,21,23).*

Skin healing occurs through re-epithelialization that ranges from weeks to months depending on the size and thickness of the area involved. Delay in healing and propensity to infection result from the systemic absorption and radiomimetic effects of mustard *(21).* Healing time depends on the severity of the lesion and may be complicated by scar formation and irregular pigmentation *(19,23,24).* Lack of an adequate animal model for sulfur mustard skin lesions hampered scientific efforts for years. However, the euthymic hairless guinea pig has been recognized most recently as demonstrating skin changes in mustard exposure similar to those in humans *(18,19,21).*

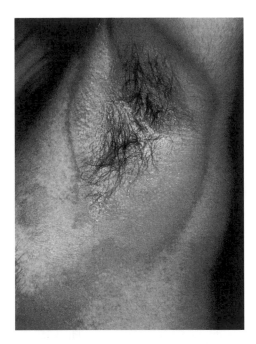

**Fig. 2.** Axillary accentuation of skin blistering and erosion in an Iraqi vesicant casualty. (Reprinted from Bennion SD, David-Bajar K. Cutaneous reactions to nuclear, biological, and chemical warfare. In: Zajtchuk R, Bellamy RF, Jenkins DP, eds. Textbook of Military Medicine, Part III: Military Dermatology. Office of the Surgeon General, Department of the Army, Falls Church, VA, 1994, pp. 96–97.)

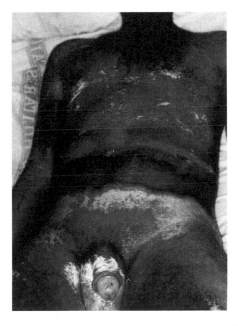

**Fig. 3.** Diffuse superficial ulcerations in a mustard casualty. Note prominent inguinal involvement and characteristic hyperpigmentation around the waist and neck regions.
(Reprinted from Bennion SD, David-Bajar K. Cutaneous reactions to nuclear, biological, and chemical warfare. In: Zajtchuk R, Bellamy RF, Jenkins DP, eds. Textbook of Military Medicine, Part III: Military Dermatology. Office of the Surgeon General, Department of the Army, Falls Church, VA, 1994, pp. 96–97.)

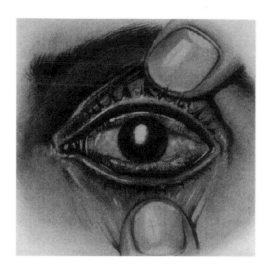

**Fig. 4.** This drawing depicts acute conjunctivitis after exposure to mustard vapor. The conjunctivae of the upper and lower lids are red and edematous. The cornea is grey and hazy, has lost its luster, and is shown as artificially dilated by atropine ointment in this drawing. (Reprinted from Joy RJT. Historical Aspect of Medical Defense Against Chemical Warfare. Reprinted, with permission, from Sidell FR, Urbanetti JS, Smith WJ, et al. Vesicants. In: Sidell FR, Takafuji ET, Franz DR, eds. Textbook of Military Medicine: Medical Aspects of Chemical and Biologic Warfare. Borden Institute, Washington, DC, 1997, p. 99.)

Blisters appearing simultaneously in large numbers of patients should alert medical personnel to search involved areas with chemical detection devices, in the absence of a known chemical attack. There is likely to be an observed effect within 1 h only when gross contact with liquid mustard occurs *(4)*.

### 1.4.2. Eye Injury

The unprotected eye is the organ most sensitive to mustard injury. Mustard penetrates the cornea more rapidly than the skin owing to the absence of a stratum corneum in the ocular epithelium; thus eye exposure is associated with a significantly shorter latency period *(16,18,19)*. Symptoms of irritation and tearing occur at concentrations of vapor 1/10th lower than that which affects the skin or airway *(19)*. Concentrations of mustard barely perceptible by odor can produce eye injury while not affecting the skin or respiratory tract *(4)*. Initially eye irritation (watering, reddening, pain, swelling of the eyelids, foreign body sensation, prolonged photophobia) occurs within 2–3 h of vapor exposure (Fig. 4) *(4)*. Within 24 h eyes may be swollen shut. The spectrum of damage to the eye is characterized by progressively worsening conjunctivitis, blepharospasm, pain, edema of the lids and conjunctivae, orange-peel roughening of the cornea, and more severe corneal injuries including dense corneal opacification and deep ulceration *(2,25)*.

Eye injuries were the most prevalent mustard casualty complaint in World War I data, 75% of which were characterized as a mild conjunctivitis and resulted in complete recovery in 1–2 wk *(2)*. Generally, the most severe eye damage is caused by liquid exposure, either through airborne droplets or self-contamination, and symptoms may become apparent within minutes of exposure *(2,25)*.

### 1.4.3. AIRWAY INJURY

Sulfur mustard vapor damages the mucosa of the upper airways in a dose-dependent fashion. Mustard has little effect on lung parenchyma *(2,5,19,26)*. Initially, catarrhal symptoms may be present: sore throat, dry cough, and pharyngeal erythema, along with a sense of chest discomfort *(27)*. Hoarseness may progress to aphonia. Symptom onset usually occurs within 4–6 h of exposure. Higher concentrations of vapor exposure result in earlier onset and more severe symptoms. In addition, any significant vapor exposure to the airway is usually associated with eye symptoms including redness, photophobia, lacrimation, and blepharospasm *(2,27)*.

Respiratory tract injuries caused by inhalation of mustard vapor affect primarily the laryngeal and tracheobronchial mucosa, with little effect on the lung parenchyma. Severe respiratory exposure will result in epithelial sloughing, significant inflammatory debris deposition, and pseudomembrane formation *(2,9)*. Pseudomembranes can peel off, requiring bronchoscopy and emergency airway management to prevent death from airway obstruction *(2)*.

Initially after vapor exposure, a nonbacterial chemical pneumonitis develops that can progress to bacterial superinfection within 4–6 d. Close assessment of sputum culture and Gram stain for evidence of bacterial infection is recommended; however, prophylactic antibiotic use is discouraged. Antibiotic therapy should be withheld until specific organisms are identified *(2)*. Deaths are usually a result of complications of bronchopneumonia and sepsis *(2)*. Pulmonary edema is not a typical feature of sulfur mustard vapor exposure *(2)*. Chronic respiratory problems may develop, but most respiratory injuries resolve within 4–6 wk *(2,18,19)*.

### 1.4.4. GASTROINTESTINAL INJURY

Nausea and vomiting are common early after sulfur mustard exposure, because of either the mild cholinergic activity *(2)* of sulfur mustard or its noxious odor, or a combination of factors. Heavy vapor exposure in the Iran-Iraq war was frequently associated with nausea and vomiting *(9,21)*. Nausea and vomiting occurring days after exposure may be a result of the radiomimetic effect of sulfur mustard and damage to the gastrointestinal mucosa. Diarrhea is very uncommon from sulfur mustard exposure *(2)*.

### 1.4.5. CNS INJURY

Mild nonspecific central nervous system (CNS) complaints such as dizziness and lethargy were common among Iranian casualties treated in European hospitals after the Iran-Iraq war *(9)*. Severe CNS effects have been described in large mustard exposures, manifested by coma, agitation, and abnormal muscular activity *(2)*.

### 1.4.6. HEMATOPOIETIC INJURY

Significant mustard absorption can result in myelosuppression within 7–10 d of exposure. Resulting leukopenia and thrombocytopenia may lead to increased risk of infection and bleeding disorders and must be monitored closely. Hematological disorders were the most serious complications among a large study of Iranian patients *(9)*. In patients with leukopenia, skin lesions became infected, most often with *Staphylococcus, Streptococcus*, or *Pseudomonas (9)*. Granulocyte colony-stimulating factor (G-CSF) can be used for treatment of mustard-induced neutropenia *(16,28)*.

## 1.5. Laboratory Analysis

There is no specific laboratory test for sulfur mustard. The necessary early medical and public health decisions required in a potential incident will be based on scene assessment and clinical judgement. Early recognition of a pattern of clinical signs and symptoms consistent with sulfur mustard exposure will be critical in guiding emergency medical care. The ability of hazardous material teams on average to detect sulfur mustard will be limited and will more likely require the resources of an analytical laboratory. The Chemical Agent Monitor (CAM) and Improved Chemical Agent Monitor (ICAM) both detect sulfur mustard vapor reliably *(29)*. This equipment may be available through military, city emergency medical services, or law enforcement operations, any of whom might be tasked with agent identification in a terrorist event. Additionally, both M-8 and M-9 chemical agent detection papers readily detect vesicants, and both are a routine part of any U.S. military agent detection system *(30)*. The U.S. military is scheduled to deploy a new chemical detection system, the Joint Chemical Agent Detector (JCAD), which will provide simultaneous detection for all major military chemical threat agents *(31)*.

Thiodiglycol, a relatively nontoxic, stable urinary metabolite of sulfur mustard with a half-life of 1.18 d, may be detectable in the urine of patients after sulfur mustard exposure *(7,19)*. Increased urinary excretion of thiodiglycol was reported in Iranian casualties cared for in Europe *(9,23)*. Detection of urinary thiodiglycol would not be a routine laboratory test available in most hospital laboratories, but it is available to military field units at the Theater Medical Lab level *(32)*.

Leukopenia, signaling severe immune system dysfunction, suggests systemic mustard exposure. Usually leukopenia begins on d 3–5 and reaches a nadir in 6–9 d *(2,9,17,19,21)*. An absolute neutrophil count below 200 cells/m$^3$ signifies a poor prognosis, as does a rapid drop in white blood cell count *(9)*. Suppression of leukocyte production is common in severe mustard exposure. In one study of 65 severe Iranian casualties treated in Europe, 29 had some degree of leukopenia *(26)*.

## 1.6. Decontamination

The first priority in treatment is to remove victims from the contaminated place and begin decontamination. Decontamination as early as possible is best and may in fact not be required in vapor exposure alone. Internal exposures (inhalation or ingestion) do not lend themselves to decontamination.

Persistent agents like mustard pose the greatest risk to rescue and medical personnel as a result of secondary exposure from handling contaminated patients or clothing. Liquid sulfur mustard may persist on skin, clothing, and equipment for many hours. For this reason, rescue personnel must clearly demarcate the contaminated zone, establish protected entry and exit points, and implement appropriate decontamination procedures *(6)*. To handle contaminated patients safely, special protective clothing must be worn. Sulfur mustard will rapidly penetrate most textiles, such as street clothing, as well as standard military fatigue uniforms, rubber, and heavy leather *(4,14)*. Specialized military protective garments contain a charcoal layer that absorbs sulfur mustard and provides approximately 6 h of protection after contamination *(30)*.

Protective clothing will significantly limit physical agility and endurance. Effectiveness is drastically reduced by the restraints of personal protective equipment (PPE), which includes special heavy protective clothing, mask, and gloves. Any personnel in protective clothing will quickly experience heat stress, reduced visibility and dexterity, and a diminished ability to communicate and operate complex mechanical systems, along with a reduced ability to perform health care duties *(30,33,34)*.

Ideally, personnel decontamination requires that the chemical agent be physically removed as rapidly as possible and chemically destroyed, while avoiding serious chemical effects to the exposed skin. Practically speaking, effective decontamination does not require chemical detoxification *(10)*. When indicated, decontamination should be performed as close to the scene of exposure as possible and ideally before patient transport.

There are many effective methods of skin decontamination. Generally speaking, removal of the toxic agent from the skin surface as quickly as possible is more important than the method of decontamination or type of decontaminant used *(34)*. Washing with 0.5% household bleach is standard in many medical systems. Soap and water can provide highly effective decontamination and can inactivate mustard on the skin. Since mustard is relatively insoluble in water, water alone as a decontaminant has limited utility *(4,16)*.

Some systems rely on the use of highly caustic chemicals and potentially dangerous solvents [e.g., Super Tropical Bleach (STB)]. U.S. military systems rely less on the use of large amounts of water, as U.S. forces must be prepared to operate in environments where large amounts of water may not be readily available *(30)*. Kits containing Fuller's earth (FE) are readily available in many countries. If water is not available, absorbent powders that could effectively bind mustard include flour, talcum powder, activated charcoal, and even earth *(21,34)*. Strong basic solutions such as ammonia and lye or chlorinated acids can also be used to decontaminate from mustard. The U.S. military has used kits: the M13 kit, containing dusting pads of FE (absorbs mustard) and chloramide powder (inactivates mustard), and the M258 kit, containing solutions of chloramide and ethanol, phenol, and sodium hydroxide. The currently fielded personnel decontamination kit, M291, contains a resin that absorbs and inactivates mustard and most major chemical agents *(30,31,35)*. European articles describe the use of anti-gas powder (calcium chloride and magnesium oxide) for decontamination *(11)*. Other substances that may be applied topically to inactivate mustard include powdered milk, albumin, activated charcoal slurry, and collagen dressings *(34)*.

Decontamination procedures are labor-intensive. A lack of adequate detection equipment often results in a large amount of effort being expended to decontaminate "clean" personnel or equipment, while insufficiently decontaminating individuals who are truly contaminated and hazardous *(36)*. All jewelry, clothing, and leather must be removed. Scrubbing and hot water are to be avoided because they promote vapor formation and may accelerate absorption. Standard household products may suffice, if used quickly, such as tissue paper, flour, talcum power, and even salad oil *(34)*. In washing, one should pay particular attention to the neck, groin, genitalia, and axillae *(9)*. Once the patients are decontaminated, there is no risk from handling them, or their tissues or body fluids *(19)*.

The U.S. military uses DS2 (70% diethylenetriamine, 28% ethylene glycol monomethyl ether, and 2% sodium hydroxide) to decontaminate equipment and moderate-sized areas, but not personnel. DS2 is effective against most chemical agents, but it is also flammable and highly corrosive and can only be applied when the user is wearing protective gear. Antifreeze, JP-4, and diesel fuel will remove sulfur mustard from hard surfaces *(30,36)*.

In warmer climates, such as the Middle East, evaporation and vapor hazard would be significant, while lessening the need for decontamination. It is highly unlikely that several days after poisoning with mustard, any clinically relevant quantities of sulfur mustard would remain present on the skin or circulating in the blood.

## 1.7. Medical Management

Protection of medical personnel is a critical aspect of mustard casualty management. Emergency responders must realize that a patient may not exhibit clinical signs or symptoms of exposure initially, even though a significant exposure may have occurred. The use of PPE by emergency responders to protect eyes, airway, and skin is essential for any one entering the contaminated area or having direct contact with contaminated victims *(6,37)*. An accident in 1956 in Northern Africa illustrates this importance. Three children were injured when a discarded mustard munition exploded. During their transport and care, nine contacts, including a physician and nurse, became exposed to sulfur mustard. Some of the exposed contacts developed severe injuries *(12)*. Another case report demonstrates the risk of medical personnel to exposure. A man who drank 5 mL of sulfur mustard died of cardiac arrest within 5 h, and gauze soaked with his blood and gastric contents was later found to cause vesication in laboratory animals *(7)*.

Chemical protective gear worn by health care providers poses significant obstacles to the evaluation and treatment of patients. Additionally, cases of skin lesions developing in persons working in chemical weapons storage facilities while wearing protective clothing have been described; however, explanations for the route of contamination were not clear *(13)*.

Chemical burns from sulfur mustard may often appear deceptively superficial on initial presentation. Mustard becomes fixed in the exposed tissues within minutes. Once fixed, its effects are irreversible. Because of the latency period involved with sulfur mustard, all patients with the potential for significant exposure must be medically monitored for up to 24 h.

Most casualties who reach medical care will survive, even after significant exposure. Sulfur mustard-related deaths in World War I were about 3% of chemical casualties *(2)*. No antidote to sulfur mustard exists. The ability to minimize the extent of injury from sulfur mustard or shorten the recovery phase of healing has not improved significantly since World War I *(19)*. Supportive therapy for sulfur mustard exposure will generally consist of eye care, skin care with attention to blister management, supplemental oxygen, bronchodilators, pulmonary toilet, and treatment of complicating infections *(2,18,19,21,38–40)*.

### 1.7.1. AIRWAY CARE

The therapeutic goal in patients with airway injury is to maintain comfort and adequate oxygenation. Underlying reactive airway disease is easily triggered; consequently, patients with bronchospasm may benefit from bronchodilators and steroid treatment *(2,21)*. Supplemental oxygen may be beneficial, depending on the extent of hyper-reactivity and underlying lung disease. Mucosal sloughing may complicate the initial toxic bronchitis picture. A casualty with severe pulmonary signs early in presentation post exposure should be intubated and mechanically ventilated. In the acute stage, bronchoscopy should be used to assess the extent of airway injury *(2,41)*. Suctioning of inflammatory necrotic debris and frequent bronchoscopy to remove pseudomembrane fragments may be necessary. A need for prolonged ventilatory support suggests a poor prognosis. A late complication of severe pulmonary injury, seen in approximately 10% of Iranian casualties treated in Europe, was progressive stenosis of the tracheobronchial tree. In these patients bronchoscopy proved vital for diagnostic purposes and therapeutic dilation. Bronchoscopic dilation, stent placement, and Nd:YAG laser therapy were all necessary to manage progressive stenosis *(42)*.

### 1.7.2. Skin Care

Sulfur mustard is lipophilic and penetrates skin rapidly *(7,21)*. Moisture on skin enhances mustard absorption. By the time skin lesions develop, mustard is already absorbed and fixed to tissue (or evaporated), so that decontamination is of little utility to the casualty but may prevent exposure of rescue personnel from contamination.

The first symptoms of skin contamination are pruritis and a stinging, burning pain over the involved area. Vesicles may appear as late as 7–12 d after exposure *(7,9)*. The care of mustard skin lesions is generally the same as that for second-degree thermal burns *(21)*. Fluid replacement is of less magnitude, however, and medical personnel should resist the temptation to overhydrate these burn patients. Blisters smaller than 1 cm should be left intact, kept clean, and treated daily with a topical antibiotic ointment (silver sulfadiazine, bacitracin, or Neosporin®). Large blisters (larger than 1 cm) should be unroofed, debrided, cleaned, and covered with a topical antibiotic *(20,21)*. Large blisters should be drained because the fluid in the vesicle will solidify and impede healing *(14)*. Daily debridement and cleansing of wounds is necessary. Biosynthetic dressings may aid in re-epithelialization *(2,18,21,43)*. A whirlpool bath is a useful means of cleansing multiple or large areas *(2)*. Skin lesions take weeks to months to heal, depending on the depth and extent of skin injury.

Additional anecdotal therapies that have been reported to ameliorate the toxic effects of mustard exposure include cooling the skin, applying trichloroacetic acid crystals, and ingestion of vitamin E *(11,21)*.

### 1.7.3. Eye Care

Eye decontamination is not very effective because decontamination must occur immediately, since damage is initiated upon contact *(7)*. Management after exposure should be focused on symptomatic treatment: analgesics to ease pain and irritation, antibacterial ointment, and sterile petroleum to keep the eyelids patent. Eye injuries should be further evaluated with acuity testing, fluorescein staining, slit-lamp exam, and ophthalmologic consultation *(22)*. Eye injury has a generally good prognosis, although severe ulceration may lead to blindness *(2,7,25)*. The slightly higher incidence of eye injuries seen in Iranian casualties after the Iran-Iraq war versus World War I is probably a result of either the higher ambient temperature in the area (as well as greater vapor exposure) or the poor use of protective equipment *(7,9,21)*.

The basic principle of the management of eye injury from sulfur mustard exposure is to prevent infection and scarring. The eyes should be irrigated to remove any residual inflammatory debris or contamination. Casualties with severe injury require hospitalization. Routine management *(2,9,25)* includes:

1. Daily irrigation to remove inflammatory debris
2. Administration of topical antibiotics 3–4 times per day
3. Administration of topical mydriatics to keep the pupil dilated (and prevent synechiae formation)
4. Vaseline applied to the skin edges to prevent adherence
5. Pain control with systemic analgesics
6. Sunglasses or dim light to reduce the discomfort from photophobia
7. Consideration of topical steroids (consult an ophthalmologist)
8. Evidence of infection/panophthalmitis requires an ophthalmology consult.

## *1.8. Disposition*

Most mustard casualties are not severely injured and will survive; however, most will require some form of medical care. Patients with conventional injuries and mustard injuries will have a significantly worse prognosis than expected from the added effects of either injury alone. In general, any person with a potential chemical agent exposure involving a latency period should be observed for a period of time, up to 24 h, to ensure that the full extent of the clinical involvement is appreciated. Potential triage categories include the following:

1. Individuals with small, noncritical areas of skin involvement, mild eye irritation or conjunctivitis, or late-onset, mild upper respiratory symptoms such as cough and sore throat, if seen long enough after exposure to expect that symptoms will not progress significantly, can be discharged with symptomatic therapy and follow-up.
2. Casualties with the following injuries must be hospitalized:
   a. Life-threatening injuries such as large-area liquid mustard burns, or early-onset moderate to severe airway symptoms.
   b. A large area of skin erythema (with or without blisters)
   c. Extremely painful eye lesions or obstructed vision
   d. Moderate respiratory symptoms including dyspnea and cough.
3. Casualties with greater than 20% body surface area burns should be evacuated to a burn center.

Pain management is extremely important. Most casualties who have lost their eyesight initially will recover their full vision. There is no evidence to support the routine use of prophylactic antibiotics, systemic corticosteroids, bronchoalveolar lavage, or charcoal hemoperfusion at any stage in sulfur mustard injury *(18,19,23)*.

## *1.9. Areas of Research*

Future military research will focus on improving battlefield protective posture while preserving agility and physical endurance through a combination of topical skin protectant and lighter weight clothing, as well as attempts to extend the therapeutic window between exposure and irreversible injury *(16,35)*. The current Food and Drug Administration (FDA)-approved topical skin protectant, Skin Exposure Reduction Paste Against Chemical Warfare Agents (SERPACWA), developed by the U.S. Army to be applied before entry into contaminated areas, contains a perfluoroalkylpolyether (PFAPE) oil and polytetrafluoroethylene (Teflon polymer) *(18,21)*. This formulation provides protection against sulfur mustard after application of a thin (0.15-mm) layer *(18)*.

Clinically, it may be possible in the future during the initial latency period after exposure to disrupt the inflammatory processes and protease activation that result from cell sulfur mustard absorption before the development of clinical symptoms, or to promote DNA strand repair *(19)*. Anti-inflammatory and sulfhydryl-scavenging agents have been suggested but have not proved to be useful therapy after lesions develop *(2,18,19)*. Several potential treatment approaches are currently being evaluated, including the administration of scavenger compounds, anti-inflammatories, anti-proteases, and poly-ADP-ribose polymerase (PARP) inhibitors, along with potential roles for cytokines and antioxidants *(18,19,44–46)*. Promising research involving topical povidone-iodine is currently under investigation *(47)*. Studies have suggested that thiols or compounds containing sulfhydryl groups may decrease the toxic effects of sulfur mustard through a systemic protective effect. Sodium thiosulfate taken before mustard exposure has proved to be effective as an antidote; however, it has no effect on mustard already bound to tissue when given after exposure *(48,49)*.

### *1.10. Long-Term Effects*

Sulfur mustard is recognized as a carcinogen and mutagen. Long-term exposure has been associated with an increased incidence of head and neck malignancies; however, most studies have been retrospective and have failed to control for exposure to other carcinogenic agents. In 1975, the International Agency for Research on Cancer (IARC) classified sulfur mustard as a group I carcinogen, similar to asbestos *(4,50)*.

## 2. LEWISITE

Lewisite [dichloro(2-chlorovinyl)arsine], an organic arsenical vesicant developed by the Allies in the closing days of World War I, promotes immediate pain on contact with the skin and eyes and probably calls for immediate protective measures in casualties. It does not demonstrate the latency period of mustard agents *(4)*. Lewisite acts by inhibiting thio-containing enzymes *(48)*.

The toxicity of lewisite vapor is considered similar to that of mustard vapor, and medical personnel should follow the same general principles that they follow for mustard lesions. Erythema and vesication from lewisite occur more quickly *(2,7,21,51)*. Blisters tend to be opaque and contain trace amounts of arsenic, but at nontoxic concentrations *(2,51)*. Contamination to the eyes with lewisite tends to be less serious, because the immediate intense irritation provokes instantaneous precautionary measures. Lewisite is associated with increased capillary permeability, pulmonary edema, and lewisite shock *(2,48,51)*. Shock may result from capillary leak and intravascular volume depletion *(2,48,51)*. Lewisite is also known to be hepatotoxic and nephrotoxic at large doses *(4)*.

There is no laboratory test for lewisite exposure; however, British anti-lewisite (BAL, dimercaprol) is a highly effective antidote. It has been used therapeutically to treat heavy metal poisonings since the 1940s. Intramuscular BAL will provide some protection from dermal and systemic lewisite exposure, but BAL itself has considerable toxic properties. BAL applied topically as an ointment may also prevent or limit lewisite absorption through the skin or eyes *(2)*. Both systemic and topical BAL analogs are currently under investigation and are less toxic *(5,48)*. Lewisite has never been used on the battlefield. For this reason, medical experience with human patients is limited.

Lewisite remains a suspected carcinogen, although this has not yet been clearly established *(2,51)*.

## 3. PHOSGENE OXIME

Phosgene oxime (CX) is a solid or liquid urticant or corrosive agent, not a vesicant, and should not be confused with phosgene (CG), which is a choking or pulmonary agent. Phosgene oxime was developed after World War I in Europe. Like lewisite, it has never been deployed on the battlefield or in a terrorist scenario. Phosgene oxime affects the skin, eyes, and lungs. On the skin, it causes immediate burning and pain, suggestive of stinging nettle. A white area surrounded by erythema rapidly develops, resembling urticaria. Eventually an eschar forms on the skin *(2)*. Its mechanism of action is unknown. Lung injury is associated with pulmonary edema *(2)*. There is no antidote for phosgene oxime.

Decontamination with soap and water or mild base solution, such as sodium bicarbonate, is recommended as soon as possible. Phosgene oxime penetrates garments and rubber much more quickly than other chemical agents. Further treatment is recommended as per usual skin burn therapy *(21)*.

## REFERENCES

1. United Nations. Report of the Mission Dispatched by the Secretary-General to Investigate Allegations by the Islamic Republic of Iran Concerning the Use of Chemical Weapons. Security Council of the United Nations, New York, 1986, Report S/16433.
2. Sidell FR, Urbanetti JS, Smith WJ, et al. Vesicants. In: Sidell FR, Takafuji ET, Franz DR, eds. Textbook of Military Medicine: Medical Aspects of Chemical and Biologic Warfare. Borden Institute, Washington, DC, 1997, pp. 197–228.
3. Blewett W. Tactical weapons: Is mustard still king? NBC Defense Technol Int 1986;1:32–39.
4. Watson AP, Griffin GD. Toxicity of vesicant agents scheduled for destruction by the chemical stockpile disposal program. Environ Health Perspect 1992;98:259–280.
5. Munro NB, Watson AP, Ambrose KA, Griffin GD. Treating exposure to chemical warfare agents: implications for health care providers and community emergency planning. Environ Health Perspect 1990;89:205–215.
6. Brennan RJ, Waeckerle JF, Sharp TW, Lillibridge SR. Chemical warfare agents: emergency medical and emergency public health issues. Ann Emerg Med 1999;34:191–204.
7. Dacre JC, Goldman M. Toxicology and pharmacology of the chemical warfare agent sulfur mustard. Pharm Rev 1996;48:289–325.
8. Central Intelligence Agency Unclassified Semi-Annual Report to Congress on the Acquisition of Technology Relating to Weapons of Mass Destruction and Advanced Conventional Weapons, 1 January–30 June, 2001. Government Printing Office, Washington DC, 2001.
9. Momeni A, Enshaeih S, Meghadi M, Amindjavaheri M. Skin manifestations of mustard gas. Arch Dermatol 1992;128:775–780.
10. Trapp R. The detoxification and natural degradation of chemical warfare agents. Stockholm International Peace Research Institute, Taylor and Francis, London, 1985.
11. Aasted A, Darre MD, Wulf HC. Mustard gas: clinical, toxicological, and mutagenic aspects based on modern experience. Ann Plast Surg 1987;19:330–333.
12. Heully F, Gruninger M. Collective intoxication caused by the explosion of a mustard gas shell. Ann Med Legal 1956;36:195–204.
13. Davis KG, Aspera G. Exposure to liquid sulfur mustard. Ann Emerg Med 2001;37:653–656.
14. Ruhl CM, Park DJ, Danisa O, et al. A serious skin sulfur mustard burn from artillery shell. J Emerg Med 1994;12:159–166.
15. Alexander SF. Medical report of the Bari Harbor mustard casualties. Mil Surg 1947;101:1–17.
16. Smith WJ. Biochemical Pharmacology Branch, US Army Medical Research Institute of Chemical Defense, Aberdeen Proving Ground, MD, personal communication, 2002.
17. Somani SM, Babu SR. Toxicodynamics of sulfur mustard. Int J Clin Pharmacol Ther Toxicol 1989;27:419–435.
18. Smith KJ, Hurst CG, Moeller RB, et al. Sulfur mustard: its continuing threat as a chemical warfare agent, the cutaneous lesions induced, progress in understanding its mechanism of action, its long-term health effects, and new developments for protection and therapy. J Am Acad Dermatol 1995;32:765–776.
19. Smith WJ, Dunn MA. Medical defense against blistering chemical warfare agents. Arch Dermatol 1991;127:1207–1213.
20. Pruitt BA. Treatment of the cutaneous injury. In: Proceedings of the Vesicant Workshop, Columbia, MD, Feb., 1987, pp. 39–43. AD A188222, USAMRICD-SP-87-03, US Army Medical Research Institute of Chemical Defense, Aberdeen Proving Ground, MD, 1987.
21. Bennion SD, David-Bajar K. Cutaneous reactions to nuclear, biological, and chemical warfare. In: Zajtchuk R, Bellamy RF, Jenkins DP, eds. Textbook of Military Medicine: Military Dermatology. Borden Institute, Washington, DC, 1997, pp. 69–110.
22. Borak J, Sidell FR. Agents of chemical warfare: sulfur mustard. Ann Emerg Med. 1992;21:303–308.
23. Willems JL. Controversies regarding diagnosis and treatment of Iranian chemical war casualties brought to Europe. In: Proceedings of the 3rd Symposium Protection Against Chemical Warfare Agents, Umea, Sweden, 11–16 June, 1989, pp. 149–150.

24. Kadivar H, Adams S. Treatment of chemical and biological warfare injuries: insights derived from the 1984 Iraqi attack on Majnoon Island. Mil Med 1991;156:171–177.

25. Safarinejad MR, Moosavi SA, Montazeri B. Ocular injuries caused by mustard gas: diagnosis, treatment, and medical defense. Mil Med 2001;166:67–70.

26. Willems JL. Clinical management of mustard casualties. Ann Med Mil Belg 1989;3S:1–61.

27. Fouyn TH, Lison D, Wouters M. Management of chemical warfare injuries. Lancet 1991;337:121–122.

28. Prevention and treatment of injury from chemical warfare agents. Med Lett Drugs Ther 2002;44:1–4.

29. US Army Soldier and Biological Chemical Command (SBCCOM). Improved Chemical Agent Monitor (ICAM). http://www.sbccom.apgea.army.mil/products/icam.htm. Accessed 25 November, 2002.

30. US Department of the Army. NBC Decontamination Operations. Headquarters, DA, Washington, DC, January, 2002. Field Manual 3-5.

31. NBC Defense Systems, Aberdeen Proving Ground, MD. Obscuration and Decontaminations Systems: Joint Chemical Agent Detector (JCAD). http://www.sbccom.apgea.army.mil/RDA/pmnbc. Accessed 23 November, 2002.

32. US Department of the Army. Assay Techniques for Detection of Exposure to Sulfur Mustard, Cholinesterase Inhibitors, Sarin, Soman, GF, and Cyanide. Headquarters, DA, Washington, DC, May, 1996. Technical Bulletin Medical 296.

33. Tur-Kaspa I, Lev E, Hendler I, et al. Preparing hospitals for toxicological mass casualties events. Crit Care Med 1999;27:1004–1008.

34. Van Hooidonk C, Ceulen BI, Bock J, Van Genderen J. CW agents and the skin. Penetration and decontamination. In: Proceedings of the International Symposium on Protection Against Chemical Warfare Agents, Stockholm, Sweden, 6–9 June, 1983, pp. 153–160.

35. Harrington DG. Development of a safe and effective skin decontamination system: a progress report. In: Proceedings of the Vesicant Workshop, Columbia, MD, Feb., 1987, pp. 85–90, AD A188222, USAMRICD-SP-87-03. US Army Medical Research Institute of Chemical Defense, Aberdeen Proving Ground, MD, 1987.

36. Koslow EE. Decontamination. NBC Defense Technol Int 1987;1:28–30.

37. Golan E, Arad M, Atsmon J, et al. Medical limitations of gas masks for civilian populations: the 1991 experience. Mil Med 1992;157:444–446.

38. Chiesman WE. Diagnosis and treatment of lesions due to vesicants. BMJ 1944;2:109–112.

39. Heyndrickx A, Heyndrickx B. Treatment of Iranian soldiers attacked by chemical and microbiological war gases. Arch Belg Med Soc D Hyg Med Trav Med Leg 1984;(suppl):157–159.

40. Evison D, Hinsley D, Rice P. Chemical weapons. BMJ 2002;324:332–335.

41. Pradkash UBS. Chemical warfare and bronchoscopy. Chest 1991;100:1486–1487.

42. Freitag L, Firusian N, Stamitis G, et al. The role of bronchoscopy in pulmonary complications due to mustard gas inhalation. Chest 1991;100:1436–1441.

43. Eaglstein WH. Experiences with biosynthetic dressings. J Am Acad Dermatol 1985;12:434–440.

44. Medical Chemical Defense. Current controversies on the poly(ADP-ribose)polymerase hypothesis for sulfur mustard-induced cytotoxicity, vol. 4. US Army Medical Research Institute of Chemical Defense, Aberdeen Proving Ground, MD, 1991, pp. 1–6.

45. Smith WJ, Gross CL. Sulfur mustard medical countermeasures in a nuclear environment. Mil Med 2002;167(suppl 1):101–102.

46. Papirmeister B. International vesicant research. In: Proceedings of the Vesicant Workshop, Columbia, MD, Feb., 1987, pp. 101–119, AD A188222, USAMRICD-SP-87-03. US Army Medical Research Institute of Chemical Defense, Aberdeen Proving Ground, MD, 1987.

47. Wormser U, Sintov A, Brodsky B, Nyska A, Topical iodine preparation as therapy against sulfur mustard-induced skin lesions. Toxicol Appl Pharmacol 2000;169:33–39.

48. Greenfield RA, Brown BR, Hutchins JB, et al. Microbiological, biological, and chemical weapons of warfare and terrorism. Am J Med Sci 2002;323:326–340.

49. Callaway S, Pearce KA. Protection against systemic poisoning by mustard gas, di(2-chloroethyl) sulphide, by sodium thiosulphate and thiocit in the albino rat. Br J Pharmacol 1958;13:395–398.

50. Hay A. Effects on health of mustard gas. Nature 1993;366:398–399.

51. Goldman M, Dacre JC. Lewisite: its chemistry, toxicology, and biological effects. Rev Environ Contam Toxicol 1989;110:75–115.

# 21

## Nerve Agents

### *Jonathan Newmark,* MD, FAAN

The opinions expressed herein are the private views of the author and should not be construed as official or as representing the opinion of the Department of the Army or the Department of Defense.

#### CONTENTS

## 1. INTRODUCTION

The organophosphonate nerve agents are the deadliest of the classical chemical warfare agents. They have been used on the battlefield and also in two terrorist attacks. Since excellent antidotal therapy for these agents exists, and since it must be applied rapidly in order to save patients, physicians must familiarize themselves with the appropriate pathophysiology and the rationale for these antidotes.

Space does not permit a full discussion of many of the issues in this chapter. An excellent reference is Sidell's review *(1)*. For field use, the reference put out by the U.S. Army Medical Research Institute of Chemical Defense is also helpful *(2)*.

From: *Physician's Guide to Terrorist Attack*
Edited by: M. J. Roy © Humana Press Inc., Totowa, NJ

## 2. HISTORY

The nerve agents are the most recently developed of the four major chemical warfare agent classes. Of the five classical members of this class, four were developed by the I.G. Farben Company in Germany in the 1930s and 1940s. The laws in Nazi Germany required newly synthesized compounds to be submitted to the military for possible weaponization. Gerhard Schrader, the chemist who first synthesized tabun and sarin, obeyed the law, and the German military, recognizing the possible military uses of these compounds, erected a production facility, which began producing tabun munitions in 1942. Even though Germany produced 10,000–30,000 tons of tabun and smaller quantities of sarin during World War II and successfully put them into munitions, it never used these weapons during that war. The Allies were unaware of these weapons until the waning days of the war, when the Soviet Army captured the major production facility at Dyrenfurth, now in Poland, and the British Army captured small stocks of munitions near Hannover. Over a single weekend, British scientists at the Chemical Defence Establishment at Porton Down demonstrated that tabun was an organophosphate causing cholinergic crisis and that its effects responded to atropine.

Immediately after World War II, the Soviet Union, Britain, and the United States went into nerve agent production. None of these countries has ever used its nerve agent munitions on the battlefield, but they all have clinical experience treating accidental exposures. In the United States production ceased in the 1960s, and the offensive chemical program itself was terminated during the Carter Administration. The United States is now destroying its nerve agent and vesicant stocks in accordance with the Chemical Weapons Convention, but munitions containing these agents remain in eight different chemical storage sites in the United States. The stockpile formerly maintained by the United States in Europe and on Okinawa was successfully destroyed at the Johnston Atoll Chemical Agent Demilitarization Facility in the Pacific Ocean.

The Chemical Weapons Convention, ratified by the United States in 1995 and in force since 1997 worldwide, outlaws nerve agent munitions and places severe restrictions on the intermediates necessary for their synthesis. During the Clinton Administration the United States bombed Khartoum, capital of the Sudan, on the strength of allegations that nerve agent intermediates had been found in soil samples taken near a chemical factory there.

The nerve agents were first used on the battlefield during the first Persian Gulf War between Iran and Iraq. Iraq invaded Iran in 1981 but failed to achieve a quick battlefield success. After 3 years of conflict, Iraq turned to the chemical option and from then until 1987 used both the vesicant sulfur mustard and the nerve agents tabun and sarin against large concentrations of Iranian troops. Some authorities consider the Iraqi use of chemicals and, after 3 years of increasingly lethal long-distance artillery attacks, the threat of Iraqi chemical attacks upon Iranian cities to have been the deciding factor in Iran's decision to end the war in 1987 *(2)*. The United Nations estimate of 45,000 casualties from chemical weapons in that war almost surely underestimated the total. One observer on the ground believes that the actual number was several times that, with most of the difference coming from nerve agent casualties. It was indicated in the third United Nations report that 12,000 victims were hospitalized in Tehran and Ahwaz because of the chemical attacks. However, the number of victims was certainly several times this estimate, since most of the mild and moderate cases of nerve agent poisoning were not registered owing to the difficult circumstances *(3)*.

The Japanese cult Aum Shinrikyo (Supreme Truth) used the nerve agent sarin twice in terrorist attacks, once on a truck-mounted spray tank in Matsumoto, Japan in 1994, and then in a much larger attack on three separate subway trains in Tokyo in 1995. In the first attack, 300 casualties and 7 deaths resulted; in the second attack, 5500 people sought medical attention, of whom 1000–1500 were symptomatic and 12 died. Good first-hand descriptions from some of the patients are available in English *(5)*.

## 3. AGENTS AND PHYSICAL STATE

The organophosphate nerve agents are all liquids at standard temperature and pressure. This carries important implications for their deployment, the clinical presentation of casualties, and the decontamination of casualties.

The classic nerve agents include GA (tabun), GB (sarin), GD (soman), GF (cyclosarin), and VX (no common name). The two-letter designations are NATO codes; GC is missing from the series because it stood for gonococcus. The G series agents were originally developed in Germany, hence the letter G; V apparently originally stood for venomous, and VX was developed originally in Britain and weaponized first by the United States. A very similar compound to VX, VR, was made in the former Soviet Union (Table 1 and Fig. 1).

All the G series nerve agents are watery organic liquids that evaporate at approximately the same rate as water. From the military point of view, they qualify as nonpersistent agents, meaning that within 24 hours a puddle of any of these lying outdoors will have evaporated. Their high volatility makes a spill of any of them a serious vapor hazard. In the Tokyo subway attack, using only a 30% solution of sarin, all the patients who experienced symptoms had inhaled the vapor of sarin that had been deliberately spilled out onto the floor of a crowded subway car by puncturing a plastic bag filled with the liquid. None of them actually came in contact with the liquid. VX, an oily rather than watery organic liquid, is the exception. Its low vapor pressure makes it much less of a vapor hazard than the others, but by the same token its slowness to vaporize makes it persistent and potentially a much greater environmental hazard over time.

## 4. PATHOPHYSIOLOGY

The nerve agents, and indeed all the organophosphate insecticides, work by inhibiting cholinesterases. Circulating cholinesterases, primarily plasma butyrylcholinesterase and red blood cell acetylcholinesterase, are easily measured. It is not their inhibition that will place the patient's life at risk. It is the tissue and specifically the synaptic cholinesterases whose inhibition causes clinical effects that can rapidly lead to death. Although there may well be other effects of nerve agent intoxication, acetylcholinesterase inhibition accounts for the major life-threatening effects, and reversal of this inhibition by antidotal therapy is effective, proving that it is the central action of these poisons.

At cholinergic synapses, acetylcholinesterase, which is bound to the postsynaptic membrane, functions as a turn-off switch to regulate cholinergic transmission. Inhibition of the enzyme causes the half-life of the released neurotransmitter, acetylcholine, to build up, and end-organ overstimulation ensues. The clinician recognizes this as cholinergic crisis.

Nerve agents differ from the more commonly encountered organophosphate insecticides (malathion, parathion, and others) chiefly by their greatly increased toxicity. Sarin in vitro is 1000 times more toxic per unit weight than parathion *(6)*. VX is the most toxic

Table 1

## Chemical, Physical, Environmental, and Biological Properties of Nerve Agents

| Properties | Tabun (GA) | Sarin (GB) | Soman (GD) | VX |
|---|---|---|---|---|
| **Chemical and physical** | | | | |
| Boiling point | 230°C | 158°C | 198°C | 298°C |
| Vapor pressure | 0.037mm Hg at 20°C | 2.1 mm Hg at 20°C | 0.40 mm Hg at 25°C | 0.0007 mm Hg at 20°C |
| Density: | | | | |
| Vapor (compared to air) | 5.64.86 | 6.39.2 | | |
| Liquid | 1.08 g/mL at 25°C | 1.10 g/mL at 20°C | 1.02 g/mL at 25°C | 1.008 g/mL at 20°C |
| Volatility | 610 mg/m$^3$ at 25°C | 22,000 mg/m$^3$ at 25°C | 3,900 mg/m$^3$ at 25°C | 10.5 mg/m$^3$ at 25°C |
| Appearance | Colorless to brown liquid | Colorless liquid | Colorless liquid | Colorless to straw-colored liquid |
| Odor | Fairly fruity | No odor | Fruity; oil of camphor | Odorless |
| Solubility: | | | | |
| In water | 9.8 g/100 g at 25°C | Miscible | 2.1 g/100 g at 20°C | Miscible <9.4°C |
| In other solvents | Soluble in most organic solvents | Soluble in all solvents | Soluble in some solvents | Soluble in all solvents |
| **Environmental and biological** | | | | |
| Detectability: | | | | |
| Vapor | M8A1, M256A1, CAM, ICAD | M8A1, M256A1, CAM, ICAD | M8A1, M256A1, CAM, ICAD | M8, M9 paper ICAD |
| Liquid | M8, M9 paper | M8, M9 paper | M8, M9 paper | M8, M9 paper |
| Persistency: | | | | |
| In soil | Half-life 1–1.5 d | 2–24 h at 5–25°C | Relatively persistent | 2–6 d |
| On materiel | Unknown | Unknown | Unknown | Persistent |
| Decontamination of skin | M258A1, diluted hypochlorite, soap and water, M291 kit | M258A1, diluted hypochlorite, soap and water, M291 kit | M258A1, diluted hypochlorite, soap and water, M291 kit | M258A1, diluted hypochlorite, soap and M291 kit water, M291 kit |
| Biologically effective amount: | | | | |
| Vapor | $LCt_{50}$: 400 mg · min/m$^3$ | $LCt_{50}$: 100 mg · min/m$^3$ | $LCt_{50}$: 50 mg · min/m$^3$ | $LCt_{50}$: 10 mg · min/m$^3$ |
| Liquid | $LD_{50}$ (skin): 1.0 g/70-kg man | $LD_{50}$ (skin): 1.7 g/70-kg man | $LD_{50}$ (skin): 350 mg/70-kg man | $LD_{50}$ (skin): 10 mg/70-kg man |

Abbreviations: CAM, chemical agent monitor; ICAD, individual chemical agent detector; $LCt_{50}$, vapor or aerosol exposure necessary to cause death in 50% of the population exposed; $LD_{50}$, dose necessary to cause death in 50% of the population with skin exposure; M8A1, chemical alarm system; M256A1, detection card; M258A1, self-decontamination kit; M291, decontamination kit; M8 and M9, chemical detection papers.

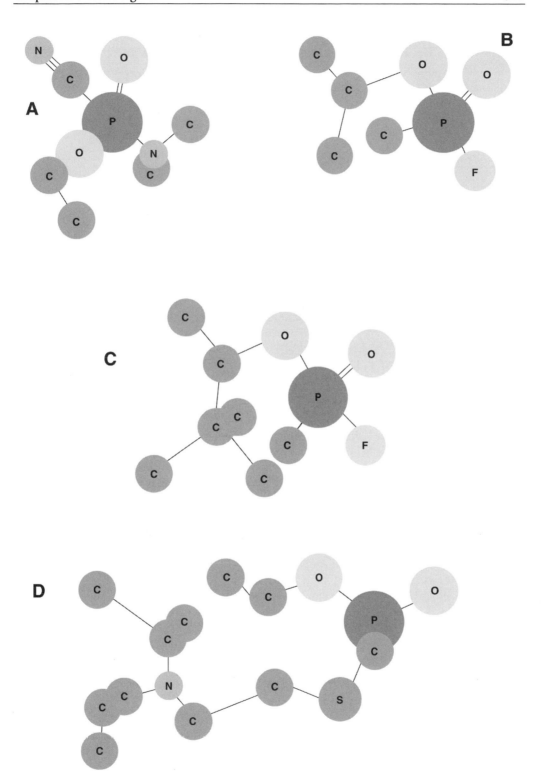

**Fig. 1.** Molecular models of **(A)** tabun (GA), **(B)** sarin (GB), **(C)** soman (GD), and **(D)** VX. (Molecular models: courtesy of Offie E. Clark, U.S. Army Medical Research Institute of Chemical Defense, Aberdeen, MD.)

substance known in neurobiology, save for the biological toxins, such as botulinum toxin, which would never be synthesized from scratch; it is fair to say, therefore, that VX is the most toxic substance that could be synthesized *de novo*. The toxic doses (see Table 1) of these compounds are estimated in two ways, via vapor exposure (inhaled) and with liquid exposure upon intact skin. For vapor exposure, toxic doses are estimated, using Haber's law, by the product of concentration × time. The lethal vapor dose, or $LCt_{50}$, by definition is the dose of vapor exposure that would kill 50% of an exposed population. For the four classic nerve agents, these doses are:

| | |
|---|---|
| Tabun vapor | 400 mg × min/m$^3$ |
| Sarin vapor | 100 mg × min/m$^3$ |
| Soman vapor | 50 mg × min/m$^3$ |
| VX vapor | 10 mg × min/m$^3$ |

In the liquid form, toxic doses are given in milligrams. The lethal liquid dose or $LD_{50}$ by definition is the amount of liquid placed on a patient's skin or ingested that would kill 50% of an exposed population. For the four classic nerve agents, these are:

| | |
|---|---|
| Tabun liquid | 1000 mg |
| Sarin liquid | 1700 mg |
| Soman liquid | 350 mg |
| VX liquid | 6-10 mg |

To picture this graphically, the amount of VX liquid it would take to kill half an exposed population, if placed on the skin of all of them, forms a drop just large enough to cover the space between two adjacent columns on the Lincoln Memorial on the back of a U.S. penny. In the old U.S. offensive munitions program 20,000 lethal doses could easily be packed into one round.

## 5. CLINICAL EFFECTS, BY EXPOSURE ROUTE

The clinical effects of nerve agent exposure are the same for both vapor and liquid routes of exposure if the dose is large enough, but the order in which symptoms appear and the speed with which they appear will differ.

Exposure of a patient to nerve agent vapor is overwhelmingly the more likely both in a battlefield and in a terrorist scenario. When this occurs, cholinergic synapses will become involved in the order in which they encounter the cholinesterase inhibitor. The most exposed cholinergic synapses on the outside of the human body are those in the pupillary muscles, which are part of the parasympathetic nervous system. Nerve agent vapor easily crosses the cornea and affects these synapses directly, producing miosis, experienced subjectively by patients as dimming of vision, or the world going black. In rare cases this produces eye pain, and in about 10% of patients nausea can ensue. Next, exocrine glands located in the nose, mouth, and pharynx become exposed to the vapor, and cholinergic synapses located there will cause increased secretions of watery fluids, causing rhinorrhea, drooling, and increased salivation. Next, vapor interacts with exocrine glands in the upper airway, causing increased secretions of watery fluids into the respiratory passages, or bronchorrhea, and also interacts with smooth muscle located in the upper airways, causing bronchospasm. Not only does this bronchospasm become easily audible, but, combined with bronchorrhea, it can cause respiratory distress and shortness of breath. In the extreme, the patient may become hypoxic.

Once the vapor has penetrated, passively, to the alveoli, it easily crosses the alveolar-capillary membrane and enters the bloodstream, where, incidentally, it will inhibit the circulating cholinesterases. Although this effect is asymptomatic, it can easily be picked up by a blood draw for cholinesterase level; the practical problem here is that patients' baseline cholinesterase levels vary so widely that it is difficult to interpret this level. Of the two commonly available tests (red blood cell acetylcholinesterase and circulating plasma butyrylcholinesterase), the former is a better guide for nerve agent poisoning. More importantly from the clinical standpoint, the bloodstream passively carries the nerve agent easily to organs where further clinical symptoms develop.

Usually the first organ system to become symptomatic from bloodborne nerve agent exposure is the gastrointestinal tract. Cholinergic synapses here cause increased motility and peristalsis, with clinical symptoms and signs of abdominal cramping, abdominal pain, nausea, vomiting, and diarrhea.

After the gastrointestinal tract has become involved, nerve agent will affect the heart, distant exocrine glands, muscles, and brain. Because there are cholinergic synapses on both the vagal (parasympathetic) and sympathetic sides of the nervous supply to the heart, it is impossible to predict in an individual case how the heart rate and blood pressure will respond to nerve agent challenge.

Cholinergic synapses innervate all exocrine glands in the body. Those not affected locally by nerve agent (vapor, as in this instance, or liquid) will be affected once the agent is bloodborne. Clinical effects from neuroglandular overstimulation will include oversecretion in the salivary, nasal, respiratory, and sweat glands—the patient will be wet all over.

Bloodborne nerve agent will interact with neuromuscular junctions at all skeletal muscles. This will cause initial fasciculations, painless but visible muscle contractions that do not move a joint, followed by frank twitching, which does move joints and can be confused with tonic-clonic jerks. If the process goes on long enough, eventually ATP in the muscle cells will be depleted and flaccid paralysis will ensue, but it is important to remember that this is never the initial presentation of neuromuscular problems from nerve agent poisoning, as it is with botulinum toxin poisoning.

In the brain, the cholinergic system is the most widely distributed of all the neurotransmitter systems. Bloodborne nerve agent exposure will rapidly overstimulate all the cholinergic synapses. Large doses will cause rapid loss of consciousness, seizures, and central apnea, which can lead to respiratory death within minutes. If respiration is supported, a form of status epilepticus unresponsive to most commonly used anticonvulsants may ensue. If nerve agent-induced status lasts for 45 minutes or more, neuronal death and permanent brain dysfunction may occur. In a very mild nerve agent exposure, insufficient to cause the full-blown syndrome, patients may experience weeks or months of irritability, sleep disturbance, and mild neurobehavioral dysfunction.

The time from exposure to development of the full-blown severe nerve agent syndrome via the vapor route can be minutes or even seconds when the dose is large. Patients may go from fully functional to helpless, seizing, apneic, and unconscious within seconds; in this situation, failure to treat rapidly will ensure that the patient will die. On the other hand, with vapor inhalational exposure there is no depot effect; agent is not trapped in the body, and rapid treatment will produce rapid improvement without subsequent deterioration. If the effects of nerve agent poisoning do not kill the patient, the circulating half-life of the nerve agents is very short.

The sequence of clinical effects from nerve agent liquid exposure on intact skin differs both in the order of affected organs and also in the time course from that caused by vapor inhalation. If nerve agent liquid contacts intact skin, a certain percentage will vaporize off (insignificant in the case of VX), and the rest will begin to travel through the skin, where it will interact with cholinergic receptors in the sweat glands and cause localized sweating. Below the dermis it will encounter local cholinergic synapses in the muscles locally, producing local fasciculations. Since muscle is a well-vascularized organ, at this point the bloodstream will passively take up the agent and convey it to the organs mentioned above, causing first gastrointestinal discomfort and then, roughly simultaneously, respiratory problems (bronchorrhea, bronchospasm, and dyspnea), heart rate changes, generalized fasciculations and twitching, loss of consciousness, seizures, and central apnea. The time course, however, will differ greatly from that seen in vapor inhalational exposure. For even a large, lethal liquid drop, the time course from surface to systemic exposure through the bloodstream will probably be up to 30 minutes, and for a small, far less than lethal, drop it could take place in up to 18 hours.

An additional difference between the two routes of exposure lies in the ability of liquid exposure to cause clinical worsening hours after exposure. Application of proper antidotal therapy in this situation may improve the patient's clinical status, but this may worsen hours later as the agent, which was on its way through skin and muscle, gets into the bloodstream.

Another difference between vapor and liquid exposure lies in the presence of miosis. The pupillary muscle lies relatively well insulated from the circulating bloodstream. Consequently, although in a vapor-exposed patient miosis is usually the first sign and is essentially an invariable one, in a liquid-exposed patient miosis is usually the last sign seen and in a small exposure may not be present. Clinically this observation implies that miosis is a poor guide to exposure if the liquid route is suspected.

In a terrorist scenario the liquid exposure route may be particularly important when a conventional munition is combined with a liquid nerve agent. When assessing a patient with a conventional wound, such as shrapnel from a conventional bomb, bear the possibility in mind that it was contaminated with nerve agent and treat the patient as a possible liquid exposure.

Unless the nerve agent is removed by specific therapy (usually an oxime), its binding to cholinesterase is irreversible. Cholinesterase activity recovers as new enzyme is synthesized. In red blood cells this occurs at the rate of red cell turnover, about 1% per day. Plasma butyrylcholinesterase, although not as accurate a surrogate for tissue cholinesterase inhibition as red cell cholinesterase, recovers more quickly and is a more accurate guide to recovery of tissue enzyme activity.

## 6. DIFFERENTIAL DIAGNOSIS

Although cholinergic crisis has many causes, if it is caused by acute exposure to a toxin, as in a terrorist attack or a military weapon, the differential diagnosis is extremely narrow. The only weaponized agent that can cause the same rapid deterioration of function and death as nerve agents is cyanide. Acute cyanide poisoning can also cause seizure, coma, and death, but it does not cause cholinergic crisis, and in particular cyanide casualties are not cyanotic (because of highly oxygenated venous blood) and do not manifest miosis, increased secretions, or neuromuscular twitching.

## 7. ACUTE THERAPY OF NERVE AGENT POISONING

The principles of nerve agent treatment have not changed since they were first elucidated by the British in 1945. Acute nerve agent poisoning is treated by decontamination of the patient, respiratory support, and three antidotes: an anticholinergic, an oxime, and an anticonvulsant. Depending on the clinical situation, these may be applied in different orders; in most acute cases all will go on almost simultaneously.

## 8. DECONTAMINATION

We decontaminate nerve agent casualties to prevent further absorption of the agent, further spread of the agent on the casualty, and (especially) spread of the agent to those taking care of the patient. Decontamination of the patient is rarely the first step in treatment, but in a hospital situation it must be borne in mind. Formally, decontamination of vapor is not actually necessary, but in the Tokyo subway attack, in which patients were evaluated in hospitals without having first removed their clothes, sarin vapor trapped in the patients' clothing caused miosis in 10% of emergency room personnel. Decontamination of liquid is accomplished in the field using the U.S. military M291 skin decontamination kit, which contains an Ambergard resin capable of pulling liquid out of the skin; civilian agencies are now stockpiling this product. At the hospital level, soap and copious amounts of water should suffice, but in any event decontamination should ideally be done before the patient enters the hospital facility to avoid contaminating other patients and emergency staff. Decontamination of a wound is not a major problem, as surrounding tissue will quickly absorb liquid agent. Irrigation with a sterile fluid should suffice, although the runoff should be sequestered for later full decontamination with bleach solution. Attention must be paid to extracting potentially contaminated clothing and other foreign material in the wound, which may serve as a depot for liquid agent.

## 9. RESPIRATORY SUPPORT

Ventilatory support may be required for patients with acute nerve agent poisoning, because of airway difficulties from bronchorrhea and bronchospasm or from central apnea. A death from nerve agent poisoning is almost always a respiratory death. The period of time during which patients require such support is much shorter, however, than that in severe organophosphate insecticide poisoning. This may seem counterintuitive, since the nerve agents are far more toxic, but the explanation is that nerve agents are not very lipid-soluble and thus they do not disappear into the body's fat stores. This implies that ventilatory support will probably not be necessary for long periods (hours at most, not days) while antidotal therapy is being applied, assuming that the heart is still beating.

Because of the bronchospasm that is part of the nerve agent toxicity syndrome, ventilation will be complicated by increased resistance and by increased secretions. If the heart is still beating, these can be most quickly treated with systemic atropine; within seconds, ventilation will become far easier. As a clinical rule, when the heart is still beating, atropine should be given before ventilation, since without atropine on board ventilation will be difficult owing to bronchospasm and to copious respiratory secretions.

# 10. ANTIDOTAL THERAPY

## *10.1. Atropine*

Almost any cholinergic blocker can in theory be used as a nerve agent antidote, but worldwide atropine is the choice for this purpose, because of its stability over wide temperature ranges and its rapid effectiveness in the intramuscular route, which is crucial for field care, and because inadvertent administration of the drug usually does not cause much central nervous system dysfunction, as is seen with some other anticholinergic drugs. Atropine rapidly reverses the effects of nerve agent on muscarinic cholinergic receptors. It has little effect at nicotinic cholinergic synapses. From the practical standpoint this means that the neuromuscular and some sympathetic effects of nerve agents are poorly treated by atropine, but since the life-threatening effects of nerve agents, particularly the respiratory ones, are mediated by muscarinic receptors, atropine is life-saving acutely.

In the field, military personnel are given MARK I kits, which contain 2 mg atropine autoinjectors. Civilian personnel are now stocking this Food and Drug Administration (FDA)-approved product, so it is likely that an emergency physician will see a patient who has been treated with this form of atropine. It is not possible to give part of an autoinjector, so the initial loading dose will be a multiple of this injector; for mild, moderate, and severe casualties field personnel are trained to give 2, 4, or 6 mg as the loading dose, with retreatment every 5–10 min until the patient's breathing and secretions improve. During the Iran-Iraq war, where oxime was not always available and evacuations were often performed without confidence that the patient would see a physician soon, much larger initial doses were given.

When the patient reaches a level of medical care at which iv drugs can be given, atropine may be given via the iv route with the same clinical signs for titration. Again, during the Iran-Iraq war, 50–100 mg of atropine was occasionally given, but if the patient is continually monitored it is likely that lower totals will be needed. In any case, the high doses used by the Iranians may have resulted from low oxime supplies *(4)*. In contrast to organophosphate insecticides, because of the lack of sequestration of nerve agent in the body's lipid stores, the total amount of atropine needed and the total time to get ahead of the toxicity syndrome for the patient will both be much less in the case of nerve agent poisoning. Although organophosphate poisoning patients may require 1000–2000 mg of atropine over several days, even severely poisoned nerve agent patients should require total amounts in the hundreds of milligrams at most, and over probably no more than hours to a day. There is no upper bound to atropine therapy in an individual patient, using either the im or iv route.

Pediatric atropine autoinjectors (0.5 and 1.0 mg) have been developed for the Israeli medical community and were FDA approved in March, 2003. When caring for a child too small for an autoinjector, iv access must be obtained before using systemic atropine. An FDA-approved atropine inhaler is available and may be helpful until iv access can be obtained in a child who is still breathing *(10)*.

In a patient who is either minimally affected by nerve agent and has miosis alone, or who was more severely affected and has recovered, and who has only residual miosis, systemic administration of atropine is inadvisable. These patients should receive atropine or homatropine eyedrops for symptomatic relief. This will produce mydriasis for about

24 h, and accommodation will be impaired either with or without therapy. Miosis may persist for weeks or even months after all other signs and symptoms have resolved.

## *10.2. Oxime Therapy*

Oximes are nucleophiles that reactivate the cholinesterase whose active site has been occupied and bound to nerve agent or organophosphate. Oxime therapy therefore restores normal enzyme function, and since enzymes are catalytic, oximes can be tremendously helpful in ameliorating the cholinergic crisis caused by nerve agents. The limitation of oxime therapy, however, lies in a second side reaction, called *aging*. In this reaction, a side chain on the nerve agent molecule falls off the complex at a characteristic rate once the nerve agent has bound to acetylcholinesterase. This leaves the remaining complex negatively charged, and oxime cannot bind to a negatively charged complex to reactivate it. The practical effect of aging differs by agent, since each agent has a characteristic speed to its aging side reaction. VX for practical purposes never ages, so that there is really no limitation to the use of oximes in VX poisoning. Sarin ages in 3–5 h and tabun over a longer period. These intervals are so much longer than the patient's expected lifespan after acute severe nerve agent toxicity that for practical purposes they may be ignored. Soman, however, because of its larger side chain, ages in 2 min, and thus after only a few minutes oxime therapy is useless in a soman-poisoned individual. In some ways, this makes soman, despite its lesser toxicity compared with VX, much harder to treat.

Countries differ in their oxime of choice. In the United States the fielded oxime is 2-pralidoxime chloride. Japan uses 2-pralidoxime iodide, which was the oxime with which Tokyo victims were treated. Iran imports obidoxime (Toxigonin) from Germany but did not have large supplies during its war with Iraq. Canada uses 2-pralidoxime chloride, but the Canadian Forces are advocating subsitution with the Hagedorn oxime, HI-6, which is not yet approved for use in either Canada or the United States. All of the oximes work via the same mechanism.

The MARK I kit in use in the United States contains an autoinjector of 600 mg of 2-pralidoxime chloride. Initial field loading doses are 1, 2, or 3 autoinjectors, or 600, 1200, or 1800 mg. Blood pressure elevation may occur after administration of 45 mg/kg, which is why field use of 2-pralidoxime chloride is restricted to 1800 mg/h; during this time, if further field treatment is given, it should be atropine alone. In the hospital setting, 2.5–25 mg/kg iv has been found to reactivate 50% or more of the inhibited enzyme. The usual recommendation is 1.0 g through slow iv drip over 20–30 min to begin. Again, no more than 2.5 g of oxime should be given within 1–1.5 h, even in the iv route, because of the strong possibility of induced hypertension. Unlike atropine, oxime therapy may improve neuromuscular functioning.

## *10.3. Anticonvulsant*

Nerve agent-induced seizures do not respond to the usual anticonvulsants used in status epilepticus. In particular, phenytoin, fosphenytoin, phenobarbital, valproic acid, carbamazepine, lamotrigine, and gabapentin are ineffective at doses used for status epilepticus in usual practice. Only two drug classes are effective against these seizures. Anticholinergics, if given within the first 20 min of seizure onset in animals, are actually effective anticonvulsants in this situation. Atropine, which is the mainstay of therapy for nerve agents, serves this function to a degree. The other major drug class that can stop nerve agent-induced seizures is the benzodiazepines.

Diazepam is the only benzodiazepine approved by the FDA for use against seizures in humans. Because of this, diazepam, in the form of a 10-mg autoinjector for im use [convulsive antidote for nerve agent (CANA)] is manufactured and given to U.S. troops for this purpose. Civilian agencies are stockpiling quantities of this product, which is not used in hospital medicine. U.S. troops are instructed to give one 10-mg diazepam autoinjector to any severely poisoned nerve agent patient and to retreat as necessary for seizures. Extrapolation from animal studies indicates that most adults will actually require 30–40 mg of diazepam to stop this form of status epilepticus. In the hospital, iv diazepam may be used at about the same dose. As emergency physicians are well aware, the use of diazepam in this setting runs the risk of respiratory depression, and monitoring is mandatory. In addition, seizures can easily be confused with the neuromuscular signs of nerve agent poisoning, so an early electroencephalogram (EEG) is advised.

Several other members of the benzodiazepine class of drugs are effective against nerve agent-induced seizures and are more commonly used than diazepam as anticonvulsants. The U.S. military is required to use FDA-approved drugs only in an on-label fashion, and that is the reason why diazepam is the fielded anticonvulsant, but if a licensed physician uses them in an off-label fashion, many other members of this class are equally effective or superior. Recent studies *(7)* have shown that the best agent in this drug class is midazolam, which achieves seizure control at lower doses and faster than any of the others.

## 11. PRETREATMENT

During the second Gulf War (1990–1991), coalition forces feared that Iraq might attack using a rapid-aging nerve agent such as soman. Because of the rapid aging of this agent, the oximes are, as previously mentioned, of only limited use. Over 100,000 U.S. and allied forces were issued pyridostigmine bromide as a pretreatment. Pyridostigmine bromide, long the standard therapy for myasthenia gravis and so approved by the FDA since 1951, is a reversible inhibitor of cholinesterases. Pretreatment with this agent at a low dose, sufficient to inhibit about 25–30% of the body's store of cholinesterases, allows a soldier to survive what would have been a toxic challenge with soman, as estimated from animal studies. The FDA approved pyridostigmine bromide therapy as a pretreatment for soman in early 2003. Pyridostigmine bromide use is still U.S. and allied military doctrine for battlefield situations in which rapid-aging nerve agent attack is expected. In the civilian sector, however, no first-responder agency has chosen to pretreat its operators, and none is likely to do so. Physicians treating first responders, therefore, must expect that any who have become affected by nerve agents will not have first been treated with pyridostigmine. Once nerve agents have poisoned the patient, pyridostigmine is contraindicated, as it will merely worsen the clinical effects of nerve agents.

## 12. LONG-TERM EFFECTS OF NERVE AGENT POISONING

There is little clinical information on the EEG patterns seen in nerve agent survivors. Information in actual patients is at the case report level and is largely uncontrolled. In one study, survivors had statistically more EEG abnormalities than age-matched controls, but data from Tokyo survivors show that the EEG normalizes over months. There are no data to suggest that nerve agent toxicity, even severe enough to cause status epilepticus, predisposes to seizure disorder.

Clinical observations have shown nonspecific neurobehavioral effects lasting for weeks to months, and in some cases these are claimed to last for years.

Animal autopsy studies show that central nervous system damage, particularly if seizures have lasted for 45 minutes or more, is permanent. Chief among the pathologies seen is neuronal loss. The difficulty in interpreting this data lies in the tendency of patients with severe nerve agent exposure to have hypoxic encephalopathy as well as direct nerve agent toxicity, making it difficult to separate out the effects caused by each one.

Peripheral neuropathy and the so-called intermediate syndrome are prominent long-term effects of poisoning with organophosphate insecticides. Perhaps surprisingly, these have not been seen in nerve agent poisoning. One patient in the Tokyo subway attack subsequently developed neuropathy (8); this case appears to be unique, and causality has not been proved.

Blood cholinesterase measurements return to normal at different rates; plasma butyrylcholinesterase can normalize within weeks, whereas red blood cell cholinesterase levels may take months to normalize.

## 13. SUMMARY

The nerve agents are peculiarly attractive to terrorists because of their rapid onset of action. Patients encountering a lethal dose can seize, lose consciousness, become apneic, and die within minutes if not treated expeditiously with antidotes. Antidotal therapy is effective and can be rapidly life-saving.

### 13.1. Rapid Access to Information

Information on all the chemical warfare agent classes, including downloadable versions of all the basic references including refs. 1 and 2, can be found on the Chemical Casualty Care Division website at http://ccc.apgea.army.mil.

---

**Case Vignette**

A 35-year-old man was exposed to sarin during the Tokyo subway attack in 1995. For 7 minutes after the exposure, he was observed to have tonic-clonic convulsions and episodes of dyspnea, requiring artificial respiration. In the hospital emergency room he was cyanotic and comatose. His pupils were constricted to 1.5 mm, and he had profuse oral and nasal secretions. He was vomiting and profusely diaphoretic. In the emergency room, atropine sulfate and 2-pralidoxime iodide (the preferred Japanese oxime) were given intravenously.

The patient only regained consciousness after 8 hours. He regained full mobility 54 hours after exposure. He was disoriented and had impaired short-term memory.

An electroencephalogram showed mild slowing of alpha activity, intermittent theta bursts, and, during hyperventilation, development of delta bursts. A repeat EEG done 3 months later showed that all of these abnormalities had resolved.

Plasma butyrylcholinesterase was reduced to 6% of the laboratory's normal acutely, but returned to the normal range within 3 weeks. Red blood cell acetylcholinesterase activity returned to normal within 3 months.

CT scan and MR imaging of the brain showed no focal lesions.

Because of the patient's persistent change in mental status, despite the recovery of all systemic signs and symptoms of nerve agent poisoning, a full neuropsychological battery was conducted. Logical memory and associate learning scales from the Wechsler Memory Scale and construction of the Rey-Osterrieth complex figure suggested a defect in the ability to construct new memory. He retained retrograde amnesia for 70 days prior to his sarin exposure. An apparently permanent personality change was evident in the direction of passivity and shallow affect.

The patient's physicians conjectured that his inability to return to his previous state of functioning implied that the patient had suffered hypoxic encephalopathy on top of his nerve agent exposure. This was consistent with the observation of severe dyspnea immediately after he was poisoned and the time lag before good respiratory function had been restored.

(From ref. 9).

# REFERENCES

1. Sidell FR. Nerve agents. In: Sidell FR, Takafuji ET, Franz DR, eds. Textbook of Military Medicine: Medical Aspects of Chemical and Biological Warfare. Borden Institute, Washington, DC, 1997, pp. 129–179.
2. Chemical Casualty Care Division, USAMRICD. Medical Management of Chemical Casualties Handbook, 3rd ed. USAMRICD, Aberdeen Proving Ground, MD, 2000. Available online at: http://ccc.apgea.army.mil/products/handbooks/mmccthirdeditionjul2000.pdf.
3. Cordesman AH, Wagner AP. The Lessons of Modern War: Vol 2, The Iran-Iraq War. Westview Press, Boulder, CO, 1990.
4. Foroutan SA. Medical notes on the chemical warfare, Part V. Kowsar Med J (original in Farsi), 1997;2.
5. Murakami H. Underground. (English translation by P. Gabriel.) Vintage Books, New York, 2001.
6. Grob D, Harvey JC. Effects in man of the anticholinesterase compound sarin. J Clin Invest 1958;37:350–368.
7. McDonough J, McMonagle J, Copeland T, Zoeffel D, Shih T.-M. Comparative evaluation of benzodiazepines for control of soman-induced seizures. Arch Toxicol 1999;73:473–478.
8. Himuro K, et al. Distal sensory neuropathy after sarin intoxication. Neurology 1995;51:1195–1197.
9. Hatta K, et al. Amnesia from sarin poisoning. Lancet 1996;347:1343.
10. Rotenberg BS and Newmark J. Nerve agent attacks on children: diagnosis and management. Pediatrics, in press.

# 22 Incapacitating Agents

*Sage W. Wiener, MD,*
*and Lewis S. Nelson, MD, FACEP, FACMT*

## CONTENTS

## Case Vignette

On March 16, 1995, eight patients presented to a Bronx hospital emergency department (ED) with acute onset of agitation and hallucinations approximately 1 hour after "snorting" heroin. These patients were initially found to have lethargy and pinpoint pupils by prehospital personnel. They had been treated with intravenous naloxone en route to the hospital and became agitated and delirious. On physical examination in the ED, they were tachycardic and mildly hypertensive, with dilated pupils, dry skin and mucous membranes, and diminished or absent bowel sounds; five had urinary retention. The findings were noted to be consistent with the anticholinergic syndrome. The patients were sedated with diazepam or lorazepam, receiving supportive care and a complete medical evaluation as their signs and symptoms resolved over the next 12–24 hours.

From: *Physician's Guide to Terrorist Attack*
Edited by: M. J. Roy © Humana Press Inc., Totowa, NJ

On March 17 (the following day), the Department of Health notified local health care personnel of a potential problem with heroin contaminated by an anticholinergic agent. Between March 17 and April 5, 1995, 10 patients with very similar presentations were seen in hospital EDs in the Bronx and Manhattan. All reported using heroin, and seven reported having used heroin with the street names "Point on Point" or "Sting." Two patients were able to provide specimens of "Sting" heroin on April 5. These specimens were analyzed by gas chromatography-mass spectrophotometry (GC-MS) by the Bureau of Laboratories, New York City Department of Health (NYCDOH) and found to contain both heroin and scopolamine. The GC-MS patterns of the drug samples were more consistent with a synthetic rather than a plant-derived source of scopolamine. Once this was known, subsequent patients were treated with intravenous physostigmine, given slowly over 5–10 minutes for suspected scopolamine poisoning. Their paranoia, hallucinations, and agitation resolved, and their mental status returned to baseline *(1,2)*.

The NYCDOH issued press releases warning of scopolamine-adulterated heroin sold under the street names "Point on Point" and "Sting." As of May 27, 1995, 325 cases were ultimately reported that were consistent with anticholinergic toxicity by history and physical findings and were associated with heroin use. All cases responded to therapy with physostigmine *(1,2)*.

## 1. INTRODUCTION

Incapacitating agents are designed to cause temporary disability on the battlefield. By military definition, such agents must be highly potent, must produce their effects mainly by altering the higher regulatory activity of the central nervous system, and in effective doses must produce effects that last for hours to days without causing permanent injury or death *(3,4)*. The rationale for their use over lethal agents is twofold. Since World War I, there has been an impetus to develop more "humane" agents as international opinion has frowned on the use of lethal chemical weapons. From a strategic perspective, an incapacitated soldier on the battlefield may be a greater liability than a dead one. Each incapacitated soldier demands that resources and personnel be diverted toward his or her care rather than toward the military objective.

The ability of these agents to cause agitated delirium also makes them ideally suited for use in domestic chemical terrorism. It can be expected that the confusion and anxiety among patients presenting to emergency departments in the aftermath of such an attack would present as much of a challenge as the care of those actually exposed.

Potential incapacitating agents include anticholinergics (e.g., BZ), indoles [e.g., D-lysergic acid diethylamide (LSD)], opioids (e.g., fentanyl and related compounds), and cannabinoids, as well as nonchemical agents such as noise, high-intensity photostimulation (bright lights), microwave bombardment, and olfactory assault *(4)*.

## 2. POTENTIAL AS WARFARE AGENTS

Many of these agents were evaluated by the U.S. Joint Non-Lethal Weapons Directorate (JNLWD) at Aberdeen Proving Grounds, MD. Although much of this work is unclassified, it has been withheld by the U.S. National Academies of Science. These agents (except for BZ and related glycolate anticholinergics) are considered by military experts to be unlikely to see use on a modern battlefield owing to a variety of factors. Most nonchemical incapacitating agents are either too dangerous for use (such as microwave bombardment and photostimulation, which may cause retinal damage) or are likely to be ineffective against a determined enemy (such as noise and olfactory assault). American military analysts rejected the development of opioids because of difficulties with dispersal and their narrow safety ratio; it would be difficult to ensure delivery of an effective but nonlethal dose. Cannabinoids and indoles are also felt to be difficult to deliver in reliably effective doses *(4,5)* and have a limited duration of effect. We focus here on BZ (and related compounds), because its high safety ratio renders it the most likely of these agents to be used.

It is possible, however, that this assumption may not hold true in chemical terrorism scenarios for several reasons. Terrorists are likely to be less concerned with the distinction between lethal and incapacitating agents and might be more likely to use compounds that are lethal to many of those exposed. It is also likely that the route of exposure and method of distribution might be different in a terrorist attack than on the battlefield. In warfare, inhalation of an outdoor aerosol is the usual means of delivery, whereas in a terrorist attack the agent could be used to contaminate food, water, or the ventilation system of a building. These differences may very well alter the choice of agent.

This assessment was borne out when Russian authorities reportedly used fentanyl (or possibly a more potent derivative thereof such as carfentanil) in an attempt to rescue hostages held in a Moscow theater in 2002. The agent was delivered through the ventilation system of the theater, rapidly incapacitating the captors and their hostages. However, 116 hostage fatalities and hundreds of prolonged hospitalizations, presumably owing to hypoxic brain injury, also reportedly occurred *(6,7)*. Metabolites of halothane were detected in the serum of two German victims, leading to some controversy over the actual agent used *(8)*. Halothane seems a reasonable explanation for the incredibly rapid incapacitation seen, although it would not explain the miosis that led physicians on the scene to suspect a nerve agent and administer atropine. If fentanyl or a derivative was in fact the agent used, it was undeniably effective at neutralizing the hostage-takers, although it can no longer be considered an incapacitating agent because of its high lethality (at least in the absence of prompt airway management, ventilation, and/or antidotal therapy with naloxone).

## 3. HISTORICAL AND CONTEMPORARY USE

Some of the earliest historical accounts of chemical weapon use involve anticholinergic compounds. Goodman conducted an unpublished review of the history of these agents in 1961. Maharbal, a soldier in Hannibal's army in 184 BC, used mandrake (containing hyoscyamine and scopolamine) to poison the wine of African rebels, returning later to kill them in their sleep *(5,9)*. In the 11th century, Duncan, the king of Scotland, poisoned invading Norwegians with wine tainted by "sleepy nightshade" *(10–12)*. In 1672, the Bishop of Münster unsuccessfully used grenades containing belladonna in his assault on Gröningen, demonstrating one of the persistent difficulties in deploying chemical weapons when the wind blew the drug back toward his own forces *(4,5)*. In 1676, Governor Berkeley of Virginia sent a group of soldiers to Jamestown to quell the Bacon Rebellion. The soldiers gathered the plant now known as *Jamestown (or Jimson) weed*,

*Datura stramonium*, for a salad and suffered anticholinergic delirium. A record from the time tells of how they "turn'd natural Fools upon it for several Days" and describes in detail the extensive impairment of these soldiers *(13,14)*. In 1881, French troops in North Africa were incapacitated by dates poisoned with *Hyoscyamus falezlez* by local resistance forces *(5,15–17)*. In 1908, French forces again succumbed to anticholinergic poisoning in Hanoi, when their dinner was tainted with *Datura*, allegedly by two indigenous officers and an artilleryman in conspiracy with pro-Chinese ex-river pirates *(18,19)*.

In the years following World War II, the United States government and the Soviet Union both became very interested in incapacitating agents, and the United States settled on BZ as the most suitable agent. By 1966, the U.S. Army Chemical Corps had successfully weaponized this agent and stockpiled arms capable of delivering it *(4,5)*. Production of BZ ended when it was realized that it had unpredictable effects on front-line troops *(20)*, and the agent never saw operational use, despite suggestions to the contrary in the film *Jacob's Ladder (5)*. The United States signed the Geneva Convention Against Chemical Weapons in 1975, 50 years after it was first adopted by most nations *(4)*. Demilitarization of existing stockpiles began in the late 1980s, and by 1988, only a few remaining grams of BZ were thought to exist *(4,20)*. Interestingly, the United States has deployed an incapacitating agent in the form of noise, with questionable efficacy. Loud, irritating rock music was played during the assault on President Noriega's forces in Panama in 1989 and again in the attack on the Branch Davidian compound in Waco, Texas in 1993 *(4)*.

In the 1990s, the spectre of BZ reappeared, as similar agents were stockpiled by Yugoslavia and Iraq, and in some cases, they may have been used by these countries. It has been proved that the Yugoslav Federal Army used irritants and anticholinesterase agents in 1991, and it is alleged to have used anticholinergic agents against civilians fleeing Srebrenica for free territory in Bosnia in 1995 *(21,22)*. Anticholinergic incapacitating agents were suspected based on clinical findings, although physical evidence has been lacking *(5)*. One analysis concluded that the hallucinations these people experienced may have been owing to the consequence of multiple stresses: artillery attacks, exhaustion because of lack of sleep, starvation, thirst, and the effects of drinking unpurified water, although chemical weapons could not be ruled out *(21)*. Iraq was accused by the British Ministry of Defense of having stockpiled a glycolate anticholinergic compound known as Agent 15, which is thought to be either identical or similar to BZ *(5)*. Iraq used chemical weapons against the Kurds in Northern Iraq, but there is no conclusive evidence that incapacitating agents were ever used.

BZ is currently classified as a Schedule 2 compound by the Chemical Weapons Convention (officially, the Convention on the Prohibition of the Development, Production, Stockpiling and Use of Chemical Weapons and on Their Destruction) of 1993. Schedule 2 compounds are high-risk precursors and toxic compounds with moderate commercial use that will be restricted 3 years after the treaty enters into effect *(23)*. One hundred forty-six nations have signed this agreement. The United States signed it in 1993 and ratified it in 1997.

## 4. PHYSICOCHEMICAL CHARACTERISTICS

BZ is known chemically as 3-quinuclidinyl benzilate [Chemical Abstract Service (CAS) registry number 6581-06-2] or QNB. It is a synthetic glycolic acid ester and exists as an odorless white crystalline solid. Because its vapor pressure is very low (0.5 m/m$^3$

at 70°C), it must be dispersed as an aerosol. BZ is only slightly soluble in water but is soluble in dilute acids and organic solvents such as propylene glycol. Its environmental half-life is 3–4 wk in moist air at 25°C. It is also heat-stable, with a half-life in solution of over 2 h at 235°C and a flash point of 246°C, allowing it to be dispersed by heat-producing munitions (explosives) *(5,24)*.

## 5. TOXICODYNAMICS/TOXICOKINETICS/TOXICITY

BZ is a competitive muscarinic cholinergic receptor antagonist. Muscarinic cholinergic receptors bind the neurotransmitter acetylcholine within the central nervous system, at postganglionic parasympathetic targets and on sweat glands *(25)*. In the central nervous system, BZ is approximately 25 times more potent than atropine and 3 times more potent than scopolamine *(4,26)*. This is owing both to its greater ability to cross the blood-brain barrier and to its higher affinity for the muscarinic cholinergic receptors prevalent in the central nervous system (M1 subtype) *(27,28)*. It has no known effect on nicotinic acetylcholine receptors. Although all known preparations of BZ have been racemic mixtures, the R-stereoisomer has the greater affinity for muscarinic receptors *(29)*.

BZ is 80% bioavailable when delivered orally and 40–50% as effective by inhalation as it is parenterally. The onset of effect after inhalational exposure is about 60 min. When dissolved in a propylene glycol vehicle, it can be absorbed transdermally, resulting in serum levels equal to 5–10% of a similar parenteral dose. When delivered topically, BZ has a particularly delayed onset of effect, possibly as much as 24–36 h when cleaned off within 1 h *(3,30)*. Generally, peripheral effects are seen initially, with progression to central effects over the following 4–12 h. Although the half-life of BZ in vivo remains unstudied *(20)*, the observed duration of effect has been as long as 96 h *(4,5)*. Metabolism is presumed to be both hepatic and renal, with excretion of both unchanged drug and metabolites in urine *(5)*.

BZ has a large safety ratio. In mice, the $LD_{50}$ (defined as the dose at which 50% of those exposed will die) is 18–25 mg/kg *(20)*. The $LCt_{50}$ (the concentration time product at which 50% of those exposed will die) in humans is estimated at 200,000 mg × min/m³ *(5)*. The $ICt_{50}$ (the concentration time product at which 50% of those exposed will be incapacitated) is reportedly between 100 and 112 mg × min/m³ *(5,24)*, whereas the $ID_{50}$ (the dose at which 50% of those exposed will be incapacitated) is reported as 6.2 μg/kg *(4)* or 0.5 mg *(26)*. The Army field drinking water standards permit exposure of soldiers to 0.5μg/kg/d. This NOAEL (no observed adverse effect level) is based on an unpublished study done by Major James S. Ketchum in 1963 *(20)*. Four healthy male volunteers were exposed to daily doses of 0.5 μg/kg of BZ intramuscularly for 5 consecutive days and again 3 days later. At the end of the exposure period, the subjects complained of rash, malaise, dysphagia, or low-grade fever, none of which was considered by the researchers to be caused by BZ *(20)*.

It is important to consider that although BZ is currently the best known antimuscarinic incapacitating agent, it is possible that clandestine research could lead to other similar agents with different toxicokinetics and different toxicodynamics.

## 6. CLINICAL MANIFESTATIONS

Medical students are often taught the mnemonic "mad as a hatter, hot as a hare, red as a beet, dry as a bone, full as a flask, and blind as a bat" when learning about the anticholinergic toxidrome. These correspond to the clinical effects of delirium, agitation and hallucination, (central effects), hyperthermia, flushing, anhidrosis and drying of mucosal secretions, urinary retention, and mydriasis (peripheral effects). Tachycardia with normal or slightly elevated blood pressure is also expected (also a peripheral effect), although in a patient with a delayed presentation, the heart rate may also be normal owing to centrally mediated effects (5). These symptoms are essentially the opposite of those expected in patients exposed to nerve agents (i.e., organophosphorus cholinesterase inhibitors).

Anticholinergic patients have difficulty communicating, both because of delirium and because of profound desiccation of the oral mucosa. "Woolgathering" behavior, or picking at small imaginary objects has often been described with anticholinergic intoxication. This may be related to the fact that hallucinations are characteristically of the Lilliputian type, meaning they typically involve miniature objects and people (5). It is said that the subjects of these hallucinations tend to get smaller and smaller over time (5). These may be distinguished from hallucinations owing to indole-type agents (e.g., LSD) and cannabinoids (e.g., marijuana derivatives) both by the pronounced peripheral effects of anticholinergic agents and by the presence of delirium, which is typically absent in pure hallucinogenic agents (26). This delirium may be associated with agitated or even violent behavior, and patients may be exceedingly difficult to control. It should be noted that late in the course of anticholinergic poisoning, the peripheral effects may resolve while the centrally mediated delirium remains. Synesthesia, or crossing of sensory perceptions, may be considered diagnostic of serotonergic (i.e., indole-type) exposure.

## 7. DIAGNOSIS

BZ can be detected in urine by gas chromatography with mass spectroscopy in the research laboratory setting (31), but this is unlikely to be available in a timely fashion in clinical practice. There is not yet any reliable field laboratory or bedside assay for BZ, so diagnosis in individual patients depends on recognition of the clinical manifestations of the anticholinergic toxidrome, as described above. It is likely that in a chemical terrorism scenario large numbers of patients may present simultaneously, possibly to different hospitals. Poison control centers and other public health institutions will probably be instrumental in recognizing epidemic poisoning, as was demonstrated in New York City in the Case Vignette described earlier. At that time, even before the heroin adulterant was identified as scopolamine, local health care personnel were alerted to the existence of this problem with an anticholinergic agent (1,2). Interestingly, Osama bin Laden has reportedly threatened to send a new "super potent heroin" to the United States in an effort to create more addiction and havoc than the form presently available (32). If this scenario were to occur today, it is likely that chemical terrorism would be an immediate consideration and that appropriate authorities would be quickly notified.

## 8. TREATMENT

### 8.1. Decontamination

In a military setting, it may be too late for decontamination to be very effective by the time symptoms become manifest, as providers are likely to have already been exposed during the long latent period (5). In the civilian setting, appropriate triage and decontamination will be an absolute priority, particularly if the agent has been delivered in a propylene glycol vehicle to enhance transdermal absorption. The first and most important step toward decontamination is the careful removal of contaminated clothes. This alone removes most of the contaminant in most exposures. The patient should then be washed in large volumes of water. Soap may be used, if available, but copious water is believed to be sufficient *(26)*. Patients should ideally be decontaminated before transfer to the nearest hospital facility to prevent exposure to prehospital and hospital personnel *(33)*. Unlike the situation on the battlefield, however, civilian patients are likely to disperse after their exposure. Because of the delayed onset of signs and symptoms and the mobility of the civilian population, patients may present at widely scattered sites, making the establishment of central decontamination areas problematic.

## 8.2. Restraint

Soft physical restraints are an important element of the management of these patients and would be expected to be particularly significant in the setting of a mass exposure, potentially enabling a few providers to care for large numbers of patients safely. Once patients are safely restrained, rapid conversion to sedation is preferred, because physical restraint of agitated patients may worsen hyperthermia and increase the risk of rhabdomyolysis. In the military setting or if civilian authorities are exposed, it would also be critical to disarm these patients, as they may be dangerous to themselves and others as delirium worsens *(30)*.

## 8.3. Cooling

Hyperthermia is an important cause of morbidity and mortality in anticholinergic poisoning and is a key mediator of many of the potentially significant sequelae, such as rhabdomyolysis. With temperatures greater than 41.1°C (106°F), the patient is at great risk for end-organ injury so sedation of psychomotor agitation along with rapid cooling with fans, cool mist, ice, and/or submersion baths should be instituted *(34)*. There is no role for antipyretics in this setting, as these agents work by lowering the hypothalamic set point, which is not elevated in anticholinergic-mediated hyperthermia *(35)*.

## 8.4. Physostigmine

Physostigmine was recognized as an anticholinergic antagonist by Fraser in 1863 *(36)* and was first used as an antidote to anticholinergic poisoning by Kleinwachter in 1864 *(37)*. As a carbamate acetylcholinesterase inhibitor with good penetration across the blood–brain barrier *(38,39)*, physostigmine is effective in reversing anticholinergic delirium, as well as the anticholinergic peripheral effects of over 600 agents *(40)*. In 1968, Duvoisin and Katz *(41)* revisited this antidote, advocating its wider use in reversing anticholinergic poisoning. In the 1970s, physostigmine was found to be effective at waking patients intoxicated by many agents with and without anticholinergic effects *(36)*. Its ability to reverse non-anticholinergic delirium is felt to be owing to its activity as a nonspecific analeptic, possibly through a cholinergic effect on the reticular activating system *(42)*.

Enthusiasm for physostigmine waned after several case reports of asystole associated with its administration in the setting of tricyclic antidepressant poisoning *(43)*. Many are now reluctant to use this agent even in clear cases of anticholinergic poisoning. In fact, one review of incapacitating agents (from a non-peer-reviewed source) advises against using physostigmine for BZ intoxication *(33)*. It is important to remember, however, that pure anticholinergic agents such as BZ are fundamentally different from complex drugs like tricyclic antidepressants. In addition to their antimuscarinic action, tricyclic antidepressants have sodium channel-blocking effects and α-1-adrenergic antagonist effects, causing cardiac toxicity and hypotension owing to peripheral vasodilation. Both of these effects may potentially have contributed to asystole in the cases reportedly caused by physostigmine administration. In a chemical terrorism attack, the large numbers of patients presenting with the anticholinergic toxidrome should make tricyclic antidepressant poisoning less of a consideration.

Most recent evidence suggests that physostigmine is beneficial when used in the proper setting. When patients present with both peripheral anticholinergic effects as well as central anticholinergic delirium, after tricyclic antidepressant intoxication has been ruled out by electrocardiography (QRS complex less than 100 ms) and physostigmine is given slowly and titrated to effect, this agent can be useful and safe *(36)*. Relative contraindications include asthma or other bronchospastic disease, peripheral vascular disease, intestinal or bladder obstruction, intraventricular conduction defects, and atrioventricular block *(36)*. A retrospective study of 52 patients suggested that physostigmine is as effective as benzodiazepines in treating anticholinergic toxicity *(44)*. Physostigmine has been studied by the U.S. military for the treatment of BZ intoxication and shown to be effective in several volunteers *(45,46)*.

Physostigmine is active by the intravenous, intramuscular, and oral routes *(47)*. In civilian clinical practice, the intravenous route is generally preferred, although military sources have recommended intramuscular and even oral treatment, particularly when treating large numbers of casualties *(4)*. The intravenous dose is 1–2 mg in adults and 0.02 mg/kg in children (with a maximum of 0.5 mg) infused over 5–10 min. Slow administration allows the infusion to be stopped if the patient develops signs of cholinergic toxicity (e.g., salivation, lacrimation, urination, defecation, emesis, bradycardia, bronchospasm, bronchorrhea, or muscle weakness, a nicotinic effect). Additional doses may be given after 10–15 min if anticholinergic signs and symptoms persist. Atropine should be available at the bedside when physostigmine is given, in case of life-threatening cholinergic toxicity (bronchorrhea, bronchospasm, or bradycardia) *(36)*. Physostigmine has an onset of effect in 10–15 min and a half-life of 16 min, although its duration of action may be as much as five times longer *(48)*. In treating a long-acting agent such as BZ, multiple doses would be necessary. Physostigmine should not be confused with pyridostigmine, an agent used as prophylaxis against nerve agent exposure. Pyridostigmine is also a carbamate cholinesterase inhibitor, but it does not cross the blood–brain barrier and so would not be expected to have any role in the reversal of anticholinergic delirium.

### *8.5. Sedation*

If supplies of physostigmine are limited, or if specific contraindications to its use are present, it is reasonable to sedate patients with agitated delirium from anticholinergic agents. Benzodiazepines would be the drugs of choice in this situation.

## 9. COMPLICATIONS AND PERSISTENT SEQUELAE

There are no known permanent or chronic effects specifically related to BZ. However, significant psychiatric and psychological sequelae should be expected, such as post-traumatic stress disorder (PTSD). A recent survey found that the prevalence of PTSD in New York City after the September 11 attack is as much as 11%, higher than that in other cities *(49)*. Potential medical complications of anticholinergic poisoning include ileus and consequences of heat stroke such as rhabdomyolysis and disseminated intravascular coagulation *(33)*. The treatment of these entities is similar to their treatment when they have other causes.

## 10. SPECIAL POPULATIONS

### 10.1. Children

There have been no published studies on the effect of BZ on children. There are some data, however, on the effect of other anticholinergic agents. During the Persian Gulf War, atropine autoinjectors were distributed to the Israeli population in preparation for a possible nerve gas attack. Children were the victims in 116 of 240 cases of unintentional self-administration of atropine during the war. Although some children did get sick, there were no fatalities or significant morbidity *(50)*. This suggests that children are able to tolerate at least a modest overdose with these agents. There are reports of sporadic outbreaks of anticholinergic poisoning in adolescents associated with the use of Jimson weed (*Datura stramonium*). Typically, a small group of these patients will present with anticholinergic poisoning after using the plant recreationally. Effects are generally similar to those seen in adults. Usually the patients will have prolonged delirium, and several deaths have been reported *(51)*.

### 10.2. The Elderly

The elderly are exquisitely sensitive to the central effects of anticholinergic drugs. There may be both pharmacodynamic (age-related limitation in cholinergic transmission) and pharmacokinetic (more limited drug metabolism and elimination) alterations compared with younger patients. Also, many of these patients (nearly 60%) are already prescribed drugs with anticholinergic activity. Pre-existing constipation may make these patients more susceptible to paralytic ileus. Pre-existing visual problems are likely to be exacerbated by exposure to BZ, and patients with narrow-angle glaucoma are at particular risk. Furthermore, coexisting cardiovascular disease is expected to compromise the ability of these patients to tolerate the tachycardia associated with anticholinergic poisoning *(52)*.

### 10.3. Pregnant Women

Atropine and scopolamine cross the placenta in humans, at least in late pregnancy. Studies of perinatal atropine administered to pregnant women demonstrate atropine levels in the umbilical artery equal to 50% of umbilical venous levels *(53–55)*. Studies of the effects of BZ administered to pregnant woman have not been reported. Given the ability of widely different anticholinergic agents to cross the blood–placenta barrier, especially scopolamine, it is reasonable to assume that BZ will have effects on the fetus as well. There are no data on fetal effects when exposure occurs in early development. As in all cases, the appropriate care of the mother is the most important step toward ensuring the best possible outcome for the fetus. Fetal monitoring would seem a reasonable adjunct to the care of these patients. Scopolamine (termed *twilight sleep*) has been used in the past as an amnestic adjunct for anesthesia during labor In one case series, 15 of these patients were reversed with physostigmine as they progressed to delivery and then treated with meperidine and diazepam. None of the women suffered adverse effects and 5-min Apgar scores were 8–10 in all children *(56)*.

## 11. CHALLENGES

Chemical agents used in terrorist attack are likely to result in major problems for health care systems independent of any physical illness caused. Terrorism exists to instill fear, and chemical weapons are well suited to this purpose. In the aftermath of a chemical attack, it can be expected that hospital emergency departments will be overwhelmed with the worried well. At the same time, they will probably be working with insufficient staffing. A survey of hospital staff in Israel during the Gulf War revealed that only 42% of hospital staff would show up at work in the event of a chemical attack *(57)*. Appropriate education of hospital staff as well as preparation (in terms of equipment, procedures, and training) to ensure their safety will be important in addressing these challenges.

## 12. PREVENTION

### *12.1. Detection*

No field detector is currently available for the detection of these agents. Research done for the U.S. demilitarization program to detect contamination of surrounding areas may now be employed to detect evidence of clandestine development or testing of these agents. In declassified military research from 1983, there was great difficulty in reliably detecting BZ in air and water samples *(58)*. In 1990, BZ was shown to be detectable in complex media such as soil using supercritical fluid chromatography in the laboratory *(59)*. These methods will potentially be important in enforcing the Chemical Weapons Convention and preventing the proliferation of these agents.

### *12.2. Personal Protective Equipment*

On the battlefield and for chemical demilitarization, the Department of the Army Technical Manual recommends maximum protection, including either a demilitarization protective ensemble (DPE) or a combination of an M9 mask and hood, M3 butyl rubber suit, M2A1 butyl boots, butyl (M3 or M4) or neoprene gloves, and unimpregnated underwear *(24)*.

In the civilian realm, decontamination prior to transport to the hospital will be key. Although there is no evidence-based rationale for any specific type of personal protective equipment (PPE), it would seem prudent that prehospital personnel involved in decontaminating victims wear the civilian equivalent of the military equipment above (level C protection).

### *12.3. Pretreatment*

During the Persian Gulf War, U.S. soldiers were pretreated with pyridostigmine as prophylaxis against potential nerve agent exposure. Physostigmine has not been used for this purpose because the doses required would cause significant central nervous system cholinergic effects, such as vomiting *(5)*. The effectiveness of pretreatment with pyridostigmine as protection against centrally acting anticholinergic agents remains unstudied, but pretreatment is unlikely to be effective because of its inability to penetrate the blood-brain barrier, as discussed earlier. There is at least some anecdotal evidence to support this; in Israel during the Gulf War, one soldier who had been pretreated with pyridostigmine presented with anticholinergic illness after injecting himself with atropine from his nerve gas antidote kit *(25)*.

## 13. SUMMARY

BZ, an antimuscarinic agent with a large safety ratio, is considered the most likely incapacitating agent to be used. Opioids such as fentanyl are too lethal to be considered incapacitating agents. Diagnosis of BZ intoxication in an individual patient depends on clinically recognizing the anticholinergic toxidrome. Poison centers will be instrumental in recognizing mass exposure, particularly because of delayed onset of effect. Treatment centers on decontamination, supportive care such as restraint, sedation, and cooling, and specific therapy with physostigmine. It is likely that emergency departments will be overwhelmed with the worried well, so efficient triage is essential. Psychiatric and psychological effects are likely to be a significant problem long after recovery from the actual exposure. The best way currently available to prevent these attacks is to keep these agents out of the hands of potential adversaries and terrorists. Technologies to detect contamination with these agents in soil, air, and water will aid in this effort.

## REFERENCES

1. Hamilton RJ, Perrone J, Hoffman R, et al. A descriptive study of an epidemic of poisoning caused by heroin adulterated with scopolamine. J Toxicol Clin Toxicol 2000;38:597–608.
2. CDC. Scopolamine poisoning among heroin users—New York City, Newark, Philadelphia, and Baltimore, 1995 and 1996. MMWR 1996;45:457–460.
3. US Army. Incapacitating agents. In: NATO Manual FM8-285/NAVMED P-5041/AFM 160-11. Department of the Army, Falls Church, VA, 1990.
4. Ketchum JS, Sidell FR. Incapacitating agents. In: Sidell FR, Takafuji ET, Franz DR, eds. Textbook of Military Medicine: Medical Aspects of Chemical and Biologic Warfare. Borden Institute, Washington, DC, 1997, pp. 287–305.
5. U.S. Army Medical Research Institute of Chemical Defense. Incapacitating agents, BZ, Agent 15. In: Medical Management of Chemical Casualties Handbook, 3rd ed. Chemical Casualty Care Division, Aberdeen Proving Ground, MD, 2000, pp. 129–149.
6. Meyers SL. Hostage drama in Moscow: Russia responds; Putin vows hunt for terror cells around the world. NY Times October 29, 2002;A1.
7. Kommersant, Moscow [Russian]. Some Russian doctors say Moscow theater hostages may never fully recover. BBC Worldwide Monitoring October 30, 2002.
8. Mitchell S. Experts dispute Russia gas label. United Press International October 30, 2002.
9. Frontinus SJ, Bennet CH, trans. The Strategems. William Heinemann, London, 1925. Quoted in: Goodman E. The Descriptive Toxicology of Atropine. Unpublished manuscript, Edgewood Arsenal, MD, 1961. Cited in: Ketchum JS, Sidell FR. Incapacitating agents. In: Sidell FR, Takafuji ET, Franz DR, eds. Textbook of Military Medicine: Medical Aspects of Chemical and Biologic Warfare. Borden Institute, Washington, DC, 1997, pp. 287–305.
10. Buchanan G, Watkins J, trans. The History of Scotland. Henry Fisher, Son, and P. Jackson, London, 1831. Cited in: Goodman E. The Descriptive Toxicology of Atropine. Unpublished manuscript, Edgewood Arsenal, MD, 1961. Cited in: Ketchum JS, Sidell FR. Incapacitating agents. In: Sidell FR, Takafuji ET, Franz DR, eds. Textbook of Military Medicine: Medical Aspects of Chemical and Biologic Warfare. Borden Institute, Washington, DC, 1997, pp. 287–305.
11. Lewin L. Die Gifte in der Waltgeschichte. Julius Springer, Berlin, 1920, pp. 537–538. Cited in: Goodman E. The Descriptive Toxicology of Atropine. Unpublished manuscript, Edgewood Arsenal, MD, 1961. Cited in: Ketchum JS, Sidell FR. Incapacitating Agents. In: Sidell FR, Takafuji ET, Franz DR, eds. Textbook of Military Medicine: Medical Aspects of Chemical and Biologic Warfare. Borden Institute, Washington, DC, 1997, pp. 287–305.

12. Mitchell TD. Materia Medica and Therapeutics, 2nd ed. JB Lippincott, Philadelphia, 1857, p. 233. Cited in: Goodman E. The Descriptive Toxicology of Atropine. Unpublished manuscript, Edgewood Arsenal, MD, 1961. Cited in: Ketchum JS, Sidell FR. Incapacitating agents. In: Sidell FR, Takafuji ET, Franz DR, eds. Textbook of Military Medicine: Medical Aspects of Chemical and Biologic Warfare. Borden Institute, Washington, DC, 1997, pp. 287–305.

13. Lewis WH, Elvin-Lewis MPF. Medical Botany: Plants Affecting Man's Health. John Wiley & Sons, New York, 1977, p. 424.

14. Jennings RE. Stramonium poisoning: a review of the literature and report of two cases. J Pediatr 1935;6:657–664.

15. Leder R. Sahara. Hanover House, Garden City, NY, 1954, pp. 151 ff. Cited in: Goodman E. The Descriptive Toxicology of Atropine. Unpublished manuscript, Edgewood Arsenal, MD, 1961. Cited in: Ketchum JS, Sidell FR. Incapacitating agents. In: Sidell FR, Takafuji ET, Franz DR, eds. Textbook of Military Medicine: Medical Aspects of Chemical and Biologic Warfare. Borden Institute, Washington, DC, 1997, pp. 287–305.

16. Skolle J. Azalei. Harper and Brother, New York, 1956, pp. 22 ff. Cited in: Goodman E. The Descriptive Toxicology of Atropine. Unpublished manuscript, Edgewood Arsenal, MD. 1961. Cited in: Ketchum JS, Sidell FR. Incapacitating agents. In: Sidell FR, Takafuji ET, Franz DR, eds. Textbook of Military Medicine: Medical Aspects of Chemical and Biologic Warfare. Borden Institute, Washington, DC, 1997, pp. 287–305.

17. Cornewin C. Des Plantes Veneneuses. Librarie de Firmin-Didot et Cit, Paris, 1893, p. 473. Cited in: Goodman E. The Descriptive Toxicology of Atropine. Edgewood Arsenal, MD. Unpublished manuscript, 1961. Cited in: Ketchum JS, Sidell FR. Incapacitating agents. In: Sidell FR, Takafuji ET, Franz DR, eds. Textbook of Military Medicine: Medical Aspects of Chemical and Biologic Warfare. Borden Institute, Washington, DC, 1997, pp. 287–305.

18. Lewin L. Gifte and Vergiftungen. Georg Stilke, Berlin, 1929, p. 809. Cited in: Goodman E. The Descriptive Toxicology of Atropine. Unpublished manuscript, Edgewood Arsenal, MD, 1961. Cited in: Ketchum JS, Sidell FR. Incapacitating agents. In: Sidell FR, Takafuji ET, Franz DR, eds. Textbook of Military Medicine: Medical Aspects of Chemical and Biologic Warfare. Borden Institute, Washington, DC, 1997, pp. 287–305.

19. The Times. London, 3 July 1908:8; 9 July 1908:7. Cited in: Goodman, E. The Descriptive Toxicology of Atropine. Unpublished manuscript, Edgewood Arsenal, MD, 1961. Cited in: Ketchum JS, Sidell FR. Incapacitating agents. In: Sidell FR, Takafuji ET, Franz DR, eds. Textbook of Military Medicine: Medical Aspects of Chemical and Biologic Warfare. Borden Institute, Washington, DC, 1997, pp. 287–305.

20. The National Academy of Sciences. Guidelines for chemical 3-quinuclidinyl benzilate. In: Guidelines for Chemical Warfare Agents in Military Field Drinking Water 2000, pp. 15–18, 55–65. Available at http://www.nap.edu/openbook/N1000954/html/15.html. Accessed on 10/4/2002.

21. Hay A. Surviving the impossible: the long march from Srebrenica. An investigation of the possible use of chemical warfare agents. Med Confl Surviv 1998;14:120–155.

22. Plavsik F, Petrovecki M, Fuchs R, et al. [The chemical war in Croatia]. [Serbo-Croatian] Lijnecnicki Vjesnik 1992;114:1–5.

23. The Henry L Stimson Center. Chemicals controlled by the chemical weapons convention. 2002. Available at http://www.stimson.org/cbw/?sn=CB2001121898. Accessed on 10/4/2002.

24. U.S. Army Center for Health Promotion and Preventive Medicine. Detailed facts about psychedelic agent 3-quinuclidinyl benzilate (BZ). The Deputy For Technical Services' Publication: Detailed Chemical Fact Sheets. 1998. Available at: http://chppm-www.apgea.army.mil/dts/dtchemfs.htm. Accessed on 10/4/2002.

25. Brown JH, Taylor P. Muscarinic receptor agonists and antagonists. In: Hardman JG, Limbird LE, Gilman AG, eds. Goodman & Gilman's The Pharmacological Basis Of Therapeutics, 10th ed. McGraw-Hill, New York, 2001, pp. 155–173.

26. Suchard JR. Chemical and biological weapons. In: Goldfrank LR, Flomenbaum NE, Lewin NA, Howland MA, Hoffmann RS, Nelson LS, eds. Goldfrank's Toxicologic Emergencies, 7th ed. McGraw-Hill, New York, 2002, pp. 1527–1551.

27. Gibson RE, Rzeszotarski WJ, Jagoda EM, et al. 3-Quinuclidinyl 4-iodobenzilate: a high affinity, high specific activity radioligand for the M1 and M2 acetylcholine receptors. Life Sci 1984;34:2287–2296.

28. Eglen RM, Watson N. Selective muscarinic agonists and antagonists. Pharmacol Toxicol 1996;78:59–68.

29. Rzeszotarski WJ, McPherson DW, Ferkany JW, et al. Affinity and selectivity of the optical isomers of 3-quinuclidinyl benzilate and related muscarinic antagonists. J Med Chem 1988;31:1463–1466.

30. McKee CB, Collins L, Keetley J, et al. The Medical NBC Battlebook, USACHPPM Tech Guide 244. U.S. Army Center for Health Promotion and Preventive Medicine, 2000, pp. 5-1–5-55.
31. Byrd GD, Paule RC, Sander LC, et al. Determination of 3-quinuclidinyl benzilate (QNB) and its major metabolites in urine by isotope dilution gas chromatography/mass spectrometry. J Anal Toxicol 1992;16:182–187.
32. Meier B. "Super" heroin was planned by bin Laden, reports say. NY Times. October 4, 2001;B3.
33. Holstege CP, Baylor M. CBRNE—incapacitating agents, 3-quinuclidinyl benzilate. EMedicine 2002. Available at: http://www.emedicine.com/emerg/topic912.htm. Accessed on 10/4/2002.
34. Vassallo SU, Delaney KA. Thermoregulatory principles. In: Goldfrank LR, Flomenbaum NE, Lewin NA, Howland MA, Hoffmann RS, Nelson LS, eds. Goldfrank's Toxicologic Emergencies, 7th ed. McGraw-Hill, New York, 2002, pp. 261–281.
35. Dinarello CA, Wolff SM. Pathogenesis of fever in man. N Engl J Med 1978;298:607–612.
36. Howland MA. Antidotes in depth: physostigmine. In: Goldfrank LR, Flomenbaum NE, Lewin NA, Howland MA, Hoffmann RS, Nelson LS, eds. Goldfrank's Toxicologic Emergencies, 7th ed. McGraw-Hill, New York, 2002, pp. 544–547.
37. Nickalls RWD, Nickalls EA. The first use of physostigmine in the treatment of atropine poisoning. Anaesthesia 1988;43:776–779.
38. Taylor P. Anticholinesterase agents. In: Hardman JG, Limbird LE, Gilman AG, eds. Goodman & Gilman's The Pharmacological Basis of Therapeutics, 10th ed. McGraw-Hill, New York, 2001, pp. 175–191
39. Atack JR, Yu QS, Soncrant TT, et al. Comparative inhibitory effects of various physostigmine analogs against acetyl- and butyrylcholinesterases. J Pharmacol Exp Ther 1989;249:194–202.
40. Daunderer M. Physostigmine salicylate as an antidote. Int J Clin Pharmacol Ther Toxicol 1980;18:523–535.
41. Duvoisin RC, Katz R. Reversal of central anticholinergic syndrome in man by physostigmine. JAMA 1968;206:1963–1965.
42. Nilsson E. Physostigmine treatment in various drug-induced intoxications. Ann Clin Res 1982;14:165–172.
43. Pentel P, Peterson CD. Asystole complicating physostigmine treatment of tricyclic antidepressant overdose. Ann Emerg Med 1980;9:588–590.
44. Burns MJ, Linden CH, Graudins A, et al. A comparison of physostigmine and benzodiazepines for the treatment of anticholinergic poisoning. Ann Emerg Med 2000;35:374–381.
45. Ketchum JS. The Human Assessment of BZ. Chemical Research and Development Laboratory, Edgewood Arsenal, MD, 1963. Technical Memorandum 20-29. Cited in: Ketchum JS, Sidell FR. Incapacitating agents. In: Sidell FR, Takafuji ET, Franz DR, eds. Textbook of Military Medicine: Medical Aspects of Chemical and Biologic Warfare. Borden Institute, Washington, DC, 1997, pp. 287–305.
46. Ketchum JS, Tharp B, Crowell E, et al. The Human Assessment of BZ Disseminated Under Field Conditions. Edgewood Arsenal, MD, 1967. Edgewood Arsenal Technical Report 4140. Ketchum JS, Sidell FR. Incapacitating agents. In: Sidell FR, Takafuji ET, Franz DR, eds. Textbook of Military Medicine: Medical Aspects of Chemical and Biologic Warfare. Borden Institute, Washington, DC, 1997, pp. 287–305.
47. Gibson M, Moore T, Smith CM, et al. Physostigmine concentrations after oral doses. Lancet 1985;i:695–696.
48. Asthana S, Greig NH, Hegedus L, et al. Clinical pharmacokinetics of physostigmine in patients with Alzheimer's disease. Clin Pharmacol Ther 1995;58:299–309.
49. Schlenger WF, Caddell JM, Ebert L, et al. Psychological reactions to terrorist attacks—findings from the national study of Americans' reactions to September 11. JAMA 2000;288:581–588.
50. Amitai Y, Almog S, Singer R, et al. Atropine poisoning in children during the Persian Gulf crisis—a national survey in Israel. JAMA 1992;268:630–632.
51. CDC. Jimson weed poisoning—Texas, New York, and California, 1994. MMWR 1995;44:41–44.
52. Mintzer J, Burns A. Anticholinergic side-effects of drugs in elderly people. J R Soc Med 2000;93:457–462.
53. Kanto J, Lindberg R, Pihlajamaki K, et al. Placental and blood-CSF transfer of intramuscularly administered atropine in the same person. Pharmacol Toxicol 1987;60:108–109.
54. Onnen I, Barrier G, d'Athis P, et al. Placental transfer of atropine at the end of pregnancy. Eur J Clin Pharmacol 1979;15:443–446.
55. Kivalo I, Saarikoski S. Placental transmission of atropine at full-term pregnancy. Br J Anaesth 1977;49:1017–1021.
56. Smiler BG, Bartholomew EG, Sivak BJ, et al. Physostigmine reversal of scopolamine delirium in obstetric patients. Am J Obstet Gynecol 1973;116:326–329.

57. Shapira Y, Marganitt B, Roziner I, et al. Willingness of staff to report to their hospital duties following an unconventional missile attack: a state-wide survey. Isr J Med Sci 1991;27:656–658.
58. Vigus ES, Deiner A. The determination of trace quantities of BZ (3-quinuclindinyl benzilate) in air and water. Technical Report ARCSL-TR-83031, Project C23. Aberdeen Proving Ground, MD, 1983.
59. Elizy MW, Ferguson FE, Bossle PC, et al. Supercritical fluid application for the analysis of lewisite (L) and 3-quinuclidinyl benzilate (BZ). Technical Report CRDEC-TR-132. Aberdeen Proving Ground, MD, 1990.

# 23    Riot Control Agents

*Richard J. Thomas, MD, MPH,*
*and Philip A. Smith, PhD*

The opinions or assertions contained herein are those of the authors and are not to be construed as official or as representing the position of the Department of the Navy or the Department of Defense.

## CONTENTS

## 1. INTRODUCTION

Exposure to riot control agents (RCAs) produces generally unpleasant, but nonpersistent medical effects *(1 3)*. Persons exposed to these inhalational or dermal contact type chemicals experience acute (but transient) adverse symptoms. This chapter will discuss the classification of riot control agents, their nomenclature and identification, and their management options. In particular, treatment options for the most widely used riot control agents in the United States will be discussed. Excluded from this discussion are chemical agents specifically used to cause damage to lung tissue and that primarily cause pulmonary edema, collectively called pulmonary or choking agents *(1)*. These include chloropicrin (PS), chlorine (Cl), phosgene (CG), and diphosgene (DP), which are discussed by Padilla in Chapter 18 of this text *(4,5)*.

Some authors have documented their concerns about the margin of safety of RCAs in uncontrolled exposures *(6–9)*. The initial presentation of patients exposed to these agents is nonspecific, which poses early management dilemmas for law enforcement personnel,

From: *Physician's Guide to Terrorist Attack*
Edited by: M. J. Roy  © Humana Press Inc., Totowa, NJ

first-level health care providers, physicians, and colleagues in medical treatment facilities when they are attempting to develop a therapeutic course of action.

## 2. HISTORY

The use of irritating chemical agents is believed to date back to as early as the 2nd century BC, when the Romans reportedly used such methods to harass an opponent *(7)*. In 1914, the French introduced gases to military conflict early in World War I, beginning with chloroacetone release in hand and rifle grenades *(10)*. In April 1915, chlorine gas released from over 5700 canisters by the Germans at Ypres, Belgium led to ocular, skin, and pulmonary injuries in over 3000 soldiers within one 18,000-man allied division in just one day *(7,11)*. More than 30 chemical agents were fielded in World War I, with limited military success in changing the course of the war *(7,12)*.

The painful first-hand memories of blinded soldiers from World War I, as well as the public's residual images, did more to limit the use of chemical agents than did the prewar Declaration on the Use of Projectiles the Object of Which is the Diffusion of Asphyxiating or Deleterious Gases of July 29, 1899 *(13)*. A second attempt to develop a worldwide ban on these agents was signed by 38 nations in July 1925 with the Geneva Convention's Protocol for the Prohibition of the Use in War of Asphyxiating, Poisonous or Other Gases, and of Bacteriological Methods of Warfare *(14)*. The United States later ratified this treaty in 1975; however, the U.S. interpretation of the treaty held that non-lethal chemicals such as RCAs were not defined as chemical warfare agents. Also in 1975, President Gerald Ford signed Executive Order 11850, "Renunciation of certain uses in war of chemical herbicides and riot control agents," which precluded first use of these agents by the U.S. military except for specified defensive operations *(15)*.

One of the first RCAs was α-chloroacetophenone [North Atlantic Treaty Organization (NATO) abbreviation CN], developed in 1871. This RCA was used by law enforcement and military personnel from the 1920s to the 1950s *(6,7)*. Beginning in the mid-1960s, CN was sold as a commercial product under the trade name Mace™ *(1)*, which was marketed for personal protection. Newer formulations contain a mixture of CN and pepper spray (capsaicin, NATO abbreviation OC) *(7)*. In 1959, ortho-chlorobenzylidenemalonitrile (NATO abbreviation CS) became the standard U.S. Army riot control and irritant agent *(7)*, three decades after Corson and Stoughton synthesized the agent in 1928 *(16)*. Noting the intensity of the irritant effects to the eyes and nose, they also realized that most of these symptoms could be avoided with the use of a gas mask *(16)*.

## 3. WHAT IS "TEAR GAS"?

To call RCAs "tear gas" is a misnomer. A gas is a general term describing dispersed molecules without definite shape or volume *(17)*. The more descriptive terms "riot control" or "harassing agents" apply to a group of chemicals that are solids or liquids at room temperature and are dispersed in a fume or smoke by a heat-generating process, or deployed as a spray using a propellant or industrial solvent *(5)*. Included under the general term "riot control agents" is a collection of chemical agents that share common adverse effects including ocular pain, spasm of the eyelids (blepharospasm), intense tearing (lacrimation), and copious vasomotor nasal secretions. There is a direct irritant effect on the skin and tissues of the oropharynx and respiratory tract, resulting in cough and chest tightness.

Similar signs and symptoms may occur in persons who are exposed in special situations to obscurant smokes, including ocular and nasal symptoms that can decrease vision and increase a sense of disorientation *(18)*.

Thus, agents that cause these acute irritant symptoms generally fall into three categories: (1) widely used RCAs (discussed in this chapter); (2) other currently lesser used RCAs; and (3) obscurants or smokes. A thorough review of the pharmacology and toxicology of both the widely and less commonly used RCAs listed in Table 1 has recently been published by Olajos and Salem *(19)*.

Nomenclature for these agents may vary for a single agent, e.g., a chemical name such as α-chloroacetophenone; a commercial or trade name such as Mace; or the one- or two-letter NATO designation such as that for α-chloroacetophenone (CN). The origin of the current NATO designation system listed in Table 1 dates back to 1928 with a standardization project of seven agents begun by the U.S. Army Chemical Warfare System including α-chloroacetophenone *(5)*.

## 4. EMPLOYMENT OF RIOT CONTROL AGENTS

The desired effect of RCAs on the target population is that the cumulative signs and symptoms are so intense and unpleasant that a rapid and unplanned escape is the most immediate behavioral reaction. Thus, these agents are useful for both law enforcement and military personnel. In the law enforcement setting, they can be used to quell a civil disturbance or to provide cover for a law enforcement unit that has lost control of a civil demonstration, prison population, or other uprising in an area. In the military setting, RCAs are frequently used as a training aid in a "confidence chamber" (a fixed structure or tent) to demonstrate to trainees that properly worn equipment can protect them from exposure. These agents are also periodically used in outdoor field settings to test the reaction time of military personnel, in quickly and correctly donning their military gas masks.

Both of these groups can employ the tactical use of riot control agents to keep antagonists away during the departure and/or reassembly of the police or military unit at another site, or to cause a dispersal or retreat. This denial of geography to an adversary can be very effective, particularly if members of the exposed population do not posses appropriate personal protective devices.

Hypothetically, an unusually dangerous scenario of RCA use would be in conjunction with exposure to a so-called weapon of mass destruction such as a chemical nerve or blister agent, a "dirty bomb" releasing a low-level radiological exposure, or a biological weapon release. The acute exposure effects caused by riot control agents include disorientation, rapid breathing, and the desire to escape without regard to other personal safety and exposure considerations. These could serve to confuse both the target population and the responders, thereby increasing vulnerability to the secondary and more dangerous attack.

## 5. RIOT CONTROL AGENT EXPOSURE HAZARDS

The toxicology of the three commonly encountered RCAs (CS, CN, and OC) as pure compounds, or mixtures (in the case of OC), are well documented. The estimated lethal concentration to 50% of a test organism population ($LC_{50}$) for CS is greater than that for CN *(19)*. In comparing $LC_{50}$ values, if all other factors (for example, slope of the experi-

Table 1
Riot Control and Some Related Chemical Agents

| Chemical name | NATO designation | CAS number | Molecular weight[a]/ Vapor pressure[b] |
|---|---|---|---|
| Widely used riot control agents | | | |
| 2-Chlorobenzylidene malonitrile | CS | 2698-41-1 | 188/0.00034 |
| (ortho-Chlorobenzylidene malononitrile) | | | |
| Chloroacetophoneone | CN | 532-27-4 | 154/0.005 |
| (2-chloro-1-phenylethanone) | | | |
| Capsaicin | OC | NA[c] | NA[c]/NA[c] |
| Lesser used riot control agents | | | |
| 1-Methoxy-1,3,5-cycloheptatriene | CH | None | 122/1.3 |
| Dibenz-(b,f)-1,4-oxazepine | CR | 257-07-8 | 195/0.000059 |
| 10-Chloro-5,10-dihydrophenarsazine[d] | DM | 578-94-9 | 277/Negligible |
| Obscurants or smokes | | | |
| Zinc oxide | HC | | |
| Phosphorous smokes—3 types | | | |
| (White-most common, red, black) | WP | | |
| Sulfur triozide/chlorosulfoninc acid | FP | | |
| (50%/50% mixture) | | | |

[a]Molecular weight of compound composed of most abundant stable isotopes, rounded to nearest whole number
[b]mm Hg
[c]OC is composed of a complex mixture with variable composition
[d]This is a vomiting agent

mental dose-response curve from which the $LC_{50}$ data are obtained) are the same, and both species have similar dose-response characteristics, then a higher $LC_{50}$ value is an indication of lower lethality. CS is also a more potent agent in eliciting the intended effects of an RCA compared with CN. These observations provided the impetus for CS to replace CN in many uses.

The toxicology of OC is complicated by its nature. Although it is a "natural product," this does not necessarily make OC any safer compared with synthetic RCAs such as CS and CN. In fact, the exact composition of commercially available OC can vary widely from one lot to another, and its activity is expressed in terms of Scoville heat units (ability to cause intense pain with exposure to the tongue) (20).

Although the intended effects from exposure to RCAs have already been discussed, the possibility for unintended consequences should also be taken into consideration. Such consequences are always potentially present. What these consequences are exactly is less clear, and this has led to some controversy regarding the claimed "benign" nature of exposure to RCAs. Exposure to oleoresin of capsicum has been blamed in several deaths following its use to subdue unruly prisoners in police custody (20–22), although its role (if any) in these cases has not been proved. Unintended health outcomes have also been attributed to CS exposure under certain conditions such as extended duration of exposure (9,23,24) or dose (particularly in indoor settings) (8,21,22,25).

Dispersion of RCAs (or other organic compounds) at high temperature can lead to formation of degradation byproducts. Smith et al. (26,27) and Kluchinsky et al. (28)

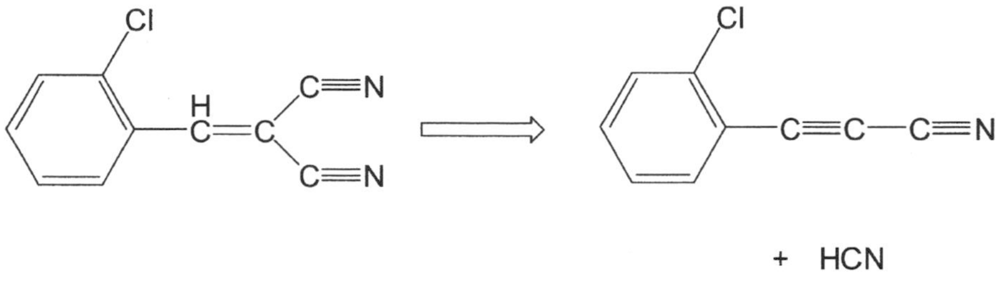

**Fig. 1.** Thermal degradation of the CS riot control agent to 3-(2-chlorophenyl)propynenitrile, with concurrent production of hydrogen cyanide.

showed that through the dispersion of CS from small hand-tossed canisters (grenades) with temperatures around 700°C, more than 20 organic compounds were dispersed along with the CS. Several of these compounds are a potential cause for concern in terms of human exposure, with acrylonitrile being the most significant *(27)*. In terms of inorganic degradation products from high-temperature CS dispersion, hydrogen cyanide is probably the most significant *(26,28)* The chemical pathway leading to hydrogen cyanide production is shown in Fig. 1. No known literature exists regarding the identification of thermal degradation products with high-temperature dispersion of RCAs other than CS.

In addition to unintended exposures that may result with high-temperature dispersion, the possibility that the heated canisters themselves could start a structural or outdoor fire should also be considered. A final concern is that thermal burns can also occur if people come into contact with the hot canisters, even minutes following dispersion.

## 6. DETECTION

Because RCAs are controlled items, not generally available to the public in large quantities, exposures frequently result from officially sanctioned use. Upon exposure, the effects to personnel are obvious and transient, creating little need by authorities to investigate. For these reasons, there has been no need to employ field detection methods for RCAs.

Official detection methods are limited to laboratory-based analysis such as the U.S. Occupational Safety and Health Administration (OSHA) method S154 for CS. As an example concerning the low priority placed on methods to quantify RCAs, this method uses older technology (liquid chromatography) and was originally validated in 1979 but is no longer considered validated according to current standards.

Field detection of riot control agents using gas chromatography/mass spectrometry (GC/MS) is possible. Smith et al. *(26)* demonstrated that CS and numerous degradation products were detected using solid phase microextraction of air that was contaminated by thermal CS dispersion. This was followed by analysis using a moveable GC/MS system. Volatility considerations dictate that detection and identification of intact CS is probably not possible using current backpack-portable field GC/MS systems, although the more volatile degradation products associated with thermal degradation of CS (such as 2-chlorobenzaldehyde) are detectable using such a system *(26)*.

Currently, neither type of these GC/MS systems would probably be available immediately following the use of riot control or other chemical agents in most foreseeable circumstances. Likewise, significant training and experience would be needed to employ such a system successfully, which would detect and identify unknown chemical compounds in a nonlaboratory setting, thus limiting the realistic usefulness of GC/MS methods in this role.

The rapid onset of intense symptoms provides what are probably the most important clues that exposure has occurred from this class of agents. In typical settings in which RCAs are released under governmental authority, the identity of the agent would most likely be available to first-care responders and other health care providers by contacting the organization(s) that employed the agent.

## 7. DECONTAMINATION

In most situations, the inherent confusion that occurs when RCAs are employed may prevent the exposed population from immediately identifying the single or mixed agent present.

This lack of specific information requires decontamination teams and first-level health care providers to develop a crude syndromic approach. In most settings, the intended behavior action—unplanned and rapid departure from an area owing to the intensity of adverse symptoms—reduces the continued exposure levels. In describing a proposed decontamination process, it will be assumed that the decontamination station and affected personnel are not in direct danger from potential adversaries and that, in the confusion of the exposure incident area, those who need care will be directed to the decontamination station first. It should be understood, however, that this may not be realistic in some terrorist incidents. For example, in the 1995 Tokyo subway attack that occurred during the peak of morning rush hour, affected individuals rapidly departed the exposure area and made their own way to various health care settings without decontamination, triage, or further transportation. This resulted in secondary contamination at the nearest medical facility where 641 patients were treated, and 23% of the hospital staff subsequently reported new-onset physical symptoms (29).

In a scenario in which decontamination and treatment of victims of riot control exposure occurs, several echelons of care should ideally be established:

1. Treatment for personnel with life-threatening injuries must be started prior to decontamination—this can be expedited by prompt removal of all contaminated clothing. Prior to complete decontamination, medical and first-responder personnel, properly protected to prevent secondary exposure cases, should perform immediate life-saving measures (i.e., the ABCs: airway, breathing, and circulation) in a designated "dirty zone." Decontamination should be completed as soon as a severely injured casualty is stabilized before movement to the "clean zone."
2. Treatment of persons whose injuries require immediate care after decontamination, or whose level of exposure is high and symptoms may be progressive if decontamination is not promptly started.
3. Treatment of those who would benefit from decontamination and a more thorough medical assessment.

Persons exposed to RCAs often improve with removal from the direct exposure site. Because these agents are particulates, irritation of skin, eyes, and mucous membranes may continue until the affected area has been completely cleaned. As best documented with CS exposure, these RCA symptoms are intensified in hot, humid climates or on skin areas wet from sweating (6,7). Use of water or saline to decontaminate patients from pepper spray (OC) may simultaneously put them at risk for hypothermia owing to the dual effects of: 1) neurogenic cooling mediated by the hypothalamus, via reflex sweating and vasodilation; and 2) the direct cooling effect of the liquid on the skin *(20)*.

It should be noted that the use of decontamination solutions that contain hypochlorite (household bleach) should be avoided if exposure to CS is suspected. Punte et al. *(30)* showed that the use of hypochlorite-containing solutions for CS decontamination led to production of severe vesication in human volunteers. Harrison and Inch *(31)* later showed that reaction of CS with hypochlorite readily leads to production of an epoxide compound derived from CS, which has been shown to be a strong vesicant.

## 8. EVALUATION AND TREATMENT CONSIDERATIONS

Clinical observations concerning the treatment and subsequent outcomes of exposure to RCAs has primarily been in the form of case reports, case series, and review articles. (The review articles generally draw on clinical observations, anecdotal reports, and interpretations of previously published studies.) The sporadic nature of the need for care from RCA exposure does not lend itself to formal clinical trials comparing either two approaches or treatment versus no-treatment/placebo. In fact, in some settings, the rigorous standards of a randomized clinical trial could preclude recruitment of appropriate numbers of participants in each study arm. This would also be complicated by the inherent ethical problems of obtaining informed consent after being exposed to a RCA and presenting for care.

Treatment in a mass-casualty scenario involves developing a triage system of care using whatever resources and interventions are readily available to provide the best care for the most patients. This treatment process may either coincide with or begin before complete decontamination takes place. This type of treatment, as described earlier, should occur prior to complete decontamination, in the event that immediate life-saving measures are necessary, whether by law enforcement, first-care providers, or other medical personnel properly protected to prevent secondary exposure cases *(4,26)*. Decontamination should then be completed as soon as a severely injured casualty is stabilized.

The movement of exposed personnel outside the exposure zone, into an area of fresh air, along with the removal of contaminated clothing, may be all that is required to care for lesser exposed patients.

### 8.1. CS, CN, and Pepper Spray Effects on the Eyes

The eye is the organ system most sensitive to RCAs. Contact with any of these agents produces corneal and conjunctival burning and leads to tearing and blepharospasm *(3,27,32,33)*. More severe injuries can occur if the exposed person is in close proximity to an RCA canister being released in a riot situation or comes in direct contact with a liquid or particulate spray that is released from commercially sold defensive weapons. There is the additional risk of ocular injury through blunt trauma from flying particles if a person is close to the point of release of these agents. The spasm causes the lids to close and produces a transient "blindness" *(34)*. Even a small amount placed in the eyes can cause an inability to open for upward of 2 min *(35)*. Controlled studies on exposure to CS in animals and to CS or OC in human volunteers demonstrated a transient conjunctivitis without corneal damage *(35–37)*. In other human exposure studies in the 1960s, visual acuity was not affected if the exposed individual was able to keep his or her eyes open throughout the exposure *(38)*. Ocular symptoms may improve by moving the affected individual to fresh air. However, treatment experience with persistent symptoms of exposure to RCAs (primarily CS, OC, and CN) has led to varied treatment approaches.

Most authors recommend thoroughly irrigating the eyes with a cool fluid such as saline *(32,39)* or water *(20)*, although the use of water can transiently worsen symptoms of irritation. A single application of a local anesthetic may be indicated for severe ocular symptoms *(6,29)*. One physician at a British Eye Hospital recommended blowing dry air across the eyes versus irrigation as the "preferred treatment" to resolve symptoms *(40)*. Other authors have cautioned against this procedure because of possible downwind contamination to medical personnel using this method *(2,41)*. Persistent complaints of eye irritation should prompt a slit-lamp evaluation for retained crystals or more serious eye injury *(39)*. One 1968 pathology case series documented the events leading to enucleation (loss of an eye) in 13 men after exposure to commercial tear gas pen defensive weapons containing CN. Effects of the blast injury from release of the explosive propellant, fragments of wadding striking the eye, and the CN agent itself appear to be additive risk factors that potentially lead to this tragic outcome *(42)*.

## 8.2. CS, CN, and Pepper Spray Effects on the Skin

Exposure to RCAs may result in skin effects such as irritant dermatitis *(7,43)*, allergic dermatitis *(44)*, and burns *(45)*. The onset of irritant symptoms on the skin usually occurs after the intense irritation effects in the eye and mucous membrane, possibly owing to the stratum corneum barrier properties *(43)*. The focus by both the patient and health care providers in controlling symptoms in the eyes and mucous membranes may lead to prolonged dermal exposure if the patient is not properly decontaminated. This delay could lead to late-onset erythema and vesicle formation occurring within 12–72 h after exposure *(2)*. This pattern of slow onset of symptoms is similar to that seen after exposure to nitrogen mustard *(7)*. Primary irritant symptoms, described as "prickly skin," may begin just minutes after exposure to CS and may be potentiated by wet skin from sweat or water, abrasions, and high humidity *(7)*. As with ocular exposure to CS, a sensation of burning may be worsened with the application of water to the skin, particularly if decontamination is delayed following exposure. An aqueous solution of 6% sodium bicarbonate, 3% sodium carbonate, and 1% benzalkonium chloride may lessen the intense stinging of affected skin areas *(7,43)*. Like CS and CN, pepper spray has a primary irritant effect but also has a neurogenic inflammation component affecting sensory neurons of the skin and airways *(19,20)*.

Allergic contact sensitization was described in an early case report from repeat exposure to CN in a routine military training exercise prior to World War II *(46)*. Eczematous dermatitis with a marked edema has been reported in civilians in Korea after recurrent exposures to CS in civil disturbances *(44)*. Although it was not substantiated, the Korean authors felt that CS was not a potent sensitizing agent and would require more recurrent and heavy exposure than CN in order to develop a contact dermatitis *(44)*. The concomitant use of OC may augment the sensitization process to other agents such as CS and CN *(20)*.

The most severe outcome from exposure to RCA is an acute skin burn injury, which could potentially result from the irritant properties of the RCA and/or the thermal effect of a hot particulate spray exiting an RCA canister at temperatures greater than 700°C *(47)*. Zekri et al. *(45)* published a case series of patients who had burns as a side effect of CS exposure during civil disturbances in a refugee detention center in Hong Kong. They described 91 patients treated for superficial or split-thickness burns with a total body surface area from 1 to 8%. Only two patients in this case series required more extensive care because of deeper burns. The authors describe three potential causes of burns from CS canisters: (1) flame generated from the canisters during initial deployment; (2) direct contact with the hot canister; and (3) the effect of the chemical powder coming in direct contact with the skin (45). Burns were also the most common complaint (52%) among Hong Kong detainees who were evaluated by the British Red Cross after CS exposure in a civil disturbance (24).

### 8.3. CS, CN, and Pepper Spray Effects on the Upper and Lower Respiratory Tracts

RCAs can cause acute irritation to the mucous membranes and upper respiratory tract, resulting in rhinorrhea, sneezing, and hyersalivation (7). Here again, these symptoms may improve with movement into fresh air. Decontamination with cool isotonic saline for periorbital irritation may be preferable to soap and water for the reasons described earlier.

Acute lung effects may include chest burning and tightness. The severity of the symptoms may be dependent on the proximity of the affected individual to the RCA canister release point. The sympathetic discharge and resultant hyperventilation from being in a chaotic riot situation may potentiate the amount of RCA actually entering the lung. Cough was the second most common complaint (38%) among Hong Kong detainees evaluated by the British Red Cross after CS exposure in a civil disturbance (24). Lung symptoms in most exposed individuals improve within 30 min. Patients with prolonged dyspnea should be considered for hospitalization and observed for hypoxia, particularly if exposed to RCAs in high concentrations or for prolonged periods, as some underlying lung diseases may be exacerbated by CS exposure. Thomas et al. (9) documented an overexposure of CS in military personnel in a field setting that occurred in 1996. This exposure was retrospectively estimated to be 1–4 min at close range to the point of canister release and resulted in a presentation of profound hypoxia 48–96 h after exposure that only became apparent with strenuous exercise. A chest computed tomography scan of the most seriously affected individual was compatible with a picture of interstitial pneumonitis. All affected individuals returned to their normal lung function within 1 wk, as documented by cycle ergometry (9). This clinical presentation is compatible with animal studies in four species attempting to calculate $LC_{50}$. Animals who died did so within 2 d with marked inflammation and hemorrhage of the trachea extending to the peripheral lung fields. Normal lungs were found in animals that survived for 14 d (7).

Pepper spray has both the direct irritant effects described above and the additional direct effects on sensory nerve endings in the lung, prompting coughing that has been reported not only in case reports from riot exposures, but also by employees working with culinary peppers (20).

### 8.4. Persistent and/or Serious Complications

There have been case reports of persistent lung symptoms following unusual RCA exposures. Pipkin (48) reported a cluster of influenza A cases in the British Royal Marines shortly after a brief exposure to CS in military training. One Royal Marine had persistent shortness of breath during exercise for 2 mo after his influenza episode (48). Roth and

Franzblau *(49)* reported a reactive airways picture at 3 yr of follow-up after a prison guard overturned a mattress that had been previously been sprayed with a combination CS and OC product. Hill et al. *(8)* described a persistent, multisystem reaction to a CS "spray" product that occurred when guards overpowered an unruly 30-yr-old prisoner in an indoor exposure. Within 8 d, the prisoner presented with an interstitial pneumonitis picture, erythroderma, and hepatitis with jaundice, which required systemic corticosteroids. The skin rash symptoms resolved over 6–7 mo, but reactive airway asthma-like symptoms were present 1 yr later. The authors felt this demonstrated a multisystem hypersensitivity rather than a direct toxic insult to the involved tissues *(8)*.

Park and Giammona *(25)* documented a severe pneumonitis requiring hospitalization for 28 d in a 4-mo-old infant exposed to CS in a house where CS canisters were released to subdue an unruly adult. Sanford *(1)* reviewed CN animal studies from the 1960s, as well as anecdotal reports of human fatalities from the use of CS during the Vietnam War era, without a definitive conclusion.

Several authors have described deaths in detainees exposed to pepper spray (OC) during apprehension *(20–22)*. A death under restraint is often a multifactorial event, with underlying behavioral conditions, concomitant use of drugs such as cocaine contributing to an excited state (even to the point of delirium), restraint, and use of force that could have an additive effect leading to asphyxia. In a small number of cases, the use of pepper spray to subdue a detainee appears to be a factor in the cause of death. The additive effects of pepper spray directly irritating lung tissue and causing laryngospasm and bronchospasm, potentially leading to a respiratory arrest in some individuals, may be important contributing effects when pepper spray is used in a fatal apprehension incident.

## 9. CONCLUSIONS

The clinical outcomes after exposure to RCAs depend on multiple factors. These include:

- The tactical situation and method of employment
- The single agent or combination of agents released
- The formulation of RCA used (including solvents and combustion byproducts of the dispersion process
- The ability of exposed personnel to quickly exit an area or to don personal protective equipment
- Underlying medical conditions and previous exposure to a sensitizing agent such as CS and CN
- Weather conditions such as temperature and humidity
- Access to early decontamination and treatment.

The summation of these factors and actual duration of exposure result in a dose-response relationship that may be unique to an individual compared with others in close proximity during a release of RCAs. Although these agents are generally considered safe, they have a potential to cause serious harm if personnel do not carefully consider the method of employment, or with unusual circumstances. The Himsworth Report to the British Home Office after the 1969 Londonderry, Northern Ireland riots recommended that RCAs should be studied using the methodology for new drug development, rather than for weapons; this call has still not been answered *(23)*.

## ACKNOWLEDGMENTS

The authors wish to thank Ms. Karen Dutro of Freelance Ink (Williamsburg, VA), for her editorial review of this manuscript.

## REFERENCES

1. Sanford JP. Medical aspects of riot control (harassing) agents. Annu Rev Med 1976;27:421–429.
2. Weir E. The health impact of crowd-control agents. Can Med Assoc J 2001;164:1889–1892.
3. Fraunfelder FT. Editorial: is CS gas dangerous? BMJ. 2000;320:454–459.
4. Padilla, RE. Pulmonary toxic agents. In: Roy MJ, ed. Physician's Guide to Terrorist Attack. Humana Press, Totowa, NJ, 2003, pp. 253–262.
5. Department of Defense. Treatment of Chemical Agent Casualties and Conventional Military Chemical Injuries: FM8-285: Part 1. Chemical Agent Casualties, 1995, p. V-1. Accessed June 25, 2002, at http://www.vnh.org/FM8285/Chapter/chapter5.html.
6. Hu H, Fine J, Epstein P, Kelsey K, Reynolds P, Walker P. Tear gas: harassing agent or toxic chemical weapon? JAMA 1989;262:660–663.
7. Sidell FR. Riot control agents. In Sidell FR, Takafuji ET, Franz DR, eds, Textbook of Military Medicine: Medical Aspects of Chemical and Biological Warfare. Borden Institute, Washington, DC, 1997:307–316.
8. Hill A, Silverberg N, Mayorga D, Baldwin H. Medical hazards of the tear gas CS: a case of persistent, multisystem, hypersensitivity reaction and review of the literature. Medicine 2000;79:234–240.
9. Thomas RJ, Smith PA, Rascona DA, Louthan JD, Gumpert BC. Acute pulmonary effects from CS "tear gas" (ortho-chlorobenzylidenemalononitrile): a unique exposure outcome unmasked by strenuous exercise following a military training event. Mil Med 2002;167:136–139.
10. Sargent EV, Kirk GD, Hite M. Hazard evaluation of monochloroacetone, Am Ind Hyg J 1986;47:375–378.
11. Love D. The Second Battle of Ypres, Apr. 1915. 2001. http://www.worldwar1.com/sf2ypres.htm. Accessed June 25, 2002.
12. Smart JK. History of chemical and biological warfare: an american perspective. In: Sidell FR, Takafuji ET, Franz DR, eds, Textbook of Military Medicine: Medical Aspects of Chemical and Biological Warfare. Borden Institute, Washington, DC, 1997, pp. 14–15.
13. Yale University Law School (The Avalon Project, 2002). Declaration on the Use of Projectiles the Object of Which is the Diffusion of Asphyxiating or Deleterious Gases of July 29, 1899. http://www.yale.edu/lawweb/avalon/lawofwar/dec99-02.htm. Accessed June 25, 2002.
14. Albright A, Shackelford M. The Hague Convention (17 June 1925) Protocol for the Prohibition of the Use in War of Asphyxiating, Poisonous or Other Gases, and of Bacteriological Methods of Warfare. Brigham Young University, 2001. http://www.lib.byu.edu/~rdh/wwi/hague/hague13.html. Accessed July 27, 2002.
15. Ford G. (1975) Presidential Executive Order 11850 "Renunciation of certain uses in war of chemical herbicides and riot control agents." http://envirotext.eh.doe.gov/data/eos/ford/19750408.html. Accessed June 25, 2002.
16. Corson BB, Stoughton RW. Reaction of alpha, beta-unsaturated dinitriles. J Am Chem Soc 1928;50:2825–2837.
17. Urbanetti JS. Toxic inhalational injury. In: Sidell FR, Takafuji ET, Franz DR, eds. Textbook of Military Medicine: Medical Aspects of Chemical and Biological Warfare. Borden Institute, Washington, DC, 1997:247–249.
18. Matarese SL, Matthews JI. Zinc chloride (smoke bomb) inhalational lung injury. Chest 1986;89:308–309.
19. Olayos EJ, Sale H. Riot control agents: pharmacology, toxicology, biochemistry, and chemistry, J Appl Toxicol 2001;21:355–391.
20. Smith CG, Stopford W. Health hazards of pepper spray. NC Med J 1999;60:268–273.
21. Steffee CH, Lantz PE, Flanagan LM, Thompson RL, Jason DR. Oleoresin capsicum (pepper) spray and "in custody deaths" Am J Forensic Pathol 1995;16:185 192.
22. Pollanen MS, Chaisson DA, Cairns JT, Young JG. Unexpected death related to restraint for excited delirium: a retrospective study of deaths in police custody and in the community. Can Med Assoc J 1998;158:1603–1608.
23. Himsworth H, Thompson RHS, Dornhorst AC. Report of the Enquiry into the Medical and Toxicological aspects of CS (Orthochlorobenzylidenemalononitrile). Great Britain Home Office, Her Majesty's Stationary Office, London, 1969:1–11.

24. Anderson PJ, Lau CS, Taylor WR, Critchley JA. Acute effects of the potent lacrimator o-chloro-benzylidene malonitirile (CS) tear gas, Human Exp Toxicol 1996;15:461–465.
25. Park S, Giammona ST. Toxic effects of tear gas on an infant during prolonged exposure, Am J Dis Child 1972;123:24–46.
26. Smith P, Kluchinsky T, Savage P, et al. Traditional sampling with laboratory analysis and solid phase microextraction sampling with field gas chromatography/mass spectrometry by military industrial hygienists. AIHA J 2002;63:284–292.
27. Smith P, Sheely M, Kluchinsky T. Solid phase microextraction with analysis by gas chromatography to determine short term hydrogen cyanide concentrations in a field setting. J Separation Sci 2002; 25:917–921.
28. Kluchinsky T, Sheely M, Savage P, Smith P. Formation of 2-chlorobenzylidenemalononitrile (CS riot control agent) thermal degradation products at elevated temperatures. J Chromatogr A 2002;952:205–213.
29. Ohbu A, Yamashina A, Takasu N, et al. Sarin poisoning on Tokyo subway. South Med J 1997;90:587–593.
30. Punte CL, Owens EJ, Gutentag PJ. Exposures to ortho-chlorobenzylidene malononitrile. Arch Environ Health 1963;6:72–80.
31. Harrison JM, Inch TD. A novel rearrangement of the adduct from CS-epoxide and dioxan-2-hydroper-oxide. Tetrahedron Lett 1981;22:679–682.
32. Blaho K, Stark M. Is CS spray dangerous? CS is a particulate spray, not a gas. BMJ 2000;321:46.
33. Hu H. Toxicodynamics of riot control agents (lacrimators). In: Somani SM, ed, Chemical Warfare Agents. Academic Press, Washington DC, 1992, pp. 271–288.
34. Rengstorff RR, Mershon MM. CS in water II. Effects on human eyes. Mil Med 1971;136:149–152.
35. Rengstorff R, Mershon MM. CS in trioctyl phosphate; effects on human eyes. Mil Med 1971;136:152–153.
36. Rengstorff R, Mershon MM. CS in water I. Effects of massive doses sprayed into the eyes of rabbits. Mil Med 1971;136:146–148.
37. Zollman TM, Bragg RM, Harrison DA. Clinical effects of oleoresin capsicum (pepper spray) on the human cornea and conjunctiva. Ophthalmology 2000;107:2186–2189.
38. Rengstorff R, Mershon MM. The effect of riot control agent CS on visual acuity. Mil Med 1969;134: 219–221.
39. Scott RAH. Illegal "Mace" contains more toxic CN particles. BMJ 1995;311:871.
40. Yih JP. CS gas injury to the eye. Blowing dry air to the eye is preferable to irrigation. BMJ 1995;311:276.
41. Gray JP. CS gas is not CS spray—formulation is important [Letter]. BMJ 2000;320:458–459.
42. Levine RA, Stahl CJ. Eye injury caused by tear-gas weapons. Am J Ophthalmol 1968;65:497–508.
43. Weigand DA. Cutaneous reaction to the riot control agent CS. Mil Med 1969;134:437–440.
44. Ro YS, Lee CW. Tear gas dermatitis allergic contact sensitization due to CS. Int J Dermatol 1991;30: 576–577.
45. Zekri AM, King WW, Yueng R, Taylor WR. Acute mass burns caused by o-chlorobenzylidene malonitirile (CS) tear gas. Burns 1995:21:586–589.
46. Queen FB, Stander T. Allergic dermatitis following exposure to tear gas (CN). JAMA 1941;117:1879–1880.
47. Kluchinsky TA, Savage PB, Sheely MV, Thomas RJ, Smith PA. Identification of CS-derived compounds formed during heat dispersion of CS riot control agent. J Microcolumn Separation 2001;13:186–190.
48. Pipkin C. Does exposure to CS gas potentiate the severity of influenza? [Letter]. J R Nav Med Serv 1990;76:188–189.
49. Roth VS, Franzblau A. RADS after exposure to a riot-control agent: a case report [Letter]. J Occup Environ Med 1996;38:863–865.

# IV ADDITIONAL CONSIDERATIONS

# 24 Radiation Effects

## Vijay K. Singh, *PhD*, and Thomas M. Seed, *PhD*

### CONTENTS

## 1. INTRODUCTION

### 1.1. Definition of Radiation Threats

At the outset, it is important to define some terminologies. A "nuclear weapon detonation" is propelled, not by conventional chemical reactions, but rather by an atomic chain reaction, in which a massive amount of energy is released in a confined space in an instant of time. This energy release manifests in several different forms, such as initial nuclear radiation, residual nuclear radiation, thermal radiation, and blast and shock waves *(1)*. Because of the massive explosive power of even small nuclear weapons, large-scale destruction of buildings and human deaths are likely. In contrast, a "radiological dispersal device" (RDD), commonly referred to as a "dirty bomb," has less impact as a weapon; radioactive materials are dispersed through the use of chemical explosives. The RDD is designed mainly to cause chronic radiation injuries and create delayed radiation sickness, panic, and fear among military and civilian populations. To predict the level of exposure or injury an RDD might cause is difficult, because radiation dose depends on many factors, such as the physical and chemical forms of the radioactive material, the size and type of explosive, and proximity to the blast. Most likely, the most severe, immediate effects of a dirty bomb would be the disruption from the evacuation, the fear and panic in the general population, the subsequent cleanup of contaminated property, and the

From: *Physician's Guide to Terrorist Attack*
Edited by: M. J. Roy © Humana Press Inc., Totowa, NJ

associated economic costs. The long-term health effects of an RDD may not be immediately predictable but clearly might produce chronic injuries and late-arising pathologies.

## 1.2. Uses and Misuses of Radiation Sources

Around the world, radioactive sources have been used beneficially for decades to
diagnose and treat illnesses, to monitor oil wells and water aquifers, to irradiate food for
eliminatation of microbes, and for many other purposes. Millions of sources have been
distributed worldwide during the past 50 years, with hundreds of thousands now produced, used, and stored.

Terrorists face essentially no barrier to the acquisition of a wide range of radioactive
materials. The radioactive materials needed to build a "dirty bomb" can be found in
almost any country in the world, and more than 100 countries may not have adequate
regulatory control and monitoring programs necessary to prevent or even detect the theft
of these materials (2).

By far the most vulnerable radiation sources are medical and industrial. Worldwide,
more than 20,000 sites have significant radioactive sources, and more than 10,000 radiotherapy units for medical care are in use. More than 12,000 industrial sources for radi-
ography are supplied annually, and about 300 operating irradiator sites contain radioactive
sources for industrial applications. About 135,000 licensees of medical and industrial
radiation sources in the United States have more than 1.8 million sources in use (2,3).

"Orphaned" radiation sources pose a significant international problem. In February
2002, a team from the Republic of Georgia, supported by the International Atomic Energy
Agency (IAEA), successfully recovered two unshielded and unsecured radioactive stron-
tium-90 sources that had seriously injured three men in December 2001 (2,3). In June
2002, IAEA experts were asked to assist Georgian officials to continue the search for lost
strontium-90 sources thought to be remaining from the former Soviet military. The
situation in Georgia may indicate the serious safety and security concerns about orphaned
sources elsewhere in the world.

## 2. NATURE OF INJURY INDUCTION BY IONIZING IRRADIATION

Common forms of ionizing radiation (IR) include electromagnetic radiation (X-rays
and $\gamma$-rays, neither of which contain mass or charge) and particulate radiation, including
electrons, protons, neutrons, and alpha particles. Electrons have a small mass ($9.1 \times 10^{-31}$ kg)
and negative charge, and protons have a relatively large mass (approximately 2000 times
that of an electron) and are positively charged. The mass of neutrons is approximately
equivalent to that of protons; an alpha particle consists of the helium nucleus (two protons
+ two neutrons, four times the mass of neutron) (4).

Beta particles are very light (i.e., comparable to the mass of electrons) charged particles
that are found primarily in fallout radiation. These electron-like particles can be accelerated to nearly the speed of light, but they will decelerate within relatively short distances following tissue penetration.

In contrast, sufficiently energetic protons have more tissue-penetrating power, but,
with final deceleration, they abruptly stop (in an area known as the Bragg peak) and
deposit large amounts of energy that creates intense ionizations at microlocales within
tissues.

The amount of ionization deposited along a track of radiation defines the extent of linear energy transfer (LET). X-rays and gamma rays are examples of low-LET radiation, characterized by tracks with sparse ionization (or energy deposited) densities; alpha particles and fission neutrons are examples of high-LET radiation tracks with high ionization densities.

It is now well recognized that free radicals formed by the radiolysis of cellular aqueous milieu, and their interaction with one another and with oxygen, are primary mediators of radiation injury *(5)*. Wide variation in individual radiation responses may relate to differing individual abilities to detoxify radiation-induced free radicals. These detoxification mechanisms are the net effects of endogenous antioxidant enzymes, thiols (free and protein-bound), and several exogenous antioxidant nutrients, such as selenium, vitamin E, carotenoids, flavinoids, and vitamin C *(6)*.

Other special features of IR that may predict a biological response include:

1. *Quality*: $^{90}$Sr and $^{239}$Pu, for example, are both bone-seeking radioisotopes but with markedly different potencies for inducing osteogenic sarcoma, as a result of their low or high LET status.
2. *Half-life*: The half-life of $^{131}$I is 8 days, but that of $^{239}$Pu is 24,000 years, for example, which translates into enormous differences in the committed dose to a given tissue.
3. *Dose rate*: The time-dependent rate at which energy is transferred. From animal studies, it has been suggested that IR delivered at a high dose rate is more carcinogenic than that delivered at a low dose rate, although data in humans are still insufficient to ascertain precise values for the magnitude of these effects *(5,7,8)*.
4. *Dose*: The accumulated energy deposited over time of exposure.

Acute radiation syndrome (ARS) is characterized by the differential response of the body's vital organ systems to various intensities of IR exposure. There are in fact at least four distinct syndromes—hematopoietic, gastrointestinal, cutaneous and neurovascular—that are dependent on the total dose, the dose rate, and the time *(9–11)*. Each follows a similar clinical pattern, which is divided into three phases: (1) an initial or prodromal phase occurring during the first few hours following exposure; (2) a latent phase, which shortens with increasing dose; and (3) the manifest phase.

The prodromal phase is characterized by the onset of nausea, vomiting, and malaise. The time of nausea and vomiting relates to the amount of radiation dose one received. Oral prophylaxis with 5-HT$_3$ inhibitor-based antiemetics will diminish these prodromal responses considerably, but in doing so, they limit the reliability and usefulness of nausea and emesis as indicators of acute IR exposure. Attending physicians and nurses need to keep this limitation in mind when recording symptoms and taking clinical histories.

The latent phase follows the prodromal phase, when the exposed individual will be relatively symptom-free. The length of the latent phase varies with the exposure intensity and setting. The latent phase may range from several weeks to several months or more. It is shorter for gastrointestinal syndrome (GIS), lasting a few days to a week, and shortest for the neurovascular syndrome, lasting only a few hours.

The illness phase presents with the clinical symptoms associated with the manifest pathologies of the major organ systems injured (marrow, intestine, skin, or neurological and vascular systems). Patients receiving 2–6 Gy of whole-body irradiation will have depression of bone marrow function and pancytopenia. Changes within the peripheral blood profile occur at 24 hours post irradiation. Blood levels of lymphocytes decline most rapidly and erythrocytes least rapidly. Other blood cell types (e.g., leukocyte subsets, neutrophils, and monocytes) decline more slowly than lymphocytes. The time of onset of blood cytopenias and extent of marrow suppression vary considerably in patients.

The GIS is elicited by doses of gamma rays that are generally much higher (≥8 Gy) than those causing the hematopoietic syndrome. However, lower radiation doses may also cause GIS under certain circumstances. GIS has serious clinical implications, especially when it is accompanied by marked reduction in the bone marrow's blood-forming capacity and suppression of the body's innate immune response.

The clinical phase of GIS occurs earlier than hematopoietic syndrome. Important clinical manifestations of GIS include severe fluid losses, hemorrhage, and diarrhea.

The cutaneous radiation syndrome (CRS) occurs as a direct result of a time-dependent cascade of IR-elicited inflammatory and proliferative responses within exposed skin. These responses can be initiated over a wide range of IR doses (i.e., from relatively low doses of approximately 1–2 Gy up to tens of Gy) and, depending on the area and volume of skin exposed and the IR dose delivered, the severity of clinically relevant pathologies can vary widely as well. During the initial triage, grades of CRS can be assigned by the extent and duration of early arising erythremic rash, e.g., grade 1, minimal transient rash through grade 4, severe, sustained rash over 40% of the body. As with the other better defined syndromes, the four major stages (i.e., prodromal, manifestation, chronic, and late stages) occur sequentially in time as a function of IR exposure intensity (dose and dose rate) and quality of radiation. Each stage can be selectively diagnosed and given specific treatments.

The neurovascular syndrome is associated with very high, acute doses of radiation. The lower limit is probably 20–40 Gy. After the short latency period, the clinical course is marked by a steadily deteriorating state of consciousness with eventual coma and death. Convulsions may also occur *(12)* (Table 1).

## 3. JUDGING DOSE AND ESTIMATING SEVERITY OF INJURIES SUSTAINED

Of all the possible features of a given radiation exposure, the three parameters most critical for eliciting an effect on tissues of the body are: (1) total dose, (2) dose rate, and (3) radiation quality. The relative contribution of each of these parameters to the strength and nature of the IR-elicited bioresponse depends largely on tissue type and organ system; for example, rapidly self-renewing tissues with high cell turnover rates are more strongly affected by dose rate than slowly renewing or non-renewing tissues, which are more strongly dependent on total dose than on dose rate.

Regardless, direct measurement of absorbed radiation dose remains the cornerstone of dosimetry. In cases of acute IR exposures, regardless of cause, estimates of absorbed dose are invariably considered useful in order to assess the level of potential injury, to make an accurate prognosis, and to develop appropriate treatment strategies. It is generally accepted that differences in absorbed dose as small as approximately 10% can translate into significant differences in the elicited pathobiological responses and that these differences might require different treatment strategies.

The technical aspects of dose reconstruction can be, and often are, complex and time-dependent, involving extensive evaluation of the nature of the radiation source, the exposure conditions and pathways, and the populations involved. Mathematical model-

Table 1
Effect of Distance (in Kilometers) from Detonation Epicenter Relative to Casualty Type

| Injury type | Severity of injury | Distance from epicenter (1-kt weapon) (km) |
| --- | --- | --- |
| Ionizing radiation | 50% reduction in performance | 0.600 |
| Ionizing radiation | 50% lethality | 0.800 |
| Blast | 50% lethality | 0.140 |
| Thermal | 50% casualty rate, second-degree burns | 0.369 |

Data from ref. *12*.

ing is frequently employed, and time is generally not a critical issue. However, in cases of acute radiation exposure, accidental or otherwise, treatment decisions need to be made quickly, based primarily on the patient's presenting symptomatology, as well as crude estimates of exposure intensities and conditions.

### 3.1. Biological Indicators (Dosimetry)

The capacity to develop radiation dose estimates both rapidly and accurately following an unplanned radiation exposure is essential for an effective triage and for making appropriate medical decisions for the radiation injury *(13,14)*. Crude estimates of absorbed dose can be obtained from clinical presentations and from hematological profiles (Fig. 1). The latter typically will be the most useful piece of information available to the practicing physician.

A select few biological markers have also been used successfully to indicate the type and intensity of a given exposure. For example, the dicentric chromosome marker is widely and successfully used as a quantitative indicator of genetic damage and, in turn, the extent of acute exposure.

Biomarkers can be subdivided according to their applications. The analysis of chromosomal aberrations in peripheral blood lymphocytes is a biological dosimetry method that is widely used to assess radiation dose. Many types of chromosomal aberrations may appear in lymphocytes following exposure to radiation.

The landmark observation of Bender and Gooch *(15)* that the formation of dicentric chromosome aberrations correlates with dose represented a major change in how IR dose could be assessed. Now, the dicentric chromosome is a well-accepted biomarker for IR exposure and currently is used to estimate radiation dose in accidental radiation exposures. In contrast to many of the other cytogenetic-based assays, the dicentric assay is quite specific for ionizing radiation and associated molecular damage related to DNA strand breakage.

The background frequency of dicentric chromosomes of peripheral blood lymphocytes for the general population is approximately 1 in 1000–2000 metaphases. Human T-lymphocytes have variable life spans but generally are long-lived (i.e., life spans ranging from months to years). However, there are minor, short-lived subpopulations capable of surviving for a few days to a few weeks.

The frequency of dicentrics following a given IR exposure, consequently, remains stable only for a limited period (i.e., a few weeks). Therefore, in interpreting results of the dicentric assay from a radiation accident case, one must consider the postexposure

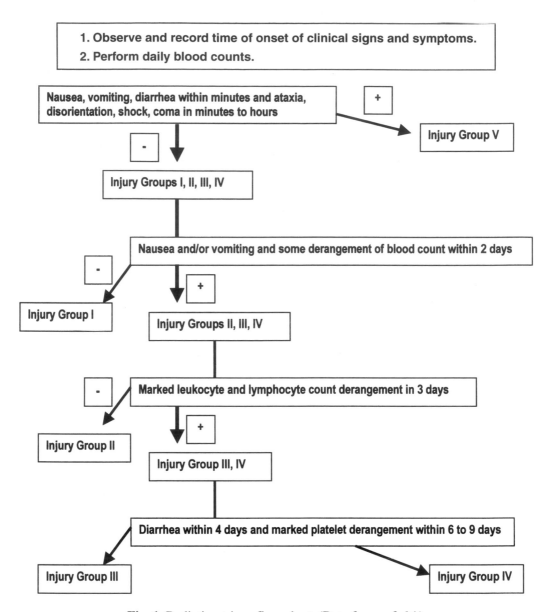

**Fig. 1.** Radiation triage flow chart. (Data from ref. *14.*)

period in order to estimate the dose of the original exposure. In general, the dicentric assay is considered reliable for up to 60 days post exposure and for only a limited exposure range, approximately 0.1–5 Gy. Similarly, the extent of exposure (volume of lympho-hematopoietic tissue exposed) should be considered as well.

After a partial-body exposure, irradiated lymphocytes from the exposed portion of the body rapidly mix in the circulation with blood from nonirradiated portions, and equilibrium is reached quickly within 24 hours. By recording not only the dicentric frequency for the lymphocyte population at large (i.e., percentage of lymphocytes bearing dicentric lesions) but also the distribution (i.e., number of dicentric lesions per cell) of dicentrics, the magnitude of partial-body exposure (per given blood/tissue volume) can be roughly estimated. Also note that the slope and shape of the dose-response curve for dicentrics is steep and nearly linear for high-LET radiation, but for low-LET radiation, the response curve assumes a linear-quadratic form *(16)*.

In cases of accidental exposures in which prolonged times have elapsed between exposure and testing, cytogenetic assays of stable chromosomal aberrations are commonly used. This assay process, *retrospective biodosimetry*, includes various types of cytogenetic endpoints, usually reciprocal translocations and chromosome-specific deletions.

These radiation-associated genetic lesions can be of a generic nature (covering the entire genome) or can be specific to individual chromosomes. Regardless of the specific endpoint, dose estimates can be derived through application of appropriate mathematical models, albeit with significant levels of uncertainty *(17)*. In contrast to older, more laborious and time-consuming cytogenetic assays such as Giemsa banding, newer fluorescence *in situ* hybridization (FISH) assays can be performed easily and rapidly.

Alternative assays are also available for dose estimation, with some benefits not readily available with more conventional translocation-based assays. For example, the *premature chromosome condensation* (PCC) assay can be used for very high doses (0.1–9 Gy, low LET) because it is based on the quantitation of induced breaks within interphase chromosomes of radiation-exposed blood lymphocytes.

Another alternative cytogenetic assay involves determination of the frequency of micronuclei within blood leukocytes of the exposed individual. The frequency of micronuclei is roughly radiation dose-dependent and therefore can be used as a crude biodosimeter. However, micronuclei represent more a reflection of intense myelosuppressive stress rather than specific ionizing radiation exposure. This type of nonspecificity of the lesion-inducing physicochemical agent is a common confounder in attempting to make use of many of biomarker/bioindicator assays for ionizing radiation exposures and associated injuries.

Finally, persistent free radicals formed in solid matrix biomaterials (dental enamel, nails, hair, and so on) from an exposed victim can be detected via electron-spin resonance. These measurements can provide reliable biophysical dose estimates as well as partial-body exposure information.

### 3.2. Molecular Dosimetry

Several new tools are being tested. Some important techniques include:

1. DNA single-strand breaks (ssb) and base alterations formed following exposure to IR *(18)*. Dose-response relationships for ssb and altered-base yields and the effect of repair at various times post exposure are well known for various nucleated blood cell components and can be used for dose assessment (G. vander Schans, personal communication, NATO TG/006).
2. Changes in gene and protein expression induced by radiation exposure. The sensitivity of the gene expression bioassay appears to be adequate for low radiation doses *(19)*, as observed in scenario 2 (*see* Subheading 5.2. below).
3. Expression of apoptotic gene *(20)*, oncogene or tumor suppressor genes *(21)*, and cytokine genes *(22)* used as biomarkers for radiation injury.
4. Chromosomal *(23)* and mitochondrial DNA mutations *(24)* used as biomarkers of exposure.

The list of radiation-responsive genes is growing as new molecular biology techniques (gene chips) permit screening for more target sequences.

### 3.3. Physical Dosimetry

Physical dosimetry should be subordinate to relevant clinical observations when treatment decisions are to be made. Nevertheless, physical dosimetry is most useful in complementing and confirming dose estimates based on clinical and biological response indicators. Physical dosimeters come in many forms and include both personal and environmental monitoring devices. When used properly, these devices can provide critically important information to the attending physician about the intensity, quantity, and quality of radiation exposure and can be useful for diagnosis and development of treatment plans.

Upon presentation, radiation casualties require both clinical and radiological examinations. Whole-body surveys, including collection of biosamples (blood, urine, and so on) should be done in cases of suspected isotopic contamination. The essential, basic instrumentation to perform these initial surveys includes Geiger-Mueller counters (with broad paddle probes for surveying the patient's body for external isotopic contamination) as well as liquid scintillation counting devices for analyzing the collected biosamples in order to roughly gauge the extent of internal contamination. Follow-up evaluation should then be done with whole-body counting to determine total-body burden and nuclear spectroscopy to identify the contaminating isotopic species.

## 4. ANTICIPATING AND PREPARING FOR MEDICAL SEQUELAE OF A NUCLEAR OR RADIOLOGICAL EVENT

### 4.1. Preventive Issues and Measures

Medical care and management of patients exposed to IR either accidentally or through adversarial actions are among the least emphasized aspects of modern medical education. The end of the Cold War dramatically reduced the likelihood of strategic nuclear weapons being used, but terrorism has made the use of nuclear or radiological weapons more real and probable than ever.

Our citizenry expects that the government, local authorities, and medical facilities will have full capacity to handle such contingencies and a full range of medical response plans to decrease the morbidity and mortality from the use of these weapons.

Some aspects of radiological terrorism, such as the use of RDDs or planted point sources, have relatively little medical impact, with few casualties and limited severity of physical injuries. However, the likelihood that terrorists will use these simple devices is significantly higher than for the more sophisticated, complex nuclear devices. Furthermore, one can anticipate that the psychological effects of such low-impact devices, e.g., RDDs, will have a profound effect on the medical system. Terrorists could no doubt easily gain access to sufficient radiological materials, to construct and to deploy RDDs, but they face significant barriers in obtaining and using more powerful nuclear devices.

If a more powerful device is detonated, prompt and effective treatment of casualties is critical. Fortunately, treatment regimens for radiation casualties do exist and are both effective and practical. The United States has significant training experience, especially with the Department of Energy's Accident Response Group (ARG), with its Nuclear

Emergency Search Teams (NEST), and the Medical-Radiobiology Advisory Team (M-RAT) of the Armed Forces Radiobiology Research Institute.

The medical management of radiation and combined injuries has three stages: triage, emergency care, and definitive care. Effective quality care can be provided both for limited casualties at a well-equipped facility and for many casualties with an efficient evacuation system. Recommendations for treatment of a few casualties may not apply to treatment of mass casualties because of limited resources.

Emergency care of the radiological casualty is provided on the basis that all life-threatening injuries are attended to first. As acute, treatable radiation injuries are by nature not immediately life-threatening, they should be attended to only after taking care of the primary, life-threatening injuries. In short, the attending physician has some leeway in terms of time in trying to manage the radiation-associated injuries. Primary treatment modalities include blocking/decorporation agents (in the case of radioisotopic contamination), antiemetics, and maintenance of fluids and electrolytes. Triage and definitive treatments are described just below.

The adage "an ounce of prevention is worth a pound of cure" is certainly relevant to trying in develop appropriate countermeasures to current nuclear/radiological threats. Keeping radioactive materials secured, protected, controlled, and accounted for is imperative, especially for radiation sources that might be crafted into usable weapons. It seems obvious that all the nuclear-capable countries of the world need to be increasingly diligent in attempting to safeguard their nuclear/radiological sources by developing and implementing effective regulations, controls, and security. Such regulatory steps would certainly help in limiting access to and fabrication of improvised nuclear/radiological devices by unfriendly, terror-bent forces throughout the world.

### 4.2. The Triage

With multiple casualties, responders must sort and prioritize victims by the severity of their injuries from trauma, burns, or radiation *(25)* (Fig. 2). Triage is extremely important in casualty situations that require allocation of limited medical resources to victims who require treatment and have the best chance of survival. However, prioritizing casualties by injury will depend on the availability of medical personnel and essential supplies.

Because a potentially treatable radiation exposure inflicts no immediately life-threatening hazard, the more serious injuries not associated with radiation (for example, trauma, burn injuries) must be treated first. Nevertheless, if radioactive materials are known or suspected to have contaminated a patient, appropriate decontamination must be undertaken as soon as possible. This treatment includes removal of clothing and body washing, to remove contaminating nuclides as quickly as possible.

The earliest clinical symptoms of acute, whole-body irradiation are upper and lower gastrointestinal disturbances (for example, nausea, vomiting, and diarrhea) and fatigue and weakness. These symptoms are ranked both by the intensity of exposure and the time following exposure (*see* Table 2 for additional details) *(26–29)*.

Note that radiation-exposed individuals respond quite differently depending on their inherent radiosensitivities, physiological conditions, and a host of other confounding factors (for example, the use of antiemetics). This individual variability is illustrated by the wide range of doses, e.g., 58–329 cGy, required to cause the fatigue and weakness syndrome in 10–90% of exposed individuals *(27)*.

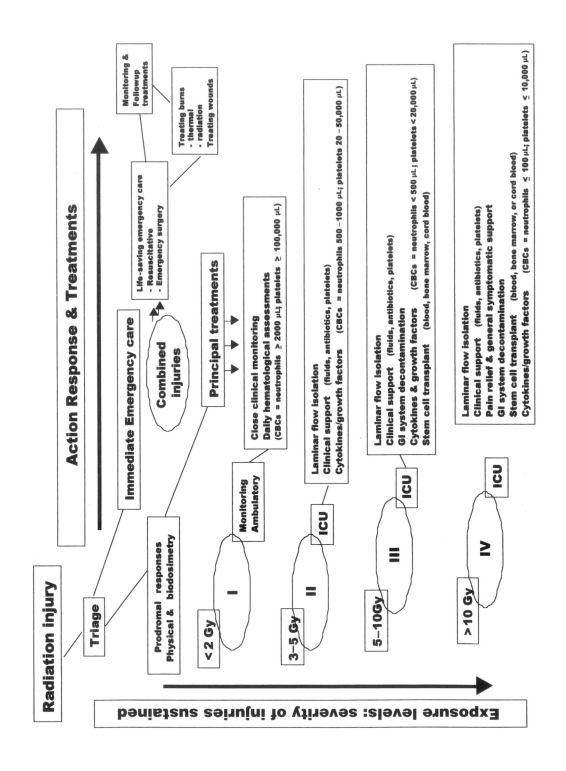

**Fig. 2.** Flow diagram suggests a sequence of triage and emergency and definitive care procedures for radiation casualties and injuries of increasing severities. Increasingly severe injuries (groups I–IV) of four primary organ systems of concern are shown: starting at the top left and extending down are the four levels of injury; to the right of each severity level is the brief listing of definitive treatments for hematopoietic system injuries. The organ systems of concern and the parameters of injury used to indicate severity include the following (as listed by Dainiak in ref. 41):

(1) *Hematopoietic system injury*: severity level I. lymphocytes >1500 mm³, granulocytes >2000 mm³, platelets >100,000 mm³; severity level II, lymphocytes 1000–5000 mm³, granulocytes 1000–2000 mm³, platelets 50,000–100,000 mm³; severity level III, lymphocytes 500–1000 mm³, granulocytes 500–1000 mm³, platelets 50,000–100,000 mm³; and severity level IV, lymphocytes <500 mm³, granulocytes <500 mm³, platelets <20,000 mm³; (2) *Gastrointestinal system injury*: severity level I, 2–3 stool/d with minimal abdominal pain; severity level II, 4–6 stools/d with moderate pain; severity level III, 7–9 stools/d with severe pain; severity level IV, ≥10 stools/d with excruciating pain; (3) *Cutaneous system injury*: severity level I, minimal transient rash; severity level II, moderate rash, ~10% body surface; severity level III, marked rash, ~10–40% of total body surface, with oncholysis; and severity level IV, severe persistent rash >40% body surface, with oncholysis; (4) *Neurovascular system injury*: severity level I, mild nausea with vomiting 1 time/d, blood pressure >100/70, normal neurological exam; severity level II, nausea and vomiting 2–3 times/d, blood pressure 100/70, focal neurological deficits and memory loss; severity level III, nausea and vomiting, 6–10 times/d, blood pressure 90/60 and >80, palpable prominent neurological deficits and major intellectual impairment; and severity level IV, refractory nausea and vomiting, blood pressure <80, loss of consciousness, memory loss. Presence of gastrointestinal system level IV, cutaneous system level IV, and neurovascular system level IV indicates probable death. Supportive therapy alone is indicated (fluids, blood components, antibiotics, pain treatment, counseling). Diagram derived in part from refs. 10, 25, and 26.

349

Table 2
Radiation Triage Categories, Survival Probabilities,
Clinical Responses, and Laboratory Indices[a]

| Triage category (group) | % Cases[b] | Est. dose | Survival probability[c] | Prodromal responses[d] (time to response in h) | Laboratory indices[e] | | |
|---|---|---|---|---|---|---|---|
| | | | | | Lymphs. | Retics. | Amylase |
| Ia | ~70 | ~1 | Certain | Variable; >6 | ~2000 | ~50000 | ~2500 |
| IIb | ~15 | ~3 | Probable | ~3–6 | ~800 | ~20000 | ~2200 |
| II | ~9 | ~5 | Possible | ~2–4 | ~300 | ~10000 | ~1500 |
| III | ~5 | ~11 | Improbable | ~1 | ~100 | ~5000 | ~500 |
| IV | <1 | ~14 | Nil | ~0.5 | <10 | <50 | ~100 |

[a]Parameters and values listed were taken from refs. *26* and *28*.

[b]Percentages of cases based on 588 radiation accident cases taken from the International Computer Database for Radiation Exposure Case Histories (ICDREC) *(29)*.

[c]Survival probability based on 60-plus d of survival following acute radiation exposure and injury.

[d]Prodromal responses are measured in terms of time (h) following initial exposure and encompass nausea, vomiting, fatigue, and weakness.

[e]Laboratory indices: lymphs. (lymphocytes) per $mm^3$ blood measured at 36 h after exposure; retics. (reticulocytes) per $mm^3$ blood measured at 48 h after exposure; and amylase (serum amylase) in units per L of blood.

Because combined-injury patients have other traumatic, chemical, or biological injuries in conjunction with their radiological insult, they generally fare clinically much worse and have poorer prognoses than do patients with single types of injury (e.g, radiation injury alone). In mass casualty situations in which medical resources are severely constrained, this situation (i.e., poorer prognoses of the combined injured) is still further amplified.

We know little about how best to manage combined injuries from the effects of weapons of mass destruction, but a few basic principles are as follows:

1. Acute radiological injury predisposes the victim to subsequent infection.
2. The medical effects of biological weapons will be devastating if the extent of radiation exposure and consequent injury is significant. Specifically, anticipate higher rates of infection and more virulent disease courses.
3. Combined chemical and radiation exposures may produce higher numbers of more serious injuries at much lower exposure levels than expected from single-agent exposures. This pathology has been amply demonstrated experimentally for relatively low doses of ionizing irradiation and neurotoxic chemical weapon agents *(30)*.

## 4.3. Decontamination Protocols and Monitoring

Patients contaminated by external radionuclides can be decontaminated effectively and easily without significantly interfering with the required medical care. In general, 90–95% of the gross, external contaminates can be eliminated simply by removing outer clothing, shoes, and hats and by thoroughly but gently washing the body with soap.

Vigorously flush open, contaminated wounds with water and, if necessary, scrub and surgically trim them to limit internalization of isotopes. Remove contact lenses.

In the second phase of decontamination, rewash and wipe the patient's face and hands and any other areas that may have been exposed. This cleaning will provide significant decontamination.

The third phase of decontamination, washing or clipping the hair and washing the scalp, is required only if the patient is without headgear or monitoring indicates that the hair is contaminated. After decontamination, it is very important to resurvey.

Evaluate externally contaminated patients for internal contamination. Collect nasal swab specimens from both nostrils before facial decontamination and collect and analyze baseline stool, urine, and sputum samples. If this evaluation confirms internal contamination and the contaminating species of nuclide is identified, one must consider appropriate procedures to reduce body burdens: the use of purging and blocking agents, chelation therapy, and so on *(31,32)* (*see* Table 3 for additional treatment details).

### 4.4. Clinical Support

Following a radiation incident, seriously injured persons should receive essential emergency care (either on-site or at a first aid station) with the immediate goal of stabilization. This treatment should occur prior to transport to the primary medical center, where definitive medical care will be provided. Emergency care should include but not be limited to: administration of intravenous fluids, dressing and bandaging burns and wounds, splinting broken bones, applying resuscitative procedures, and providing ventilatory support *(33)*.

The major medical concerns that drive various elements of clinical support include fluid loss and electrolyte imbalances, uncontrolled bleeding, and infections and sepsis *(9)*. These treatment measures, as well as prevention and management of infection, comprise the essentials of clinical support and therapeutic intervention for those injured by radiation.

Because of the well-recognized quantitative relationship between the degree of neutropenia and the increased risk of infectious complications *(34)*, antibiotic prophylaxis should be considered in afebrile patients at the highest risk of infection (with blood neutrophil counts of $\leq$ 500/mm$^3$). Caution should be used, however, when placing the patient on a prophylactic antibiotic regimen, because early suppression of dominant, antibiotic-sensitive bacterial flora can (and will) give way to the outgrowth of more resistant, more difficult to manage, bacterial strains. On the other hand, for patients whose clinical profiles indicate that they have received substantial exposures (1–2 Gy) and are at relatively high risk of infection and sepsis, antibiotic prophylaxis is clearly indicated and justified.

Similarly, if estimated radiation doses are sufficiently high to cause GI damage and associated bacterial translocation, the physician will need to assume an even larger effect on the blood-forming system in terms of level of injury and degree of suppression. In such cases, it is important to consider more aggressive use of broad-spectrum antibiotics, administered both orally and parenterally for the purpose of eliminating unwanted oral and gut flora and providing a bacteriostatic or bacteriocidal shield against tissue-translocating, blood-invading bacteria. Naturally or therapeutically elicited restorations of normal bone marrow and epithelial barrier functions will help to minimize this occurrence.

The management of established or suspected infection (neutropenia and fever) in irradiated persons resembles that of other febrile neutropenic patients *(35)*. Broad-spec-

Table 3
Therapies for Internally Deposited Radionuclides

| Nuclide | Therapeutic agent | Regimen | Comments |
|---|---|---|---|
| Uranium | Na-bicarbonate | Oral, iv infusions | Monitor urine, need to keep alkaline<br>Treat chemical nephrotoxicity |
| Transuranics<br>Americium<br>Californium<br>Curicum<br>Neptunium<br>Plutonium | Ca-DTPA/Zn-DTPA | iv infusions<br>1 g/100–250 mL<br>5% glucose-water | Ca-EDTA may substitute, but is less effective; DFOA may be used in high Pu dose given over 30-min exposures |
| Rare earths<br>Cerium<br>Lanthanum<br>Promethium<br>Scandium<br>Yttrium | Ca-DTPA/Zn-DTPA | iv infusions, nebulizer<br>1 g/100–250 mL<br>5% glucose-water<br>given over 30 min | Ca-EDTA may substitute, but less effective; consider lavaging and purgative |
| Cesium | Prussian blue | Oral, 1–3 g × 3/d | Lavage and purgatives |
| Cobalt | Penicillamine |  | Stomach lavage and purgative |
| Iodine | KI or NaI, or SSKI | Oral, 300 mg on d 1<br>100 mg on d 2, 3, 4,<br>and so on | Early (<12 h) administration critical |
| Phosphorus | Aluminum hydroxide |  | Stomach lavage, oral dosing with high-dose exposures |
| Radium | Magnesium sulfate<br>Alginates<br>Calcium |  | No effective treatment after absorption; consider lavaging |
| Strontium | Ammonium chloride<br>Aluminum phosphate<br>gel, strontium<br>lactate | Oral, 100 mL | Barium sulfate, alginates as alternatives; consider lavaging early |
| Tritium | Forced fluids/water | 3–10 L/d × 7 d |  |

Data from refs. *31* and *32*.

trum empiric therapy with high doses of one or more antibiotics should be initiated at the onset of fever. The attending physician should consider first the oral use of a second-generation quinolone, such as ciprofloxacin, or a third-generation quinolone, such as levofloxacin. Both provide broad coverage against a wide range of Gram-negative and Gram-positive organisms.

Ciprofloxacin may be administered orally, 500–700 mg every 12 h for 3–4 wk. Use of a second antibiotic such as the fourth-generation cephalosporin cefeprime, holds the advantage of higher efficacy against *Pseudomonas* and Enterobacteriaceae but would require twice-daily (1000–2000 mg) intravenous infusion. Intravenous aminoglycosides such as gentamicin also may be useful for Gram-negative coverage. Antibiotics should be continued for 7 d.

Sufficiently intense radiation exposures can result in severe thrombocytopenia days to weeks following exposure. Hemorrhagic complications may result when blood platelet levels fall below critical threshold values ($50,000/mm^3$). Clinical management includes periodic platelet transfusions, for example, once per week from random platelet donors in order to maintain blood platelet levels above a critical threshold.

If the patient becomes immunologically refractory to the random-donor platelet infusions, platelets must be from HLA-compatible donors. For patients requiring surgery, preoperative platelet levels may need to be increased to 50,000 or 75,000 $mm^3$, to minimize hemorrhagic complications.

Before using platelet-enriched plasma preparations, the transfusates must be depleted of white cells both to minimize allosensitization and to minimize the risk of transmitting viral infections (for example, cytomegalovirus). The preparations also must be treated with high doses (approximately 20 Gy) of gamma rays before transfusion, to sterilize the remaining immunocompetent cells that might foster a graft-versus-host response.

In principle, radiation-induced thrombocytopenia can be treated with recombinant cytokines/hematopoietic growth factors [interleukin-11 (IL-11), IL-6, IL-3] to stimulate megakaryocytopoiesis and, in turn, platelet production. The Food and Drug Administration (FDA) has approved Neumega® (IL-11) for treatment of idiopathic and chemotherapy-induced severe thrombocytopenia but not for radiation-induced thrombocytopenia *per se*.

Fluid and electrolyte replacement is fundamental to managing patients with acute radiation syndrome to compensate for excessive water loss, mainly from damage to the gastrointestinal mucosa but also injury to other organ systems (for example, the skin). Intravenous infusion of lactated Ringer's solution or an equivalent balanced salts solution should be administered as needed.

### 4.5. Treatments: Cytokines/Growth Factors

The use of cytokines and growth factors in treating radiation injury has focused on enhancing recovery from acute radiation syndrome. A number of new growth factors have shown significant in vivo and in vitro preclinical efficacy. The FDA recently approved some of them, some are in various phases of clinical trials, and others are moving through preclinical evaluations *(36)*.

Four recombinant growth factors, plus a single cytokine (interleukin) currently have FDA approval for use in humans in treating clinical sequelae of acute bone marrow suppression. These recombinants include: (1) granulocyte colony-stimulating factor (rhuG-CSF) (called Neupogen® or commonly filigrastim and produced by Amgen); (2) a sustained-release formulation of G-CSF (called Neulasta® or commonly pegfilgrastim, again produced by Amgen); (3) granulocyte/macrophage CSF (GM-CSF; called Leukine® or sargramostim and produced by Immunex/Amgen); (4) erythropoietin (rhuEpo) (called Epogen® or Epogen alpha®, produced by Amgen; and (5) IL-11 (called Neumega® or oprelvekin, produced by Genetics Institute).

Although the administration of all of these growth factors/cytokines ably serves to enhance bone marrow function following a suppressive radiation exposure event, each of these growth factors/cytokines does this in a selective and often specific manner. For example, rhuG-CSF (Neupogen) selectively stimulates marrow progenitors committed to granulocyte production, whereas rhu-GM-CSF stimulates a slightly more primitive progenitor having bipotential commitments to both granulocyte and monocyte production. Epo (Epogenr), by contrast, targets solely erythroid progenitors, whereas IL-11 (Neumega) enhances proliferative and differentiative functions of megakaryocytes, i.e., the cells that manufacture blood platelets, which are critical for hemostasis.

The efficacious nature of these recombinants in treating acute myelosuppression of various etiologies has been clearly and consistently demonstrated both in clinical settings and experimentally as well. However, because these remarkable therapeutics have been approved by the FDA for very specific indications, it is not uncommon (in fact it is often the rule) for these agents to be administered off-label by the attending physician for the benefit of the patient. In this regard, none of these recombinants have been approved by the FDA specifically for accidental radiation exposures. Therefore, these drugs would have to be administered at the discretion of the attending physician off-label to individual irradiated patients who are in therapeutic need. Although at first glance, this restriction seems to be a minor one, it presents a substantial handicap to public health officials responsible for stockpiling these essential pharmaceuticals and for maintaining medical readiness for mass casualty nuclear/radiological events.

In terms of administering myelopoietic growth factors/cytokines (G-CSF/GM-CSF/ IL-11) to irradiated patients, each growth factor/cytokine generally is administered daily by either subcutaneous injection or intravenous infusion (Table 4) and should continue at least until critical blood levels are restored [for example, absolute neutrophil count (ANC) > 1000/mm$^3$; platelets > 20,000/mm$^3$; hematocrit > 36%) (25). Treatment should be initiated as soon as possible following acute irradiation. Treatment should be administered only if radiation exposure is suspected to be of sufficient magnitude to cause severe neutropenia (≤500/mm$^3$) or thrombocytopenia (<20,000/mm$^3$) and to have potential health-compromising consequences (such as increased risks of infections and bleeding complications) (33,37).

The recombinant growth factor erythropoietin (Epogen) is available but is considered of limited therapeutic use during early myelosuppressive phases of the evolving acute radiation syndrome. During this early period, the degree of anemia is generally not severe enough to be immediately life-threatening. Later in the course, as blood leukocyte and platelet levels are restored, significant anemia can occur, which can be effectively alleviated by administration of recombinant erythropoietin.

The beneficial role of G-CSF and GM-CSF in reducing the duration and degree of neutropenia cannot be overestimated. It has been determined that the longer the duration of severe neutropenia, the higher the risk of secondary infections. An additional benefit of cytokines is their ability to increase functional capacity of neutrophils and thereby contribute to the prevention of infection as an active part of cellular host defense (25,38).

G-CSF and GM-CSF are currently in widespread clinical use for treating acute neutropenia. Both of these agents are potent but selective stimulators of the granulopoietic arm of the hematopoietic system and serve not only to increase blood neutrophil counts but also to enhance the maturation and function of these vital defense cells. Both agents have high therapeutic ratios, they can be administered and monitored with relative ease, and they can effectively minimize risk of infection resulting from a radiation exposure-compromised lymphohematopoietic system.

Table 4

Recommended Schedule and Dosing for Therapeutic Recombinant Cytokines
and Growth Factors, Following Acute Radiation Exposures Suspected
to Result in Either Severe Febrile Neutropenia or Thrombocytopenia[a]

| Cytokine or growth factor | Trade name | Dosing[b] | Route[b] | Schedule[b] | Treatment |
|---|---|---|---|---|---|
| rhuG-CSF | Neupogen | 2.5–5.0 µg/mg | sc or iv | Daily | ~14 d or ANC levels >10,000/mm$^3$ |
| rhuG-CSF-sr | Neulasta | 6.0 mg | sc | 1× | 1 d |
| rhuGM-CSF | Leukine | 5.0–10.0 µg/kg | sc or iv | Daily | ~14 d or ANC levels >1500/mm$^3$ |
| rhu IL-11 | Neumega | 50 µg/kg | sc | Daily | ~21 d or PTL levels >50,000/mm$^3$ |
| rhu-epo | Epogen | 150 U/kg | sc or iv | 3×/wk | ~8 wk or until hematocrit >36% |

[a]All recombinants listed have been approved by the FDA for either idiopathic or chemotherapy-induced myelosuppression. These agents have *not* been approved for the specific indication of radiation-induced myelosuppression.

[b]Dosing and schedule listed were taken from refs. *25, 33, 37* and manufacturer's inserts.

Abbreviations: ANC, absolute neutrophil count; epo, erythropoietin; G-CSF, granulocyte colony-stimulating factor; GM-CSF, granulocyte/macrophage colony-stimulating factor; IL-11 interleukin-11.

The predominant side effect noted with administration of G-CSF is medullary bone pain, which may be observed shortly after initiation of G-CSF treatment and again just before onset of neutrophil recovery from nadir. G-CSF may exacerbate pre-existing inflammatory conditions. The most common side effects with administration of GM-CSF are fever, nausea, fatigue, headache, bone pain, and myalgias. It is not clear whether side effects of G-CSF or GM-CSF differ markedly when conventional doses are administered.

In addition to the above recombinant cytokines, a new generation of chimeric growth factors is being developed. Three products (myelopoietin, promegapoietin, and progenipoietin) are in preclinical evaluation *(36)*. All are the result of recombinant technology and do not exist in nature. They are engineered as chimeric molecules formed by the combination of two hematopoietic receptors with agonist arms linked by a common bridging scaffold.

Myelopoietin features IL-3 and G-CSF ligands linked to stimulate hematopoietic progenitors bearing IL-3 and G-CSF surface receptors. Promegapoietin links IL-3 and MPL ligands, and progenipoietin combines flt-3 (an early-acting hematopoietic cytokine) and G-CSF ligands *(39)*. All three chimeric molecules exhibit an enhanced capacity to minimize the duration and severity of the initial myelosuppression that follows acute, potentially lethal, high-dose exposure to radiation. The long-term consequences of using these recombinant molecules to establish a fully reconstituted and stable hematopoietic system are not yet known.

The most promising new growth factors in the context of enhancing the viability of irradiated hematopoietic stem cells are flt-3L, c-kitL, and c-mplL. These growth factors, along with IL-3, maintain viability, suppress apoptosis, and promote clonal growth of primitive murine and human hematopoietic progenitor cells. There is also evidence that they may have synergistic effects.

## *4.6. Stem Cell Transplants*

One dilemma physicians may face is whether to consider bone marrow transplantation to ensure the best chance of survival for severely irradiated patients. Bone marrow transplants may be beneficial in patients whose radiation dose estimate exceeds the $LD_{50/60}$ (50–60 lethal dose) for a human receiving a full complement of clinical support that includes cytokine therapy.

Patients considered for allogeneic bone marrow transplants should meet the following conditions: availability of HLA-matched marrow donors; low absolute lymphocyte counts ($<0.1 \times 10^3/mm^3$ at approximately 36 h post exposure); high radiation dose estimates that exceed 7–8 Gy total-body irradiation; absence of significant radionuclide contamination (internalized and fixed nuclide); and the absence of other injuries or disease states that would preclude survival regardless of clinical management (i.e., the "expectant" patient) (25).

Evidence exists that hematopoietic stem cells are mobilized effectively from bone marrow into peripheral blood by treatment with high doses of hematopoietic growth factors (for example, recombinant human G-CSF) and that these mobilized blood stem cells can serve for transplantation purposes. Blood stem cells are efficient in providing both reliable and rapid hematopoietic engraftments and, in turn, higher output of granulocytes and platelets (40).

## *4.7. Follow-up*

Late or delayed health effects occur after exposure to ionizing radiation. Generally, late effects are proportional to the intensity, duration, and quality of the irradiation. Delayed effects appear months to years after irradiation and involve almost any body tissue or organ system. Possible delayed consequences of radiation injury include carcinogenesis, cataract formation, chronic radiodermatitis, decreased fertility, genetic mutations, and a shortened life span (41).

The Hiroshima, Nagasaki, and Russian experiences have not shown significant genetic effects in humans (41). The frequency and severity of late-developing disease entities are exposure-dependent, regardless of their stochastic or deterministic nature. Exposed individuals must be monitored periodically for clinical signs of evolving disease, with attention to tissues and organ systems known to be at risk and dose and dose distribution. The clinical information obtained as time passes following exposure is informative both on behalf of the patient and from an epidemiological standpoint.

Few "early markers" of late-arising radiation-induced disease prove to be prognostically useful. Notable exceptions include the aberrant hybrid *BCR-ABL* gene formed by an early chromosomal translocation; the 5q-chromosomal deletion associated with preclinical evaluation of mutagen-induced myeloid leukemia (42); abnormally elevated plasma levels of transforming growth factor-α (TGF-α) as a marker of evolving tissue fibrosis (43); and *BRCA1* and *BRCA2* mutations in radiosensitive, repair-deficient breast cancer patients (44).

The advent of gene and protein arrays brings renewed hope for the development of preclinical marker profiles based on expressed gene and protein profiles (45,46).

## 5. RADIATION EXPOSURE SCENARIOS

### *5.1. Scenario 1: Planting a Contained Radiation Source in a Public Place*

A terrorist group gains access to a number of strong $^{60}Co$ gamma ray sources from old radiotherapy units and plants them under benches situated in well-used public parks in several major cities. A week following the placement, the group announces what it has done, and the newspapers report it as a potential serious health hazard to those who might have been near the sources. Local panic ensues, and hospitals near the parks begin to attract patients claiming to have been near the various planted radiation sources.

Who needs to be examined and treated for radiation injuries sustained? What are the casualty management protocols?

### 5.1.1. BASIC STEPS IN CASUALTY CARE AND MANAGEMENT

1. Perform triage for presenting patients based on a combination of (a) clinical histories (time and distance from an affected park bench); and (b) presenting clinical symptoms (presence or absence of clinical indicators suggesting acute radiation illness, namely, severity and frequency of upper and lower GI disturbances, extent of weakness, disorientation, presence of localized erythemic wheals on the skin).
2. Collect blood and run a standard battery of hematology and clinical chemistry assays. (*Note*: sequential blood samples should be taken whenever possible.)
3. Request physical dose reconstruction support from medical center health physicists. (*Note*: this support will be useful only if (a) the radiation source has been recovered and its strength determined and (b) the patient can provide reasonably accurate descriptions of the time and distance from the source).
4. Segregate patients into treatment categories according to estimated radiation dose received. (*Note*: dose estimates need to be derived from a combination of clinical symptoms, hematological profiles, and possibly reconstructed dose estimates.)
5. Asymptomatic patients, with normal hematological profiles and with low estimated exposures (<1 Gy), would not receive additional treatments but only reassurance of good health and encouragement to return for follow-up examinations.
6. Patients presenting with significant clinical signs of substantial radiation exposure (for example, upper GI distress, erythemic skin wheals), plus markedly deranged blood profiles (for example, lymphocyte counts in the range of $1000/mm^3$ several days following exposure), and with rough physical dose estimates of 2–4 Gy would be administered recombinant hematopoietic growth factor (rhu-G-CSF/Neopogen) along with a broad-spectrum antibiotic such as a second-generation quinolone, e.g., ciprofloxacin.
   General clinical support would be provided as needed, including fluids, electrolytes, and platelets. Inflammatory skin lesions would be treated topically with linoleic or nonatrophogenic-based creams and systematically with antihistamines *(47)*.
7. Patients presenting with more severe clinical symptoms (for example, recurrent vomiting, diarrhea, weakness, and disorientation) and with marked deranged blood profiles (for example, early, severe pancytopenia) need to be managed aggressively in intensive care (and, if possible, with reverse-phase isolation) not only with full clinical support, prophylactic antibiotics, and growth factor therapies as indicated above, but also with consideration of marrow transplantation.

## 5.2. Scenario 2: Detonation of a Radiological Dispersal Device

A terrorist group gains access to a small amount (approximately 1 pound) of depleted uranium (DU) and fabricates a small RDD by placing the DU into a small container packed with C4 explosive. The device is placed in a backpack, carried into a shopping mall, and left under a table in the food court area.

A terrorist detonates the device through remote control during lunchtime at midweek. The first responders find the food court area filled with dust and a small number of casualties. Two persons are unconscious, one without a pulse and the second with a pulse and shallow breathing. First responders initiate resuscitation for the first victim and perform an initial evaluation of the second.

A dozen or so other people with a range of cuts and abrasions are scattered throughout the dining area. At first glance, none of them appears to have life-threatening injuries.

All casualties and, to a lesser extent, the first responders are covered with dust and debris from the explosion. Within 15–20 minutes of the explosion, the local emergency medical crews arrived on the scene. With no advance notice or warning, neither the first responders nor the responding emergency medical team suspected a radiological event and did no radiation monitoring.

### 5.2.1. Basic Steps in Casualty Care and Management

1. An emergency paramedical team arrives and quickly assesses the clinical status of the victims. The paramedics give the critically injured emergency first aid and then take care of remaining injured. After they treat all injured persons and deem them stable, the injured are prepared for transportation to a local medical center for further evaluation or treatment.
2. Upon arrival at the local medical center, the patients are monitored with a hand-held radiac. Upon detection of radioisotopic contamination, the hospital staff calls for health physics support to determine the offending isotope of uranium (i.e., $^{235}$U-depleted, a fairly benign species harboring only approximately 60% of the radioactivity of naturally occurring uranium). The health physicist relays to the attending physician and the nursing staff the major health risks associated with DU exposure. (DU exposure presents more of a chemical hazard than a radiological hazard. Nevertheless, the staff exercises due caution and takes appropriate medical steps.)
3. Patients are moved to an adjoining empty storage area for decontamination. Contaminated clothing is removed, and full body washes are performed. Radiac surveys ensure that external DU contamination has been minimized. Patients are provided with clean gowns and subsequently moved into the hospital for further evaluation and treatment.
4. Patients are examined clinically, both for blast-associated injuries and DU-associated toxicity. Blood and urine samples must be taken periodically to assess hematological and clinical chemistry profiles.
5. Special attention is paid to kidney and liver function, because uranium is a nephrotoxic and hepatotoxic heavy metal. (*Note*: urinary levels of uranium of 100 µg/dL or more can cause kidney failure.) Appropriate assays include: urinalysis, 24-h urine assays for uranium content, blood urea nitrogen (BUN), creatinine, $\beta_2$-microglobulin, and liver function assays.
6. Additional treatment options include selective use of: (a) blocking, diluting, or purging agents to minimize gastrointestinal absorption; or (b) lavaging of stomach or lungs to reduce uranium concentrations directly.

## 5.3. Scenario 3: Detonation of a Low-Yield Nuclear Weapon

Terrorists smuggle a suitcase-sized, small-yield (1-KT) nuclear weapon into the United States. The weapon is placed in shrubbery bordering the stairs leading up to the U.S. Capitol on the National Mall in Washington, DC, and detonated remotely late one sunny Friday afternoon in autumn.

Congress is not in session, and crowds on the mall, in the Capitol, and surrounding buildings are limited. Nevertheless, the extent of destruction and loss of life is massive. The nuclear emergency response operational center for the Washington area identifies within minutes the nuclear nature of the explosion and quickly locates its epicenter. With real-time analysis, the center estimates and projects the extent and direction of fallout plumes over time.

### 5.3.1. Basic Steps in Casualty Care and Management

1. Casualty estimates: approx 7000 immediate fatalities; 1000–3000 combined injuries; approximately 140,000 radiation casualties, about half (66,000) with treatable, recoverable injuries; 53,000 casualties (approximately 38%) require intensive care and monitoring and consume medical resources. The remaining 13% are expectant and would receive only palliative care (48).

2. Determining radiological conditions and mapping the site is critical. In contrast to the first two scenarios, the first responders and secondary medical emergency crews must wait until radiological conditions are determined.

   Through whatever communications possible, all survivors within several hundred kilometers of the blast's epicenter and within reach of the fallout plume must seek shelter. Shelters should be as airtight as possible, with windows and doors closed and sealed and air ventilation systems turned off.

   Emergency crews, unprepared for existing radiological hazards, are at significant risk of potentially lethal exposure soon after detonation. After the radiological conditions are mapped, crews can be prepared with protective clothing, respiratory devices, and radiological monitors to proceed. Survivors are located, provided with essential first aid, and transported out of the area to local medical centers.

3. For triage, attend first those victims with serious, life-threatening blast and thermal injuries and second those with radiological injuries.

4. Decontaminate victims adjacent to and downwind from the primary medical facility, following previously published guidelines (37). The decontamination site must accommodate both ambulatory and litter patients who are contaminated.

   Medical aides, properly outfitted in anticontamination garments and with respiratory devices, will assist in removing patients' clothing and begin body washing. Patients will be monitored with a radiac and high-activity body areas rewashed until activity levels decline to acceptably low levels. After decontamination, patients will receive clean hospital gowns and move into the medical center proper for further assessment and clinical care.

5. For clinical assessment, conduct full clinical examinations and treat primary, nonradiological injuries first. Re-examine injuries treated in the field and manage them accordingly.

   For secondary management of radiation injuries, start with an initial assessment of clinical symptoms, coupled with radiation dose reconstruction, based on the patient's relative location at the time of the blast, subsequent exposure to the plume, and extent of body contamination.

   Collect and assess urine samples for the type and extent of contaminating isotopes. Collect serial blood samples, and establish conventional blood and clinical chemistry profiles.

6. Treatment: Base all treatment decisions on the patient's clinical profiles and status, coupled with supporting physical dosimetry information. Basic treatment options for external radiation exposure of groups I–IV (Figs. 1 and 2) are as follows:

   a. Group Ia patients with minimal doses (<0.7 Gy), lacking overt symptoms and with normal hematological and clinical chemistry profiles, require no additional treatment, only reassurance of good health.

    b. Group Ib patients with mild doses (approximately 0.7–2 Gy) that are not life-threat-ening and that have only slight derangement of hematological or clinical chemistry profiles require continuous clinical monitoring and subsequent administration of recombinant hematopoietic growth factor(s) (Neupogen/rhuG-CSF and possibly Neumega/rhuIL-11), if severe neutropenia or thrombocytopenia develop, and a broad-spectrum antibiotic (Cipro®/ciprofloxacin), if patient becomes febrile.

    c. Group II patients with moderately high, potentially fatal doses (approximately 3–5 Gy) are placed in intensive care with reverse isolation and full clinical support (fluids, blood cell replacement, antibiotics). Recombinant growth factors (GFs) should be administered daily until blood profiles return to safe ranges, along with prophylactic administration of broad-spectrum antibiotics as indicated previously.

    d. Group III patients with high, potentially lethal doses (approximately 5–10 Gy) must be clinically managed like group II, except under intensive care, in reverse-phase isolation, and with full clinical support, blood cell replacement, and administration of GF and antibiotic therapies. Bone marrow transplantation warrants consideration as an additional therapeutic option for the more heavily exposed patients (approximately 8–10 Gy);

    e. Group IV patients with supralethal doses (>10 Gy) must be considered expectant under mass casualty conditions and should receive palliative treatment alone in most cases. If casualty numbers are limited and resources and facilities are available, pro-cedures to salvage these patients would be comparable to those for Group III patients, including stem cell (blood or marrow) transplants.

7. Treatment for internally deposited radionuclides: Isotope species and the extent of contamination dictate treatment protocols. If treatments are initiated promptly, they are likely to be effective. The goal is to reduce body burdens as much and as safely as possible *(49)*.

Principal treatment strategies include reduction of isotopic intake and absorption, and enhancement of isotopic elimination or excretion (Table 3). Two major fallout isotopes of concern are $^{90}$Sr and $^{137}$Cs. To treat $^{90}$Sr contamination, administer stable strontium (strontium lactate) either orally (300 mg, two to five times daily) or by intravenous infusion (600 mg/d with 500 mL 5% glucose-water over a 4-h period). To treat $^{137}$Cs contamination, administer Prussian blue (1–3 g orally, three times daily).

Specific treatments for other less likely contaminating radioisotopes may be obtained from Gusev et al. *(11)*. In cases of emergency, contact the Radiation Emergency Assistance Center/Training Site (REAC/TS), Oak Ridge, TN, for assistance and guidance (Tel. # 424-576-3131).

## REFERENCES

1. Glasstone S, Dolan PJ. The effects of nuclear weapons. Department of the Army Pamphlet, No. 50-3. Headquarters, Department of the Army, Washington, DC, 1977.
2. Inadequate control of world's radioactive sources. Available at www.iaea.org/worldatom/Press/P_release/2002/prn0209.shtml.
3. Levi MA, Kelly HC. Weapons of mass disruption. Sci Am 2002;287:77–81.
4. Alt AL, Forcino CD, Walker RI. Nuclear events and their consequences. In: Walker RI, Gerveny TJ, eds. Text Book of Military Medicine: Medical Consequences of Nuclear Warfare. TMM Publications, Office of the Surgeon General, Falls Church, VA, 1989, pp. 1–14.
5. Hall E J. Radiology for radiologists. JB Lippincott, Philadelphia, 1994.
6. Kumar KS, Vaishnav YN, Weiss JF. Radioprotection by antioxidant enzymes and enzyme mimetics. Pharmacol Ther 1988;39:301–309.
7. Goldman M, Rosenblatt LS, Book SA. Lifetime radiation effects research in animals: an overview of the status and philosophy of studies at University of California-Davis Laboratory for Energy-Related Health

Research. In: Thompson RC, Mahaffey JA, eds. Life-Span Radiation Effects Studies in Animals: What Can They Tell Us? CONF-830951. Office of Scientific and Technical Information, US Department of Energy, Washington, DC, 1986, pp. 53–65.

8. Fritz TE, Seed TM, Tolle DV, Lombard LS. Late effects of protracted whole-body irradiation of beagles by cobalt-60 gamma rays. In: Thompson RC, Mahaffey JA, eds. Life-Span Radiation Effects Studies in Animals: What Can They Tell Us? CONF-830951. Office of Scientific and Technical Information, US Department of Energy, Washington, DC, 1986, pp. 116–141.

9. Cerveny TJ, MacVittie TJ, Young RW. Acute radiation syndrome in humans. In: Walker RI, Gerveny TJ, eds. Text Book of Military Medicine: Medical Consequences of Nuclear Warfare. TMM Publications, Office of the Surgeon General, Falls Church, VA, 1989, pp. 15–36.

10. Dainiak N. Hematologic consequences of exposure to ionizing radiation. Exp Hematol 2002;30:513–528.

11. Gusev IA, Guskova AK, Mettler FA, eds. Medical Management of Radiation Accidents. CRC Press, Boca Raton, FL, 2001.

12. Glasstone S, Dolan PJ, eds. The effects of Nuclear Weapons. Headquarters, Department of the Army, Washington, DC, 1977.

13. Blakely WF, Brooks AL, Loft RS, van der Schans GP, Voisin P. Overview of low-level radiation exposure assessment: biodosimetry. Mil Med 2002;167(suppl 1):20–24.

14. Wald N. Alterations of hematological parameters by radiation. In: Proceedings of Triage of Irradiated Personnel, 1998. Presented at the Armed Forces Radiobiology Research Institute Workshop, 1996, Bethesda, MD.

15. Bender MA, Gooch PC. Somatic chromosome aberrations induced by human whole-body irradiation: the "Recuplex" criticality accident. Radiat Res 1996;29:568-582.

16. Mettler FA, Upton AC. Medical Effects of Ionizing Radiation, 2nd ed. WB Saunders, Philadelphia, 1995.

17. Anspaugh LR, Akleyev AV, Degteva MO, Straume T, Napier BA. Interpretation of results of FISH assays when zero or only a few translocations are observed. In: Chronic Radiation Exposure: Possibilities of Biological Indication. Russian Federation, Chelyabinsk, Russia, 2000:112.

18. Ward JF. The complexity of DNA damage: relevance to biological consequences. Int J Radiat Biol 1994;66:427–432.

19. Amudson SA, Do KT, Fornace AJ. Induction of stress genes by low doses of gamma rays. Radiat Res 1999;152:225–231.

20. Maity A, Kao GD, Muschel RJ, McKenna WG. Potential molecular targets for manipulating the radiation response. Int J Radiat Biol Phys 1997;37:639–653.

21. Anderson A, Woloschak, GE. Cellular proto-oncogene expression following exposure of mice to gamma rays. Radiat Res 1992;130:340–344.

22. Beetz A, Messer G, Oppel T, van Beuningen D, Peter RU, Kind P. Induction of interleukin-6 by ionizing radiation in human epithelial cell line: control by corticosteroids. Int J Radiat biol 1997;72:33–43.

23. Forrester HB, Yeh RF, Dewey WC. A dose response for radiation-induced intrachromosomal DNA rearrangements detected by inverse polymerase chain reaction. Radiat Res 1999;152:232–238.

24. Kubota N, Hayashi JI, Inada T, Iwamura Y. Induction of a particular deletion in mitochondrial DNA by X-rays depends on the inherent radiosensitivity of the cells. Radiat Res 1998;148:395–398.

25. MacVittie TJ, Weiss JF, Browne D. Consensus summary on the treatment of radiation injuries. In: MacVittie TJ, Weiss JF, Browne D, eds. Advances in the Treatment of Radiation Injuries. Pergamon Press, New York, 1996.

26. Kindler H, Densow D, Fliedner TM. Prediction of clinical course through serial determinations. In: Reeves G, Jarrett DG, Seed TM, King GL, Blakely WF, eds. Triage of Irradiated Personnel. AFRRI Special Publication 98-2. Armed Forces Radiobiology Research Institute, Bethesda, MD, 1998, pp. B6–B9.

27. Anno G. Fatigability and weakness as clinical indicators of exposure. In: Reeves G, Jarrett DG, Seed TM, King GL, Blakely WF, eds. Triage of Irradiated Personnel. AFRRI Special Publication 98-2. Armed Forces Radiobiology Research Institute, Bethesda, MD, 1998, pp. B12–B21.

28. Wald N. Alterations of hematological parameters by radiation In: Reeves G, Jarrett DG, Seed TM, King GL, Blakely WF, eds. Triage of Irradiated Personnel. AFRRI Special Publication 98-2. Armed Forces Radiobiology Research Institute, Bethesda, MD, 1998, pp. B1–B5.

29. Densow D, Kindler H, Baranov AE, Tibken B, Hofer EP, Fliedner TM. Criteria for the selection of radiation accident victims for stem cell transplantation. Stem Cells 1997;15(suppl 2):287–297.

30. Knudson GB, Elliott TB, Brook I, et al. Nuclear, biological and chemical combined injuries and countermeasures on the battlefield. Mil Med 2002;167(suppl 1):95–97.

31. Hubner KF, Fry SA, eds. The Medical Basis of Radiation Accident Preparedness. Elsevier, Amsterdam, 1979.

32. Voelz GL. Assessment and treatment of internal contamination: general principles. In: Gusev IA, Guskova AK, Mettler FA, eds. Medical Management of Radiation Accidents. CRC Press, Washington, DC, 2001, pp. 319–343.
33. NATO Handbook on the Medical Aspects of NBC Defense Operations AMEDP-6(B), 01 Feb. 1996.
34. Boxer L, Dale DC. Neutropenia: causes and consequences. Semin Hematol 2002;39:75–81.
35. Brook I, Elliott TB, Ledney GD, Knudson GB. Management of postirradiation sepsis. Mil Med 2002;167(suppl 1):105–106.
36. MacVittie TJ, Farese AM. Cytokine-based treatment of radiation injury: potentiation benefits after low-level radiation exposure. Mil Med 2002;167(suppl 1):68–70.
37. Jarrett DG. Medical Management of Radiological Casualties Handbook. Armed Forces Radiobiology Research Institute, Bethesda, MD, 1999.
38. Buchsel PC, Forgey A, Grape FB, Hamann SS. Granulocyte macrophage colony-stimulating factor: current practice and novel approaches. Clin J Oncol Nurs 2002;6:198–205.
39. Seed TM, Fry SA, Neta N, Weiss JF, Jarrett DG, Thomassen D. Prevention and treatments: summary statement. Mil Med 2002;167(suppl 1):87–93.
40. Chen Y, Huang X, Xu L, et al. A pilot study of G-CSF mobilized allogeneic bone marrow cells plus peripheral blood stem cells transplantation for malignant hematological diseases. Zhonghua Yi Xue Za Zhi 2002;82:1306–1309.
41. BEIR V. Health effects of exposure to low levels of ionizing radiation. Committee on the Biological Effects of Ionizing Radiations, Board on Radiation Effects Research, Commission on Life Sciences. National Academy Press, Washington, DC, 1990.
42. Le Beau MM, Albain KS, Larson RA, et al. Clinical and cytogenetic correlations in 63 patients with therapy-related myelodysplastic syndromes and acute nonlymphocytic leukemia: further evidence for characteristic abnormalities of chromosomes no. 5 and 7. J Clin Oncol 1986;4:325–345.
43. Anscher MS, Kong FM, Sibley G, et al. Using plasma TGFB1 as a marker to select patients for radiotherapy dose escalation. In: Moriarty M, Motherstill C, Edington M, Ward JF, Fry RJM, eds. Radiation Research, vol 2. Proceeding of the 11th ICRR, Dublin, 1999. Allen Press, Lawrence, KS, 2000, pp. 638–640.
44. Nascimento PA, da Silva MA, Oliveira EM, Suzuki MF, Okazaki K. Evaluation of radioinduced damage and repair capacity in blood lymphocytes of breast cancer patients. Braz J Med Biol Res 1999;34:165–176.
45. Biodosimetry Assessment Tool. Armed Forces Radiobiology Research Institute, Bethesda, MD, 2002.
46. Blakely W, Prasanna PGS, Miller AC. Update on current and new developments in biological dose-assessment techniques. In: Ricks RC, Berger ME, O'Hara FM, eds. The Medical Basis for Radiation-Accident Preparedness: The Clinical Care of Victims. Parthenon Publishing Group, Washington, DC, 2001, pp. 23–32.
47. Peter RW, Gottlober P. Management of cutaneous radiation injuries: diagnosis and therapeutic principles of the cutaneous radiation syndrome. Mil Med 2002;167(suppl 1):110–112.
48. Hazard Prediction and Assessment Capability, version 4.0, program estimates, Defense Threat Reduction Agency, June 1, 2001, Alexandria, VA.
49. Terrorism with Ionizing Radiation General Guidance: Pocket Guide, Employee Education System for the Office of Public Health Environmental Hazards. Department of Veterans Affairs, Washington, DC, 2001.

# 25

## Explosives

*John M. Wightman,* EMT-T/P, MD, MA, FACEP, FACFE,
*and Barry A. Wayne,* EMT-T, MD, FAAEM, FACFE

The opinions or assertions contained herein are the private views of the authors and are not to be construed as official or as reflecting the views of the Department of the Navy, the Department of the Air Force, or the Department of Defense.

### CONTENTS

## 1. INTRODUCTION

Intentional bombings occur throughout the world on an almost daily basis. Many are simple acts of vandalism, such as pipe bombs in mailboxes. Others are targeted to destroy specific structures or kill specific individuals. Although these crimes could be considered acts of terror, this chapter focuses on injuries seen in victims of explosions intended to affect as many people as possible. Conventional explosives remain the most common form of terrorist attack, because they are easy to buy or steal, do not require sophisticated equipment or operator training to employ, can be transported and concealed easily, and are capable of causing widespread damage with a single attack. Moreover, bombs can be activated remotely in either distance or time, thus allowing the perpetrators to be removed from the incident scene for safety, escape, or alibi purposes. They can also turn individuals into human weapons, as the epidemic of suicide bombers in Israel demonstrated in 2002.

In the modern medical literature, many articles have described terrorist attacks with conventional explosives *(1–11)*. Subsequent authors have pooled data from individual incidents to draw a more generalized picture of the epidemiological patterns of injuries sustained by victims *(12–18)*. Severe head injury is the most frequent cause of death in many reports *(11,13,16,19,20)*. Other common causes of mortality include penetrating neck and torso trauma from flying debris *(2,12,16)*, traumatic amputations *(2,8,21)*, and

From: *Physician's Guide to Terrorist Attack*
Edited by: M. J. Roy © Humana Press Inc., Totowa, NJ

crushing injuries owing to collapse of buildings *(4,11,22)*. Injuries found in victims initially surviving terrorist bombings usually include penetrating and blunt soft tissue trauma, closed and open fractures, flashburns, and occasional internal injuries *(1–17,23)*. Burns dominate after detonation of an incendiary device *(9,24)*. Despite the fact that victims of explosions are not commonly encountered by medical providers in the civilian out-of-hospital and in-hospital settings, the vast majority of injuries are due to penetrating, blunt, and thermal trauma. A large number of casualties generated at one time may severely stretch medical resources in any setting *(25,26)*, but these types of injuries are usually obvious or easily detected by providers experienced in the management of gunshot wounds, falls from heights, fires, and other conventional trauma. On the other hand, detonation of high-order explosives can result in additional injuries, which may be clinically occult immediately after detonation. Primary blast injury (PBI) occurs as a direct result of changes in atmospheric pressure induced by the energy of a high-order explosion *(27–29)*. The physics and pathophysiology of this mechanism of injury have been recently reviewed *(30)*.

In brief, explosives generate gasses under extremely high pressures, which then compress the surrounding air faster than thermal motion can disperse its individual molecules. This leads to a thin region of high-pressure air, which expands away from the point of detonation at an initially supersonic speed. The region of high pressure is called a blast wave and the magnitude of maximum change over ambient air pressure is called the peak overpressure. PBI occurs when this band of overpressure contacts a body, thus creating a pressure differential between the blast wave and tissues. Bands of overpressure in blast waves also create winds from these regions of high pressure to adjacent areas of low pressure. These winds are brief in duration, but their magnitude can be hundreds of miles per hour. High-speed winds can accelerate objects into people (causing secondary blast injury) or people into objects (causing tertiary blast injury) *(30)*.

## 2. CLINICAL INDICATORS

The initial evaluation of victims of intentional bombings begins with ensuring the safety of the incident scene, so as not to place medical resources (e.g., personnel, equipment, and so on) at undue risk of loss. Secondary devices or follow-on attacks are a common tactic used to cause injury to emergency responders. Once entry into the affected area is cleared by the on-scene commander, the first three steps include an overall scene survey, communication of additional resources anticipated, and triage of surviving casualties. Many Emergency Medical Services (EMS) systems have adopted various modifications of the Simple Triage and Rapid Treatment (START) methodology for mass-casualty incidents *(31,32)*. It is important to select one triage system for all situations in order to simplify training and improve retention of skills, but the START algorithm was initially developed for response to earthquakes. Although there are similarities to bombings, with building collapses, fires, and victims distributed over a relatively large geographical area, more casualties with penetrating trauma will be seen following high-order explosions, so control of external hemorrhage must be the first priority for identification and intervention.

### 2.1. Penetrating Trauma

Penetration of the body surface by flying debris is usually easy to detect by complaints of pain and the detection of holes in clothing and external wounds. However, many victims of secondary blast injuries (i.e., those caused by ballistic objects) have multiple wounds, not all of which they may be able to localize verbally. Bleeding is relatively common, but life-threatening external exsanguination is not. Eyes are frequently injured, so visual complaints should be investigated and the eyes inspected to rule out penetration *(16)*.

## 2.2. Blunt Trauma

Blunt trauma occurs by secondary and tertiary mechanisms, as well as by falling debris from a damaged building or other structure. The initial evaluation of these injuries is no different following an explosion than they would be following similar nonblast mechanisms of injury, except that they will more frequently occur in the setting of a multiple- or mass-casualty event.

## 2.3. Primary Blast Injury

Pressure differentials between a blast wave contacting the surface of a victim's body and that body's underlying tissues generate a force directed inward relatively perpendicular to the surface. The resulting high acceleration over a very short duration creates an internal stress wave. Just as sound travels at different speeds through air and water, this stress wave moves at different velocities as it passes through organs and tissues of different densities. Shearing forces are then generated at tissue planes, particularly where tissue interfaces with air. When the tensile strengths of tissues are exceeded *(27)*, tearing results in bleeding or abnormal communications *(29,30)*.

Tympanic membranes (TMs), lungs, and bowel are the most common air-containing organs affected through PBI. Usually the TMs are simply ruptured, but fractures and dislocations of the auditory ossicles do occur *(33–35)*. Temporary or permanent hearing loss can result but does not require intervention immediately after a bombing occurs *(3,35–38)*. TM rupture does not appear to be an independent marker for increased likelihood of pulmonary or gastrointestinal PBI *(30,39)*.

Bleeding in the lungs can range from subpleural petechiae of no respiratory consequence, to pulmonary contusions of various sizes, to frank lung lacerations with hemothorax *(40–42)*. Indicators of the latter two include dyspnea, respiratory difficulty, and decreased breath sounds on physical examination *(30)*. Abnormal communications can manifest as hemoptysis, arterial air embolism (AAE), or pneumothorax *(43)*. Massive hemoptysis is an immediate airway problem. AAE can present as any one or a combination of infarction syndromes such as stroke, heart attack, spinal level, or others. Like hemothorax, pneumothorax is indicated by dyspnea, respiratory difficulty, and decreased breath sounds on physical examination. Massive hemothorax and tension pneumothorax are suspected by the combination of asymmetrical breath sounds and shock. Shock can also result from the inability to oxygenate circulating hemoglobin or following persistent blood loss into the airways, pleural space, or elsewhere *(29,30)*.

Bleeding from the bowel wall can result in contusion or hematoma formation, hematochezia, or hemoperitoneum *(40,41)*. Abdominal or testicular pain, tenesmus, and rectal bleeding are each indicators of bowel injury. Obstruction with bilious emesis could be caused by a hematoma in the bowel wall. Abnormal communications result in perforation or fistula formation *(29)*. Perforation can occur acutely or up to a week after the bowel has been stretched through PBI *(44)*. In either case, manifestations of peritonitis will occur hours to days after exposure to the blast wave *(45)*.

Another form of PBI not involving air-containing structures is traumatic amputations. Stress waves shatter long bones and blast winds rip off the distal part of the neck or limb *(46)*. These injuries are easily identified but commonly fatal *(2,8,21)*, although some victims can survive with early intervention *(12,14,22,47)*.

## 2.4. Crushing Injuries

Blunt trauma to muscles and blood vessels (brief but intense), microvascular compression (prolonged but less intense), or systemic hypoxia or hypoperfusion can result in acute traumatic ischemia (ATI) of tissues. A victim who is slammed against a wall by the force of an explosion is an example of the first mechanism. A body or body part pinned beneath rubble is an example of the second mechanism. Pulmonary PBI, blunt chest injury, or the limited oxygen remaining in small air spaces within a collapsed building may lead to hypoxia. External and internal hemorrhage often results in global hypoperfusion and regional ischemia of skin, muscle, and gut.

Early recognition of crushing injuries and ATI may allow prevention of life-threatening sequelae. An understanding of the pathophysiology provides a means to gauge the appropriate entry point for various interventional strategies and therapeutic modalities. A heightened index of suspicion is required to detect the early subtle findings found in these cases. Mechanisms similar to those noted above and prolonged immobilization following the injury are common features.

Although any tissue can be affected, muscle and nerve within myofascial compartments are at particular risk. Suspicion of such a condition can be corroborated clinically by noting pain out of proportion to the apparent extent of trauma, paresthesias in the distribution of peripheral nerves running through the affected compartments, or eliciting pain with passive stretch of any involved muscles. Confirmation occurs with actual pressure measurements in a hospital *(48)*. Although the utility of capillary refill in a field setting has been called into question, it may provide a useful screening tool for detecting asymmetry and for serial checks before transportation. An affected limb may not appear to be diffusely swollen until the onset of significantly increased intracompartmental pressure that exceeds capillary perfusion pressure. An intact pulse distal to the affected area does not indicate that muscle and nerve tissues are being adequately perfused. Blood will simply shunt through collateral channels around tissue compartments with high pressure. Areas of skin that are pale or hyperemic should prompt an extended evaluation. Palpation of the entire body should be done to determine whether there are areas of tenderness, crepitus, ecchymosis, swelling, or firm muscular bundles.

## 2.5. Thermal Trauma

Like penetrating injuries, thermal trauma is readily evident on the external surfaces of the body. Flashburns are extremely common *(3)*, but these are superficial and of little immediate consequence except when they affect the eyes. Victims caught in the fireball of a high-order explosion are usually close enough to the blast to be killed by multiple mechanisms of injury *(30)*, so they will not probably require medical resources. However, individuals can be caught in buildings, vehicles, or vegetated areas ignited by the fireball, but not fatally wounded by flying debris or the blast wave because of intervening barriers or other protection. Additionally, incendiary devices are designed to produce thermal trauma, and multiple burn casualties can consume large amounts of medical resources *(9,24)*.

## *2.6. CBR Release*

The recognition of chemical, biological, or radiological (CBR) contamination and the management of casualties produced by these agents are discussed in other chapters. Reports of immediate incapacitation of casualties after a small detonation should raise a suspicion for release of a blood agent or nerve agent. Low-order explosions with little if any fireball, minimal physical destruction in the vicinity, or unexpected clouds or odors should raise the suspicion of a "dirty bomb" possessing CBR activity. The blast itself may not have been the intended or only threat. Chemical release is much more likely to be secondary to explosive targeting of industrial chemical stores than prepackaged agents typically used for chemical warfare.

## *2.7. Toxic Inhalations*

Even if there is no CBR release, explosions do create toxic hazards both directly and indirectly. Direct toxic hazards are most commonly the nitrogenous byproducts of high-order detonations, such as nitric and nitrous oxides. Indirect toxic hazards include byproducts of combustion, such as smoke and carbon monoxide, and burning substances, such as cyanide from some plastic materials. However, recognition of smoke inhalation or carbon monoxide toxicity is no different after an explosion than following a conventional fire in a structure.

## 3. INITIAL MANAGEMENT

Out-of-hospital management begins with triage of victims and early communication with the overall incident commander in order to mobilize additional resources to the site and prepare hospitals for receipt of casualties.

## *3.1. Triage and Transportation*

The primary goal of triage in the field is to differentiate victims with more immediate or potentially serious problems from those with less serious problems for both out-of-hospital treatment and transportation to a definitive-care facility. Once any individual casualty is identified as having a life-threatening condition, the decision to intervene in the field or transport to a hospital must be made based on available resources and time estimates. A modified START methodology for mass-casualty situations works well *(32)*, because it uses a familiar airway–breathing–circulation–disability (A–B–C–D) approach, and each parameter assessed is easy to determine in the field. However, its primary limitation is that it does not specifically address the importance of stopping external hemorrhage. Therefore, further modification to X–A–B–C–D is preferred, where X signifies that eXternal hemorrhage is stopped with direct pressure at any time in the algorithm.

Exsanguinating eXternal hemorrhage must be controlled immediately. Direct pressure can be applied by medical personnel or rapidly demonstrated to untrained bystanders or "walking wounded" to apply to themselves or others. If direct pressure is either inadequate or cannot be maintained with the resources at hand, a tourniquet should be applied to bleeding extremities.

Following a high-order detonation with many victims, the likelihood of a wound causing Airway compromise is relatively remote. Airway problems will more commonly be caused by position in casualties with depressed levels of consciousness from head injury or shock. Rescuers should begin by checking all individuals who cannot walk to a rapidly established Casualty Collection Point (CCP). Those who can walk should initially be considered DELAYED until a more detailed evaluation can be performed.

If no spontaneous breathing is evident during the first "look, listen, and feel" assessment, the airway should be opened by any means for which there is time, personnel, and equipment. This may often be accomplished by simply rolling the victim into the "recovery position" (left lateral decubitus with the hips and knees partially flexed). If the casualty does not begin unassisted breathing after this intervention, he or she should be considered UNSALVAGEABLE at that moment in time, and the rescuer should move on to the next victim. If the casualty does breathe spontaneously, the airway must be maintained and the victim considered IMMEDIATE.

Any victims maintaining their own airway are next evaluated for adequacy of *B*reathing. Casualties complaining of dyspnea at rest, or who appear to be in respiratory distress, as well as those breathing too slowly (i.e., $\leq 10$ breaths/min), too fast (i.e., $\geq 30$ breaths/min), or too shallowly (i.e., not expanding the chest wall), should be placed in the IMMEDIATE category for evaluation of the cause when resources allow. A rapid assessment for tension pneumothorax, and needle thoracentesis if suspected, could be lifesaving during this phase of triage. If these abnormal parameters are not present, it is unlikely that the casualty has a major disturbance of circulation, and he or she should be considered DELAYED.

If the victim cannot respond to questioning or breathing cannot be sufficiently assessed, both radial pulses should be palpated simultaneously to evaluate the adequacy of *C*irculation. Absence of one pulse indicates vascular compromise in one limb. Absence of both pulses indicates systemic vascular compromise. If neither carotid pulse can be palpated, the casualty should be considered UNSALVAGEABLE at that moment in time, and the rescuer should move on to the next victim. If both radial pulses are absent but at least one carotid pulse is present, the casualty should be considered in or at risk for shock and then placed in the IMMEDIATE triage category.

*D*isability is assessed by having a casualty with adequate bilateral radial pulses follow a few simple commands. If the victim cannot follow commands, he or she should be considered IMMEDIATE, because of the possibility of significant closed head injury. If the victim can follow commands, he or she should be considered DELAYED.

On their first pass through all casualties, rescuers cannot spend sufficient time with each individual to rule out all potentially serious problems. Therefore, no victims are placed in the MINIMAL category initially. With regard to limb-threatening injuries, orthopedic and vascular surgery has made enormous progress in the past two decades, and extremities, which may have once been unsalvageable, can now be stabilized, debrided, and reconstructed. As a result, many physicians will go to extraordinary lengths to attempt to save a limb when sufficient resources are available. However, it should be realized, particularly in the case of mass-casualty incidents or disasters, that amputation of a nonviable limb may be the only procedure capable of preventing the life-threatening sequelae of the crush syndrome *(49)*. Sight-threatening injuries are very common following a detonation that accelerates glass and other debris to high speeds. However, in the absence of corrosive materials, there is little treatment feasible to provide in the out-of-hospital setting that can be expected to improve outcomes. As a result, most of these casualties will be DELAYED for field treatment but may have a high priority for transportation to definitive care.

Once individuals with immediately life-, limb-, or sight-threatening conditions are managed to the extent resources allow, all remaining potentially salvageable casualties should be more carefully evaluated for serious problems that could develop in a more delayed fashion. This second-pass triage can then sort patients into IMMEDIATE, DELAYED, and MINIMAL categories. Application of geographical triage will allow easier delegation of resources and begins the process of preparing casualties for transportation.

Triage for transportation to definitive care is somewhat different from triage for field treatment, because the parameters for decision making are less physiological and more resource-based. In most mass-casualty situations, not all victims should be transported to the same hospital. This will simply turn a mass-casualty event in the field to a mass-casualty event at the destination. Evacuation decisions must be based on the time frame within which definitive care must be initiated for an individual casualty's problems, transportation resources available at any given moment in time, and capabilities of the receiving facility. Transportation resources include vehicle type (e.g., ground or air), staffing expertise (e.g., basic or advanced), and equipment appropriateness (e.g., adult or pediatric). Capabilities of the receiving facility include qualifications of the emergency department (ED) staff and ancillary personnel, availability of surgeons and anesthesiologists experienced in trauma, blood supplies, and resources for intensive care after initial management. Travel time, current workload, and numbers of open beds should also be considered. Special considerations for rotary-wing evacuation of casualties with injuries of air-containing structures following a high-order blast should be no different from those following conventional blunt or penetrating trauma, except that the likelihood of these injuries is increased.

### 3.2. Emergent Problems

Receipt of casualties into the ED will depend on how many are expected, based on information from EMS personnel at the scene and proximity of the hospital to the incident site. Many casualties will not wait for ambulance transportation and will walk or drive to the closest facility (26). Hospital disaster plans must be frequently reviewed, and personnel must be trained on a regular basis to bring order to chaos. Once a casualty arrives in the ED, he or she should be reassessed, and initial management should be instituted as described above.

Unless a victim has a depressed level of consciousness from head injury or shock, the need for airway intervention will be unlikely. On the other hand, when massive hemoptysis from pulmonary PBI is present, the attendant medical provider must be able to selectively intubate the mainstem bronchus of the least injured lung (50). If a double-lumen endotracheal tube or Univent tube is not available or the operator is not skilled in their use, a standard endotracheal tube should be passed orally until only the hub extends out of the mouth and the cuff should be inflated (51). Virtually all of these will pass into the right mainstem bronchus. If more blood passes around the tube than through the tube, the left lung is the source of heavier bleeding and the right lung is relatively protected. If the opposite is true, the left lung will have to be selectively intubated blindly. The highest percentage chance of accomplishing this will be to pass the orotracheal tube through the larynx, then turn the casualty's head to the right and turn the tube 180° so the natural curve of the tube points toward the left lung before advancing it fully. If the casualty's other injuries preclude neck motion, the tube can be turned 90° to the left before advancing it *(51)*. If this is still unsuccessful, the tube can be turned counterclockwise in 90° increments from 90° to 180° to 270° and then back to 0° in order to place the bevel into the left side.

Tension pneumothorax is relatively common after moderate to severe PBI of the lungs *(43)*, and it should be assumed to exist in any victim with decreased or absent breath sounds in one hemithorax and clinical manifestations of shock *(30)*. Needle thoracentesis should follow emergently. Although severe pulmonary contusions and hemothoraces might present with a similar clinical picture, needle thoracentesis will probably not be harmful, and these conditions often require tube thoracostomy anyway. If sufficient air cannot be removed to relieve the tension, a thoracostomy placing a large-bore tube will have to be performed, possibly under field conditions. If the tension still persists with a functioning large-bore chest tube, the existence of a bronchopleural fistula should be assumed. Options for management include: (1) placement of additional tube thoracostomies sufficient to evacuate as much air out of the affected hemithorax as is coming into it; or (2) selective bronchial intubation of the opposite lung as described above *(30)*. Bilateral tension pneumothoraces caused by bronchopleural fistulae have been described *(43)*.

Blood in the pulmonary interstitium following blunt trauma or PBI inhibits diffusion of gasses between the alveoli and capillaries. It also makes the lungs less compliant and, therefore, more difficult to ventilate. Using positive-pressure ventilation (PPV) to overcome the greater airway resistance places the casualty at risk for barotrauma and volutrauma with sequelae such as pneumothorax or AAE. The risk of AAE increases with increased airway pressures associated with PPV, decreased pulmonary venous pressures associated with blood loss, or a combination of both *(52)*. Hence, spontaneous (i.e., negative-pressure) ventilations are preferred whenever possible *(50)* or airway pressures must be kept low if PPV is absolutely required *(43)*.

Shock will most frequently be owing to tension pneumothorax, profound hypoxia, or hemorrhage *(30)*, but tension pneumoperitoneum has been described *(53)*. Bleeding is more commonly caused by penetrating and blunt trauma than PBI-induced hemothorax, hemoperitoneum, or hematochezia *(54)*. One notable exception to this is victims exposed to an underwater detonation: fragments do not move far, but the blast wave can be propagated great distances to affect the abdomen more than the lungs in casualties treading water *(27,30,55)*. Resuscitation for hypovolemic shock must be tempered by the potential presence of cerebral or pulmonary injury, which could be worsened by injudicious fluid administration. Standard boluses with 2 L of crystalloid fluids run as rapidly as possible have the potential for increasing lung edema in patients with pulmonary contusion following blunt trauma *(56,57)*. Therefore, initial fluid resuscitation should be in smaller (e.g., 500-mL) boluses with more frequent assessments of end-organ function (e.g., improving mental status) and markers of untoward effects (e.g., diminishing pulmonary function) *(30)*.

Two additional causes of shock include: (1) AAE to the heart, brain, or spinal cord *(23)*; and (2) dehydration or the "crush syndrome" following entrapment in a collapsed structure followed by delayed access to care *(58)*. AAE is initially managed with 100% oxygen *(50)* and possibly positioning the victim in a semi-left-lateral decubitus position (i.e., halfway between lateral and prone) *(30)*. The crush syndrome is initially managed by adequate volume resuscitation *(59)* modified by the guidelines above.

## 4. CONTINUED CARE

Once patients are evaluated and initially managed in the ED (or alternative site in a disaster situation), a triage process must again be applied to determine those who must go to surgery, those who need additional care in an intensive care unit (ICU) or on a hospital ward, and those who can be discharged home. If the resources needed for a particular patient are not available at the receiving facility, he or she should be stabilized as best as possible and transferred to a higher level of care.

### 4.1. Ventilation Management

Although spontaneous, negative-pressure respirations are desired, positive pressure may be required to maintain oxygenation and should be instituted when truly necessary. Prior to endotracheal intubation and manual or mechanical ventilation, administration of 100% oxygen and decompression of any pneumothorax should be performed. If this is unsuccessful in improving oxygen saturation and the casualty's situation is less critical, techniques using continuous positive airway pressure (CPAP) (60) or biphasic positive airway pressure (BiPAP) may be attempted.

One group of investigators has proposed a classification system for blast lung injuries. They used chest radiographic infiltrate patterns and arterial blood-gas (ABG) analyses to assign categories of mild, moderate, and severe (43). Patients with mild lung injury did not require PPV for a respiratory problem. On the other hand, mechanical ventilation was necessary for all casualties with moderate or severe lung injury. The methods and durations of PPV were frequently different, however (Table 1) (43), because severe pulmonary contusions of this nature often behave like the acute respiratory distress syndrome (ARDS), with markedly increased shunts and decreased compliance. The latter increases susceptibility to barotraumas and volutrauma (61). Permissive hypercapnia has been specifically described for use in patients with blast lung injury (62).

### 4.2. Arterial Air Embolism

The goal in managing suspected AAE is to keep the patient alive until he or she can receive hyperbaric oxygen (HBO) therapy. The mainstay of temporizing management includes placing the patient on 100% oxygen, minimizing airway pressures, prevention or correction of hypovolemia, and prevention of decreased atmospheric pressure by ground or air transportation with significant altitude changes. It may be possible to reduce the risk further by positioning the victim with the head at the same level as the heart to prevent cerebral AAE and in a semi-left-lateral decubitus position (i.e., halfway between lateral and prone) to prevent coronary AAE by positioning the coronary arteries at their lowest point relative to the aorta (30).

### 4.3. Internal Injuries

Hospital-based trauma teams should not have to substantially alter the processes by which they rule in or out internal hemorrhage following blunt or penetrating trauma. In patients manifesting shock, if external bleeding has been controlled and tension pneumothorax or AAE can be reasonably excluded or treated, continued fluid or blood requirements should be assumed owing to internal hemorrhage (29,30). Plain chest

Table 1
Severity Categories for Primary Blast Injury of the Lung[a]

|  | Mild | Moderate | Severe |
|---|---|---|---|
| Radiographic infiltrates | Unilateral | Asymmetrical bilateral | Diffuse bilateral |
| PFR (mmHg) | >200 | 60–200 | <60 |
| PPV requirement | Unlikely for respiratory problem | Highly likely but conventional methods usually | Universal and unconventional methods common |
| PEEP requirement (cmH$_2$O) | <5 if PPV needed | 5–10 usually needed | >10 commonly needed |
| Bronchopleural fistula | No |  | Yes |

[a]The categories are as reported by Pizov et al. (43) and reproduced from Wightman and Gladish (30). They may help predict the necessity for use of positive-pressure ventilation (PPV) and positive end-expiratory pressure (PEEP). PFR is the $p_aO_2$-to-$F_IO_2$ ratio, where $F_IO_2$ is expressed as a fraction of 1.

radiographs provide the most effective screening for life-threatening injuries in the chest that are not readily apparent on physical examination. Focused abdominal sonography for trauma (FAST) or diagnostic peritoneal tap and lavage (DPTL) can be used in the ED to determine whether free intraperitoneal fluid (FIF) is present or absent. FIF noted on FAST examination would preclude the need for DPTL. Computed tomography (CT) can be used in stable patients who are not hemodynamically compromised, but DPTL is more sensitive at detecting bowel injury than is CT. Each trauma team will have to employ the screening and diagnostic modalities in which they have the most confidence.

Internal injuries are usually repaired by surgeons, embolized by interventional radiologists, or observed in an environment in which immediate treatment can be instituted if the patient's condition deteriorates. Some early literature on the management of blast injuries suggested that surgery in the immediate postinjury phase resulted in higher mortality owing to tension pneumothorax and AAE when accomplished in the presence of blast lung injury (52,63,64). This is less likely to be the case with modern preoperative evaluations, anesthesiological techniques, and intraoperative monitoring. Several authors, particularly in the UK, have recommended bilateral prophylactic chest tubes prior to inhalational anesthesia and PPV (54,65,66). When practicable, regional or spinal anesthesia may be safer (52,54,64).

### 4.4. Crush Syndrome

Following crushing mechanisms of injury, ATI of muscle cells results in lack of substrate and oxygen, which translates into a decrease in available ATP and cellular acidosis. As the level of energy available within the cell decreases, the cells lose their ability to perform normal homeostatic mechanisms, such as the maintenance of the cellular membrane. A leaking cell membrane causes an influx of ions, the eventual derangement of intracellular organelles, and eventual cellular death with rhabdomyolysis. Upon lysis of muscle cells, there is a release of mediators of inflammation, promoting vasoconstriction, platelet aggregation, and vascular permeability, which cause further edema and decreased tissue perfusion, continuing the destructive cycle. Cellular death also results in the release of lactate, potassium, phosphate, and myoglobin. This aspect of acute traumatic rhabdomyolysis is responsible for the initiation of the crush syndrome, manifested by profound weakness, renal failure, circulatory collapse, cardiac dysrhythmia, and death *(67–68)*.

Any affected limbs should be immobilized with padded splints in a position that will enhance local circulation and permit ongoing neurovascular examinations. Supplemental oxygen should be provided to keep the hemoglobin saturation greater than 95%, and blood should be transfused to keep the hemoglobin greater than 10 g/dL. Continuous cardiac monitoring and pulse oximetry should be performed whenever possible. Apart from any labs needed for specific concomitant injuries, blood should be drawn for a complete blood count (CBC) with platelets, blood urea nitrogen (BUN), creatinine, electrolytes, phosphorus, calcium, and creatine kinase (CK). A urinanalysis and urine myoglobin determination should also be obtained. Urine myoglobin should be obtained on freshly produced urine, not the pretrauma specimen that the bladder initially contains. If urine myoglobin is not readily available, the urine can be dipped for hemoglobin. If it is positive, and there are no red blood cells (RBCs) on the microscopic examination, the test should be considered positive for myoglobin in this context.

Traditional trauma management dictates that a patient be given 2 L of warmed crystalloid at a wide-open rate. With a patient who may have pulmonary parenchymal injuries, this may be a dangerous practice. Initial fluid resuscitation should be done with 250-mL aliquots of body temperature normal saline every 15 min until urine is produced. If urine is not produced despite a resuscitated systolic arterial pressure greater than 90 mmHg, furosemide 40–120 mg iv may be given either alone or with 20 g of mannitol (although, in general, mannitol should not be given to anuric patients) *(68)*. Furosemide causes renal vasodilation, decreased oxygen demands by the kidney and increased renal intratubular flow. The goal is a urine output greater than 2 mL/kg/h. Alkalinization of the urine, to prevent precipitation of the myoglobin in the glomeruli, is advocated in most standard emergency medicine texts. The usual procedure is to add 50 mEq of sodium bicarbonate solution to 1 L of 0.45% (half-normal) sodium chloride. The goal is a urinary pH of 7.55 or greater. It should be realized that alkalinization may exacerbate the hypocalcemia that is sometimes associated with rhabdomyolysis.

Frequent neurological and vascular checks are essential to detect developing processes that may have been occult to the examiner initially. Serial laboratory exams of potassium, CK, and urine myoglobin should likewise be obtained, particularly if the initial results are normal in a clinical context that strongly suggests the possibility of ATI. There will ordinarily be a time delay between the injury, the onset of ATI, and the appearance of abnormal laboratory findings. Specimens that are obtained soon after the injury can be anticipated to be normal or nearly so. This should not cause the physician to cease to look for evidence of developing ATI. HBO therapy has recently been shown to be effective in extremity ATI in a double-blind trial *(69)* and should be considered for these patients when it is available.

### 4.5. Delayed Presentation

Because trapped victims may have to be extricated from a collapsed structure, transportation may be delayed in overwhelming mass-casualty situations, and some casualties may not seek medical attention immediately; health care providers should anticipate the possibility of patients presenting for medical care after delays of hours to days. Mental health problems may present weeks, months, or years later.

Extricated victims may have been trapped in a small space for hours or days. They may not only have their original blast injuries, but also crush injuries causing local and humoral problems, irritatation of the respiratory system by smoke and dust, prolonged hypoxia from low $F_IO_2$ in small spaces and breathing uncirculated air for prolonged periods, exposure to toxins and hazardous materials, and lack of water and food. These patients can have advanced pathophysiological derangements when they finally present for definitive care (58).

Casualties with open wounds or initially minor eye or ear problems may present with established infections. Breaches in the skin could lead to cellulitis, abscess formation, parasite infestation, deep-space infections such as gas gangrene or necrotizing fasciitis, and even systemic sepsis. Delayed eye infections may include keratitis or endophthalmitis. Retention of foreign bodies is always a possibility after any secondary or tertiary penetrating injury. PBI of the eye may cause a hyphema. PBI of the ear causing TM rupture may increase susceptibility to myringitis or otitis if water or other foreign material enters the ear canal.

## 5. DISPOSITION

Casualties from an explosion should be admitted or discharged based on two sets of considerations: (1) conventional penetrating, blunt, and thermal trauma; and (2) potential manifestations of primary blast injury. Obviously, any patient requiring airway support, ventilatory assistance, hemodynamic stabilization, or an extensive surgical procedure must be admitted to an intensive care unit after initial interventions. If the resources required are not available at the receiving facility, the patient will have to be transferred to a more capable hospital (30).

All patients with suspected ATI from a crushing mechanism require admission for intravenous fluid therapy, repeated determinations of serum potassium, CK, and myoglobin, as well as close clinical monitoring for the onset of compartment syndromes. Frequent neurological and vascular examinations must be performed at least hourly for the first 4 h after admission. The treatment of hyperkalemia, hypercalcemia, hypophosphatemia, and myoglobinuria associated with rhabdomyolysis is discussed in standard texts.

Patients with chest complaints, any degree of dyspnea, or a significant electrocardiographical, radiographical, or ABG abnormality should be admitted overnight for observation (30). Virtually all pulmonary contusions will manifest in the first day. Significant ones are more likely to be evident in the first hour (39). Recognition of abdominal symptoms or signs are an also an indication for observation, even if initial diagnostic studies return negative results; the duration should be at least 2–3 d (30), because manifestations of bowel injury may be delayed (44,64).

Isolated rupture of the TM can be managed on an outpatient basis with referral to an otorhinolaryngologist within 3 d to unfold torn TM edges if necessary, and then to follow for possible cholesteatoma formation. If significant debris in the external canal requires irrigation, this should be accomplished by the consultant during the initial visit to prevent infection (70,71). Most perforations will heal without surgical repair (36).

## REFERENCES

1. Caro D, Irving M. The Old Bailey bomb explosion. Lancet 1973;1:1433–1435.
2. Waterworth TA, Carr MJT. An analysis of the post-mortem findings in the 21 victims of the Birmingham pub bombings. Injury 1975;7:89–95.

3. Waterworth TA, Carr MJT. Surgery of violence: report on injuries sustained by patients treated at the Birmingham General Hospital following the recent bomb explosions. BMJ 1975;2:25–27.
4. Brismar B, Bergenwald L. The terrorist bomb explosion in Bologna, Italy, 1980: an analysis of the effects and injuries sustained. J Trauma 1982;22:216–220.
5. Adler J, Golan E, Golan J, et al. Terrorist bombing experience during 1975-79: casualties admitted to the Shaare Zedek Medical Center. Isr J Med Sci 1983;19:189–193.
6. Frykberg ER, Tepas JJ, Alexander RH. The 1983 Beirut Airport terrorist bombing: injury patterns and implications for disaster management. Am Surg 1989;55:134–141.
7. Katz E, Ofek B, Adler J, et al. Primary blast injury after a bomb explosion in a civilian bus. Ann Surg 1989;209:484–488.
8. Rignault DP, Deligny MC. The 1986 terrorist bombing experience in Paris. Ann Surg 1989;209:368–373.
9. Gomez Morell PA, Escudero Naif F, Palao Domenech R, et al. Burns caused by the terrorist bombing of the department store Hipercor in Barcelona: part 1. Burns 1990;16:423–425.
10. Hodgetts TJ. Lessons from the Musgrave Park Hospital bombing. Injury 1993;24:219–221.
11. Mallonee S, Shariat S, Stennies G, et al. Physical injuries and fatalities resulting from the Oklahoma City bombing. JAMA 1996;276:382–387.
12. Hadden WA, Rutherford WH, Merrett JD. The injuries of terrorist bombing: a study of 1532 consecutive patients. Br J Surg 1978;65:525–531.
13. Hill JF. Blast injury with particular reference to recent terrorist bombing incidents. Ann R Coll Surg (Engl) 1979;61:4–11.
14. Pyper PC, Graham WJH. Analysis of terrorist injuries treated at Craigavon Area Hospital, Northern Ireland, 1972-1980. Injury 1983;14:332–338.
15. Frykberg ER, Tepas JJ. Terrorist bombings: lessons learned from Belfast to Beirut. Ann Surg 1988;208:569–576.
16. Mellor SG, Cooper GJ. Analysis of 828 servicemen killed or injured by explosion in Northern Ireland 1970–1984: the Hostile Action Casualty System. Br J Surg 1989;76:1006–1010.
17. Abenhaim L, Dab W, Salmi LR. Study of civilian victims of terrorist attacks (France 1982–1987). J Clin Epidemiol 1992;45:103–109.
18. Coupland RM, Meddings DR. Mortality associated with use of weapons in armed conflicts, wartime atrocities, and civilian mass shootings: literature review. BMJ 1999;319:407–410.
19. Cooper GJ, Maynard RL, Cross NL, Hill JF. Casualties from terrorist bombings. J Trauma 1983;23:955–967.
20. Scott BA, Fletcher JR, Pulliam MW, Harris RD. The Beirut terrorist bombing. Neurosurgery 1986;18:107–110.
21. Hull JB, Bowyer GW, Cooper GJ, Crane J. Pattern of injury in those dying from traumatic amputation caused by bomb blast. Br J Surg 1994;81:1132–1135.
22. Hull JB. Traumatic amputation by explosive blast: pattern of injury in survivors. Br J Surg 1992;79: 1303–1306.
23. Quintana DA, Parker JR, Jordan FB, Tuggle DW, Mantor PC, Tunell WP. The spectrum of pediatric injuries after a bomb blast. J Pediatr Surg 1997;32:307–310; discussion, 310–311; errata, 932.
24. Jimenez-Hernandez FH, Lliro Blasco E, Leiva Oliva R, et al. Burns caused by the terrorist bombing of the department store Hipercor in Barcelona: part 2. Burns 1990;16:426–431.
25. Frykberg ER, Hutton PM, Balzer RH. Disaster in Beirut: an application of mass casualty principles. Mil Med 1987;152:563–566.
26. Hogan DE, Waeckerle JF, Dire DJ, Lillibridge SR. Emergency department impact of the Oklahoma City terrorist bombing. Ann Emerg Med 1999;34:160–167.
27. Stuhmiller JH, Phillips YY, Richmond DR. The physics and mechanisms of primary blast injury. In: Bellamy RF, Zajtchuk R, eds. Conventional Warfare: Ballistic, Blast, and Burn Injuries. Office of the Surgeon General of the United States Army, Washington DC, 1991, pp. 241–270.
28. Iremonger MJ. Physics of detonations and blast-waves. In: Cooper GJ, Dudley HAF, Gann DS, Little RA, Maynard RL, eds. Scientific Foundations of Trauma. Butterworth-Heineman, Oxford, 1997, pp. 189–199.
29. Wightman JM, Wayne BA. Blast and crushing injuries. In: Tintinalli JE, Kelen GD, Stapczynski JS, eds. Emergency Medicine: A Comprehensive Study Guide, 6th ed. McGraw-Hill, New York, in press.
30. Wightman JM, Gladish SL. Explosions and blast injuries. Ann Emerg Med 2001;37:664–678.
31. Benson M, Koenig KL, Schultz CH. Disaster triage: START, then SAVE—a new method of dynamic triage for victims of a catastrophic earthquake. Prehosp Disast Med 1996;11:117–124.
32. Garner A, Lee A, Harrison K, Schulz CH. Comparative analysis of multiple-casualty incident triage algorithms. Ann Emerg Med 2001;38:541–548.

33. Singh D, Ahluwalia KJS. Blast injuries of the ear. J Laryngol Otol 1968:82;1017–1028.

34. Sudderth ME. Tympanoplasty in blast-induced perforation. Arch Otolaryngol 1974;99:157–159.

35. Roberto M, Hamernik RP, Turrentibe GA. Damage to the auditory sytem associated with acute blast trauma. Ann Otol Rhinol Laryngol 1989;98(suppl 140):23–34.

36. Pahor AL. The ENT problems following the Birmingham bombings. J Laryngol Otol 1981;95:399–406.

37. Walby AP, Kerr AG. Hearing in patients with blast lung. J Laryngol Otol 1986;100:411–415.

38. Garth RJN. Blast injury of the auditory system: a review of the mechanisms and pathology. J Laryngol Otol 1994;108:925–929.

39. Leibovici D, Gofrit ON, Shapira SC. Eardrum perforation in explosion survivors: is it a marker of pulmonary blast injury? Ann Emerg Med 1999;34:168–172.

40. Rössle R. Pathology of blast effects. In: German Aviation Medicine: World War II. Office of the Surgeon General of the United States Air Force, Washington DC, 1950, pp. 1260–1273.

41. Sharpnack DD, Johnson AJ, Phillips YY. The pathology of primary blast injury. In: Bellamy RF, Zajtchuk R, eds. Conventional Warfare: Ballistic, Blast, and Burn Injuries. Office of the Surgeon General of the United States Army, Washington DC, 1991, pp. 271–294.

42. Mayorga MA. The pathology of primary blast overpressure injury. Toxicology 1997;121:17–28.

43. Pizov R, Oppenheim-Eden A, Matot I, et al. Blast lung injury from an explosion on a civilian bus. Chest 1999;115:165–172.

44. Paran H, Neufeld D, Shwartz I, et al. Perforation of the terminal ileum induced by blast injury: delayed diagnosis or delayed perforation? J Trauma 1996;40:472–475.

45. Cripps NPJ, Cooper GJ. Risk of late perforation in intestinal contusions caused by explosive blast. Br J Surg 1997;84:1298–1303.

46. Hull JB, Cooper GJ. Pattern and mechanism of traumatic amputation by explosive blast. J Trauma 1996;40(suppl 3):S198–S205.

47. Hull JB. traumatic amputation by explosive blast: pattern of injury in survivors. Br J Surg 1992;79: 1303–1306.

48. Stack LB. Compartment syndrome evaluation. In: Roberts JR, Hedges JR, eds. Clinical Procedures in Emergency Medicine, 3rd ed. WB Saunders, Philadelphia, 1998, pp. 932–946.

49. Complications of Trauma, WorldOrtho Inc, 1997, p. 1 (accessed via www.worldortho.com on 18 August 2002).

50. Ost D, Corbridge T. Independent lung ventilation. Clin Chest Med 1996;17:591–601.

51. Kubota H, Kubota Y, Toyoda Y, et al. Selective blind endotracheal intubation in children and adults. Anesthesiology 1987;67:587–589.

52. Ho AM-H, Ling E. Systemic air embolism after lung trauma. Anesthesiology 1999;90:564–575.

53. Oppenheim A, Pizov R, Pikarsky A, et al. Tension pneumoperitoneum after blast injury: dramatic improvement in ventilatory and hemodynamic parameters after surgical decompression. J Trauma 1998;44:915–917.

54. Mellor SG. The pathogenesis of blast injury and its management. Br J Hosp Med 1988;39:536–539.

55. Huller T, Bazini Y. Blast injuries of the chest and abdomen. Arch Surg 1970;100:24–30.

56. Richardson JD, Franz JL, Grover FL, et al. Pulmonary contusion and hemorrhage: crystalloid versus colloid replacement. J Surg Res 1974;16:330–336.

57. Fulton RL, Peter ET. Physiosologic effects of fluid therapy after pulmonary contusion. Am J Surg 1984;148:145–151.

58. Barbera JA, Macintyre A. Urban search and rescue. Emerg Med Clin North Am 1996;14:399–412.

59. Hofmeister, EP, Shin, AY. The role of prophylactic fasciotomy and medical treatment in limb ischemia and revascularization. Hand Clin 1998;14: 457–464.

60. Uretzky G, Cotev S. The use of continuous positive airway pressure in blast injury of the chest. Crit Care Med 1980;8:486–489.

61. Batistella FD. Ventilation in the trauma and surgical patient. Crit Care Clin 1998;14:731–742.

62. Sorkine P, Szold O, Kluger Y, et al. Permissive hypercapnia ventilation in patients with severe pulmonary blast injury. J Trauma 1998;45:35–38.

63. Desaga H. Blast injuries. In: German Aviation Medicine: World War II. Office of the Surgeon General of the United States Air Force, Washington DC, 1950, pp. 1274–1293.

64. Weiler-Ravell D, Adatto R, Borman JB. Blast injury of the chest: a review of the problem and its treatment. Isr J Med Sci 1975;11:268–274.

65. Phillips YY, Zajtchuk JT. The management of primary blast injury. In: Bellamy RF, Zajtchuk R, eds. Conventional Warfare: Ballistic, Blast, and Burn Injuries. Office of the Surgeon General of the United States Army, Washington DC, 1991, pp. 295–335.

66. Maynard RL, Coppel DL, Lowry KG. Blast injury of the lung. In: Cooper GJ, Dudley HAF, Gann DS, Little RA, Maynard RL, eds. Scientific Foundations of Trauma. Butterworth-Heineman, Oxford, 1997, pp. 214–224.

67. Mubarak SJ, Owen CA. Compartment syndrome and its relation to the crush syndrome: a spectrum of disease. Clin Orthop 1975;113:81–89.

68. Better OS. Rescue and salvage of casualties suffering from the crush syndrome after mass disasters. Mil Med 1999; 164:366–369.

69. Bouachour G, Cronier P, Couello JP, et al. Hyperbaric oxygen therapy in the management of crush injuries: a randomized double-blind, placebo-controlled, clinical trial. J Trauma 1996;41:333–339.

70. Kerr AG, Byrne JET. Concussive effects of bomb blast on the ear. J Laryngol Otol 1975;89:131–143.

71. Garth RJN. Blast injury of the ear. In: Cooper GJ, Dudley HAF, Gann DS, Little RA, Maynard RL, eds. Scientific Foundations of Trauma. Butterworth-Heineman, Oxford, 1997, pp. 225–235.

# 26 Psychological Impact of Terrorist Incidents

## Timothy J. Lacy, MD and David M. Benedek, MD

The opinions or assertions contained herein are the private views of the author and are not to be construed as official or as reflecting the view of the Department of the Army, Department of the Air Force, or the Department of Defense.

### Contents

## 1. INTRODUCTION

The psychological effect of terrorism is fear, chaos, and social disruption. Terrorist attacks may take the form of conventional assaults with firearms and explosives or more unconventional weapons such as biological or chemical agents, nuclear weapons, bombs contaminated with radioactive materials, "truck" bombs, and even hijacked airplanes. Significant psychological and behavioral reactions to such an attack are predictable. After an attack, primary care and emergency physicians will see many patients who have acute stress-related emotional and physical symptoms or exacerbations of pre-existing health concerns. The large number of behavioral or psychological casualties will have a significant impact on health care delivery.

From: *Physician's Guide to Terrorist Attack*
Edited by: M. J. Roy © Humana Press Inc., Totowa, NJ

## 2. IMPACT OF PSYCHOLOGICAL CASUALTIES
## ON HEALTH CARE DELIVERY

After a terrorist attack, many individuals will seek care who either had no exposure to the agent of terror or who mistake symptoms of arousal and anxiety for exposure to a toxic agent. Behavioral casualties may overwhelm emergency rooms and hospitals. For example, an Israeli study analyzed 1059 Emergency Room (ER) visits after SCUD missile attacks during the Persian Gulf War. Of the patients seen, 20% were direct casualties (injured by missiles or debris), and 80% were psychological or behavioral casualties *(1,2)*. After the Tokyo sarin attack, 5510 people sought medical attention at more than 200 hospitals and clinics in Tokyo within several hours of the incident. Approximately 25% of those seen were hospitalized; the remainder had no signs of exposure and were sent home *(3)*. Delayed psychiatric casualties will present to primary care clinics that will be ill-prepared for an influx of new patients *(4)*. With such an influx of new patients, medical personnel may experience a decreased level of performance and a high rate of "burn-out" owing to stress and fatigue. Making matters worse, medical and rescue workers may resist treatment for themselves, as they did after the Oklahoma City bombing *(5)*.

## 3. BEHAVIORAL RESPONSES TO A TERRORIST ATTACK

The psychological and behavioral reactions to terror attacks may be separated into group and individual responses. The range and types of psychological reactions will most likely be similar regardless of the type of attack.

### *3.1. Group Responses*

Collective or group responses to terrorist attacks include symptoms of emotional distress, misattribution of physical symptoms leading to acute and chronic syndromes, and social symptoms such as loss of confidence in government, anger at governmental authority figures, fear of contagion and disease spread, scapegoating, paranoia, social isolation, and demoralization *(6–8)*. Three specific group responses merit further discussion: mass panic, acute outbreaks of medically unexplained symptoms, and chronic cases with medically unexplained physical symptoms.

Mass panic is characterized by intense contagious fear, leading individuals to behave with reference only to self. There may be mass flight in a desire to escape or, alternatively, people may become behaviorally "frozen" or paralyzed. Mass panic leads to a loss of social organization and social roles as well as substantial community chaos. One might anticipate that mass panic would be a common problem after a devastating attack. However, panic did not follow the Tokyo sarin attack, the Israeli SCUD missile attacks, the Oklahoma City bombing, or the Hiroshima and Nagasaki nuclear attacks. Mass panic is actually rare following disasters. Instead, pro-social, adaptive, and helpful behavior is the norm *(6)*. The risk of mass panic is reduced by providing accurate knowledge, even if the information is disturbing, along with advanced training and disaster and terror simulation. Governmental transparency and honesty are essential for maintaining the public trust. Mass panic is more likely when the situation is high risk, when there is a belief that there is a small chance of escape from the agent, when the treatment resources are available but limited, or when there is no perceived effective response from authority figures that have lost credibility. One example of mass panic is seen in the plague outbreak in Surat, India, in which 600,000 people (75% of the city's population including

80% of the physicians) fled the city in one night by all available means *(9)*. In Dehli, some 1200 km away, people began to panic and hoard tetracycline. They used any available material as a mask against infection. India was quarantined by surrounding states, and the country lost $2–3 billion in 2–3 weeks.

Of the potential psychological responses to terror attacks, the physiological responses to stress create the greatest initial burden to primary care. In response to terror and trauma, individuals experience a number of symptoms of arousal and anxiety as a normal survival reaction. Many individuals may mistakenly attribute these physiological reactions to the effect of some toxic agent or medical illness. These symptoms may affect an entire group of people and present as mass outbreaks of medically unexplained symptoms (OMUS), sometimes called "mass hysteria" or "mass psychogenic illness" *(10)*. These outbreaks are manifested by "contagious" physical symptoms in a group of people with no identifiable cause. They rapidly affect an entire group and spread by sight and sound whether on-site or via media and are characterized by rapid onset and rapid remission *(11–18)*. Frequent symptoms include hyperventilation, dyspnea, dizziness, nausea, headache, syncope, abdominal distress, and agitation. Symptoms may or may not mimic the reported effects of an infectious or chemical agent. Common settings are schools, factories, sporting events, and other social groupings. One type of OMUS outbreak involves inaccurate reports of "poisonous gas" *(13,18)*. For example, in 1973 a ship containing 50 drums of a harmless organophosphate defoliant docked in Auckland, New Zealand. Workers noticed a foul odor and saw the word "poison" on the drums. Miscommunication about the ship's cargo ensued, and as concern mounted, a crisis developed. Even though no one was physically affected by the organophosphates, 643 people sought urgent medical care for symptoms consistent with anxiety and somatoform reactions *(19,20)*.

An example of a panicked population with medically unexplained symptoms is seen in the case of a radiation accident in Goiania, Brazil in 1987 *(21)*. Two scavengers broke into an abandoned medical clinic and stole a medical device for its scrap metal value. It was broken open and sold to a junk dealer. The junk dealer noticed that the powder inside the device glowed in the dark and he shared it with his family and friends. The glowing powder initially fascinated people, but they soon developed nausea, vomiting, diarrhea, and anorexia. The junk dealer's wife notified authorities, who identified the material as cesium 137, a radioactive isotope. Authorities set up a radiological screening post in a nearby soccer stadium and announced that anyone concerned about contamination could come for a free screening. Ten percent of the city (125,800) immediately came forward for screening. The ratio of concerned, anxious, and panicky people requiring attention to those actually contaminated was approximately 500:1. Of the first 60,000 people reporting for screening 5000 had somatoform reactions that mimicked the symptoms of radiation exposure.

Although these acute outbreaks remit rapidly, entire groups of people may develop physical symptoms that become chronic. Medically unexplained physical symptoms (MUPS) have occurred after World War I, Vietnam, the Three-Mile Island nuclear catastrophe in 1979, industrial exposures at Love Canal in the 1970s and 1980s, and military activities in the Balkans and the Persian Gulf *(22)*. MUPS are usually termed somatoform disorders, a label that may alienate patients and lead physicians to ignore genuine physical complaints. These patients may eventually become quite disabled, be convinced of the medical nature of their symptoms, and search desperately for a cure. Physicians, on the other hand, may adopt a position of diagnostic skepticism and send patients the message that their symptoms are "not real." This amounts to a doctor patient "stand-off" in which the doctor stops searching for potential medical problems and the patient becomes more invested in finding a cause for his/her suffering. This tension between doctor and patient may lead to substandard medical care (22).

The mass media plays an important role in the light of these behaviorally "contagious" group responses. Mass media communication either can serve as a "vector" for propagating distress and misperceptions, or can be an effective tool for educating the public and promoting responsible behaviors. Physicians may be the "frontline" experts interviewed by reporters and, depending on their conduct, may either fuel panic or calm and reassure the public (6).

### 3.2. Individual Responses to Traumatic Stress

Our understanding of individual psychological reactions to terror attacks is drawn primarily from military and disaster psychiatry. Although individual patterns of response to large scale traumatic events vary, several phases generally emerge over time (7).

#### 3.2.1. PHASE ONE, THE IMMEDIATE RESPONSE

Strong emotions, disbelief, numbness, fear, and confusion are common in the immediate aftermath of an attack. Signs and symptoms of anxiety and autonomic arousal are considered normal responses to an abnormal event (Table 1). Biological responses immediately following a traumatic event include the release of stress hormones such as corticotropin-releasing factor, adrenal corticotropic hormone, and peripheral catecholamines. Furthermore, areas of the brain related to perception of threat are activated. These changes usually result in improved performance that is generally adaptive in the aftermath of a terrorist attack. However, as stress persists, behavior and thinking may become narrowly focused, with a loss of flexibility. Thinking may eventually become disorganized, resulting in either a fight-or-flight response or a "freeze" response (22). During this phase, the risk of mass panic or acute outbreaks of medically unexplained symptoms is at its peak.

#### 3.2.2. PHASE TWO, INTERMEDIATE RESPONSE: ADAPTATION, AROUSAL, AND AVOIDANCE

Phase two of the traumatic response occurs from one week to several months after the event. Intrusive symptoms such as recollections of the event with increased autonomic arousal (e.g., startle response, hypervigilance, insomnia, and nightmares) are common. Increased visits to primary care for somatic symptoms such as dizziness, headache, fatigue, and nausea are also commonly seen. Clinics may be overwhelmed with patients reporting new somatic symptoms or a worsening of existing health problems. Stress may even precipitate early labor in pregnant women or cause fetal distress. Some may develop psychiatric disorders during this phase. Additionally, anger, irritability, apathy, grief and mourning, and social withdrawal are common.

#### 3.2.3. PHASE THREE, LONG-TERM RESPONSE: RECOVERY, IMPAIRMENT, AND CHANGE

Phase three may last for up to a year or more. During this stage, victims may experience feelings of disappointment and resentment if initial hopes for aid and restoration are not met. The sense of community may be weakened as individuals focus on their personal needs. Some individuals may experience continued post-traumatic psychiatric symptoms as well as extended grief and mourning for years after the attack. Fortunately, most will rebuild their lives and focus on the future.

Table 1
Symptoms of Anxiety and Autonomic Arousal

Anorexia
Chest pain/tightness
Diaphoresis
Diarrhea
Dizziness
Dry mouth
Dyspnea
Faintness
Flushing
Hyperventilation
Light-headedness
Muscle tension/aches
Nausea
Pallor
Palpitations
Paresthesias
Tachycardia
Urinary frequency
Vomiting

## 4. PSYCHIATRIC DISORDERS

After traumatic stress, most people will experience acute symptoms that dissipate over time. However, some will develop psychiatric disorders, most commonly post-traumatic stress disorder (PTSD), which occurs in as many as 30% of individuals exposed to extreme emotional trauma *(7,23–25)*. The cardinal features of PTSD include intrusive re-experiencing of the trauma via nightmares and/or flashbacks, avoidance of reminders of the trauma along with emotional numbing, and persistent symptoms of autonomic hyperarousal. The best predictor of PTSD is the degree of exposure to the traumatic event. Those whose lives are directly threatened, who are physically injured, or who are exposed to extremely horrifying or grotesque events are at greatest risk *(7)*. However, all who have exposure to the event are at potential risk, including immediate victims, family members and friends, rescue workers, health care workers, and any others in the local community. The effects of a terrorist attack may even be experienced at a distance. In a study conducted just 3 days after the September 11 attacks, 560 adults and their children from across the country were randomly contacted by telephone and given a modified PTSD questionnaire designed to elicit symptoms of post-traumatic stress. Of those who responded, 90% had at least one symptom, and 44% adults had "substantial" symptoms of stress. Forty-seven percent of the children had "substantial" symptoms of stress. Stress symptoms were positively correlated with the amount of television terror attack coverage watched and negatively correlated with distance from the World Trade Center. Prior psychiatric disorder made no statistical difference *(26)*.

PTSD symptoms may persist for months or even years after the traumatic event *(24)*. Other psychiatric problems such as depression, somatoform disorders, other anxiety disorders such as panic disorder, and generalized anxiety, bereavement, and grief often arise as individuals struggle with the loss and pain associated with the event. Furthermore, there may be increased reports of substance use and domestic violence.

## 5. REACTIONS TO BIOLOGICAL AND CHEMICAL ATTACK

Several unique features of biological and chemical agents make them especially terrifying *(8,25)*. Like radiation, they are frequently invisible and odorless. With certain agents, exposed or infected individuals may initially develop symptoms of common illnesses and therefore avoid early detection. Most of these agents are unfamiliar to American doctors, and treatment may not be readily available. Some agents cause gross deformities such as the lesions of smallpox or the severe blisters of mustard gas. The unseen and mysterious nature of these agents may lead to situations like the medically unexplained physical symptoms mentioned above or the so-called "gas hysteria" seen during World War I, in which there were twice as many gas hysteria cases as there were actual gas exposure cases *(25)*. Even protective measures can be problematic. The protective MOPP gear worn during chemical and biological attacks increases one's sense of isolation, decreases intragroup communication, and may increase the incidence of psychiatric casualties *(27,28)*. Other likely syndromes include conversion reactions with respiratory features and "gas mask phobia," which was a significant problem during the Persian Gulf War *(27)*.

The behavioral response to biological agents will differ from that of chemical agents *(8)*. There is usually a time delay between initial exposure to a biological agent and the development of symptoms. The "first responders" to a biological attack will be ER staff, clinics, and public health officials rather than the firemen and emergency medical technicians who are the first responders to a chemical attack. If the attack is covert, it may not even be identified as such but may appear to be a natural outbreak. On the other hand, the responsibility for a natural outbreak may be claimed by terrorists in order to further their agenda. Furthermore, people may fear the contagious spread of disease across a region or nation, especially when there is uncertainty about the attack or questions about the effectiveness of treatment. Attempted quarantine, infection control, vaccination, and treatment programs may be accompanied by unfounded rumor and also present an opportunity to do real harm. This may create a public opinion backlash against government and public health officials.

## 6. PREVENTING PSYCHOLOGICAL CASUALTIES

A lack of social preparedness makes community chaos and behavioral problems more likely after a terror attack *(29)*. Prevention must therefore be directed at improving preparedness. Robust communication systems must be in place to provide communities with realistic information about both the nature of the threat and the appropriate actions to take in response. Hospitals and communities must develop emergency and disaster plans and repeatedly practice them. Simulated exercises should involve all relevant medical, psychiatric, and other personnel *(7)*. Sufficient logistical facilities must be in place, and all plans and facilities must be adequately funded. Funding and planning reduce the community's sense of helplessness before and after an attack. If leaders, first responders, and other community members are prepared for their roles prior to a terrorist event, then after the attack, energies can be directed toward providing social support to victims instead of wasting time sorting out roles and responsibilities. Conversely, poorly planned or executed responses increase feelings of individual and community helplessness and confusion and lead to psychological and behavioral casualties. The development and practice of a well-supported disaster plan may be the single most important "psychological" intervention.

Table 2
Neuropsychiatric Effects of Chemical Agents

| Agent | Syndrome, symptoms, and comments |
|---|---|
| Organophosphates (nerve agents such as sarin, soman, VX, and tabun) | Depression, irritability, and sleep disturbance<br>Impaired cognition<br>Delirium<br>Psychosis |
| Atropine (treatment for organophosphates) | Blurred vision, tachycardia, dry mouth, anhydrosis, urinary retention, cognitive impairment, psychosis, and delirium (disorientation, delusions, hallucinations) |
| Cyanide | Early symptoms of cyanide exposure are anxiety, confusion, giddiness, and hyperventilation |
| Blistering agents, mustard gas, and Phosgene | No direct neuropsychiatric effects, but they are insidious agents with a delayed time of onset (several hours), which is terrifying; cause blindness and burns<br>Psychic distress over disfigurement.<br>Phosgene inactivates charcoal and causes a frightening suffocating sensation like lungs filling with fluid. |
| Mycotoxins (fungal toxins) | Produce terrifying rapid symptoms of vomiting, tissue necrosis, and failure of blood coagulation<br>In natural outbreaks, ergots and other mycotoxins are thought by some to be responsible for St. Vitus dance and "tarantism" (psychosis with somatization) |

Data from ref. 20.

## 7. AFTER THE ATTACK

### 7.1. Initial Assessment and Treatment

Immediately after a terrorist attack, hospitals, clinics, and ERs may be overwhelmed with persons seeking medical treatment. Patients may present with physical injuries, symptoms that reflect either the direct effect of a biological or chemical agent or with psychological reactions. Biological and chemical agents directly affect the central nervous system and cause symptoms such as lethargy, anxiety, depression, disorientation, and psychosis (Tables 2 and 3) (25,30). The treating or triaging physician must distinguish between the psychological symptoms of hyperarousal and the medical symptoms of a toxic exposure. This may be the most difficult task since the psychological symptoms often mimic the symptoms of toxic exposure. Nevertheless, swift diagnosis and prompt treatment minimize both medical and neuropsychiatric complications and also decrease the opportunity for the psychological symptoms to "spread" to other frightened victims. Once a medical diagnosis is made, individuals who require medical treatment should be treated like any other ER patients. Those who have completed treatment or who require no medical treatment fall into two groups: those who are emotionally distressed and those who are not. Those who are adequately reassured by being medically cleared may be discharged with education and reassurance. However, those who are emotionally upset by the trauma require further treatment.

The mainstay of treatment for emotionally distressed individuals is rest, reassurance, education, and support. They should be placed in a location where any disruptive behaviors can be monitored (Fig. 1). This location should be sufficiently removed from high-

Table 3
Neuropsychiatric Syndromes or Symptoms in Selected Biological Agents

| Biological Agent | Syndrome or symptoms | Comment |
|---|---|---|
| Anthrax | Meningitis | May be rapidly progressive |
| Brucellosis | Depression, irritability, headaches | Fatalities associated with CNS involvement |
| Q fever | Malaise, fatigue Encephalitis, hallucinations | In 1/3 of patients In advanced cases |
| Botulinum toxin | Depression | Owing to lengthy recovery |
| Viral encephalitides | Depression, cognitive impairment | Other mood changes also |
| All biological agents | Delirium | Acutely impaired attention, memory, and perceptual disturbances |

Data from refs. *3* and *18*.

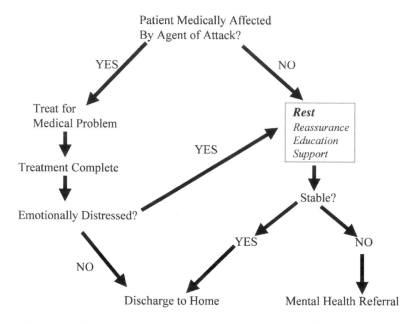

**Fig. 1.** Flow chart depicting assessment and treatment of patients affected by a terrorist attack.

tempo triage activity, yet close enough to the main ER to permit further medical treatment if needed. Patients should be reassured that symptoms of autonomic arousal and anxiety are normal responses to an abnormal situation, and they should be encouraged to resume their usual routines as soon as possible. This reassurance, combined with support and rest, is often enough to diminish symptoms.

## 7.2. Medications

Although most patients will respond to a conservative and supportive approach, some may require medications for agitation, psychosis, or insomnia *(30,31)*. Antipsychotic medications such as haloperidol are effective in low doses for delirium or psychosis resulting from toxic agents (Table 4). Although newer antipsychotics may have fewer

Table 4
Selected Medications for Emergency Use After a Terrorist Attack

| Medication | Dosage | Indication |
| --- | --- | --- |
| Antipsychotics | | |
|   Haloperidol | 1–5 mg bid-tid (po, im, iv) | Psychosis, agitated delirium |
| Anticholinergics | | |
|   Diphenhydramine | 25–50 mg bid-qid (po or slow iv push in emergencies) | Motor side effects of antipsychotics |
|   Benztropine | 1–2 mg bid-qid (po or slow iv push in emergencies) | |
| Benzodiazepines | | |
|   Diazepam | 2–10 mg tid-qid (po, im, iv) | Anxiety, panic |
|   Lorazepam | 1–2 mg bid-tid (po, im, iv) | |
|   Clonazepam | 0.5–1 mg bid-tid (po) | |
| Antiadrenergics | | |
|   Propranolol | 10–20 mg bid-tid (po) | Hyperadrenergic states: |
|   Clonidine | 0.1–0.2 mg bid-tid (po) |   diaphoresis, goose-flesh, anxiety, hyperstartle response, hypervigilance |
| Soporifics | | |
|   Trazodone | 25–50 mg QHS (po) | Insomnia |
|   Zolpidem | 5–10 mg QHS (po) | |
|   Zaleplon | 5–10 mg QHS (po) | |

side effects, haloperidol is almost universally available; it may be used in po, im, or iv forms, and it is therefore still the first choice in emergencies. Side effects of antipsychotic use include parkinsonism, akathisia (restlessness), and dystonias. These side effects are problematic and could even be lethal, as in the case of laryngeal dystonias. Anticholinergic medications such as benztropine or diphenhydramine are useful for treating these side effects. Benzodiazepines like lorazepam, diazepam, or clonazepam may be used for severe anxiety or insomnia. These medications should be used as short-term measures to ameliorate acute distress, and patients should be told this. Lorazepam and diazepam are quick acting and come in po, im, and iv formulations that make them quite versatile. Clonazepam, on the other hand, has the advantage of a gradual onset of action and a long half-life, decreasing its addictive potential. Patients treated with benzodiazepines should be cautioned about sedation and possible impairment in driving and decision making. β-blockers like propranolol and α-agonists like clonidine, via their antiadrenergic action, may also be helpful in the short term for decreasing agitation. Trazodone, zolpidem, or zaleplon are often the preferred choices for insomnia because they preserve sleep architecture. Although the above medications may be helpful for acute distress, psychosis, and insomnia, no medications have yet been shown to prevent the development of posttraumatic psychiatric disorders.

## 8. TREATING MEDICALLY UNEXPLAINED SYMPTOMS

In the case of acute OMUS, a few additional measures are required. Lengthy incident scene investigations and elaborate searches for the offending agent may worsen and prolong the event. Therefore, if you are called to the site, try to keep the investigation low profile. The involved group should be informed about the scope of the problem, and the role of the offending agent should be minimized. Leaders and physicians should be calm, authoritative, supportive, and nonconfrontational. Individuals should be separated in order to minimize the spread of symptoms by sight and sound. Repetitive questioning about symptoms and use of language suggestive of infection or exposure should be avoided *(12,13)*.

The treatment of chronic MUPS is more problematic. These conditions may persist for years after a traumatic event and may frustrate patient and physician alike. The physician must be respectful and empathic, and must validate the patients' concerns. A supportive and collaborative approach, hopefully involving a team of caregivers, combined with minimizing unnecessary medical tests and procedures, is essential *(22)*.

## 9. DEBRIEFING

Group debriefing techniques have been used in the aftermath of natural disasters and terrorist events. Debriefings offer affected persons an opportunity to join others in a group review of the traumatic event, share emotional reactions, and give some structure to their chaotic experience. Most debriefing models are designed for use with first responders such as firemen and emergency medical technicians, but debriefing has also been used for victims. There is no convincing evidence that such debriefings reduce the incidence of PTSD or other psychiatric disorders. In fact, encouraging the expression of intense emotions immediately after a recent trauma may be harmful and may even retraumatize some individuals *(32–34)*. Nevertheless, debriefings may be of some benefit in fostering group cohesion and helping individuals deal with the post-attack chaos. Debriefings may help sustain performance, reduce the sense of isolation, and facilitate identification of those who need further mental health treatment *(32,35)*.

If group debriefings are conducted, it is important that the group be composed of persons linked socially by working relationships or friendships rather than haphazardly assembled groups of people who just happen to be at the terror scene at the same time. Open and frank discussions among care providers, rescue workers, terror responders, and victims may foster a sense of cohesion and reduce individual isolation. The focus of the debriefing should be the creation of a cognitive historical narrative of the event, i.e., "what happened." Debriefings should not be quasi-psychotherapy sessions. Participants should be allowed to express their feelings about what happened if they choose, and such emotions should be supported. However, any attempt to extract the "real" or "underlying" emotions is strongly discouraged. Those with prior abusive experience, minimal ability to regulate affect, limited ego functioning, or serious pre-existing mental illness may be harmed by being "forced" to participate in highly emotional, mandatory debriefings.

In the immediate aftermath of an attack, the most important intervention is to take care of the victims' physical needs. Blankets, bandages, food, and rest are much more important than group debriefing sessions. Victims need to know that they are being cared for, and after a terrorist attack this does not mean talking, it means safety. Previous experience with emergency operations in response to terrorist hoaxes has shown that neglect of comfort issues and lack of respect for the dignity or privacy of those subjected to quarantine or decontamination are among the most distressing aspects of these operations.

## 10. THE PHYSICIAN AND COMMUNITY RESOURCES

In the wake of an attack, additional community and regional resources will be required *(7)*. These resources include the Red Cross, community mental health centers, social workers, and hospice care providers, as well as teachers and religious officials. Schools, churches, synagogues, and mosques may serve as additional locations for debriefings, support, reassurance, rest, and education. Incorporation of these resources into the local disaster and terror response plan strengthens the community's social organization, enlists a larger portion of the community in responding positively to the attack, and decreases the burden on primary care facilities. Additionally, by including these agencies in the disaster planning process, post-attack confusion is substantially decreased. Well-intentioned, but often poorly trained, volunteers will arrive on the scene after any disaster or terrorist attack. Such offers of help can unintentionally create more confusion and make an already difficult situation worse. In addition to personal liaison with various agencies, several Internet sites provide useful information. Sites sponsored by the Red Cross (www.redcross.org), the Centers for Disease Control and Prevention (www.cdc.gov), and the Uniformed Services University for the Health Sciences (www.usuhs.mil/psy/ disasteresources.html) provide excellent printable handouts and articles free of charge. These handouts can be kept in emergency rooms and clinics and are good educational sources for both patients and providers.

## REFERENCES

1. Carmeli A, Liberman N, Mevorach L. Anxiety-related somatic reactions during missile attacks. Isr J Med Sci 1991;27:677–680.
2. Karsenty D, Shermer J, Alshech I, et al. Medical aspects of the Iraqi missile attacks on Israel. Israel J Med Sci 1991; 27:603–607.
3. Sidell FR. Chemical agent terrorism. Ann Emerg Med 1996;28:223–224.
4. Stephenson J. Medical, mental health communities mobilize to cope with terror's psychological aftermath. JAMA 286:1823–1825.
5. Anteau CM, Williams LA. What we learned from the Oklahoma City bombing. Nursing 1998;28:52–55.
6. Glass TA, Schloch-Spana M. Bioterrorism and the people: how to vaccinate a city against panic. CID 2002;34:217–223.
7. Ursano RJ, Fullerton CS, Norwood AE. Psychiatric dimensions of disaster: patient care, community consultation, and preventive medicine. Harv Rev Psychiatry 1995;3:196–209.
8. Holloway HC, Norwood AE, Fullerton CS, et al. The threat of biological weapons: prophylaxis and mitigation of psychological and social consequences. JAMA 1997;278:425–427.
9. Ramalingaswami, V. Psychosocial effects of the 1994 plague outbreak in Surat, India. Mil Med 2001;166(suppl 2):29–30.
10. Pastel R. Outbreaks of medically unexplained physical symptoms after military action, terrorist threat, or technological disaster. Mil Med 2001;166(suppl 2):44–46.
11. Levine RJ. Mass hysteria: diagnosis and treatment in the emergency room. Arch Intern Med 1984;144:145–146.
12. Elkins GR, Gamino LA, Rynearson RR. Mass psychogenic illness, trance states, and suggestion. Am J Clin Hypnosis 1988;30:267–275.
13. Gamino LA, Elkins GR, Hackney KU. Emergency management of mass psychogenic illness. Psychosomatics 1989;30:446–449.
14. Modan B, Swartz TA, Tirosh M, et al. The Arjenyattah Epidemic, a mass phenomenon: spread and triggering factors. Lancet 1983;2:1472–1474.
15. Wason S, Bausher JC. Epidemic "mass" hysteria. Lancet 1983;2:731–732.
16. Seden BS. Adolescent epidemic hysteria presenting as a mass casualty, toxic exposure incident. Ann Emerg Med 1989;18:892–895.

17. Struewing JP, Gray GC. An epidemic of respiratory complaints exacerbated by mass psychogenic illness in a military recruit population. Am J Epidemiol 1990;132:1120–1129.
18. Rockney RM, Lemke T. Casualties from a junior-senior high school during the Persian Gulf War: toxic poisoning or mass hysteria? J Dev Behav Pediatr 1992;13:339–342.
19. DiGiovani C. Domestic terrorism with chemical or biological agents: psychiatric aspects. Am J Psychiatry 1999;156:1500–1505.
20. McLeod WR. Merphos poisoning or mass panic? Aust NZ J Psychiatry 1975;9:225–229.
21. Salter CA. Psychological effects of nuclear and radiological warfare. Mil Med 2001;166(suppl 2):17–18.
22. Engel C. Outbreaks of medically unexplained physical symptoms after military action, terrorist threat, or technological disaster. Mil Med 2001;166 (suppl 2):47–48.
23. Shalev AY. Acute to chronic: etiology and pathophysiology of PTSD—a biopsychosocial approach. In: Fullerton CS, Ursano RJ, eds. Posttraumatic Stress Disorder. American Psychiatric Press, Washington, DC, 1997, pp. 209–240.
24. North, CS, Nixon, SJ, Shariat, S, et al. Psychiatric disorders among survivors of the Oklahoma City bombing. JAMA 1999;282:755–762.
25. Jones FD. Neuropsychiatric casualties of nuclear, biological, and chemical warfare. In: Zajtchuk R, Bellamy RF, eds. Textbook of Military Medicine, Part I. War Psychiatry. The Office of the Surgeon General, Department of the Army, United States of America, TMM Publications, Washington, DC, 1995, pp. 85–111.
26. Schuster M, et al. A national survey of stress reactions after the September 11, 2001, terrorist attacks. N Engl J Med 2001;345:1507–1512.
27. Ritchie EC. Psychological problems associated with mission oriented protective gear. Mil Med 2001;166(suppl 2):83–84.
28. Fullerton CS, Ursano RJ. Health care delivery in the high-stress environment of chemical and biological warfare. Mil Med 1994;159:524–528.
29. Lerner M. The Belief in a Just World: A Fundamental Delusion. Plenum Press, New York, 1980.
30. Franz DR, Jahrling PB, Friedlander AM, et al. Clinical recognition and management of patients exposed to biological warfare agents. JAMA 1997;278:399–411
31. Holloway HC, Benedek DM. The changing face of terrorism and military psychiatry. Psychiatr Ann 1999;29:363–374.
32. Rafael B. Conclusion: debriefing—science, belief, and wisdom. In: Raphael B, Wilson JP, eds. Psychological Debriefing: Theory, Practice, and Evidence. Cambridge University Press, New York, 2000, pp. 351–359.
33. Kaplan Z, Iancu I, Bodner E. A review of psychological debriefing after traumatic stress. Psychiatr Serv 2001;52:824–827.
34. Gavin Y. Psychologists question "debriefing" for traumatized employees. BMJ 2001;320:140.
35. Barker M. Calming the aftershocks. Occup Health Safety 2001;70:28–33.

# 27 Conclusions

## Michael J. Roy, MD, MPH, FACP

The opinions or assertions contained herein are the private views of the author and are not to be construed as official or as reflecting the view of the Department of the Army or the Department of Defense.

### CONTENTS

## 1. INTRODUCTION

Terrorism may be defined as the deliberate or threatened use of violence to coerce governments and/or societies in the pursuit of a political, religious, or ideological agenda. For a group or government seeking to influence an economically and militarily more powerful opponent, biological, chemical, and radioactive agents (weapons of mass destruction) may have particular appeal, since they are often relatively inexpensive and unsophisticated, may engender disproportionate fear, and have the potential to level the playing field rapidly. Although a number of nations have engaged in the development and stockpiling of biological and chemical arsenals, they have largely refrained from their use. Terrorist groups and criminals have demonstrated a growing interest in biological and chemical agents, have not stopped short of using them, and have sometimes caused transient disruptions through fear; however, the use of such agents has been largely unsuccessful, for one reason or another. Unfortunately, it is virtually inevitable that a rogue group or nation will at some point cause significant numbers of casualties through the use of weapons of mass destruction.

The preceding chapters have described how to respond to a terrorist attack and then detailed an approach to the diagnosis and management of victims of particular agents. This information may be sufficient to prepare physicians for most circumstances, but there are several additional elements to consider. First, how can terrorist-induced injuries be distinguished from influenza and other common illnesses that may be occurring in the general population simultaneously? Second, how should a victim be managed if he or she

From: *Physician's Guide to Terrorist Attack*
Edited by: M. J. Roy © Humana Press Inc., Totowa, NJ

is exposed to more than one agent? Third, physicians need to be attuned to the psycho logical sequelae of terrorist attacks not only in the victims, but also in their family members and friends and even other members of the general population. Finally, prevention and readiness efforts must be redoubled in order to minimize physical and psychological casualties most effectively.

## 2. DIFFERENTIATION FROM COMMON ILLNESSES

The mail-disseminated anthrax cases that occurred in the fall of 2001 drew considerable attention to efforts to distinguish the clinical presentation of anthrax from that of influenza and influenza-like illnesses. The most useful clinical signs in this case are the presence of dyspnea and nausea or vomiting, each of which are present in most anthrax victims but usually absent in viral syndromes, and rhinorrhea and sore throat, which are common in influenza and viral upper respiratory infections, but uncommon with anthrax. The chest radiograph can also be very helpful. Mediastinal widening is pathognomonic for anthrax, pleural effusions are common, and infiltrates may also be seen. Interstitial infiltrates may bee seen with influenza, but the chest radiograph will usually be normal.

There is less experience to draw on in distinguishing other bioterrorist agents from common viral processes, but there will usually be red flags to guide management. Given the current world climate, it is prudent when more than one patient presents with serious illness of unclear etiology to ask about attendance at recent sporting events or other large public gatherings, as well as recent food and water sources. Inhalational tularemia is likely to have a longer latency period than anthrax, typically 3–5 days, and the initial fever and upper respiratory symptoms are indistinguishable from those of influenza. However, the initial symptoms then rapidly progress to bronchopneumonia and/or pleuritis, although not so fulminant as anthrax, so there is still generally a good response to initiation of antibiotics at this point. Inhalational plague is likely to be characterized by a latency period (and rapidity of progression) that is somewhere between that of anthrax and that of tularemia. Dyspnea and gastrointestinal symptoms are as common with plague as they are with anthrax, helping to distinguish it from influenza and other viral processes. Multilobar consolidation or infiltrates are characteristic of plague. Inhalation of ricin toxin may be characterized by primary pulmonary symptoms, and the key differentiating features have been described in the corresponding chapter. Brucella and Q fever each may involve a number of different organ systems, resulting in a broad range of clinical presentations, but each also characteristically has a subacute, albeit chronic, course, with far lower mortality than other potential bioterrorist agents. Thus they are less likely to be employed by terrorists, and also physicians have the luxury of time in trying to make diagnoses.

Smallpox may initially be indistinguishable from a severe case of influenza, marked as they both are by fever, severe fatigue, headache, and backache. The clear delineating factor will be the characteristic skin lesions, which require differentiation from varicella, utilizing features described in the corresponding chapter. Mycotoxins are often likely to produce a wide range of symptoms beyond simple skin irritation, and the rapidity of onset is likely to make differentiation from chemical agents more problematic than differentiation from smallpox. The differentiation of other biological agents, such as botulinum toxin and staphylococcal enterotoxin B, has been well described in the corresponding chapters. Distinction of chemical or radiological exposure is unlikely to be subtle, owing to the large number of casualties and the rapid onset of symptoms that can be expected.

Table 1
Pharmacological Therapy for Agents of Bioterrorism

| Agent | Treatment | Postexposure prophylaxis |
|---|---|---|
| *Bacillus anthracis* (inhalational) (combination therapy advised for clinical illness) | **iv ciprofloxacin** **iv doxycycline** iv penicillin iv levofloxacin iv ofloxacin iv rifampin iv gentamicin iv erythromycin iv chloramphenicol iv tetracycline | **po ciprofloxacin** **po doxycycline** **po amoxicillin** po levofloxacin po ofloxacin |
| *Francisella tularensis* or *Yersinia pestis* | **iv streptomycin** **iv gentamicin** iv ciprofloxacin (other quinolones probably effective too) iv chloramphenicol | **po doxycycline** **po ciprofloxacin** **iv doxycycline** |
| *Brucella* (various species) (use at least two drugs) | **iv doxycycline** **iv rifampin** iv trimethoprim-sulfamethoxazole iv gentamicin | **po doxycycline** **po rifampin** |
| *Coxiella burnetii* | **Doxycycline** **Tetracycline** Macrolides Quinolones Rifampin | **Doxycycline** **Tetracycline** |
| Botulinum toxin | **Antitoxin** | **Toxoid** |
| T-2 mycotoxins | Supportive ?Steroids | NA |
| Staphylococcal enterotoxin B | Supportive | NA |
| Ricin | Supportive | **Toxoid** |
| Smallpox | NA | **Vaccination** Cidofovir |
| Viral hemorrhagic fevers | Ribavirin antibody for some | NA |
| Viral encephalitides | Supportive | NA |

NA, not available; treatments of choice appear in bold type.

# 3. EXPOSURE TO MORE THAN ONE AGENT

The potential use of two or more agents simultaneously must be considered. For biological agents, either doxycycline or ciprofloxacin is effective not only against anthrax (the agent requiring most urgent treatment) but also against many of the other bacterial pathogens that have predominant pulmonary signs and symptoms. Physicians should have a reference (such as Table 1) available and should also be aware of the two antibiotics that cover many of the most serious biological threats. With the exception of botulinum antitoxin for botulism, most of the biological agents that are not responsive to doxycycline or ciprofloxacin are treated primarily by supportive care. This may make it less likely for a terrorist to decide to employ two biological agents together. Use of a chemical agent or a toxin that would have a relatively immediate effect, along with a biological agent that would have delayed onset, might not make strategic sense either, as this would significantly raise medical awareness before the biological agent manifests symptoms. Utilization of radiation, such as a "dirty bomb," in conjunction with a biological agent, might inactivate the biological agent, in addition to raising medical awareness, again perhaps not making strategic sense, although it remains possible that a terrorist might hope for a "one-two punch." Smallpox is probably the most feared of all biological agents and may represent the "second punch" with the greatest effect as well. If anthrax, botulinum, or another biological agent were released in conjunction with smallpox, victims would receive treatment for the first agent to manifest, and, during the course of treatment, probably while still hospitalized, might then have the onset of smallpox. This would pose a significant risk for secondary infection of medical personnel (although the vaccination program for medical personnel should mitigate this risk), other hospitalized patients, and friends and family members visiting the hospital. Although there may not be a good method for diagnosing smallpox prior to the onset of symptoms, awareness of this possibility may at least lead physicians to consider the diagnosis during the febrile phase of smallpox, before skin lesions develop.

## 4. PREVENTIVE MEASURES

Preventive measures can be taken to limit the significance and scope of some terrorist attacks. This begins with individual provider education and includes readiness achieved through group training such as mass-casualty exercises. Training and provider education efforts should incorporate lessons learned from prior events, as described in the first chapter of this text. Paramount among these lessons is the need for training of first responders from multiple services (the military, fire departments, police departments, physicians, and other emergency personnel) to try to limit the inevitable traffic jams, communication problems, and command and control issues that hinder response and treatment efforts. One of the most important preventive measures is one in which all physicians can participate: ensuring that immunizations are up to date for as much of the general population as possible. Limiting the number, and severity, of influenza cases through immunization is particularly helpful, both by decreasing the likelihood that influenza will be confused with anthrax or other bioterrorism-induced illnesses and by decreasing the strain on medical resources from conventional illnesses at a time when they are needed for unconventional illness and injury. Much the same argument can be made for pneumococcal vaccination. Immunization against smallpox, anthrax, tularemia, and other agents of bioterrorism may also be administered in the face of terrorist use or legitimate threat.

## 5. ROLE OF THE PHYSICIAN
## IN TREATING PSYCHOLOGICAL SEQUELAE

In sheer numbers, at least, regardless of the scope of a terrorist event, individuals with functional impairment owing to psychological sequelae, ranging from somatic symptoms that mimic true exposure to post-traumatic stress disorder, will far exceed the direct victims of the terrorist agent. The previous chapter describes many historical examples of this and outlines the role that physicians may play in evaluating, reassuring, and treating these symptoms. For the average physician not directly involved as a first responder, this is likely to be the most important role and, in fact, arguably the most important purpose of the medical community in general, in terms of preventing impaired function on a societal level. This is particularly true in light of recent studies that have documented significant and often persistent symptoms of post-traumatic stress in a sizeable percentage of the population not in the immediate vicinity of the event. Although the likelihood of persistent distress is greater the closer one is to the site of a terrorist event, even viewing at a distance the news of an attack repeatedly on television can clearly be associated with impairment. Seventeen percent of Americans outside New York City acknowledged symptoms of post-traumatic stress disorder 2 months following the September 11 attacks, and 5.8% had persistent symptoms at 6 months *(1)*. Persistent symptoms of distress have been reported in victims of mail-disseminated anthrax *(2)* and in a strikingly high 60% of those presenting for evaluation after the sarin attack in the Japanese subway *(3)*.

Those with persistent symptoms have reduced productivity, miss more work, have greater difficulty in interpersonal relationships (including an increase in domestic disputes and violence), increase their consumption of tobacco and alcohol products, and make more visits to health care professionals. Because a terrorist attack is likely to occur in the context of an otherwise mundane or pleasurable event, aspects of life such as opening mail or going to the theater or to a sports event may suddenly become triggers for bothersome symptoms. Physicians should expect physical and psychological manifestations of distress after a terrorist attack; they should assure patients that symptoms like this are common and can occur in anyone—they often improve over time, but if they persist, effective treatment is available. It is important to encourage patients to talk about their symptoms, whether to you as their physician or to mental health professionals, counselors, chaplains, or other sources of support. Owing to the nature of the symptoms, which are frequently somatic, patients are likely to seek the help of their physicians first more often than not, providing a valuable opportunity for physicians to provide early reassurance and intervention.

## REFERENCES

1. Silver RC, Holman EA, McIntosh DN, Poulin M, Gil-Rivas V. Nationwide longitudinal study of psychological responses to September 11. JAMA 2002;288:1235–1244.
2. Sun LH. Anthrax patients' ailments linger. Washington Post, April 20, 2002.
3. Ohbu S, Yamashina A, Takasu N, et al. Sarin poisoning on Tokyo subway. South Med J 1997;90:587–593.

# Index